# Obesity and Cardiovascular Disease

# Fundamental and Clinical Cardiology

Editor-in-Chief
Samuel Z. Goldhaber, M.D.
Harvard Medical School
and Brigham and Women's Hospital
Boston, Massachusetts, U.S.A.

# Obesity and Cardiovascular Disease

*Edited by*

**Malcolm K. Robinson, M.D.**
*Brigham and Women's Hospital*
*Harvard Medical School*
*Boston, Massachusetts, U.S.A.*

**Abraham Thomas, M.D., M.P.H.**
*Brigham and Women's Hospital*
*Harvard Medical School*
*Boston, Massachusetts, U.S.A.*

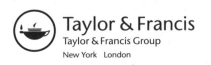

Taylor & Francis
Taylor & Francis Group
New York   London

Published in 2006 by
Taylor & Francis Group
270 Madison Avenue
New York, NY 10016

© 2006 by Taylor & Francis Group, LLC

International Standard Book Number-10: 1-57444-863-3 (Hardcover)
International Standard Book Number-13: 978-1-57444-863-4 (Hardcover)
Library of Congress Card Number 2005046609

### Library of Congress Cataloging-in-Publication Data

Obesity and cardiovascular disease / edited by Malcolm K. Robinson, Abraham Thomas.
        p. ; cm. -- (Fundamental and clinical cardiology ; 58)
    Includes bibliographical references and index.
    ISBN-13: 978-1-57444-863-4 (alk. paper)
    ISBN-10: 1-57444-863-3 (alk. paper)
    1. Obesity--Complications. 2. Cardiovascualr system--Diseases. I. Robinson, Malcolm K. II.
Thomas, Abraham, 1965- III. Fundamental and clinical cardiology ; v. 58.
    [DNLM: 1. Obesity--complications. 2. Cardiovascular Diseases--etiology. WD 210 O11214 2006]

RC628.O2262 2006
616.3'98--dc22                                                                              2005046609

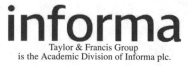

Taylor & Francis Group
is the Academic Division of Informa plc.

**Visit the Taylor & Francis Web site at
http://www.taylorandfrancis.com**

# Series Introduction

Taylor & Francis Group has focused on the development of various series of beautifully produced books in different branches of medicine. These series have facilitated the integration of rapidly advancing information for both the clinical specialist and the researcher.

My goal as Editor-In-Chief of the Fundamental and Clinical Cardiology Series is to assemble the talents of world-renowned authorities to discuss virtually every area of cardiovascular medicine. In the current monograph, Drs. Robinson and Thomas have edited a much-needed and timely book which addresses the pandemic of obesity and metabolic syndrome. Future contributions to this series will include books on molecular biology, interventional cardiology, and clinical management of such problems as coronary artery disease and ventricular arrhythmias.

Samuel Z. Goldhaber, M.D.
*Professor of Medicine*
*Harvard Medical School*
*Boston, Massachusetts, U.S.A.*

# Preface

Over 65% of adults in the United States are overweight or obese with over 60 million Americans meeting the National Institutes of Health definition of frank obesity. These figures are even more startling when one realizes that the number of obese individuals has increased by 50% in the past decade. Although cardiovascular disease remains the number one proximate cause of death in the United States, it is now estimated that obesity or "overnutrition" may be equivalent to smoking as the leading cause of preventable death in the United States. Not surprisingly, there is a significant association between obesity and cardiovascular disease. Thus obesity and cardiovascular disease are major public health concerns. These conditions afflict millions and cost billions of dollars to treat.

This text was developed out of a growing imperative for all clinicians to understand and address two of the major health problems of our time. Obesity and cardiovascular disease are frequently seen daily, and often concomitantly, in many clinical practices. The book is intended for students, medical generalists, and specialists alike who wish to gain understanding of the epidemiology of obesity and cardiovascular disease, while reviewing the current understanding of pathological changes that occur in the obese.

The book starts with an overview of the epidemiology of the obesity epidemic and its relationship to cardiovascular disease. Chapters 1 to 8 outline our current understanding of genetics and the pathophysiological changes in the obese that lead to the development of heart disease and vascular dysfunction. Obesity-related syndromes are reviewed as well. Chapters 9 to 17 present expected improvement in cardiovascular risk factors with weight reduction in the obese, and address specific treatment strategies for managing the obese patient with cardiovascular disease. Whenever possible, the authors have included recommendations on medical management issues that may be of specific relevance to the obese patient. Finally, given the huge public health implications of overnutrition; the concluding chapter discusses public health initiatives and obesity prevention strategies.

All too often patients are treated for cardiovascular disease without concerted effort to address significant weight issues. This book provides the rationale as well as approach to management of a complex and common group of patients, emphasizing the need to treat both cardiovascular disease *and* obesity. The effect of such a combined treatment strategy may be synergistic. We believe this text will be a valuable tool for anyone who provides care for obese patients with cardiovascular disease.

A new book does not succeed without the hard work of many individuals. We would like to thank all the authors who have contributed their time and effort to make this new text a valuable resource. In addition, there are a few individuals who are essential to the successful completion of such a project, but work behind the scenes. We would like to thank specifically two individuals—Barbara Hodges and Kris Mogensen—who are also co-authors of this book. With their administrative and editorial assistance, Barbara and Kris have helped bring this book from its inception to its finish and have made the journey much easier than it would have been without their help.

*Malcolm K. Robinson*
*Abraham Thomas*

# Contents

# Contributors

**Caroline Apovian**  Boston University School of Medicine and Center of Nutrition and Weight Management, Boston Medical Center, Boston, Massachusetts, U.S.A.

**Alain D. Baron**  Indiana University School of Medicine, Indianapolis, Indiana, and Amylin Pharmaceuticals, Inc., San Diego, California, U.S.A.

**Shari S. Bassuk**  Division of Preventive Medicine, Brigham and Women's Hospital, Harvard Medical School, Boston, Massachusetts, U.S.A.

**Kenneth L. Baughman**  Advanced Heart Disease Section, Cardiovascular Division, Department of Medicine, Brigham and Women's Hospital, Harvard Medical School, Boston, Massachusetts, U.S.A.

**George L. Blackburn**  Beth Israel Deaconess Medical Center and Harvard Medical School, Center for the Study of Nutrition Medicine, Boston, Massachusetts, U.S.A.

**Kelly D. Brownell**  Department of Psychology, Yale University, New Haven, Connecticut, U.S.A.

**Supawan Buranapin**  Boston University School of Medicine, Boston, Massachusetts, U.S.A.

**Yvon C. Chagnon**  Psychiatric Genetic Unit, Laval University Robert-Giffard Research Center, Beauport, Québec, Canada

**Zara Cooper** Department of Surgery, Brigham and Women's Hospital, Harvard Medical School, Boston, Massachusetts, U.S.A.

**Natalie M. Egan** Program for Weight Management, Brigham and Women's Hospital, Boston, Massachusetts, U.S.A.

**Cesar E. Escareno** Department of Surgery, Brigham and Women's Hospital, Harvard Medical School, Boston, Massachusetts, U.S.A.

**Robert B. Fogel** Division of Sleep Medicine, Brigham and Women's Hospital, Boston, Massachusetts, U.S.A.

**Andrew B. Geier** Department of Psychology, University of Pennsylvania, Philadelphia, Pennsylvania, U.S.A.

**Michael M. Givertz** Advanced Heart Disease Section, Cardiovascular Division, Department of Medicine, Brigham and Women's Hospital, Harvard Medical School, Boston, Massachusetts, U.S.A.

**J. Efren Gonzalez** Metabolic Support Service and the Department of Surgery, Brigham and Women's Hospital, Harvard Medical School, Boston, Massachusetts, U.S.A.

**Jenny Hegmann** Program for Weight Management, Brigham and Women's Hospital, Boston, Massachusetts, U.S.A.

**Barbara B. Hodges** Baystate Medical Center, Springfield, Massachusetts, U.S.A.

**Danny O. Jacobs** Department of Surgery, Duke University Medical Center, Durham, North Carolina, U.S.A.

**Tulika Jain** Department of Internal Medicine and the Donald W. Reynolds Cardiovascular Clinical Research Center, University of Texas Southwestern Medical Center, Dallas, Texas, U.S.A.

**Lalita Khaodhiar** Beth Israel Deaconess Medical Center and Harvard Medical School, Center for the Study of Nutrition Medicine, Boston, Massachusetts, U.S.A.

**Nikheel S. Kolatkar** Division of Endocrinology, Diabetes, and Hypertension, Brigham and Women's Hospital, Harvard Medical School, Boston, Massachusetts, U.S.A.

**David B. Lautz** Department of Surgery, Brigham and Women's Hospital, Harvard Medical School, Boston, Massachusetts, U.S.A.

**JoAnn E. Manson** Division of Preventive Medicine, Brigham and Women's Hospital, Harvard Medical School, Boston, Massachusetts, U.S.A.

**Christos S. Mantzoros** Division of Endocrinology, Diabetes and Metabolism, Department of Medicine, Beth Israel Deaconess Medical Center and Harvard Medical School, Boston, Massachusetts, U.S.A.

**Kieren J. Mather** Indiana University School of Medicine, Indianapolis, Indiana, U.S.A.

**Karen C. McCowen** Beth Israel Deaconess Medical Center and Harvard Medical School, Boston, Massachusetts, U.S.A.

**Darren K. McGuire** Department of Internal Medicine and the Donald W. Reynolds Cardiovascular Clinical Research Center, University of Texas Southwestern Medical Center, Dallas, Texas, U.S.A.

**Kathy McManus** Department of Nutrition, Brigham and Women's Hospital, Boston, Massachusetts, U.S.A.

**Kris M. Mogensen** Metabolic Support Service, Brigham and Women's Hospital, Boston, Massachusetts, U.S.A.

**Sanjay R. Patel** Case Western Reserve University, Cleveland, Ohio, U.S.A.

**Jorge Plutzky** Department of Internal Medicine and the Donald W. Reynolds Cardiovascular Clinical Research Center, Harvard Medical School, Boston, Massachusetts, U.S.A.

**Aruna D. Pradhan** Advanced Heart Disease Section, Cardiovascular Division, Department of Medicine, Brigham and Women's Hospital, Harvard Medical School, Boston, Massachusetts, U.S.A.

**Douglas A. Raynor** The State University of New York, Geneseo, New York, U.S.A.

**Vincent Ricchiuti** Division of Endocrinology, Diabetes and Hypertension, Department of Medicine, Brigham and Women's Hospital, Harvard Medical School, Boston, Massachusetts, U.S.A.

**Malcolm K. Robinson**   Metabolic Support Service and the Department of Surgery, Brigham and Women's Hospital, Harvard Medical School, Boston, Massachusetts, U.S.A.

**Greeshma K. Shetty**   Division of Endocrinology, Diabetes and Metabolism, Department of Medicine, Beth Israel Deaconess Medical Center and Harvard Medical School, Boston, Massachusetts, U.S.A.

**Abraham Thomas**   Division of Endocrinology, Diabetes, and Hypertension, Brigham and Women's Hospital, Harvard Medical School, Boston, Massachusetts, U.S.A.

**Asha Thomas-Geevarghese**   Columbia University, College of Physicians and Surgeons, New York, New York, and Medstar Research Institute, Washington, D.C., U.S.A.

**Gordon H. Williams**   Division of Endocrinology, Diabetes, and Hypertension, Brigham and Women's Hospital, Harvard Medical School, Boston, Massachusetts, U.S.A.

**Rena R. Wing**   The Miriam Hospital/Brown Medical School, Providence, Rhode Island, U.S.A.

# 1

# Overview of the Obesity Epidemic and Its Relationship to Cardiovascular Disease

Shari S. Bassuk and JoAnn E. Manson
*Division of Preventive Medicine, Brigham and Women's Hospital, Harvard Medical School, Boston, Massachusetts, U.S.A.*

## PREVALENCE AND OVERALL HEALTH IMPACT OF OVERWEIGHT AND OBESITY

The prevalence of obesity has increased dramatically in recent years. Obesity, or excess body fat, is usually operationally defined in terms of body mass index (BMI), calculated by dividing an individual's weight in kilograms (kg) by the square of height in meters (m). The World Health Organization (WHO) and the U.S. National Institutes of Health (NIH) define overweight as a BMI of 25 to 29.9 $kg/m^2$ and obesity as a BMI of 30 $kg/m^2$ or greater. By this definition, nearly two in three U.S. adults (64.5%) are overweight or obese (1). Although the percentage of adults classified as overweight but not obese has been stable since the 1960s, the prevalence of obesity doubled between 1980 and 2000, rising from 14.5% to 30.5%, and that of severe obesity (i.e., BMI $\geq$40 $kg/m^2$) more than tripled, increasing from 1.3% to 4.7% during this period (1,2). The proportion of U.S. children and adolescents who are overweight is also increasing. In 2000, the prevalence of overweight among those aged 2 to 5 years, 6 to 11 years, and 12 to 19 years was 10.4%, 15.3%, and 15.5%, respectively, as compared with 7.2%, 11.3%, and 10.5% in 1994 (3). Similar trends are occurring in many developed and developing countries. Worldwide, an

*1*

estimated 135 million people were obese in 1995; that number is projected to jump to 300 million by 2025 (4).

Although viewed more as a cosmetic rather than a health concern by the general public and some health care professionals, excess weight is a major risk factor for chronic disease and other medical complications. Recent epidemiologic research has quantified the impact of overweight and obesity on premature mortality, cardiovascular disease (CVD), type 2 diabetes mellitus, respiratory disorders, osteoarthritis, gallbladder disease, certain types of cancer, and other adverse outcomes (5). Direct, dose-dependent relationships between increasing BMI and lifetime risks of cardiovascular and other conditions have been observed in nationally representative samples, such as the National Health and Nutrition Examination Surveys (NHANES) (6) and the Behavioral Risk Factor Surveillance System surveys (7), and in large cohorts followed for lengthy periods, such as the Nurses' Health Study (NHS) (8), the Health Professionals Follow-up Study (HPFS) (8), and the Framingham Heart Study (9) (Table 1). Data from the national Healthcare for Communities survey indicate that, in the United States, obesity is associated with greater morbidity and poorer health-related quality of life than smoking, problem drinking, or poverty (10). One conservative estimate, derived from five long-term prospective cohort studies, is that obesity accounts for 300,000 deaths each year in the United States (11) and will likely overtake smoking as the primary cause of preventable death if current trends continue (12). Data from the Framingham Heart Study (13) and NHANES III (14) indicate that even a moderate amount of excess weight confers a noticeable diminution in life expectancy and that, as degree of overweight increases, a striking and steady contraction of life span occurs. For example, in the Framingham Heart Study, 40-year-old, overweight but not obese nonsmokers without a history of CVD lived an average of three years less than their normal-weight counterparts, and obese 40-year-olds lived six to seven years less than those with normal weight (13). In NHANES III, the number of years of life lost due to severe obesity (BMI $\geq 45 \, \text{kg/m}^2$) was estimated to be eight years for 20- to 30-year-old white women and 13 years for their male counterparts (14). The direct medical costs of obesity comprise 5.5% to 7% of total health care expenditures in the United States (15). The substantial morbidity and mortality associated with overweight and obesity underscore the pressing need to educate the public and medical communities about the hazards of excess weight and to remove the barriers to healthy eating and greater physical activity.

Indeed, the alarming increase in the prevalence of obesity, along with a concurrent rise in that of type 2 diabetes, threatens to undermine the advances in the prevention and treatment of CVD that are thought to be responsible for the striking decline in cardiovascular mortality that occurred during the latter half of the 20th century in the United States and other

**Table 1** Relative Risks and Prevalence Ratios of Selected Cardiovascular Risk Factors and Conditions in the Nurses' Health Study (NHS),[a] the Health Professionals Follow-up Study (HPFS),[a] and the Third National Health and Nutrition Examination Survey (NHANES III)[b]

| | Diabetes | Hypertension | High cholesterol level | Coronary heart disease |
|---|---|---|---|---|
| **NHS** | | | | |
| *Women aged 40–65 years at baseline* | | | | |
| BMI (kg/m²) | | | | |
| 18.5–21.9 (referent) | 1.0 | 1.0 | 1.0 | 1.0 |
| 22.0–24.9 | 2.2 | 1.4 | 1.3 | 1.2 |
| 25.0–29.9 | 8.1 | 2.1 | 1.3 | 1.5 |
| 30.0–34.9 | 17.8 | 2.6 | 1.0 | 1.7 |
| ≥35.0 | 30.1 | 2.9 | 0.8 | 1.7 |
| **HPFS** | | | | |
| *Men aged 40–75 years at baseline* | | | | |
| BMI (kg/m²) | | | | |
| 18.5–21.9 (referent) | 1.0 | 1.0 | 1.0 | 1.0 |
| 22.0–24.9 | 1.8 | 1.5 | 1.3 | 1.1 |
| 25.0–29.9 | 5.6 | 2.4 | 1.6 | 1.7 |
| 30.0–34.9 | 18.2 | 3.8 | 1.5 | 2.2 |
| ≥35.0 | 41.2 | 4.2 | 1.6 | 2.4 |

*(Continued)*

**Table 1** Relative Risks and Prevalence Ratios of Selected Cardiovascular Risk Factors and Conditions in the Nurses' Health Study (NHS),[a] the Health Professionals Follow-up Study (HPFS),[a] and the Third National Health and Nutrition Examination Survey (NHANES III)[b] (Continued)

| | Diabetes | Hypertension | High cholesterol level | Coronary heart disease |
|---|---|---|---|---|
| **NHANES III** | | | | |
| *Women aged <55 years/≥55 years* | | | | |
| BMI (kg/m²) | | | | |
| 18.5–24.9 (referent) | 1.0/1.0 | 1.0/1.0 | 1.0/1.0 | 1.0 |
| 25–29.9 | 3.82/1.81 | 1.65/1.16 | 1.90/1.23 | 1.30 |
| 30–34.9 | 2.49/2.49 | 3.22/1.24 | 1.67/1.10 | 1.58 |
| 35–39.9 | 10.67/3.24 | 3.90/1.42 | 1.71/1.19 | 1.74 |
| ≥40 | 12.87/5.76 | 5.45/1.41 | 1.68/0.91 | 2.98 |
| *Men aged <55 years/≥55 years* | | | | |
| BMI (kg/m²) | | | | |
| 18.5–24.9 (referent) | 1.0/1.0 | 1.0/1.0 | 1.0/1.0 | 1.0 |
| 25–29.9 | 3.27/1.77 | 1.62/1.11 | 1.28/1.18 | 0.97 |
| 30–34.9 | 10.14/2.56 | 2.52/1.35 | 1.34/1.17 | 1.59 |
| 35–39.9 | 7.95/4.23 | 4.50/1.47 | 1.37/0.85 | 1.14 |
| ≥40.0 | 18.08/3.44 | 4.60/1.66 | 1.45/0.88 | 2.22 |

[a]Table values are relative risks after 10 years of follow-up, adjusted for age, smoking status, and race/ethnicity. For the NHS, the data are based on a cohort of 77,690 women aged 40–65 years at start of the 10-year follow-up. For the HPFS, the data are based on a cohort of 46,060 men aged 40–75 years at start of the 10-year follow-up.

[b]Table values are prevalence ratios, adjusted for age, smoking status, and race/ethnicity. The data are based on a cross-sectional analysis of 16,884 men and women aged 25 years and older. For all conditions except coronary heart disease, prevalence ratios are reported within four gender–age subgroups (men aged <55 years, men aged ≥55 years, women aged <55 years, and women aged ≥55 years). For coronary heart disease, prevalence ratios were similar in those aged <55 years and those aged ≥55 years; therefore, the data are stratified only by gender for this outcome.

*Abbreviations*: BMI, body mass index.

*Source*: Data from Refs. 6, 8.

developed countries. Since the late 1960s, reductions in CVD mortality have averaged 2% each year in the United States. Nevertheless, CVD is expected to remain the number one killer in the Western world for the foreseeable future, and the long-standing secular decline in cardiovascular mortality may be reaching a plateau. Although age-adjusted death rates from coronary heart disease (CHD) declined more than 3% per year between 1970 and 1990, the yearly rate of decline in CHD mortality fell below 3% between 1990 and 2000 (16). For stroke mortality, there has been an even more marked deceleration of the annual rate of decline. After falling at a rate of 4.9% per year between 1970 and 1980, and 3.5% per year between 1980 and 1990 (17), age-adjusted stroke mortality declined less than 2% per year from 1990 to 2000 (16). In addition, congestive heart failure mortality more than doubled between 1970 and 2000 (16).

## METHODOLOGIC ISSUES IN EPIDEMIOLOGIC STUDIES OF OBESITY AND HEALTH OUTCOMES

Many epidemiologic studies report U- or J-shaped relationships between BMI and morbidity or mortality, with disease or death rates elevated in persons with very low and high relative body weights. While extremes of adiposity or leanness are clearly deleterious, pinpointing the precise range of weights associated with optimal health or minimal mortality has been controversial, primarily because of methodologic limitations that can distort inferences about the role of weight in health outcomes (18). One such problem is the failure to consider the effects of preexisting overt or occult disease. Weight loss resulting from illness may obfuscate positive dose–response relationships between adiposity and morbidity or mortality. To reduce bias from this reverse causation, investigators may limit analyses to subjects who appear to be healthy at baseline, and they may exclude the first several years of follow-up. However, certain unrecognized conditions such as preclinical cancers, depression, alcoholism or other substance abuse, early pulmonary or cardiac failure, or diabetes are often associated with insidious weight loss beginning years before formal diagnosis. Another limitation is uncontrolled confounding by factors such as cigarette smoking. Because smoking tends to be more prevalent among lean individuals and is also a strong independent risk factor for diseases such as CVD and cancer, failure to adjust for its effect will produce artificially inflated disease or mortality rates among the lean. Although such confounding can be partly controlled by statistical methods, the best estimates are likely to be derived from studies of never smokers. A third issue is that of inappropriate statistical control for the biologic consequences of obesity, such as hypertension, dyslipidemia, or hyperglycemia. This approach eliminates some of the physiologic pathways by which obesity mediates morbidity and mortality risk, thus attenuating observed associations.

Early studies did not fully address these methodologic issues. For example, the Metropolitan Life Insurance Company tables of desirable weights were developed without information on cigarette smoking and were thus biased toward higher recommended weights. Because the full impact of smoking on health may not become apparent until after many decades of exposure, this bias may be accentuated over time. Such an effect might account for the upward revision to the weight-for-height ranges that occurred when the 1959 Metropolitan Life tables were updated in 1983.

One early investigation that did attempt to control for confounders was the American Cancer Society's Cancer Prevention Study I, a cohort of nearly one million men and women who were followed for 12 years (19). Although the analysis did not address the potential for reverse causation due to preclinical disease, it did stratify the data by smoking status. Among individuals who had never smoked, mortality was minimal at or somewhat below the cohort's average relative weight. The excess mortality observed in the lowest weight groups was more pronounced among current or ex-smokers than among never smokers, and was mainly due to cancers of the lung, bladder, and pancreas, strongly implicating smoking as the causal factor. A reanalysis of these data using BMI instead of relative weights and excluding smokers and those with a history of cancer, CVD, or recent weight loss (20), and a new analysis of a second American Cancer Society cohort of more than one million adults with 14 years of follow-up (21), showed a clearer pattern of increasing mortality with increasing weight. Among healthy people who had never smoked, the lowest mortality occurred at a BMI of 23.5 to $24.9\,kg/m^2$ for men and 22.0 to $23.4\,kg/m^2$ for women (Fig. 1). These results confirm similar observations from recent large cohort studies, including a 27-year follow-up of 19,000 middle-aged men in the Harvard Alumni Study (22), a 16-year follow-up of 115,000 middle-aged female nurses in the NHS (23), a 10-year follow-up of 40,000 middle-aged men in the HPFS (24), a 12-year follow-up of 20,000 nonsmoking Seventh Day Adventists in the Adventist Health Study (25), a 13-year follow-up of 10,000 Canadians in the nationally representative Canada Fitness Survey (26), and a 22-year follow-up of more than two million Norwegian men and women (27). In the aggregate, these studies support current guidelines that set the healthy weight range for adults at BMIs between 18.5 and $25\,kg/m^2$.

In contrast to weight in adulthood, weight in childhood has been less extensively studied as a predictor of subsequent health outcomes. However, a recent investigation of 227,000 Norwegian adolescents aged 14 to 19 years who were followed for 32 years found that a high BMI was strongly associated with premature mortality (28). Compared with those whose baseline BMI was in the 25th to 75th percentile of a U.S. reference population, males with baseline BMI in the 85th to 95th percentile and those with BMI above the 95th percentile were 30% and 80% more likely to die in early to middle

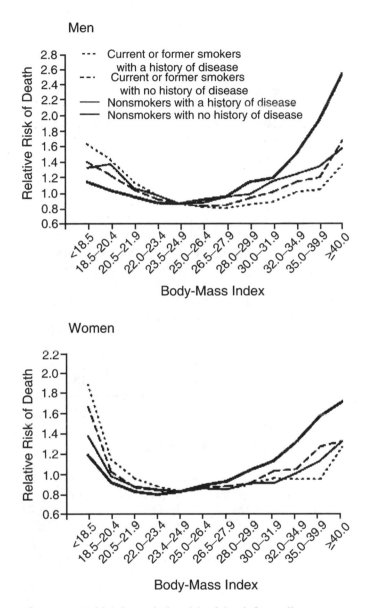

**Figure 1** Multivariate relative risk of death from all causes among men and women according to BMI, smoking status, and disease status. Subjects with a BMI of 23.5 to 24.9 kg/m² are the reference group. *Abbreviation*: BMI, body mass index. *Source*: From Ref. 21.

adulthood, respectively. The corresponding risk increases among females were 30% and 100%.

Regarding the opposite end of the age spectrum, some data suggest that the range of optimal weights shifts upward in later life. However, this finding may be an artifact of the increasing prevalence of weight loss secondary to chronic disease among older individuals, the cumulative effects of cigarette smoking, and the reduced reliability of BMI as a measure of adiposity with advancing age. Although technically a function of both fat and fat-free mass, BMI is highly correlated with fat mass in young and middle-aged adults. Among the elderly, however, weight changes often reflect losses in fat-free mass resulting from inactivity or chronic illness, thus complicating interpretation of indices such as BMI that are based only on weight and height. For example, a population-based study of 787 Swedish men who were 60 years old found that, while the 22-year mortality rate was lowest among those in the middle fifth of the BMI distribution, death rates increased in a linear fashion from the lowest to the highest quintile of percentage fat mass (29). Larger studies that relied on BMI as an indirect measure of adiposity, such as the American Cancer Society's Cancer Prevention Study I (20), the Framingham Heart Study (30), the Adventist Health Study (25), and the aforementioned study of two million Norwegians (27), indicate that although the strength of the association between body weight and mortality does decrease with age, being overweight remains predictive of premature death, and that at least up to age 75 years, a BMI under $25 \, \text{kg/m}^2$ is associated with reduced total mortality. It is also worth noting that observed age-associated reductions in the *relative* risk of mortality associated with obesity do not imply reductions in the *absolute* risk or risk difference. Rather, the absolute number of deaths attributable to obesity appears to increase with age.

Most estimates of the health effects of obesity are derived from studies of white populations of European ancestry. Data are sparse for other racial and ethnic groups. Some investigators have suggested that optimal BMI varies with the prevalence of obesity in the population in question; that is, among groups with a high prevalence of obesity, such as African Americans, Pacific Islanders, and American Indians, the adverse impact of adiposity on morbidity or mortality may occur at a somewhat higher BMI, whereas among groups with a low prevalence of obesity, such as people of Asian ancestry, the adverse impact may occur at a somewhat lower BMI. However, there is currently no compelling evidence to support the exclusion of any racial or ethnic group from the current WHO/NIH definitions of overweight and obesity (31).

One limitation that pertains specifically to studies of total mortality, as opposed to studies of disease-specific outcomes, is that they are insensitive in pinpointing the weight range associated with optimal health. There are two reasons for this insensitivity. First, obesity, similar to virtually every other risk factor, is unlikely to influence all causes of death. In large investigations of multiple health outcomes (e.g., the NHS), the relative risks associated with high BMI are generally lower for all-cause mortality than for the incidence of specific conditions such as myocardial infarction (MI), ischemic stroke, and type 2 diabetes. Similarly, although only limited data support the hypothesis that intentional weight loss reduces total mortality, such weight loss has conclusively been shown to reduce many disease-specific risks. The second reason that the use of mortality outcomes is not the best way to determine optimal weights is that mortality is only a small part of the substantial burden of disease caused by conditions such as diabetes, hypertension, angina pectoris, and total CVD.

## OBESITY AND CVD

Although linked with CVD for centuries, obesity was named a major modifiable coronary risk factor by the American Heart Association only within the last decade (32). In epidemiologic studies, obesity has been associated with an increased risk of CHD, stroke, venous thromboembolism, and congestive heart failure.

### Intermediate End Points

Cardiovascular Risk Factors

Obesity raises the risk of developing CVD partly through its effects on established vascular risk factors such as hypertension, dyslipidemia, insulin resistance, and glucose intolerance. Excess weight is also associated with several novel risk factors for CVD and diabetes, most notably elevations in thrombotic markers such as fibrinogen and plasminogen activator inhibitor-1 (33–35), and in inflammatory markers such as interleukin-6 and C-reactive protein (36–38). Independent of its effect on these established and novel risk factors, obesity also appears to have a residual impact on risk of CVD itself, a finding that is most pronounced in prospective studies with long follow-up periods. For example, the Chicago Heart Association Detection Project in Industry Study, a 25-year investigation of 40,000 male and female employees of Chicago-area companies, found that, in analyses adjusted for systolic blood pressure, serum cholesterol level, and diabetes, the association between BMI and cardiovascular mortality did not clearly emerge until after 16 years of observation (39).

Consistent with the excess CHD risk observed even among persons at the upper limit of the healthy weight range, the prevalence and incidence of some cardiovascular risk factors rises rapidly at BMIs above $20 \, \text{kg/m}^2$. For example, as shown in Figure 2, the relative risks of incident hypertension after 16 years of follow-up in the NHS were 1.00 for BMI under $20 \, \text{kg/m}^2$ (the referent category), 1.15 for BMI of 20.0 to $20.9 \, \text{kg/m}^2$, 1.35 for BMI

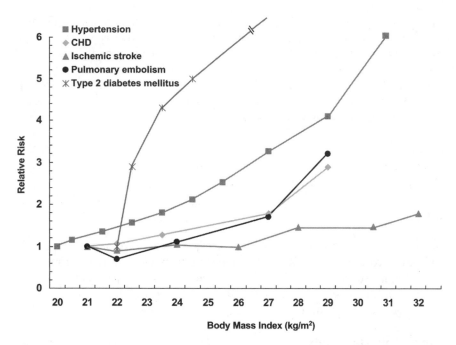

**Figure 2** Age-adjusted relative risks of hypertension, coronary heart disease, ischemic stroke, pulmonary embolism, and type 2 diabetes mellitus according to BMI up to 32 kg/m$^2$, after 14 to 16 years of follow-up of the Nurses' Health Study cohort. *Abbreviation*: BMI, body mass index. *Source*: Data from Refs. 40–44.

of 21.0 to 21.9 kg/m$^2$, 1.56 for BMI of 22.0 to 22.9 kg/m$^2$, 1.80 for BMI of 23.0 to 23.9 kg/m$^2$, and 2.12 for BMI of 24.0 to 24.9 kg/m$^2$ (40). Relative risks continued to climb with increasing degrees of overweight, reaching 6.12 for BMI of 31 kg/m$^2$ or higher. In a study of 14,000 healthy female employees of the British company Marks and Spencer, marked age-adjusted increases in systolic and diastolic blood pressure, serum total cholesterol, low-density lipoprotein (LDL) cholesterol, triglycerides, and fasting blood glucose, as well as significant decreases in high-density lipoprotein (HDL) cholesterol, were observed across seven categories of BMI ranging from less than 20 to greater than 30 kg/m$^2$ (45). The Framingham Offspring Study has also demonstrated that many men and women with BMIs between 23 and 25 kg/m$^2$ have abnormalities in serum lipids, glucose tolerance, and blood pressure compared with those with BMIs less than 23 kg/m$^2$, and that most individuals with BMIs above 25 kg/m$^2$ have such abnormalities (46); the BMI associated with the optimal cardiovascular risk profile was 22.6 kg/m$^2$ for men and 21.2 kg/m$^2$ for women. While most investigations of weight and metabolic risk factors have been conducted among Western populations, a study of 1610 rural Chinese peasants also found a striking monotonic rise in adverse lipid, glucose, and blood pressure profiles as BMI increased from $<18$ to $>24 \, kg/m^2$ (47).

Strong associations between relative body weight and cardiovascular risk factors have also been observed in children and adolescents (48–53). In the Bogalusa Heart Study, which examined 9157 Louisiana children aged 5 to 17 years, lipid, insulin, and blood pressure levels did not vary with BMI at levels below the 85th percentile of a national reference population (48). However, the probability of having an adverse lipid, blood pressure, or insulin profile was substantially higher in children with BMI above the 95th percentile than in children with BMI below the 85th percentile. Overweight children were 2.4, 3.0, 3.4, 7.1, and 12.6 times more likely than normal-weight children to have a total cholesterol level above 200 mg/dL, LDL cholesterol above 130 mg/dL, HDL cholesterol below 35 mg/dL, triglycerides of 130 mg/dL or higher, and fasting insulin at or above the 95th percentile, respectively. Overweight children were also 4.5 times more likely to have an elevated systolic blood pressure and 2.4 times more likely to have an elevated diastolic blood pressure than their normal-weight counterparts.

Few data are available regarding the long-term benefits of intentional weight loss on incidence of CVD. In small, short-term clinical trials of varying design, modest weight loss among overweight and obese individuals has been associated with favorable changes in cardiovascular risk factors, including blood pressure, glucose tolerance, lipoprotein profile, and markers of inflammation and hemostasis (54–58). In the observational Framingham Heart Study, a 2.25-kg (5 lb) weight loss (intentionality was not assessed) over 16 years lowered the sum of five cardiovascular risk factors (highest quintile of systolic blood pressure, triglycerides, blood glucose, and serum total cholesterol, plus lowest quintile of HDL cholesterol) by 48% in men and 40% in women; conversely, a 2.25-kg weight gain was associated with a 20% increase in the cardiovascular risk factor sum in men and a 37% increase in women (59). However, data from the Swedish Obese Subjects study, which examined outcomes of surgically induced weight loss in middle-aged obese individuals, suggest that, over an eight-year period, persons who had maintained significant weight loss experienced a return to baseline blood pressure, despite their maintenance of a lower weight (60). More research is needed in this area.

### Subclinical Atherosclerosis

Several recent angiographic and autopsy studies have examined the association between excess weight and subclinical atherosclerosis. In three cohorts followed from childhood to early or middle adulthood (ages 25 to 42 years)—the Muscatine (Iowa) Study (61), the Cardiovascular Risk in Young Finns Study (62), and the Bogalusa Heart Study (63)—participants with high BMI as children were significantly more likely to have high carotid intima-media thickness (IMT), measured using B-mode ultrasound, as adults. Indeed, childhood BMI was better than adult BMI at predicting IMT in these studies. In the Kuipio Ischemic Heart Disease Risk Factor Study of 774 Finnish men aged 42 to 60 years, abdominal obesity was associated with an accelerated progression of atherosclerosis, as measured by changes in IMT during four years of follow-up (64). In an autopsy study of 3000 15- to 34-year-old persons who died of external causes, obesity, as measured by BMI or by thickness of the panniculus adiposus (an indicator of subcutaneous abdominal fat), was strongly associated with the presence of coronary lesions among adolescent boys and young men, although not among similarly aged females (65). The relationship between adiposity and atherosclerosis in males remained strong even after adjustment for major coronary risk factors.

## Clinical Cardiovascular Outcomes

### CHD

Many long-term prospective cohort studies have demonstrated a strong association between excess weight and CHD, the leading cause of death in the United States. The relationship appears to be linear, and even individuals of average weight at midlife are at increased risk compared with their leaner counterparts. For example, in the NHS, even after controlling for age, smoking, menopausal status, postmenopausal hormone use, and parental history of MI, the relative risk of CHD over 14 years of follow-up was 1.19 for women with BMIs of 21 to 22.9 $kg/m^2$, 1.46 for BMIs of 23 to 24.9 $kg/m^2$, 2.06 for BMIs of 25 to 28.9 $kg/m^2$, and 3.56 for BMIs of 29 $kg/m^2$ or more, compared with women whose BMIs were less than 21 $kg/m^2$ (41). Nearly two-fifths (37%) of CHD incidence in this cohort was attributable to excess weight, defined as a BMI of 21 $kg/m^2$ or greater. Weight gain between the age of 18 and midlife was also associated in a dose-dependent fashion with increased risk of CHD. Compared with women with stable weight, women who gained 5 to 7.9 kg were 1.25 times more likely to develop CHD, and those who gained 20 kg or more were 2.65 times more likely to do so. Viewed alternatively, CHD risk increased by 3.1% for each kilogram gained. More than one-quarter (27%) of the overall incidence in this cohort could be accounted for by weight gains of 5 kg or more.

In the British Regional Heart Study, a 15-year follow-up of nearly 8000 middle-aged men, the risk of major coronary events and cardiovascular mortality increased progressively with increasing BMI, even after adjustment for age, smoking, social class, alcohol use, and physical activity level (66). An increase in body weight equivalent to 1 BMI unit from 20.0 $kg/m^2$ onwards was predictive of a 10% increase in the rate of coronary events. In a cohort of 16,000 middle-aged Finnish men and women followed for 15 years, each 1-unit increase in BMI was associated with a 4% to 5%

increase in CHD mortality (67). A 26-year follow-up of 5200 participants in the Framingham Heart Study showed that high relative weight at baseline was directly associated with CHD and coronary mortality independent of age, cholesterol level, systolic blood pressure, smoking, and other cardiovascular risk factors (9). In agreement with findings from the NHS, the proportion of CHD attributable to excess weight was estimated to be approximately 25%, and weight gain during young and middle adulthood was associated with increased risk of CVD in both men and women.

In the Framingham Heart Study, a strong association between relative weight and CHD incidence did not emerge until after eight years of observation, at which point the strength of the relationship remained fairly constant for the remainder of the 26-year follow-up (9). Similarly, in a cohort of 3983 young men (mean age at baseline, 30.8 years) who participated in the Manitoba Study, an association between BMI and CHD was not evident until after 16 years of observation, with the strongest relationship seen after 20 years (68). Among 1707 middle-aged male employees without a history of CHD or cancer in the Chicago Western Electric Company Study, the BMI–CHD mortality association appeared U-shaped during the first 14 years of follow-up, but became linear in years 15 through 22 (69). In a 30-year study of 1619 Finnish men aged 40 to 59 years, a high BMI (BMI $\geq 24.8 \, \text{kg/m}^2$) was predictive of increased CHD risk only during the third decade of follow-up (70). These data illustrate the importance of using sufficiently long follow-up periods to ensure that adverse effects of excess weight on cardiovascular outcomes are not underestimated in epidemiologic studies.

In addition to the amount of excess fat, the regional distribution of such fat also appears to influence cardiovascular health. Adipose tissue in the waist, abdomen, and upper body is more metabolically active than that in the hip, thigh, or buttocks, and abdominal fat accumulation appears to be a more important predictor than gluteofemoral fat of atherogenic dyslipidemia (specifically, the combination of elevated triglycerides, small dense LDL particles, and low HDL cholesterol), hypertension, and CHD, as well as of type 2 diabetes. Abdominal adiposity is commonly estimated using waist circumference or waist-to-hip ratio (WHR). The National Heart, Lung, and Blood Institute (NHLBI) recommends that a waist circumference of 88 cm or more (35 in. or more) in women or 102 cm or more (40 in. or more) in men, or alternatively, a WHR higher than 0.80 in women or 0.95 in men, be used as an adjunct to BMI to classify high-risk obesity (31). In NHANES III, waist circumference was more closely related to the prevalence of various cardiovascular risk factors than was BMI (71). Moreover, within BMI categories of 18.5 to 24.9, 25 to 29.9, and 30 to 34.9 $\text{kg/m}^2$, individuals whose waist circumferences were higher than the NHLBI cutoff points were more likely to have hypertension, diabetes, and dyslipidemia than those with smaller waist circumferences, although these relationships were stronger in women than in men (72). Indeed, abdominal obesity is a prominent component of the clustering of metabolic risk factors known as the metabolic syndrome, which is a powerful risk factor for diabetes and CVD (73,74). Defined by the National Cholesterol Education Program as the presence of at least three of the following: abdominal obesity, hypertriglyceridemia, low HDL cholesterol, hypertension, and fasting hyperglycemia (75), the metabolic syndrome is present in 20% to 25% of U.S. adults (76,77). The heightened sensitivity of abdominal fat cells to lipolytic agents and the subsequent direct delivery of free fatty acids and glycerol to the liver, which can induce insulin resistance, are possible pathophysiologic explanations for the observed associations (78).

A few prospective studies have found more robust associations between abdominal obesity and CHD in women than in men, although more data are needed to confirm this gender difference (79). In an eight-year follow-up of NHS participants, after adjustment for BMI and other cardiac risk factors, women in the highest WHR or waist circumference quintile had 2.5 times the risk of developing CHD as compared with women in the lowest quintiles (80). In analyses limited to women with BMI of $25 \, kg/m^2$ or less, a WHR of 0.76 or higher (vs. WHR <0.72) and a waist circumference of 76.2 cm (30 in.) or more (vs. waist circumference <71.1 cm) were each associated with an approximate doubling of CHD incidence, after adjustment for cardiac risk factors. By contrast, the Physicians' Health Study, which followed 16,164 male physicians aged 40 to 84 years for 3.9 years, indicated abdominal adiposity was not an independent predictor of CHD; after adjustment for BMI, men in the highest WHR ($\geq 0.99$) and waist circumference ($\geq 103.6$ cm) quintiles were 23% and 6% more likely to develop CHD, respectively, compared with men in the lowest quintiles (79). Neither risk increase was statistically significant. In a similar analysis using data from the HPFS, men in the highest waist circumference quintile ($\geq 40$ in.) experienced a nonsignificant 44% increase in CHD risk during three years of follow-up (81). However, some longer term studies have found that abdominal adiposity remains strongly associated with incident CHD in men after adjustment for BMI. For example, in an 11-year follow-up of 1346 middle-aged men in the Kuipio Ischemic Heart Disease Risk Factor Study, WHR added to the predictive value of BMI, whereas the converse was not observed (82). Similarly, in a 13-year follow-up of 792 Swedish men in the 54-year age group (The Study of Men Born in 1913), WHR was more closely associated with incident CVD than BMI (83).

If there is a true gender difference in the strength of the association between abdominal adiposity and CHD, the underlying cause is not known. Higher relative risks in women may result in part from the fact that they have a lower baseline risk of CHD than men. Also, in women as compared with men, there may be tighter correlations between abdominal adiposity and elevated adrenal corticosteroids and androgens, and high levels of these hormones may confer an elevated CHD risk (84).

Stroke

The clear weight-related increases in blood pressure, lipids, and blood glucose described above should be expected to lead to an elevated risk of stroke among overweight and obese individuals. However, epidemiologic data on the obesity–stroke relationship are less consistent than are data on the obesity–CHD relationship, with roughly equal numbers of positive and null findings to date. Some of the contradictory results may be due to the fact that stroke subtypes have rarely been examined, despite the fact that ischemic and hemorrhagic strokes may have differing risk factor profiles. Indeed, among women in the NHS, BMI and weight gain were strongly associated with an increased risk of total and ischemic stroke, but not hemorrhagic stroke, over a 16-year period (42). After adjustment for age, smoking, postmenopausal hormone use, and menopausal status, the relative risks of ischemic stroke increased steadily with degree of over-weight, from 1.75 among women with BMIs of 27.0 to $28.9 \, \text{kg/m}^2$, to 1.90 for BMI of 29.0 to $31.9 \, \text{kg/m}^2$, and to 2.37 for BMI of $32 \, \text{kg/m}^2$ or more, compared with women with a BMI of less than $21 \, \text{kg/m}^2$. Conversely, there was an inverse (albeit nonsignificant) relationship between excess weight and hemorrhagic stroke, with the highest risk among women in the leanest BMI category. Low serum cholesterol, which is more prevalent among lean individuals, may be associated with increased blood vessel fragility or altered endothelial function, predisposing to hemorrhagic strokes. These findings suggest that because hemorrhagic stroke is more often fatal than ischemic stroke, studies that rely on mortality end points may underestimate the impact of obesity on total stroke incidence.

On the other hand, the Physicians' Health Study, a 12-year follow-up of 21,000 U.S. male physicians, found that high BMI was associated with an elevated risk of hemorrhagic as well as ischemic stroke; indeed, the magnitude of the relative risk was similar for both outcomes (85). Compared with men with a BMI of less than $23 \, \text{kg/m}^2$, those with a BMI of $30 \, \text{kg/m}^2$ or higher had nearly twice the risk of ischemic stroke and 2.25 times the risk of hemorrhagic stroke. Other studies also suggest that excess weight increases the risk of total stroke in men. For example, in the Gothenburg Study, a 15-year follow-up of 2287 70-year-old Swedes, men in the top quartile of the sample BMI ($\geq 28 \, \text{kg/m}^2$) or WC ($\geq 99 \, \text{cm}$) distributions were 68% and 65% more likely, respectively, to experience a stroke than men in the bottom quartiles, after adjustment for vascular risk factors; such associations were not observed in women (86).

Venous Thromboembolism

Studies of the risk factors for venous thromboembolism, which have largely been conducted among samples of hospitalized patients, have generally demonstrated an association between excess weight and deep-vein thrombosis or pulmonary embolism. Two prospective studies of community-dwelling populations support this association. Among 113,000 female nurses participating in the NHS, the risk of developing primary pulmonary embolism over 16 years of follow-up was threefold higher among those with BMIs of at least $29 \text{ kg/m}^2$ as compared with those with BMIs less than $21 \text{ kg/m}^2$ (43). Among 855 60-year-old Swedish men followed for 26 years, men with waist circumferences exceeding 100 cm (corresponding to the highest decile of the distribution in the sample) were nearly four times as likely as men with waist circumferences under 100 cm to experience deep-vein thrombosis or pulmonary embolism (87).

### Congestive Heart Failure

Obesity has been linked to congestive heart failure via its impact on cardiovascular risk factors, including hypertension, dyslipidemia, and hyperglycemia, that increase risk of MI, a precursor of heart failure. Indeed, epidemiologic data indicate that about 60% of heart failure cases are attributable to preexisting CHD (88). However, obesity also appears to promote the development of heart failure independently of its effect on CHD. For example, obesity directly affects left ventricular function by increasing cardiac output and intravascular volume, which leads to elevated left ventricular filling pressure and end-diastolic volume. The resulting cardiac dilatation and left ventricular hypertrophy increase heart failure risk.

In the NHANES I Epidemiologic Follow-up Study, which followed 13,643 adults aged 25 to 74 years for 19 years, persons who were overweight (defined as BMI $\geq 27.8 \text{ kg/m}^2$ for men and BMI $\geq 27.3 \text{ kg/m}^2$ for women) were 30% more likely to develop heart failure than were their normal-weight counterparts. After adjustment for CHD history, hypertension, diabetes, and other risk factors for heart failure (88), the proportion of heart failure cases attributable to excess weight was estimated to be 8.0%. In a 10-year follow-up of 1749 New Haven, Connecticut residents aged 65 or older without CHD at baseline, persons with a BMI of $28 \text{ kg/m}^2$ or greater were 60% more likely to develop heart failure than were those with BMI of less than $24 \text{ kg/m}^2$ (89), and the association was not attenuated after adjustment for the occurrence of MI during follow-up. In these two cohorts, left ventricular function was not assessed, and heart failure was diagnosed via hospital discharge records or death certificates.

In a 14-year follow-up of Framingham Heart Study participants, overweight individuals were 34% more likely than normal-weight individuals to develop heart failure, and obese individuals were twice as likely to do so, even after adjustment for electrocardiographically measured left ventricular hypertrophy, history of MI, and other risk factors (90). There was a graded increase in the risk for incident heart failure across BMI levels; for each 1-unit increase in BMI, heart failure risk climbed by 6%. About 14% of cases of heart failure among women and 11% of cases among men were attributable to obesity. In analyses limited to patients who had undergone echocardiographic evaluation within 30 days of first hospitalization for heart failure (24% of incident cases), obesity predicted both systolic and diastolic heart failure.

## OBESITY AND DISORDERS THAT ARE ASSOCIATED WITH AN ELEVATED RISK OF CVD

### Type 2 Diabetes Mellitus

Excess weight plays a critically important role in the etiology of type 2 diabetes mellitus, which in the United States is a major risk factor for premature CHD and stroke (91,92), as well as the main cause of kidney failure, limb amputations, and new-onset blindness in adults (93). Obesity, especially abdominal obesity, causes insulin resistance and compensatory hyperinsulinemia, which in turn are implicated in the development of type 2 diabetes. The marked rise in obesity among U.S. adults during the past decade has been accompanied by a 49% increase in diabetes prevalence (93), and it is estimated that the number of individuals in the United States with diagnosed diabetes will increase by 165% between 2000 and 2050 (94). Observed increases in type 2 diabetes have been especially marked in younger age groups, which portends devastating health consequences. In a four-year follow-up of 7844 members of a health-maintenance organization, patients whose type 2 diabetes had been diagnosed at ages 18 to 44 years were 14 times more likely to suffer an MI than were age- and sex-matched control subjects (95). In contrast, patients whose type 2 diabetes had been diagnosed at ages 45 years or older had 3.7 times the risk of MI than similarly matched controls. Although part of the difference in the relative risks is due to the difference in baseline risks of type 2 diabetes in younger and older age groups, early-onset type 2 diabetes appears to be an even more deleterious disease than late-onset diabetes in terms of cardiovascular sequelae.

Data from NHANES III indicate a direct relationship between BMI and prevalence of type 2 diabetes among U.S. adults (Fig. 3) (96). Strong associations between BMI and type 2 diabetes have also been consistently observed in ethnically diverse populations, including Europeans (97), Japanese (98), Mexicans (99), and Native Americans (100). Of five "lifestyle" variables—obesity, lack of physical activity, poor diet, current smoking, and alcohol abstinence—examined in the NHS, excess body weight was by far the single most important predictor of diabetes onset among 85,000 women (101). The risk of developing type 2 diabetes over 16 years of follow-up was nearly 40-fold higher for women with a BMI of 35 kg/m$^2$ or greater and 20-fold higher for women with a BMI of 30.0 to 34.9 kg/m$^2$, as compared with women who had a BMI of 23 kg/m$^2$ or less. Even a BMI in the high "normal" range (23.0–24.9 kg/m$^2$) was associated with a

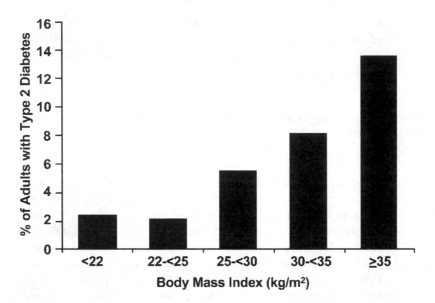

**Figure 3**  Prevalence of type 2 diabetes mellitus according to body mass index in adults aged 20 years or older, Third National Health and Nutrition Examination Survey, 1988–1994. *Source*: From Ref. 96.

nearly threefold increase in risk over that experienced by women with BMIs of 23.0 kg/m$^2$ or less. Taking women with BMIs less than 25.0 kg/m$^2$ as the reference group, the 10-year relative risk of incident diabetes was 4.6 among women with BMIs of 25.0 to 29.9 kg/m$^2$, 10.0 among those with BMIs of 30.0 to 34.9 kg/m$^2$, and 17.0 among those with BMIs of 35.0 kg/m$^2$ or greater (8). In the HPFS, taking men with BMIs less than 25.0 kg/m$^2$ as the reference group, the 10-year relative risk was 3.5 for those with BMIs of 25.0 to 29.9 kg/m$^2$, 11.2 for those with BMIs of 30.0 to 34.9 kg/m$^2$, and 23.4 for those with BMIs of 35.0 kg/m$^2$ or greater (8). In the NHANES Epidemiologic Follow-up Study, a nationally representative cohort of 8545 adults aged 18 and older followed for nine years, the incidence of diabetes climbed rapidly as BMIs increased above 22 kg/m$^2$ (102). For each 1-unit increase in BMI (about 2.7–3.6 kg for the average participant), the risk of developing diabetes increased 12%. The proportion of diabetes in U.S. adults attributable to excess weight (i.e., BMI ≥22 kg/m$^2$) was estimated to be approximately 70%, after factoring out the effects of smoking, alcohol use, cholesterol, blood pressure, and use of antihypertensive medications.

In each of these studies, weight gain during adulthood was also associated with a significant increase in risk of developing type 2 diabetes, although the magnitude of the estimates varied. In the NHANES

Epidemiologic Follow-up Study, individuals who gained 5.0 to 7.9 kg over the preceding 10 years experienced a doubling of risk over a nine-year period as compared with their stable-weight counterparts, and those who gained 20.0 kg or more had a fourfold risk increase (102). In the NHS, compared with women with stable weight, women who gained 5.0 to 7.9 kg from early to mid-adulthood also had a near doubling of risk over a 14-year follow-up, but women who gained 20.0 kg or more had more than a 12-fold risk increase (44).

Given the high prevalence of diabetes—in the United States, more than 17 million people have the disease, and an additional 16 million have blood glucose levels in the "prediabetic" range (93)—even modest reductions in risk could dramatically influence the health impact of this disorder. Although findings are not entirely consistent (103,104), metabolic benefits of weight loss have been observed in population-based observational studies (105,106). Among more than 200,000 overweight participants in the American Cancer Society's Cancer Prevention Study I, a history of intentional weight loss at baseline, as compared with a history of stable weight, was associated with a reduction in diabetes incidence of 28% in women and 21% in men over 13 years of follow-up, after adjustment for pre-baseline BMI and other metabolic risk factors (105). On average, for every 20 pounds lost, the risk of diabetes fell by 17% in women and by 11% in men. Among the 4970 overweight individuals with diabetes, intentional weight loss was associated with a 28% reduction in mortality due to diabetes or CVD and a 25% reduction in total mortality (106). The largest mortality reduction was associated with weight losses of 20 to 29 pounds (10–15% of initial weight); losses of 70 or more pounds ($\geq$30% of initial weight) were associated with a slight increase in mortality. A similar pattern of results was observed for diabetes- and CVD-related mortality.

In addition, many intervention studies in high-risk populations suggest that modest-to-moderate weight loss, either alone or combined with physical activity, improves glucose levels and insulin action among persons with type 2 diabetes (107) and lowers the risk of diabetes among overweight individuals. In the Swedish Obese Subjects study, severely obese patients (mean BMI, 41 kg/m$^2$) who received gastric surgery or conventional treatment were followed for eight years. During follow-up, the gastric surgery patients maintained an average weight loss of 20.1 kg (16% of initial body weight) and experienced a 84% reduction in diabetes risk as compared with the conventionally treated patients, whose weight did not change significantly (60). Although treatment was not randomly assigned in this study, randomized clinical trials convincingly demonstrate that even modest weight loss reduces diabetes risk. In the Da Qing Impaired Glucose Tolerance and Diabetes Study, 577 middle-aged Chinese men and women with impaired glucose tolerance were randomized to one of three treatment groups—diet only, exercise only, or diet plus exercise—or to a control group (108). Over six years, the three interventions were associated with statistically significant reductions of 31%, 46%, and 42% in diabetes risk, respectively. In the Finnish Diabetes Prevention Study, 522 middle-aged, overweight men and women with impaired glucose tolerance were randomly assigned to an intensive lifestyle intervention designed to promote healthy eating and exercise patterns or to a control group (109). Members of the diet and exercise intervention group lost significantly more weight than did the control group (3.5 kg vs. 0.8 kg) and reduced their risk of developing diabetes by 58% over a three-year interval. The U.S. Diabetes Prevention Program, a three-year follow-up of 3234 men and women aged 25 to 85 years with impaired glucose tolerance, also reported a 58% reduction in diabetes risk among the intervention group, whose members, on average, exercised 30 minutes/day and lost 5% to 7% of their body weight during the course of the trial (110). This trial oversampled older individuals, as well as members of ethnic groups that suffer disproportionately from diabetes (i.e., African, Hispanic, and Asian Americans; Pacific Islanders; and American Indians), and found that the lifestyle intervention was effective in reducing diabetes risk in all age and ethnic groups. Indeed, among people aged 60 and older, who have a nearly 20% prevalence of diabetes, the intervention was associated with a 71% reduction in diabetes risk. Another ongoing large-scale randomized intervention, the Look AHEAD (Action For Health in Diabetes) trial funded by the National Institute of Diabetes and Digestive and Kidney Diseases, should provide valuable information about the long-term (≥10 years) effects of sustained weight loss through decreased caloric intake and exercise on the risk of CVD and other chronic conditions in obese diabetic individuals (111).

## Respiratory Disorders

Excessive fat in the pharyngeal area, chest wall, and abdomen can profoundly alter pulmonary function via adverse effects on respiratory mechanics, respiratory muscle function, lung volume, and upper-airway narrowing. Sleep apnea, defined as frequent episodic airflow cessation during sleep that is often accompanied by excessive daytime sleepiness, is a common obesity-related respiratory complication, especially among men. Habitual snoring and sleep apnea were reported by more than half of men and one third of women in the Swedish Obese Subjects study (112), compared with 4% of men and 2% of women in general populations. In the Wisconsin Sleep Cohort Study, a four-year follow-up of 690 middle-aged state government employees, weight gain was a significant risk factor for sleep apnea, with a 10% weight gain associated with a sixfold increase in the risk of developing moderate-to-severe sleep-disordered breathing (113). In addition to interfering with work and social functioning, sleep apnea also appears to be an independent risk factor for hypertension, insulin resistance, and possibly CVD (114,115). Among 6400 middle-aged participants in the multi-center Sleep Heart Health Study, for example, sleep-disordered breathing was significantly associated with increased risks of heart failure, stroke, and CHD, even after adjustment for BMI (116). Weight loss significantly alleviates sleep apnea and improves nighttime breathing (117).

Obesity has been linked to the development of asthma, which is a potential, though not established, risk factor for CVD (118). In a four-year follow-up of 86,000 NHS participants, overweight women experienced a 50% increase in risk, and obese women a tripling of risk, of adult-onset asthma, compared with women with BMIs of 20.0 to 22.4 kg/m$^2$ (119). Weight gain was also associated with a significant increase in asthma risk. In a two-year follow-up of 9149 adults in the Canadian National Population Health Surveys, obese women were 90% more likely than normal-weight women to develop asthma, but a similar relationship between BMI and asthma was not observed in men (120). Additional prospective studies are needed to confirm these findings.

## Quality of Life

Health-related quality of life is a multidimensional construct, encompassing functional status as well as social and emotional feelings of well being that reflect an individual's evaluation of and reaction to health or illness. In recent years, prospective epidemiologic studies have provided clear evidence of the importance of psychosocial factors such as depression, anxiety, social isolation, and chronic life stress in the development and prognosis of CVD (121–124). In addition, other studies have established the value of regular, moderate physical activity for cardioprotection (125). Thus, to the extent that obesity adversely affects social and psychological health and curtails one's ability to engage in work- or leisure-time physical activity, it would be expected to increase the risk of CVD.

Numerous studies indicate that obese persons experience significant impairments in their health-related quality of life, with greater degrees of obesity associated with greater impairments. In NHANES III, for example, the proportion of men and women who perceived themselves to be in excellent health decreased linearly with increasing BMI among whites, blacks, and Hispanics, even in the absence of chronic disease conditions (126). The Healthcare for Communities survey, which interviewed a nationally representative sample of 9585 U.S. adults, found that obesity is associated with a poorer quality of life than smoking, problem drinking, or poverty (10).

### Social and Psychological Health

Negative stereotypes of obesity, especially of obesity in women, pervade many Western societies. Obese people are often perceived as indolent, less intelligent, dishonest, and lacking in self-control. These unfavorable attitudes can lead to discrimination in school, workplace, and other settings, resulting in diminished economic and social opportunities for obese individuals (127). Compared with their leaner counterparts, obese workers earn less money for equivalent jobs, and they are less likely to be hired in the first place. Obese women are less likely to marry than are nonobese women, and those who do marry are more likely to wed someone of a lower socioeconomic status.

Although it is plausible that chronic social stigmatization may lead to lowered self-esteem or other poor psychological outcomes in obese individuals, few population-based studies have examined the relationship between perceived weight discrimination and emotional disturbance in obese persons. Indeed, studies of obesity and psychological symptoms report inconsistent results, with some studies finding direct association and others finding no association. Several surveys suggest that the psychological ramifications of obesity are worse for women than for men. In a nationally representative sample of 40,000 U.S. adults, for example, a BMI of 30 kg/m² or more was associated with a 37% *increased* risk of past-year major depression among women but only a 37% *decreased* risk of depression among men, as compared with the risk observed among individuals with BMIs of 20.8 to 29.9 kg/m², after adjustment for age, race, education, income, and history of cardiovascular or other disease (128). Similar patterns were also observed for suicidal thoughts and behaviors. Among obese women, risks of recent suicide ideation and attempts were each elevated by about 20%, whereas among obese men, risks of suicide ideation and attempts were lower by 26% and 55%, respectively. In the Swedish Obese Subjects study, while severely obese participants of both genders reported significantly more symptoms of anxiety and depression than either chronically ill or general population samples, such associations were far more pronounced in women (129). However, appetite changes and disordered eating patterns are common manifestations of affective disorders, rendering it impossible to disentangle cause and effect in these cross-sectional studies. Among 40,000 women in the NHS, a higher BMI at baseline was not related to subsequent onset of mood symptoms during a four-year follow-up, although a weight gain of 9 kg or more was significantly correlated with concomitant increases in such symptoms (130). In the 26-year Chicago Heart Association Detection Project in Industry Study, a higher BMI in middle age was associated with poorer social functioning and mental health at older ages; baseline psychosocial measures were not available (131). Additional population-based longitudinal research is needed to clarify the nature of relationship between excess weight and psychopathology.

### Physical Functioning

In contrast to the equivocal findings for mental health outcomes, available epidemiologic data consistently implicate obesity in the development of physical disability. In the NHS, for example, both higher BMI at baseline and substantial weight gain were strongly associated with reduced daily physical functioning and vitality and a greater burden of bodily pain. The average decline in physical function experienced by women under the age of 65 who gained 9 kg or more over a four-year period was approximately three times the magnitude of that associated with cigarette smoking over the same period (130). In the four-year NHANES Epidemiologic Follow-up Study, limitations in daily activities requiring mobility occurred twice as often among middle-aged and elderly white women who were in the highest BMI tertile compared with those in the lowest tertile (132). Self-reported onset of difficulties in walking and climbing a flight of stairs also occurred 2.3 times more often in the obese among a predominantly African- and Mexican-American middle-aged population, with an overall incidence rate of 6% during a two-year follow-up (133). The Whitehall II study, a large population study of British civil servants, found that obesity without other chronic conditions predicted the onset of impaired physical functioning in both men and women, although the relative risks were higher in women (134). Steady weight gain from early to middle adulthood also predicted poor physical function in women, independent of baseline BMI.

## CONCLUSION

While the prevalence of many cardiovascular risk factors, including smoking, high cholesterol, and untreated hypertension, has fallen significantly in the United States and other developed countries since the 1960s, the prevalence of overweight and particularly obesity continues to rise and is reaching epidemic proportions in both developed and developing nations. Given the strong associations between excess weight and CHD, ischemic stroke, type 2 diabetes, and other conditions that increase the risk of CVD, this trend portends an enormous global burden of obesity-related cardiovascular morbidity and mortality in the coming years.

Adapting successful public health strategies used to educate the public about the dangers of smoking, high cholesterol, and hypertension should help with the prevention and treatment of overweight. In terms of prevention, to experience optimal health and quality of life, most adults should strive to maintain a body weight corresponding to a BMI between 18.5 and 25 kg/m$^2$, although the upper limit of the range should be somewhat lower to minimize cardiovascular risk. Even small weight gains of five or more kilograms are important signals indicating the need for adjustments in caloric intake and physical activity to prevent further weight increases. In terms of treatment, health professionals should play an active role in counseling already overweight and obese patients about the hazards of excess weight and encouraging sustained behavioral changes in the context of setting realistic goals and emphasizing the benefit of modest weight reductions. According to data compiled by the U.S. Preventive Services Task Force, high-intensity counseling and behavioral interventions typically produce sustained weight loss of 3 to 5 kg over periods of one year or more in obese persons (high-intensity is defined as two or more sessions per month for at least the first three months of a given intervention) (135). Given the soaring prevalence of overweight and obesity, helping even a small percentage of overweight or obese patients achieve a lower weight would substantially reduce cardiovascular morbidity and mortality, as would helping those already in the healthy weight range avoid future weight gain.

## REFERENCES

1. Flegal KM, Carroll MD, Ogden CL, Johnson CL. Prevalence and trends in obesity among US adults, 1999–2000. JAMA 2002; 288:1723–1727.
2. Flegal KM, Carroll MD, Kuczmarski RJ, Johnson CL. Overweight and obesity in the United States: prevalence and trends, 1960–1994. Int J Obes Relat Metab Disord 1998; 22:39–47.
3. Ogden CL, Flegal KM, Carroll MD, Johnson CL. Prevalence and trends in overweight among US children and adolescents, 1999–2000. JAMA 2002; 288:1728–1732.
4. King H, Aubert RE, Herman WH. Global burden of diabetes, 1995–2025: prevalence, numerical estimates, and projections. Diabetes Care 1998; 21: 1414–1431.
5. Willett WC, Dietz WH, Colditz GA. Guidelines for healthy weight. N Engl J Med 1999; 341:427–434.
6. Must A, Spadano J, Coakley EH, Field AE, Colditz G, Dietz WH. The disease burden associated with overweight and obesity. JAMA 1999; 282:1523–1529.
7. Mokdad AH, Ford ES, Bowman BA, et al. Prevalence of obesity, diabetes, and obesity-related health risk factors, 2001. JAMA 2003; 289:76–79.
8. Field AE, Coakley EH, Must A, et al. Impact of overweight on the risk of developing common chronic diseases during a 10-year period. Arch Intern Med 2001; 161:1581–1586.
9. Hubert HB, Feinleib M, McNamara PM, Castelli WP. Obesity as an independent risk factor for cardiovascular disease: a 26-year follow-up of participants in the Framingham Heart Study. Circulation 1983; 67:968–977.
10. Sturm R, Wells KB. Does obesity contribute as much to morbidity as poverty or smoking? Public Health 2001; 115:229–235.
11. Allison DB, Fontaine KR, Manson JE, Stevens J, VanItallie TB. Annual deaths attributable to obesity in the United States. JAMA 1999; 282: 1530–1538.
12. U.S. Department of Health and Human Services. The Surgeon General's Call to Action to Prevent and Decrease Overweight and Obesity. Rockville, MD: U.S. Department of Health and Human Services, Public Health Service, Office of the Surgeon General, 2001.

13. Peeters A, Barendregt JJ, Willekens F, Mackenbach JP, Al Mamun A, Bonneux L. Obesity in adulthood and its consequences for life expectancy: a life-table analysis. Ann Intern Med 2003; 138:24–32.

14. Fontaine KR, Redden DT, Wang C, Westfall AO, Allison DB. Years of life lost due to obesity. JAMA 2003; 289:187–193.

15. Thompson D, Wolf AM The medical-care cost burden of obesity. Obes Rev 2001; 2:189–197.

16. National Heart Lung and Blood Institute. Morbidity and Mortality: 2002 Chart Book on Cardiovascular, Lung, and Blood Diseases, 2002.

17. Cooper R, Cutler J, Desvigne-Nickens P, et al. Trends and disparities in coronary heart disease, stroke, and other cardiovascular diseases in the United States: findings of the National Conference on Cardiovascular Disease Prevention. Circulation 2000; 102:3137–3147.

18. Manson JE, Stampfer MJ, Hennekens CH, Willett WC. Body weight and longevity. A reassessment. JAMA 1987; 257:353–358.

19. Lew EA, Garfinkel L. Variations in mortality by weight among 750,000 men and women. J Chronic Dis 1979; 32:563–576.

20. Stevens J, Cai J, Pamuk ER, Williamson DF, Thun MJ, Wood JL. The effect of age on the association between body-mass index and mortality. N Engl J Med 1998; 338:1–7.

21. Calle EE, Thun MJ, Petrelli JM, Rodriguez C, Heath CW Jr. Body-mass index and mortality in a prospective cohort of U.S. adults. N Engl J Med 1999; 341:1097–1105.

22. Lee IM, Manson JE, Hennekens CH, Paffenbarger RS Jr. Body weight and mortality. A 27-year follow-up of middle-aged men. JAMA 1993; 270: 2823–2828.

23. Manson JE, Willett WC, Stampfer MJ, et al. Body weight and mortality among women. N Engl J Med 1995; 333:677–685.

24. Baik I, Ascherio A, Rimm EB, et al. Adiposity and mortality in men. Am J Epidemiol 2000; 152:264–271.

25. Singh PN, Lindsted KD, Fraser GE. Body weight and mortality among adults who never smoked. Am J Epidemiol 1999; 150:1152–1164.

26. Katzmarzyk PT, Craig CL, Bouchard C. Underweight, overweight and obesity: relationships with mortality in the 13-year follow-up of the Canada Fitness Survey. J Clin Epidemiol 2001; 54:916–920.

27. Engeland A, Bjorge T, Selmer RM, Tverdal A. Height and body mass index in relation to total mortality. Epidemiology 2003; 14:293–299.

28. Engeland A, Bjorge T, Sogaard AJ, Tverdal A. Body mass index in adolescence in relation to total mortality: 32-year follow-up of 227,000 Norwegian boys and girls. Am J Epidemiol 2003; 157:517–523.

29. Heitmann BL, Erikson H, Ellsinger BM, Mikkelsen KL, Larsson B. Mortality associated with body fat, fat-free mass and body mass index among 60-year-old Swedish men – a 22-year follow-up. The Study of Men Born in 1913. Int J Obes Relat Metab Disord 2000; 24:33–37.

30. Garrison RJ, Castelli WP. Weight and thirty-year mortality of men in the Framingham Study. Ann Intern Med 1985; 103:1006–1009.

31. National Heart Lung and Blood Institute. Clinical guidelines on the identification, evaluation, and treatment of overweight and obesity in adults—the evidence report. Obes Res 1998; 6:51S–209S.

32. Eckel RH, Krauss RM. American Heart Association call to action: obesity as a major risk factor for coronary heart disease. AHA Nutrition Committee. Circulation 1998; 97:2099–2100.

33. Sakkinen PA, Wahl P, Cushman M, Lewis MR, Tracy RP. Clustering of procoagulation, inflammation, and fibrinolysis variables with metabolic factors in insulin resistance syndrome. Am J Epidemiol 2000; 152:897–907.

34. Mavri A, Alessi MC, Bastelica D, et al. Subcutaneous abdominal, but not femoral fat expression of plasminogen activator inhibitor-1 (PAI-1) is related to plasma PAI-1 levels and insulin resistance and decreases after weight loss. Diabetologia 2001; 44:2025–2031.

35. Mertens I, Van der Planken M, Corthouts B, et al. Visceral fat is a determinant of PAI-1 activity in diabetic and non-diabetic overweight and obese women. Horm Metab Res 2001; 33:602–607.

36. Visser M, Bouter LM, McQuillan GM, Wener MH, Harris TB. Elevated C-reactive protein levels in overweight and obese adults. JAMA 1999; 282:2131–2135.

37. Festa A, R D'Agostino Jr, Williams K, et al. The relation of body fat mass and distribution to markers of chronic inflammation. Int J Obes Relat Metab Disord 2001; 25:1407–1415.

38. Rexrode KM, Pradhan A, Manson JE, Buring JE, Ridker PM. Relationship of total and abdominal adiposity with CRP and IL-6 in women. Ann Epidemiol 2003; 13:674–682.

39. Dyer AR, Stamler J, Garside DB, Greenland P. Long-term consequences of body mass index for cardiovascular mortality: the Chicago Heart Association Detection Project in Industry Study. Ann Epidemiol 2004; 14:101–108.

40. Huang Z, Willett WC, Manson JE, et al. Body weight, weight change, and risk for hypertension in women. Ann Intern Med 1998; 128:81–88.

41. Willett WC, Manson JE, Stampfer MJ, et al. Weight, weight change, and coronary heart disease in women. Risk within the 'normal' weight range. JAMA 1995; 273:461–465.

42. Rexrode KM, Hennekens CH, Willett WC, et al. A prospective study of body mass index, weight change, and risk of stroke in women. JAMA 1997; 277: 1539–1545.

43. Goldhaber SZ, Grodstein F, Stampfer MJ, et al. A prospective study of risk factors for pulmonary embolism in women. JAMA 1997; 277:642–645.

44. Colditz GA, Willett WC, Rotnitzky A, Manson JE. Weight gain as a risk factor for clinical diabetes mellitus in women. Ann Intern Med 1995; 122:481–486.

45. Ashton WD, Nanchahal K, Wood DA. Body mass index and metabolic risk factors for coronary heart disease in women. Eur Heart J 2001; 22:46–55.

46. Garrison RJ, Kannel WB. A new approach for estimating healthy body weights. Int J Obes Relat Metab Disord 1993; 17:417–423.

47. Hu FB, Wang B, Chen C, et al. Body mass index and cardiovascular risk factors in a rural Chinese population. Am J Epidemiol 2000; 151:88–97.

48. Freedman DS, Dietz WH, Srinivasan SR, Berenson GS. The relation of overweight to cardiovascular risk factors among children and adolescents: the Bogalusa Heart Study. Pediatrics 1999; 103:1175–1182.

49. Gillum RF. Distribution of waist-to-hip ratio, other indices of body fat distribution and obesity and associations with HDL cholesterol in children and young adults aged 4–19 years: The Third National Health and Nutrition Examination Survey. Int J Obes Relat Metab Disord 1999; 23:556–563.

50. Daniels SR, Morrison JA, Sprecher DL, Khoury P, Kimball TR. Association of body fat distribution and cardiovascular risk factors in children and adolescents. Circulation 1999; 99:541–545.

51. Cook DG, Mendall MA, Whincup PH, et al. C-reactive protein concentration in children: Relationship to adiposity and other cardiovascular risk factors. Atherosclerosis 2000; 149:139–150.

52. Cook DG, Whincup PH, Miller G, et al. Fibrinogen and factor VII levels are related to adiposity but not to fetal growth or social class in children aged 10–11 years. Am J Epidemiol 1999; 150:727–736.

53. Ford ES. C-reactive protein concentration and cardiovascular disease risk factors in children: Findings from the National Health and Nutrition Examination Survey 1999–2000. Circulation 2003; 108:1053–1058.

54. Stefanick ML. Physical activity and weight loss. Manson JE, Buring JE, Ridker PM, Gaziano JM, eds. Clinical Trials in Heart Disease: A companion guide to Braunwald's Heart Disease. WB Saunders: Philadelphia 2004; 315–332.

55. Neter JE, Stam BE, Kok FJ, Grobbee DE, Geleijnse JM. Influence of weight reduction on blood pressure: A meta-analysis of randomized controlled trials. Hypertension 2003; 42:878–884.

56. Esposito K, Pontillo A, Di C Palo, et al. Effect of weight loss and lifestyle changes on vascular inflammatory markers in obese women: A randomized trial. JAMA 2003; 289:1799–1804.

57. Tchernof A, Nolan A, Sites CK, Ades PA, Poehlman ET. Weight loss reduces C-reactive protein levels in obese postmenopausal women. Circulation 2002; 105:564–569.

58. Van Gaal LF, Wauters MA, De Leeuw IH. The beneficial effects of modest weight loss on cardiovascular risk factors. Int J Obes Relat Metab Disord 1997; 21:S5–S9.

59. Wilson PW, Kannel WB, Silbershatz H, D'Agostino RB. Clustering of metabolic factors and coronary heart disease. Arch Intern Med 1999; 159: 1104–1109.

60. Sjostrom CD, Peltonen M, Wedel H, Sjostrom L. Differentiated long-term effects of intentional weight loss on diabetes and hypertension. Hypertension 2000; 36:20–25.

61. Davis PH, Dawson JD, Riley WA, Lauer RM. Carotid intimal-medial thickness is related to cardiovascular risk factors measured from childhood through middle age: the Muscatine Study. Circulation 2001; 104:2815–2819.

62. Raitakari OT, Juonala M, Kahonen M, et al. Cardiovascular risk factors in childhood and carotid artery intima-media thickness in adulthood: the Cardiovascular Risk in Young Finns Study. JAMA 2003; 290:2277–2283.

63. Li S, Chen W, Srinivasan SR, et al. Childhood cardiovascular risk factors and carotid vascular changes in adulthood: The Bogalusa Heart Study. JAMA 2003; 290:2271–2276.

64. Lakka TA, Lakka HM, Salonen R, Kaplan GA, Salonen JT. Abdominal obesity is associated with accelerated progression of carotid atherosclerosis in men. Atherosclerosis 2001; 154:497–504.

65. McGill HC Jr, McMahan CA, Herderick EE, et al. Obesity accelerates the progression of coronary atherosclerosis in young men. Circulation 2002; 105: 2712–2718.

66. Shaper AG, Wannamethee SG, Walker M. Body weight: implications for the prevention of coronary heart disease, stroke, and diabetes mellitus in a cohort study of middle aged men. BMJ 1997; 314:1311–1317.

67. Jousilahti P, Tuomilehto J, Vartiainen E, Pekkanen J, Puska P. Body weight, cardiovascular risk factors, and coronary mortality. 15-year follow-up of middle-aged men and women in eastern Finland. Circulation 1996; 93: 1372–1379.

68. Rabkin SW, Mathewson FA, Hsu PH. Relation of body weight to development of ischemic heart disease in a cohort of young North American men after a 26-year observation period: The Manitoba Study. Am J Cardiol 1977; 39:452–458.

69. Spataro JA, Dyer AR, Stamler J, Shekelle RB, Greenlund K, Garside D. Measures of adiposity and coronary heart disease mortality in the Chicago Western Electric Company Study. J Clin Epidemiol 1996; 49:849–857.

70. Pekkanen J, Tervahauta M, Nissinen A, Karvonen MJ. Does the predictive value of baseline coronary risk factors change over a 30-year follow-up? Cardiology 1993; 82:181–190.

71. Zhu S, Wang Z, Heshka S, Heo M, Faith MS, Heymsfield SB. Waist circumference and obesity-associated risk factors among whites in the Third National Health and Nutrition Examination Survey: clinical action thresholds. Am J Clin Nutr 2002; 76:743–749.

72. Janssen I, Katzmarzyk PT, Ross R. Body mass index, waist circumference, and health risk: evidence in support of current National Institutes of Health guidelines. Arch Intern Med 2002; 162:2074–2079.

73. Haffner S, Taegtmeyer H. Epidemic obesity and the metabolic syndrome. Circulation 2003; 108:1541–1545.

74. Alexander CM, Landsman PB, Teutsch SM, Haffner SM. NCEP-defined metabolic syndrome, diabetes, and prevalence of coronary heart disease among NHANES III participants age 50 years and older. Diabetes 2003; 52: 1210–1214.

75. Expert Panel on Detection, Evaluation, and Treatment of High Blood Cholesterol in Adults. Executive summary of the Third Report of the National Cholesterol Education Program (NCEP) Expert Panel on Detection, Evaluation, and Treatment of High Blood Cholesterol in Adults (Adult Treatment Panel III). JAMA 2001; 285:2486–2497.

76. Ford ES, Giles WH. A comparison of the prevalence of the metabolic syndrome using two proposed definitions. Diabetes Care 2003; 26:575–581.

77. Ford ES, Giles WH, Dietz WH. Prevalence of the metabolic syndrome among US adults: findings from the Third National Health and Nutrition Examination Survey. JAMA 2002; 287:356–359.

78. Reaven GM. Banting lecture 1988. Role of insulin resistance in human disease. Diabetes 1988; 37:1595–1607.

79. Rexrode KM, Buring JE, Manson JE. Abdominal and total adiposity and risk of coronary heart disease in men. Int J Obes Relat Metab Disord 2001; 25:1047–1056.

80. Rexrode KM, Carey VJ, Hennekens CH, et al. Abdominal adiposity and coronary heart disease in women. JAMA 1998; 280:1843–1848.

81. Rimm EB, Stampfer MJ, Giovannucci E, et al. Body size and fat distribution as predictors of coronary heart disease among middle-aged and older US men. Am J Epidemiol 1995; 141:1117–1127.

82. Lakka HM, Lakka TA, Tuomilehto J, Salonen JT. Abdominal obesity is associated with increased risk of acute coronary events in men. Eur Heart J 2002; 23:706–713.

83. Larsson B, Svardsudd K, Welin L, Wilhelmsen L, Bjorntorp P, Tibblin G. Abdominal adipose tissue distribution, obesity, and risk of cardiovascular disease and death: 13-year follow-up of participants in the Study of Men Born in 1913. Br Med J (Clin Res Ed) 1984; 288:1401–1404.

84. Haffner SM. Sex hormones, obesity, fat distribution, type 2 diabetes and insulin resistance: Epidemiological and clinical correlation. Int J Obes Relat Metab Disord 2000; 24:S56–S58.

85. Kurth T, Gaziano JM, Berger K, et al. Body mass index and the risk of stroke in men. Arch Intern Med 2001; 162:2557–2562.

86. Dey DK, Rothenberg E, Sundh V, Bosaeus I, Steen B. Waist circumference, body mass index, and risk for stroke in older people: A 15-year longitudinal population study of 70-year-olds. J Am Geriatr Soc 2002; 50: 1510–1518.

87. Hansson PO, Eriksson H, Welin L, Svardsudd K, Wilhelmsen L. Smoking and abdominal obesity: Risk factors for venous thromboembolism among middle-aged men: "The Study of Men Born in 1913". Arch Intern Med 1999; 159:1886–1890.

88. He J, Ogden LG, Bazzano LA, Vupputuri S, Loria C, Whelton PK. Risk factors for congestive heart failure in US men and women: NHANES I Epidemiologic Follow-up Study. Arch Intern Med 2001; 161:996–1002.

89. Chen YT, Vaccarino V, Williams CS, Butler J, Berkman LF, Krumholz HM. Risk factors for heart failure in the elderly: a prospective community-based study. Am J Med 1999; 106:605–612.

90. Kenchaiah S, Evans JC, Levy D, et al. Obesity and the risk of heart failure. N Engl J Med 2002; 347:305–313.

91. Creager MA, Luscher TF, Cosentino F, Beckman JA. Diabetes and vascular disease: pathophysiology, clinical consequences, and medical therapy: Part I. Circulation 2003; 108:1527–1532.

92. Luscher TF, Creager MA, Beckman JA, Cosentino F. Diabetes and vascular disease: pathophysiology, clinical consequences, and medical therapy: Part II. Circulation 2003; 108:1655–1661.

93. Centers for Disease Control and Prevention. Diabetes: Disabling, Deadly, and on the Rise, 2003.

94. Boyle JP, Honeycutt AA, Narayan KM, et al. Projection of diabetes burden through 2050: impact of changing demography and disease prevalence in the U.S. Diabetes Care 2001; 24:1936–1940.

95. Hillier TA, Pedula KL. Complications in young adults with early-onset type 2 diabetes: losing the relative protection of youth. Diabetes Care 2003; 26: 2999–3005.

96. National Task Force on the Prevention and Treatment of Obesity. Overweight, obesity, and health risk. Arch Intern Med 2000; 160:898–904.

97. Sargeant LA, Wareham NJ, Khaw KT. Family history of diabetes identifies a group at increased risk for the metabolic consequences of obesity and physical inactivity in EPIC-Norfolk: a population-based study. The European Prospective Investigation into Cancer. Int J Obes Relat Metab Disord 2000; 24: 1333–1339.

98. Sakurai Y, Teruya K, Shimada N, et al. Association between duration of obesity and risk of non-insulin-dependent diabetes mellitus. The Sotetsu Study. Am J Epidemiol 1999; 149:256–260.

99. Wei M, Gaskill SP, Haffner SM, Stern MP. Waist circumference as the best predictor of noninsulin dependent diabetes mellitus (NIDDM) compared to body mass index, waist/hip ratio and other anthropometric measurements in Mexican Americans—a 7-year prospective study. Obes Res 1997; 5:16–23.

100. Lee ET, Howard BV, Savage PJ, et al. Diabetes and impaired glucose tolerance in three American Indian populations aged 45–74 years. The Strong Heart Study. Diabetes Care 1995; 18:599–610.

101. Hu FB, Manson JE, Stampfer MJ, et al. Diet, lifestyle, and the risk of type 2 diabetes mellitus in women. N Engl J Med 2001; 345:790–797.

102. Ford ES, Williamson DF, Liu S. Weight change and diabetes incidence: findings from a national cohort of US adults. Am J Epidemiol 1997; 146: 214–222.

103. Modan M, Karasik A, Halkin H, et al. Effect of past and concurrent body mass index on prevalence of glucose intolerance and type 2 (non-insulin-dependent) diabetes and on insulin response. The Israel study of glucose intolerance, obesity and hypertension. Diabetologia 1986; 29:82–89.

104. French SA, Folsom AR, Jeffery RW, Zheng W, Mink PJ, Baxter JE. Weight variability and incident disease in older women: the Iowa Women's Health Study. Int J Obes Relat Metab Disord 1997; 21:217–223.

105. Will JC, Williamson DF, Ford ES, Calle EE, Thun MJ. Intentional weight loss and 13-year diabetes incidence in overweight adults. Am J Public Health 2002; 92:1245–1248.

106. Williamson DF, Thompson TJ, Thun M, Flanders D, Pamuk E, Byers T. Intentional weight loss and mortality among overweight individuals with diabetes. Diabetes Care 2000; 23:1499–1504.

107. Goldstein DJ. Beneficial health effects of modest weight loss. Int J Obes Relat Metab Disord 1992; 16:397–415.

108. Pan XR, Li GW, Hu YH, et al. Effects of diet and exercise in preventing NIDDM in people with impaired glucose tolerance. The Da Qing IGT and Diabetes Study. Diabetes Care 1997; 20:537–544.
109. Tuomilehto J, Lindstrom J, Eriksson JG, et al. Prevention of type 2 diabetes mellitus by changes in lifestyle among subjects with impaired glucose tolerance. N Engl J Med 2001; 344:1343–1350.
110. Diabetes Prevention Program Research Group. Reduction in the incidence of type 2 diabetes with lifestyle intervention or metformin. N Engl J Med 2002; 346:393–403.
111. Ryan DH, Espeland MA, Foster GD, et al. Look AHEAD (Action for Health in Diabetes: design and methods for a clinical trial of weight loss for the prevention of cardiovascular disease in type 2 diabetes. Control Clin Trials 2003; 24:610–628.
112. Grunstein R. Obstructive sleep apnoea as a risk factor for hypertension. J Sleep Res 1995; 4:166–170.
113. Peppard PE, Young T, Palta M, Dempsey J, Skatrud J. Longitudinal study of moderate weight change and sleep-disordered breathing. JAMA 2000; 284:3015–3021.
114. Shamsuzzaman AS, Gersh BJ, Somers VK. Obstructive sleep apnea: implications for cardiac and vascular disease. JAMA 2003; 290:1906–1914.
115. Lattimore JD, Celermajer DS, Wilcox I. Obstructive sleep apnea and cardiovascular disease. J Am Coll Cardiol 2003; 41:1429–1437.
116. Shahar E, Whitney CW, Redline S, et al. Sleep-disordered breathing and cardiovascular disease: cross-sectional results of the Sleep Heart Health Study. Am J Respir Crit Care Med 2001; 163:19–25.
117. Flemons WW. Clinical practice. Obstructive sleep apnea. N Engl J Med 2002; 347:498–504.
118. Suissa S, Assimes T, Brassard P, Ernst P. Inhaled corticosteroid use in asthma and the prevention of myocardial infarction. Am J Med 2003; 115:377–381.
119. Camargo CA Jr, Weiss ST, Zhang S, Willett WC, Speizer FE. Prospective study of body mass index, weight change, and risk of adult-onset asthma in women. Arch Intern Med 1999; 159:2582–2588.
120. Chen Y, Dales R, Tang M, Krewski D. Obesity may increase the incidence of asthma in women but not in men: longitudinal observations from the Canadian National Population Health Surveys. Am J Epidemiol 2002; 155:191–197.
121. Rozanski A, Blumenthal JA, Kaplan J. Impact of psychological factors on the pathogenesis of cardiovascular disease and implications for therapy. Circulation 1999; 99:2192–2217.
122. Hemingway H, Marmot M. Evidence based cardiology: psychosocial factors in the aetiology and prognosis of coronary heart disease. Systematic review of prospective cohort studies. BMJ 1999; 318:1460–1467.
123. Rugulies R. Depression as a predictor for coronary heart disease. A review and meta-analysis. Am J Prev Med 2002; 23:51–61.
124. Wulsin LR, Singal RM. Do depressive symptoms increase the risk for the onset of coronary disease? A systematic quantitative review. Psychosom Med 2003; 65:201–210.

125. Bassuk SS, Manson JE. Physical activity and the prevention of cardiovascular disease. Curr Atheroscler Rep 2003; 5:299–307.
126. Okosun IS, Choi S, Matamoros T, Dever GE. Obesity is associated with reduced self-rated general health status: evidence from a representative sample of white, black, and Hispanic Americans. Prev Med 2001; 32:429–436.
127. Puhl R, Brownell KD. Stigma, discrimination, and obesity. In: Fairburn CG, Brownell KD, eds. Eating Disorders and Obesity. 2nd ed. New York: Guilford Press, 2002:108–112.
128. Carpenter KM, Hasin DS, Allison DB, Faith MS. Relationships between obesity and DSM-IV major depressive disorder, suicide ideation, and suicide attempts: results from a general population study. Am J Public Health 2000; 90:251–257.
129. Sullivan M, Karlsson J, Sjostrom L, et al. Swedish obese subjects (SOS)—an intervention study of obesity. Baseline evaluation of health and psychosocial functioning in the first 1743 subjects examined. Int J Obes Relat Metab Disord 1993; 17:503–512.
130. Fine JT, Colditz GA, Coakley EH, et al. A prospective study of weight change and health-related quality of life in women. JAMA 1999; 282:2136–2142.
131. Daviglus ML, Liu K, Yan LL, et al. Body mass index in middle age and health-related quality of life in older age: The Chicago Heart Association Detection Project in Industry Study. Arch Intern Med 2003; 163:2448–2455.
132. Launer LJ, Harris T, Rumpel C, Madans J. Body mass index, weight change, and risk of mobility disability in middle-aged and older women. The Epidemiologic Follow-up Study of NHANES I. JAMA 1994; 271:1093–1098.
133. Clark DO, Stump TE, Wolinsky FD. Predictors of onset of and recovery from mobility difficulty among adults aged 51–61 years. Am J Epidemiol 1998; 148:63–71.
134. Stafford M, Hemingway H, Marmot M. Current obesity, steady weight change and weight fluctuation as predictors of physical functioning in middle aged office workers: the Whitehall II Study. Int J Obes Relat Metab Disord 1998; 22:23–31.
135. U.S. Preventive Services Task Force. Screening for obesity in adults: recommendations and rationale. Ann Intern Med 2003; 139:930–932.

# 2

# Obesity and Hypertension

**Nikheel S. Kolatkar, Abraham Thomas, and Gordon H. Williams**
*Division of Endocrinology, Diabetes, and Hypertension, Brigham and Women's Hospital, Harvard Medical School, Boston, Massachusetts, U.S.A.*

## INTRODUCTION

Obesity is a highly prevalent disease in the United States and worldwide. From 1991 to 2002 in the United States, the prevalence of obesity, as defined by a body mass index (BMI) greater than $30 \, kg/m^2$, increased 74% (1). The proportion of U.S. states with greater than 15% of the population classified as obese grew from 9% to 98% (1). Hypertension, as defined by a blood pressure greater than 140/90 mmHg is also common, affecting 24% of the U.S. adult population (1). Not surprisingly, a close association exists between obesity and hypertension. In African-American women older than 50 years, the prevalence of obesity is approximately 70%, with a coincident rate of hypertension exceeding 70% (2).

The association between obesity and hypertension has been observed in similar ethnic groups living in different locations, both in industrialized and nonindustrialized societies (3). Cross-sectional data of one million Americans participating in hypertension screening independently associate obesity with hypertension (4). Longitudinal data from the Framingham Heart Study indicate that obesity confers an adjusted relative risk of 2.23 in men and 2.63 in women for the development of hypertension (5). Data from the Nurses' Health Study and the Health Professionals Study cohorts provide similar estimates (6,7). Although blood pressure is not elevated in all obese individuals, animal and human studies consistently demonstrate

33

an independent increase in blood pressure with weight gain, and a decline in blood pressure with weight loss (8–13). The dissociation between obesity and hypertension observed in some individuals may be related to lower baseline blood pressure, genetic differences, or other factors.

Although the association between obesity and hypertension is well established, the pathophysiology is not fully elucidated. Proposed mechanisms include cardiovascular dysfunction, renal structural and hemodynamic changes, activation of the renin–angiotensin–aldosterone system (RAAS) (systemic and intra-adipose tissue), natriuretic peptide effects, changes in hormonal and biochemical mediators [leptin, insulin, free fatty acids (FFA), and glucocorticoids], and nervous system changes (sympathetic nervous system activation, neuropeptides, and neurochemicals).

## CARDIOVASCULAR DYSFUNCTION

### Vascular Dysfunction

Vascular dysfunction has been observed in obese children (14). It is established that insulin resistance and elevated FFA, both highly prevalent in obesity, diminish vascular reactivity (15,16). Insulin resistance also inhibits vascular smooth muscle calcium influx and dampens vessel reactivity (17). Peroxisome proliferator–activated receptor gamma agonists, which reduce insulin resistance, decrease blood pressure in humans (18). Obesity may affect responsiveness to vasoactive peptides such as endothelin-1. Cardillo et al. observed an independent association between BMI and enhanced endothelin-dependent vasoconstrictor activity in subjects infused with an endothelin-receptor antagonist (19).

### Cardiac Dysfunction

Atrial and ventricular function are impaired in obesity. Initially, however, cardiac output increases with weight gain (20,21). Dogs fed a high-fat, sodium-controlled diet over five weeks had significant increases in mean arterial pressure (MAP), resting heart rate, and cardiac output, compared with baseline and lean controls. The initial weight-related increase in cardiac output is primarily due to increased stroke volume (from plasma volume expansion) and compensatory tachycardia (22,23). Over time, however, cardiac hypertrophy and decreased ventricular compliance develop, with myocardial steatosis and lipoapoptosis being observed in animal models (24). Rabbits fed a high-fat diet over 12 weeks become obese and develop left ventricular hypertrophy with reduced diastolic compliance, as compared to lean controls; similarly, dogs fed a high-fat diet for 12 weeks develop increased intracardiac filling pressures and impaired diastolic relaxation (25). Human observational data suggest that BMI independently correlates with left ventricular mass (26,27). Obese participants in the Framingham

Heart Study had twice the risk for development of congestive heart failure over a mean follow-up of 14 years, compared with participants of a normal BMI (28). Obese patients achieving weight reduction through either lifestyle modification or gastroplasty demonstrate improvement in systolic and diastolic function and reduction in left ventricular mass (29,30).

## RENAL STRUCTURAL AND HEMODYNAMIC CHANGES

Weight gain causes renal structural and hemodynamic changes that contribute to increased blood pressure. Excess fat encapsulating the kidney causes extrarenal compression, and deposition of fat, glycosaminoglycan, and hyaluronate in the renal medulla increases interstitial pressure (31–34). These events cause intrarenal pressure to rise, resulting in glomerular hyperfiltration, increased proximal tubular sodium reabsorption, decreased sodium delivery to the macula densa, and RAAS activation. Over time, these hemodynamic changes cause glomerular hypertrophy and glomerulosclerosis (35,36).

## RAAS ACTIVATION

### Systemic RAAS

Obesity is associated with the activation of the systemic RAAS despite an expanded plasma volume (37,38). Tuck et al. measured blood pressure, plasma renin activity (PRA), and plasma aldosterone levels in 25 obese patients over 12 weeks on a weight-reducing diet with either medium (120 mmol/day) or low (40 mmol/day) sodium intake (10). By 12 weeks, PRA and plasma aldosterone decreased independently of sodium intake, and MAP fell significantly in both groups, suggesting that the reductions in PRA and aldosterone contributed to the decline in blood pressure. Boulter et al. studied PRA and plasma aldosterone levels in obese subjects on a 10 day fast with a fixed (50 mmol/day) sodium intake (39). During the first few days, natriuresis occurred, plasma aldosterone rose, and PRA decreased. With continued fasting, however, urinary sodium excretion markedly decreased, plasma aldosterone fell, and PRA rose. Because neither blood pressure nor weight changes were recorded during the study, the significance of these short-term changes in PRA and plasma aldosterone and their potential impact on blood pressure remains unclear (40).

### Adipose Tissue RAAS

Animal and human data suggest the presence of a local RAAS within adipose tissue. Angiotensinogen (AGT) is locally secreted from adipose tissue, and AGT mRNA has been identified in periaortal brown adipose tissue and in adipocytes from arterial vessel walls, atria, and mesentery (41–43). Renin activity has been demonstrated in rat brown adipose tissue after bilateral nephrectomy, and production of angiotensin II from differentiating preadipocytes can be blocked with captopril (44,45). Angiotensin II type 1 (AT1) and type 2 (AT2) receptors have been identified in rat and human adipocytes; however, the function of these receptors is not yet known. Mice with adipose tissue–specific AGT overexpression had greater fat mass and higher blood pressure compared with wild-type animals (46). Faloia et al. studied 35 obese normotensive, 30 obese hypertensive, and 20 nonobese, nonhypertensive control subjects and found no significant difference between groups in PRA or plasma aldosterone levels (47). However, AT1 gene expression in subcutaneous adipose tissue was significantly higher in the obese hypertensives compared to the obese normotensives or controls. It has been hypothesized that an adipose tissue RAAS may act on cellular targets proximal to adipocytes, such as smooth muscle cells, sympathetic nerve fibers, and mononuclear and lymphocytic cells; however, data are lacking.

## NATRIURETIC PEPTIDE SYSTEM EFFECTS

Natriuretic peptides are produced in a variety of tissues and, along with the RAAS, regulate blood pressure via effects on plasma volume, renal sodium handling, and vascular tone (48). The natriuretic peptide system consists of atrial (ANP), brain (BNP), and C-type natriuretic peptides (CNP). Each natriuretic peptide binds to a specific receptor (NPr-A, NPr-B, and NPr-C, respectively) that shares a common structure consisting of a ligand-binding site and transmembrane domain (49). In humans and rats, adipose tissue expresses NPr-A and NPr-C, with NPr-C being highly expressed in obese humans (50). Observational studies have found that ANP and BNP independently negatively correlate with BMI (51,52). Differences in natriuretic peptide clearance via the natriuretic peptide clearance receptor (NPRC) may also contribute to the decreased natriuretic peptide levels seen in obesity. Sarzani et al. found that the cystosine variant of the alanine/cystosine polymorphism in a conserved promoter element of the NPRC was associated with lower ANP levels and higher systolic blood pressure (SBP) and MAP in obese hypertensives, compared with nonobese hypertensives (53).

## EFFECTS OF BIOCHEMICAL AND HORMONAL MEDIATORS

### Leptin

Leptin has a complex effect on blood pressure and may be a mediator in a signaling pathway between adipose tissue and the nervous system (54,55). Leptin does not have a significantly acute effect on blood pressure due to opposing pressor and depressor actions. Leptin administration in Sprague-Dawley rats over three hours increases regional sympathetic nerve activity to brown adipose tissue, the kidneys, and adrenal glands, in the absence of changes in plasma glucose or insulin, but arterial pressure does not increase (56). Acute leptin infusion increases endothelial nitric oxide production, which may offset the greater sympathetic nerve activity (57). However, the pressor effects of leptin appear to predominate chronically. Leptin infusion for 12 days in Sprague-Dawley rats significantly increases arterial pressure, despite a decrease in food intake and an improvement in insulin sensitivity, both of which would be expected to decrease arterial pressure (58).

Neuropeptide Y (NPY) may also mediate the chronic hypertensive effects of leptin. Hyperleptinemia is associated with reduced brain NPY levels, and hypothalamic NPY injection reproduces features of hypoleptine-mia in animals (59). Although administration of NPY into the vagal nucleus of the tractus solitarius or the caudal ventrolateral medulla in the sponta-neously hypertensive rat causes a reduction in blood pressure, relatively few studies have examined the effects of NPY on blood pressure (60). A human study examined the relationship between hypertension and a microsatellite polymorphism region of the leptin gene in hypertensive and normotensive subjects (61). The alleles of the polymorphism consisted of two groups with different size distributions. Investigators found that the genotype frequency of individuals homozygous for the shorter allele was significantly higher in the hypertensive subjects, independent of BMI. A study investigating three leptin receptor polymorphisms (Lys109Arg in exon 4, Gln223Arg in exon 6, and Lys656Asn in exon 14) found that indi-viduals homozygous for arginine at codon 109 (compared with Lys109 homozygotes) and those homozygous for arginine at codon 223 (compared with Gln223 homozygotes) have lower blood pressure independent of other variables (62). No differences were found relative to the Lys656Asn poly-morphism. Further human studies investigating the relationship between leptin, obesity, and blood pressure are warranted.

## Insulin

Obesity is associated with fasting hyperinsulinemia and an exaggerated insu-lin response to glycemic loading (63,64). Insulin, like leptin, also appears to have differential effects on blood pressure. Insulin infusion acutely increases renal sodium reabsorption and reduces sodium excretion. However, chronic hyperinsulinemia stimulates the sympathetic nervous system and increases plasma catecholamines (65,66). In rats, inhibition of thromboxane synthesis or angiotensin-converting enzyme (ACE) abolishes the insulin-induced rise in blood pressure, suggesting that hyperinsulinemia may increase arterial pressure via the RAAS and thromboxane metabolic pathways (67,68). This hypothesis, however, has not been observed in other animal models or in humans. In dogs and humans, experimental hyperinsulinemia does not impair renal pressure–natriuresis or increase arterial pressure (68). In fact, insulin infusions given to raise plasma concentrations of insulin to levels found in obesity actually decrease arterial pressure due to peripheral vaso-dilation. Insulin also does not appear to potentiate the hypertensive or renal effects of pressor substances such as norepinephrine or angiotensin II (69). Studies in dogs using cerebral insulin infusion to examine potential central effects of hyperinsulinemia have not demonstrated an effect on blood pressure (70). Although there may be species variation, further studies are needed to investigate the observed discrepancies between animals and humans regarding the effects of insulin on blood pressure.

## Free Fatty Acids

Obese hypertensive subjects have circulating FFA levels approximately twice those of obese normotensives (71). In rats, short-term FFA (oleic acid) infusion into the portal or systemic circulation increases blood pressure and heart rate, and adrenergic blockade abolishes these effects (72). Infusion into the portal circulation results in a greater blood pressure rise, suggesting that FFA exposure may activate hepatic afferent pathways that lead to sym-pathetic activation. FFA infusion into the cerebrovascular circulation in dogs over several days does not increase blood pressure (73). In humans, peripheral intralipid infusions over four hours significantly increased MAP and decreased elasticity indices in large and small arteries (74).

## Glucocorticoids

The phenotype of Cushing's syndrome resembles that of obesity. It is well established that glucocorticoids regulate adipose tissue differentiation, function, and distribution, and that their systemic excess results in a syn-drome of central adiposity, glucose dysregulation, dyslipidemia, and hypertension. Although obesity is also associated with the same metabolic consequences, circulating glucocorticoid levels are typically normal. How-ever, glucocorticoid action also depends on the intracellular regeneration of active glucocorticoids via the so-called "cortisone–cortisol" shuttle (75). 11β-Hydroxysteroid dehydrogenase (11β-HSD1), which generates active glucocorticoids from inactive cortisone and 11-dehydroxycorticosterone, is widely distributed and abundant in liver and adipose tissue and may serve as a tissue-specific amplifier of glucocorticoid action. Bujalska et al. studied cultured omental and subcutaneous adipose stromal cells from human subjects undergoing elective abdominal surgery (76). Investigators observed significantly higher levels of 11β-HSD1 in omental adipose tissue, sugges-ting tissue-specific amplification of glucocorticoid action in the omentum. 11β-HSD1 knockout mice exhibit an insulin-sensitive phenotype and resist visceral fat accumulation even when fed a high-fat diet (77,78). Conversely, mice with adipose tissue–specific 11β-HSD1 overexpression develop visceral obesity, insulin resistant–diabetes, dyslipidemia, increased blood pressure, increased AGT mRNA expression in mesenteric fat, and higher plasma angiotensin II and aldosterone levels (79,80). These data suggest a potential contribution of adipose tissue 11β-HSD1 expression in the pathogenesis of obesity hypertension.

## NERVOUS SYSTEM CHANGES

### Increased Sympathetic Nervous System Activity

Initial observations in obese humans of increased plasma and urinary catecholamines and an exaggerated plasma norepinephrine response to an upright posture and isometric handgrip, led to the hypothesis that sympathetic stimulation contributes to increased blood pressure in obesity (81). In obese normotensives, Grassi et al. demonstrated that postganglionic sympathetic nerve firing rates, as measured by the microneurographic technique, were twice that of lean controls (82). In dogs, combined alpha- and beta-blockade reduces arterial pressure to a significantly greater extent in obese animals compared to lean animals, and clonidine prevents onset of weight gain–induced hypertension (83). Increased renal efferent sympathetic nerve activity may contribute to the observed sympathetic activation in obesity. In dogs fed a high-fat diet, sodium retention and hypertension were significantly attenuated with bilateral renal denervation (84).

### Neuropeptides and Neurochemical Changes

Evidence from agouti yellow obese mice suggests the possible involvement of the pro-opiomelanocortin (POMC) pathway in the increased sympathetic nerve activity observed in obesity hypertension (85,86). Blockade of hypothalamic alpha–melanocyte stimulating hormone (α-MSH) receptors causes obesity in the agouti syndrome, and agouti yellow obese mice have significantly higher blood pressure, compared with lean controls (87). In Sprague-Dawley rats, acute stimulation of hypothalamic melanocortin (MC)-4 receptors by intracerebroventricular injection of melanotan II increases sympathetic nerve activity to brown adipose tissue and the kidney, but does not result in higher blood pressure (88). Transgenic mice with either targeted disruption of the prohormone convertase-2 (PC2) gene, necessary for processing of POMC into γ-MSH, or the MC3 gene, encoding the MSH receptor, develop salt-sensitive hypertension (89). Intra-abdominal γ-MSH (but not α-MSH) infusion prevents the development of hypertension in the PC2 knockout but not in the MC3 knockout, suggesting that the hypertension may be a specific consequence of impaired POMC processing into γ-MSH. In humans with a mutation at codon 183 (Ile183Asn) in the transmembrane domain of the MC3 receptor, insulin resistance and early-onset obesity has been described. Early-onset obesity has also been described in patients with MSH deficiency, due to mutations interfering with appropriate synthesis of α-MSH and POMC translation (90,91).

The relevance of these findings remains unclear because patients with MSH deficiency due to hypopituitarism have normal energy expenditure and are not uniformly obese or hypertensive (92).

## TREATMENT OF OBESITY HYPERTENSION

### Lifestyle Modification

As with obesity or hypertension alone, lifestyle modification is the recommended initial treatment for obesity hypertension. Caloric reduction and increased physical activity can result in sustained weight loss and amelioration of hypertension in some individuals. In clinical trials implementing low-calorie interventions, moderate weight reduction (10 kg) decreases blood pressure in normotensive and hypertensive subjects. A prospective study of obese adult hypertensives found that modest weight reduction was associated with a significantly lower incidence of hypertension over five years (93,94). Moderate weight loss has also been independently associated with decreased sympathetic activity, PRA, plasma aldosterone, left ventricular mass, and ventricular stroke-work (95).

### Medical Therapy

#### Antihypertensives

Many patients will require pharmacologic intervention to adequately control blood pressure even if weight loss is achieved. Although guidelines from The Joint National Committee (JNC VII) on Prevention, Detection, Evaluation, and Treatment of High Blood Pressure make no specific treatment recommendations for patients with obesity hypertension, suggestions can be made based upon clinical trials data (96,97). The Treatment in Obese Patients with Hypertension (TROPHY) trial examined the efficacy of lisinopril versus hydrochlorothiazide in 232 obese patients with hypertension in a 12-week randomized, placebo-controlled trial (98). At study end, overall blood pressure control was similar with both drugs; however, lisinopril was more effective in Caucasians, and hydrochlorothiazide was more effective in African-Americans. ACE inhibitors may reduce the incidence of type 2 diabetes mellitus as observed in subgroup analyses of the Heart Outcomes Prevention Evaluation (HOPE) trial and the antihypertensive and lipid-lowering treatment to prevent heart attack (ALLHAT) randomized trials (99,100). Similar findings have been reported for angiotensin-receptor blockers in secondary analyses of the Losartan Intervention for Endpoint Reduction (LIFE) and the Candesartan in Heart Failure Assessment of Reduction in Mortality and Morbidity (CHARM) studies (101,102). Trials using beta-blockers have noted blunting of weight reduction, or even relative weight gain. In the United Kingdom Prospective Diabetes Study (UKPDS), diabetic hypertensive subjects treated with beta-blockers gained more weight, as compared with those on ACE inhibitors, although they had equivalent cardiovascular outcomes (103). In the Trial of Antihypertensive Interventions and Management (TAIM), 878 nonobese hypertensive patients were prospectively randomly assigned to no diet change, weight loss, and a low sodium diet (104). The drug effects of placebo, chlorthalidone, or atenolol on weight change were examined in each group. At six months, the drug effect was most pronounced in the weight loss group. In this group, the mean weight reduction was 4.4 kg in the placebo arm, 6.9 kg in the chlorthalidone arm, but only 3.0 kg in the atenolol arm. These differences in drug effect persisted at 24 months. A prospective study of long-term propranolol treatment and changes in body weight after myocardial infarction observed that, at 40 months of follow-up, patients treated with propranolol had gained more weight than those given placebo, after controlling for effects of diuretics and differences in physical activity, gender, and age (105). A double-blinded randomized trial studying obesity as a determinant for the response to antihypertensive therapy in 42 Caucasian men examined the effects on blood pressure of metoprolol versus isradipine in obese and lean subjects (106). Investigators found that after accounting for age and baseline blood pressure, there was a significantly greater decline in MAP with beta-blockers in obese patients.

### Antiobesity Agents

Pharmacologic therapies used primarily to achieve weight loss can affect blood pressure and should be used judiciously in patients with obesity hypertension. There are currently two anti-obesity agents approved for long-term (one year) use by the U.S. Food and Drug Administration: sibutramine and orlistat. Sibutramine is associated with a dose-dependent increase in blood pressure and heart rate and is not generally recommended for use in the obese patient with hypertension (107). In the six-month, randomized, double-blinded, placebo-controlled Sibutramine Trial on Obesity Reduction and Maintenance (STORM), a higher proportion of patients in the treatment arm compared to placebo experienced a significant increase in blood pressure (108). Orlistat, a pancreatic lipase inhibitor, has been associated with favorable effects on lipids, glucose levels, and blood pressure in obese hypertensive patients on antihypertensive medications (109). A meta-analysis of patients from five multicenter, randomized, placebo-controlled trials revealed that, after 56 weeks, orlistat-treated patients had lost significantly more weight than those on placebo, and their mean SBP and diastolic blood pressure (DBP) were significantly reduced compared to those on placebo. These findings were confirmed in a 12-week prospective, randomized trial with primary endpoints of weight and blood pressure reduction (110). Studies of the blood pressure–lowering effects of antiobesity agents beyond two years are lacking. One-year data from the European Rimonabant in Obesity (RIO-Europe) randomized trial demonstrated that subjects receiving the 20 mg dose of rimonabant, a cannabinoid-1 receptor antagonist, had significant reductions in weight, waist circumference, insulin resistance, and triglycerides, compared with those receiving placebo. Blood pressure, however, was not significantly different between the groups (111).

### Surgical Therapy

In the Swedish Obesity Subjects (SOS) study, Sjostrom et al. prospectively followed 4047 obese subjects for up to 10 years. Of these, 1157 were treated with gastric surgery (gastric bypass, gastroplasty, or gastric banding) and 1031 were matched controls treated nonoperatively in primary healthcare settings (112–114). Two-year follow-up data were available for 3505 total subjects and 1,268 had 10 year data. The mean weight losses from baseline for subjects treated with surgery were 23% at 2 years and 16% at 10 years, compared with mean weight gains of 1% and 2%, respectively, in the controls. While the surgical group had significant reductions in SBP and DBP at 2 years, only DBP remained lower in the surgically treated group at 10 years, despite the persistent weight loss. In a study specifically examining the effect of gastric bypass surgery on hypertension, Carson et al. followed 45 subjects with diastolic hypertension (DBP > 90 mmHg) over 4 years (115). Hypertension improved or resolved in 69% at 12 months and these findings persisted to the study end. There was a significant relationship between amount of weight loss and improvement of blood pressure at the 1-, 12-, 24-, and 48-month visits. Similarly, in a study of 143 subjects undergoing laparoscopic adjustable banding compared to 120 matched diet-treated controls, Pontiroli et al. observed an approximate 15% weight reduction in both groups (116). At 1 year, the diet-treated controls had regained all of the weight lost; however, the surgically treated subjects maintained the 15% weight loss to 36 months. SBP and DBP significantly improved (4% and 5%, respectively) in the surgically treated subjects at 36 months. Finally, as part of a meta-analysis of bariatric surgery and obesity comorbidities involving 22,094 subjects from 136 studies (including 5 randomized trials), Buchwald et al. specifically examined the effect of bariatric surgery on hypertension (117). Of 4085 subjects included, hypertension improved or resolved in 78.5% with follow-up ranging from 6 to 48 months. In summary, bariatric surgery has the potential to enable subjects who have failed dietary and medical therapy to achieve significant long-term weight reduction and improvements in obesity-related metabolic derangements. However, the blood pressure reduction observed with bariatric surgery is variable and, if sustained, modest.

## SUMMARY

Obesity causes maladaptive responses in many physiologic systems, which contributes to the development of associated hypertension. Although a number of putative mechanisms have been elucidated, further work is needed. As the global prevalence of obesity increases, a better understanding of the causal relationship between obesity and hypertension has the potential to considerably aid in the prevention and treatment of hypertension, and its associated comorbidities, in obese individuals.

## ACKNOWLEDGMENT

N.K. is supported by a National Research Service Award (HL07609) from the National Heart, Lung, and Blood Institute.

## REFERENCES

1. Prevalence of overweight and obesity among adults: United States 1985–2003. Atlanta, GA: Centers for Disease Control. Accessed on May 19, 2005 (http://www.cdc.gov/nccdphp/dnpa/obesity/trend/maps/).
2. Kumanyika S. Obesity in black women. Epidemiol Rev 1987; 9:31–50.
3. Cooper RS, Rotimi CN, Ward R. The puzzle of hypertension in African-Americans. Sci Am 1999; 280(2):56–63.
4. Stamler R, Stamler J, Riedlinger WF, Algera G, Roberts RH. Weight and blood pressure. Findings in hypertension screening of 1 million Americans. JAMA 1978; 240(15):1607–1610.
5. Wilson PW, D'Agostino RB, Sullivan L, Parise H, Kannel WB. Overweight and obesity as determinants of cardiovascular risk: the Framingham experience. Arch Int Med 2002; 162(16):1867–1872.
6. Huang Z, Willett WC, Manson JE, et al. Body weight, weight change, and risk for hypertension in women. Ann Intern Med 1998; 128(2):81–88.
7. Chan JM, Rimm EB, Colditz GA, Stampfer MJ, Willett WC. Obesity, fat distribution, and weight gain as risk factors for clinical diabetes in men. Diabetes Care 1994; 17(9):961–969.
8. Rocchini AP, Moorehead C, Wentz E, Deremer S. Obesity-induced hypertension in the dog. Hypertension 1987; 9(6):64–68.
9. Rocchini AP. Cardiovascular regulation in obesity-induced hypertension. Hypertension 1992; 19(1):156–160.
10. Tuck ML, Sowers J, Dornfeld L, Kledzik G, Maxwell M. The effect of weight reduction on blood pressure, plasma renin activity, and plasma aldosterone levels in obese patients. N Engl J Med 1981; 304(16):930–933.
11. Rocchini AP, Key J, Bondie D, et al. The effect of weight loss on the sensitivity of blood pressure to sodium in obese adolescents. N Engl J Med 1989; 321(9):580–585.
12. Reisin E, Abel R, Modan M, Silverberg DS, Eliahou HE, Modan B. Effect of weight loss without salt restriction on the reduction in blood pressure in overweight hypertensive patients. N Engl J Med 1978; 298(1):1–6.
13. Su HY, Sheu WH, Chin HM, Jeng CY, Chen YD, Reaven GM. Effect of weight loss and insulin resistance in normotensive and hypertensive obese individuals. Am J Hypertens 1995; 8(11):1067–1071.

14. Rocchini AP. Adolescent obesity and cardiovascular risk. Pediatr Ann 1992; 21(4):235–240.
15. Fossum E, Hoieggen A, Moan A, Rostrup M, Nordby G, Kjeldsen SE. Relationship between insulin sensitivity and maximal forearm blood flow in young men. Hypertension 1998; 32(5):838–843.
16. Tripathy D, Mohanty P, Dhindsa S, et al. Elevation of free fatty acids induces inflammation and impairs vascular reactivity in healthy subjects. Diabetes 2003; 52(12):2882–2887.
17. Zemel MB. Nutritional and endocrine modulation of intracellular calcium: implications in obesity, insulin resistance and hypertension. Mol Cell Biochem 1998; 188(1–2):129–136.
18. Raji A, Seely EW, Bekins SA, Williams GH, Simonson DC. Rosiglitazone improves insulin sensitivity and lowers blood pressure in hypertensive patients. Hypertension 2004; 43(1):36–40.
19. Cardillo C, Campia U, Iantorno M, Panza JA. Enhanced vascular activity of endogenous endothelin-1 in obese hypertensive patients. Hypertension 2004; 43(1):36–40.
20. Vasan RS. Cardiac function and obesity. Heart 2003; 89(10):1127–1129.
21. Hall JE, Brands MW, Dixon WN, Smith MJ Jr. Obesity-induced hypertension. Renal function and systemic hemodynamics. Hypertension 1993; 22(3): 292–299.
22. Mizelle HL, Edwards TC, Montani JP. Abnormal cardiovascular responses to exercise during the development of obesity in dogs. Am J Hypertens 1994; 7: 374–378.
23. Messerli FH, Christie B, DeCarvalho JG, et al. Obesity and essential hypertension. Hemodynamics, intravascular volume, sodium excretion, and plasma renin activity. Arch Int Med 1981; 141(1):81–85.
24. Zhou YT, Grayburn P, Karim A, et al. Lipotoxic heart disease in obese rats: implications for human obesity. Lipotoxic heart disease in obese rats: implications for human obesity. Proc Natl Acad Sci USA 2000; 97(4):1784–1789.
25. Carroll JF, Huang M, Hester RL, Cockrell K, Mizelle HL. Hemodynamic alterations in hypertensive obese rabbits. Hypertension 1995; 26(3): P465–P470.
26. Hammond IW, Devereux RB, Alderman MH, Laragh JH. Relation of blood pressure and body build to left ventricular mass in normotensive and hypertensive employed adults. J Am Coll Cardiol 1988; 12(4):996–1004.
27. Pascual M, Pascual DA, Soria F, et al. Effects of isolated obesity on systolic and diastolic left ventricular function. Heart 2003; 89:1152–1156.
28. Kenchaiah S, Evans JC, Levy D, et al. Obesity and the risk of heart failure. N Engl J Med 2002; 347(5):305–313.
29. Alpert MA, Terry BE, Lambert CR, et al. Factors influencing left ventricular systolic function in nonhypertensive morbidly obese patients, and effect of weight loss induced by gastroplasty. Am J Cardiol 1993; 71(8):733–737.
30. Alpert MA, Lambert CR, Terry BE, et al. Effect of weight loss on left ventricular mass in nonhypertensive morbidly obese patients. Am J Cardiol 1994; 73(12):918–921.

31. Hall JE, Brands MW, Henegar JR, Shek EW. Abnormal kidney function as a cause and a consequence of obesity hypertension. Clin Exp Pharmacol Physiol 1998; 25(1):58–64.

32. Swann HG, Railey MJ, Carmignani AE. Functional distention of the kidney in perinephritic hypertension. Am Heart J 1959; 58:608–622.

33. Alonso-Galicia M, Dwyer TM, Herrera GA, Hall JF. Increased hyaluronic acid in the inner renal medulla of obese dogs. Hypertension 1995; 25:888–892.

34. Johnsson C, Tufveson G, Wahlberg J, Hallgren R. Experimentally-induced warm renal ischemia induces cortical accumulation of hyaluronan in the kidney. Kidney Int 1996; 50(4):1224–1229.

35. Henegar JR, Bigler SA, Henegar LK, Tyagi SC, Hall JE. Functional and structural changes in the kidney in early stages of obesity. J Am Soc Nephrol 2001; 12(6):1211–1217.

36. Fujiwara K, Hayashi K, Matsuda H, et al. Altered Pressure-Natriuresis in Obese Zucker Rats. Hypertension 1999; 33(6):1470–1475.

37. Rocchini AP, Moorehead C, DeRemer S, Goodfriend TL, Ball DL. Hyperinsulinemia and the aldosterone and pressor responses to angiotensin II. Hypertension 1990; 15(6):861–866.

38. Engeli S, Sharma AM. The renin-angiotensin system and natriuretic peptides in obesity-associated hypertension. J Mol Med 2001; 79(1):21–29.

39. Boulter PR, Spark RF, Arky RA. Dissociation of the renin-aldosterone system and refractoriness to the sodium-retaining action of mineralocorticoid during starvation in man. J Clin Endocrinol Metab 1974; 38(2):248–254.

40. Spark RF, Arky RA, Boulter PR, Saudek CD, O'Brian JT. Renin, aldosterone and glucagon in the natriuresis of fasting. N Engl J Med 1975; 292(25): 1335–1340.

41. Giacchetti G, Faloia E, Sardu C, et al. Gene expression of angiotensinogen in adipose tissue of obese patients. Int J Obes Relat Metab Disord 2000; 24(suppl 2):S142–S143.

42. Naftilan AJ, Zuo WM, Inglefinger J, Ryan TJ Jr, Pratt RE, Dzau VJ. Localization and differential regulation of angiotensinogen mRNA expression in the vessel wall. J Clin Invest 1991; 87(4):1300–1311.

43. Cassis LA, Lynch KR, Peach MJ. Localization of angiotensinogen messenger RNA in rat aorta. Circ Res 1988; 62(6):1259–1262.

44. Shenoy U, Cassis L. Characterization of renin activity in brown adipose tissue. Am J Physiol 1997; 272(3):C989–C999.

45. Harp JB, DiGirolamo M. Components of the renin-angiotensin system in adipose tissue: changes with maturation and adipose mass enlargement. J Gerontol A Biol Sci Med Sci 1995; 50(5):B270–B276.

46. Massiera F, Bloch-Faure M, Ceiler D, et al. Adipose angiotensinogen is involved in adipose tissue growth and blood pressure regulation. FASEB J 2001; 15(14):2727–2729.

47. Faloia E, Gatti C, Camilloni MA, et al. Comparison of circulating and local adipose tissue renin-angiotensin system in normotensive and hypertensive obese subjects. J Endocrinol Invest 2002; 25(4):309–314.

48. Levin ER, Gardner DG, Samson WK. Natriuretic peptides. N Engl J Med 1998; 339(5):321–328.

49. Nakao K, Ogawa Y, Suga S, Imura H. Molecular biology and biochemistry of the natriuretic peptide system. J Hypertens 1992; 10(9):907–912.
50. Dessi-Fulgheri P, Sarzani R, Tamburrini P, et al. Plasma atrial natriuretic peptide and natriuretic peptide receptor gene expression in adipose tissue of normotensive and hypertensive obese patients. J Hypertens 1997; 15(12): 1695–1699.
51. Grandi AM, Laurita E, Selva E, et al. Natriuretic peptides as markers of preclinical cardiac disease in obesity. Eur J Clin Invest 2004; 34(5):342–348.
52. Wang TJ, Larson MG, Levy D, et al. Impact of obesity on plasma natriuretic peptide levels. Circulation 2004; 109(5):594–600.
53. Sarzani R, Dessi-Fulgheri P, Salvi F, et al. A novel promoter variant of the natriuretic peptide clearance receptor gene is associated with lower atrial natriuretic peptide and higher blood pressure in obese hypertensives. J Hypertens 1999; 17(9):1301–1305.
54. Mark AL, Correia M, Morgan DA, Shaffer RA, Haynes WG. State-of-the-art lecture: obesity-induced hypertension: new concepts from the emerging biology of obesity. Hypertension 1999; 33(1S):537–541.
55. Schwartz MW, Porte D Jr. Diabetes, obesity, and the brain. Science 2005; 307(5708):375–379.
56. Haynes WG, Morgan DA, Walsh SA, Sivitz WI, Mark AL. Cardiovascular consequences of obesity: role of leptin. Clin Exp Pharmacol. Physiol 1998; 25(1): 65–69.
57. Lembo G, Vecchione C, Fratta L, et al. Leptin induces direct vasodilation through distinct endothelial mechanisms. Diabetes 2000; 49(2):293–297.
58. Shek EW, Brands MW, Hall JE. Chronic leptin infusion increases arterial pressure. Hypertension 1998; 31(1):409–414.
59. Stanley BG, Chin AS, Leibowitz SF. Feeding and drinking elicited by central injection of neuropeptide Y: evidence for a hypothalamic site(s) of action. Brain Res Bull 1985; 14(6):521–524.
60. McAuley MA, Reid JL, Macrae IM. Central cardiovascular effects of rilmenidine and neuropeptide Y in the conscious spontaneously hypertensive rat: haemodynamic and biochemical evidence for a negative interaction. Cardiovasc Pharmacol 1992; 19(6):945–952.
61. Shintani M, Ikegami H, Fujisawa T, et al. Leptin gene polymorphism is associated with hypertension independent of obesity. J Clin Endocrinol Metab 2002; 87(6):2909–2912.
62. Rosmond R, Chagnon YC, Holm G, et al. Hypertension in obesity and the leptin receptor gene locus. J Clin Endocrinol Metab 2000; 85(9):3126–3131.
63. Hall JE. Hyperinsulinemia: A link between obesity and hypertension? Kidney Int 1993; 43(6):1402–1417.
64. Anderson EA, Mark AL. The vasodilator action of insulin: implications for the insulin hypothesis of hypertension. Hypertension 1993; 21(2):136–141.
65. Meehan WP, Buchanan TA, Hsueh W. Chronic insulin administration elevates blood pressure in rats. Hypertension 1994; 23(6):1012–1017.
66. Brands MW, Hildebrandt DA, Mizelle HL, Hall JE. Sustained hyperinsulinemia increases arterial pressure in conscious rats. Am J Physiol 1991; 260(4): R764–R768.

67. Keen HL, Brands MW, Smith MJ Jr, Shek EW, Hall JE. Inhibition of thromboxane synthesis attenuates insulin hypertension in rats. Am J Hypertens 1997; 10:1125–1131.
68. Brands MW, Harrison DL, Keen HL, Gardner A, Shek EW, Hall JE. Insulin-induced hypertension depends on an intact renin-angiotensin system. Hypertension 1997; 29(4):1014–1019.
69. Hall JE, Brands MW, Zappe DH, et al. Hemodynamic and renal responses to chronic hyperinsulinemia in obese, insulin resistant dogs. Hypertension 1995; 25(5):994–1002.
70. Hildebrandt DA, Smith MJ Jr, Hall JE. Cardiovascular regulation during acute and chronic vertebral artery insulin infusion in conscious dogs. J Hypertens 1999; 17(2):252–260.
71. Stepniakowski KT, Goodfriend TL, Egan BM. Fatty acids enhance vascular alpha-adrenergic sensitivity. Hypertension 1995; 25:774–778.
72. Grekin RJ, Dumont CJ, Vollmer AP, Watts SW, Webb RC. Mechanisms in the pressor effects of hepatic portal venous fatty acid infusion. Am J Physiol 1997; 273(1):R324–R330.
73. Hall JE, Brands MW, Hildebrandt DA, Kuo J, Fitzgerald S. Role of sympathetic nervous system and neuropeptides in obesity hypertension. Braz J Med Biol Res 2000; 33(6):605–618.
74. Lopes HF, Morrow JD, Stojiljkovic MP, Goodfriend TL, Egan BM, Stoijiljkovic MP. Acute hyperlipidemia increases oxidative stress more in African Americans than in white Americans Am J Hypertens 2003; 16(5): 331–336.
75. Quinkler M, Stewart PM. Hypertension and the cortisol-cortisone shuttle. J Clin Endocrinol Metab 2003; 88(6):2384–2392.
76. Bujalska IJ, Kumar S, Stewart PM. Does central obesity reflect "Cushing's disease of the omentum"? Lancet 1997; 349(9060):1210–1213.
77. Kotelevtsev Y, Holmes MC, Burchell A, et al. 11beta-hydroxysteroid dehydrogenase type 1 knockout mice show attenuated glucocorticoid-inducible responses and resist hyperglycemia on obesity or stress. Proc Natl Acad Sci USA 1997; 94(26):14924–14929.
78. Morton NM, Paterson JM, Masuzaki H, et al. Novel adipose tissue-mediated resistance to diet-induced visceral obesity in 11 beta-hydroxysteroid dehydrogenase type 1-deficient mice. Diabetes 2004; 53(4):931–938.
79. Masuzaki H, Paterson J, Shinyama H, et al. A transgenic model of visceral obesity and the metabolic syndrome. Science 2001; 294(5549):2166–2170.
80. Masuzaki H, Yamamoto H, Kenyon CJ, et al. Transgenic amplification of glucocorticoid action in adipose tissue causes high blood pressure in mice. J Clin Invest 2003; 112(1):83–90.
81. Sowers JR, Whitfield LA, Catania RA, et al. Role of the sympathetic nervous system in blood pressure maintenance in obesity. J Clin Endocrinol Metab 1982; 54:1181–1186.
82. Grassi G, Seravalle G, Cattaneo BM, et al. Sympathetic activation in obese normotensive subjects. Hypertension 1995; 25(4):560–563.

83. Rocchini AP, Mao HZ, Babu K, Marker P, Rocchini AJ. Clonidine prevents insulin resistance and hypertension in obese dogs. Hypertension 1999; 33(1): 548–553.

84. Kassab S, Kato T, Wilkins FC, Chen R, Hall JE, Granger JP. Renal denervation attenuates the sodium retention and hypertension associated with obesity. Hypertension 1995; 25(4):893–897.

85. Boston BA, Blaydon KM, Varnerin J, Cone RD. Independent and additive effects of central POMC and leptin pathways on murine obesity. Science 1997; 278(5343):1641–1644.

86. Seeley RJ, Yagaloff KA, Fisher SL, et al. Melanocortin receptors in leptin effects. Nature 1997; 390(6658):349.

87. Mark AL, Shaffer RA, Correia ML, Morgan DA, Sigmund CD, Haynes WG. Contrasting blood pressure effects of obesity in leptin-deficient ob/ob mice and agouti yellow obese mice. J Hypertens 1999; 17(12):1949–1953.

88. Haynes WG, Morgan DA, Djalali A, Sivitz WI, Mark AL. Interactions between the melanocortin system and leptin in control of sympathetic nerve traffic. Hypertension 1999; 33(1):542–547.

89. Ni XP, Pearce D, Butler AA, Cone RD, Humphreys MH. Genetic disruption of $\gamma$-melanocyte stimulating hormone signaling leads to salt-sensitive hypertension in the mouse. J Clin Invest 2003; 111(8):1251–1258.

90. Krude H, Biebermann H, Luck W, Horn R, Brabant G, Gruters A. Severe early-onset obesity, adrenal insufficiency and red hair pigmentation caused by POMC mutations in humans. Nat Genet 1998; 19(2):155–157.

91. Lee YS, Poh LK, Loke KY. A novel melanocortin 3 receptor gene (MC3R) mutation associated with severe obesity. J Clin Endocrinol Metab 2002; 87(3): 1423–1426.

92. Mersebach H, Svendsen OL, Astrup A, Feldt-Rasmussen U. Abnormal sympathoadrenal activity, but normal energy expenditure in hypopituitarism. J Clin Endocrinol Metab 2003; 88(12):5689–5695.

93. Reisin E, Abel R, Modan M, Silverberg DS, Eliahou HE, Modan B. Effect of weight loss without salt restriction on the reduction of blood pressure in overweight hypertensive patients. N Engl J Med 1978; 298(1):1–6.

94. Stamler R, Stamler J, Gosch FC, et al. Primary prevention of hypertension by nutritional-hygienic means. Final report of a randomized, controlled trial. JAMA 1989; 262(13):1801–1807.

95. Reisin E, Frohlich ED, Messerli FH, et al. Cardiovascular changes after reduction in obesity hypertension. Ann Intern Med 1983; 98(3):315–319.

96. Chobanian AV, Bakris GL, Black HR, et al. Joint National Committee on Prevention, Detection, Evaluation, and Treatment of High Blood Pressure. National Heart, Lung, and Blood Institute; National High Blood Pressure Education Program Coordinating Committee. Seventh report of the Joint National Committee on Prevention, Detection, Evaluation, and Treatment of High Blood Pressure. Hypertension 2003; 42(6):1206–1252.

97. Snow V, Barry P, Fitterman N, Qaseem A, Weiss K. Clinical Efficacy Assessment Subcommittee of the American College of Physicians. Pharmacologic and surgical management of obesity in primary care: a clinical practice

guideline from the American College of Physicians. Ann Intern Med 2005; 142(7):525–531.

98. Reisin E, Weir MR, Falkner B, Hutchinson HG, Anzalone DA, Tuck ML. Lisinopril versus hydrochlorothiazide in obese hypertensive patients: a multicenter placebo-controlled trial. Treatment in obese patients with hypertension (TROPHY) study group. Hypertension 1997; 30(1):140–145.

99. Yusuf S, Gerstein H, Hoogwerf B, et al. HOPE Study Investigators. Ramipril and the development of diabetes. JAMA 2001; 286(15):1882–1885.

100. Furberg CD, Psaty BM, Pahor M, Alderman MH. Clinical implications of recent findings from the antihypertensive and lipid-lowering treatment to prevent heart attack trial (ALLHAT) and other studies of hypertension. Ann Int Med 2001; 135(12):1074–1078.

101. Lindholm LH, Ibsen H, Borch-Johnsen K, et al. For the LIFE study group. Risk of new-onset diabetes in the Losartan Intervention For Endpoint reduction in hypertension study. J Hypertens 2002; 20(9):1879–1886.

102. Pepine CJ, Cooper-Dehoff RM. Cardiovascular therapies and risk for development of diabetes. J Am Coll Cardiol 2004; 44(3):509–512.

103. United Kingdom Prospective Diabetes Study Group. Efficacy of atenolol and captopril in reducing risk of macrovascular and microvascular complications in type 2 diabetes. BMJ 1998; 317(7160):713–720.

104. Wassertheil-Smoller S, Blaufox MD, Oberman AS, Langford HG, Davis BR, Wylie-Rosett J. The Trial of Antihypertensive Interventions and Management (TAIM) study. Adequate weight loss, alone and combined with drug therapy in the treatment of mild hypertension. Arch Intern Med 1992; 152(1):131–136.

105. Rossner S, Taylor CL, Byington RP, Furberg CD. Long term propranolol treatment and changes in body weight after myocardial infarction. BMJ 1990; 300(6729):902–903.

106. Schmieder RE, Gatzka C, Schachinger H, Schobel H, Ruddel H. Obesity as a determinant for response to antihypertensive treatment. BMJ 1993; 307(6903): 537–540.

107. Bray GA, Ryan DH, Gordon D, Heidingsfelder S, Cerise F, Wilson K. Double-blind, randomized, placebo-controlled trial of sibutramine. Obes Res 1996; 4(3):263–270.

108. James WP, Astrup A, Finer N, et al. Effect of sibutramine on weight maintenance after weight loss: a randomised trial. STORM Study Group. Sibutramine Trial of Obesity Reduction and Maintenance. Lancet 2000; 356(9248): 2119–2125.

109. Bloch KV, Salles GF, Muxfeldt ES, Da Rocha Nogueira A. Orlistat in hypertensive overweight/obese patients: results of a randomized clinical trial. J Hypertens 2003; 21(11):2159–2165.

110. Sharma AM, Golay A. Effect of orlistat-induced weight loss on blood pressure and heart rate in obese patients with hypertension. J Hypertens 2002; 20(9): 1873–1878.

111. Van Gaal LF, Rissanen AM, Scheen AJ, Ziegler O, Rossner S. RIO-Europe Study Group. Effects of the cannabinoid-1 receptor blocker rimonabant on weight reduction and cardiovascular risk factors in overweight patients:

1-year experience from the RIO-Europe study. Lancet 2005; 365(9468): 1389–1397.

112. Sjostrom CD, Peltonen M, Sjostrom L. Blood pressure and pulse pressure during long-term weight loss in the obsess: the Swedish Obese Subjects (SOS) intervention study. Obes Res 2001; 9(3):188–195.

113. Sjostrom L, Lindroos AK, Peltonen M, et al. Swedish Obese Subjects Study Scientific Group. Lifestyle, diabetes, and cardiovascular risk factors 10 years after bariatric surgery. N Engl J Med 2004; 351(26):2683–2693.

114. Solomon CG, Dluhy RG. Bariatric surgery—quick fix or long-term solution? N Engl J Med 2004; 351(26):2751–2753.

115. Carson JL, Ruddy ME, Duff AE, Holmes NJ, Cody RP, Brolin RE. The effect of gastric bypass surgery on hypertension in morbidly obese patients. Arch Intern Med 1994; 154(2):193–200.

116. Pontiroli AE, Pizzocri P, Liberenti MC, et al. Laparoscopic adjustable gastric banding for the treatment of morbid (grade 3) obesity and its metabolic complications: a three-year study. J Clin Endocrinal Metab 2002; 87(8):3555–3561.

117. Buchwald H, Avidor Y, Braunwald E, et al. Bariatric surgery: a systematic review and meta-analysis. JAMA 2004; 292(14):1724–1737.

# 3

# Insulin Resistance, Obesity, Body Fat Distribution, and Risk of Cardiovascular Disease

**Greeshma K. Shetty and Christos S. Mantzoros**

*Division of Endocrinology, Diabetes and Metabolism, Department of Medicine, Beth Israel Deaconess Medical Center and Harvard Medical School, Boston, Massachusetts, U.S.A.*

## INTRODUCTION

The escalating prevalence of obesity is thought to be multifactorial, involving behavioral, genetic, and environmental factors. Obesity is associated with insulin resistance and the metabolic syndrome, and is a known risk factor for cardiovascular disease (CVD). Adipose tissue is no longer considered an inert accumulation of fat, but rather a dynamic endocrine organ in which adipocytes generate and secrete many hormones and cytokines. These inflammatory cytokines, known as adipokines, play an important role in insulin resistance and the metabolic syndrome and may mediate the effect of obesity in CVD. Identification and research involving these adipokines has elucidated pathways linking obesity with insulin resistance and CVD. Current treatments of obesity involve lifestyle modifications, such as modifications in diet and exercising, medications that either suppress appetite/increase satiety or decrease nutrient absorption, and surgical intervention for appropriately selected patients. To understand and treat obesity and its complications, it is critical to appreciate the redundancy in the various signaling pathways.

Hopefully, recent discoveries in the energy homeostasis model will enhance the therapeutic armamentarium in the near future for this rapidly growing disease.

## OBESITY/FAT DISTRIBUTION/INFLAMMATORY MARKERS

Obesity is a growing epidemic—most recent estimates state that 30% of U.S. adults are obese and another 35% are overweight (1). Moreover, the global scope of this disease is alarming, because it appears that no age, race, gender, or socioeconomic status provides immunity from its expanding prevalence. Thus, research efforts on its etiology, pathophysiologic consequences, and treatment have been intensified recently.

### Defining Obesity

The body mass index [(BMI), calculated as the weight in kilograms divided by the square of the height in meters] is used to diagnose being overweight (BMI of $25.0$–$29.9 \, \text{kg/m}^2$) and obese (BMI $\geq 30.0 \, \text{kg/m}^2$) (2). It is believed that the BMI is a better indicator of adiposity than the weight-for-height tables, even though neither assessment directly measures body fat (3). The correlation between BMI and body fatness is age and sex dependent, but independent of ethnicity (4). A limitation to BMI is that it does not account for fat distribution, degree of muscularity, or bone density, all of which are independent predictors of health risk (5). Quantifying fat mass by dual energy X-ray absorptiometry scans or other methods may be the ideal obesity indicator, but because this is currently difficult to perform, for practical purposes the BMI is the method used clinically. Obesity and overweight independently confer an increased risk of mortality and this risk begins to rise at a BMI greater than $25 \, \text{kg/m}^2$ (6). In the Nurses' Health Study, BMI values above $22 \, \text{kg/m}^2$ were associated with an increased risk of diabetes (7), illustrating that some of these comorbidities are associated with increasing BMI levels below that established for the diagnosis of overweight, but increase significantly at BMI values above 25. Life-insurance data and epidemiological studies confirm that increasing degrees of overweight and obesity are important predictors of decreased longevity (8). Increased weight is associated with numerous comorbidities such as type 2 diabetes mellitus, hypertension, dyslipidemia, congestive heart failure (CHF), stroke, colon cancer, endometrial and breast cancer, infertility, osteoarthritis, and obstructive sleep apnea. Moreover, obesity is notable for elevated fasting insulin levels and exaggerated insulin response to oral glucose loads (9). The INTERnational study of SALT and blood pressure (INTERSALT) study reported that a 10-kg increase in weight was associated with a 3.0-mmHg rise in systolic blood pressure and a 2.3-mmHg rise in diastolic blood pressure (10). Finally, increasing BMI is associated with increases in total cholesterol, triglycerides, and low-density lipoprotein (LDL), and a decrease in high-density lipoprotein (HDL) (11).

## Body Fat Distribution

Recent evidence suggests that the specific location of weight gain is even more important than overall obesity as a predictor of risk. More specifically, central distribution of body fat (the ratio of waist-to-hip circumference $> 0.90$ in women and $>1.0$ in men) is associated with a higher risk of morbidity and mortality than a more peripheral distribution of body fat and may be a better indicator of the risk of morbidity than absolute fat mass (12). When comparing similar-weight patients, patients with central (abdominal or visceral) obesity have a greater risk for insulin resistance, hyperinsulinemia (13), glucose intolerance (14), type 2 diabetes mellitus (15), hypertension (16), hyperlipidemia, coronary heart disease, stroke, and hormone-dependent cancers of the breast and endometrium (17–19).

## Genetic Factors in the Etiology of Obesity

Obesity does run in families and it appears that certain genes have a "permissive-role" to nongenetic factors in the development of the disease. Twin studies have suggested that the heritability of fat mass ranges between 40% and 70% with a concordance of 0.7 to 0.9 between monozygotic twins compared to 0.35 to 0.45 between dizygotic twins (20,21). The permissive-gene hypothesis is also supported by twin studies in which the twin pairs were exposed to periods of positive and negative energy balance, which resulted in weight and fat deposition changes that had greater similarity within pairs than between pairs (22). The exact genetic contribution to obesity has yet to be completely understood, but the discovery of the ob gene and its gene product leptin (23) has sparked an explosion of research in this area. This has resulted in the discovery of several monogenic obesity syndromes, which present with childhood morbid obesity, such as: congenital leptin deficiency, leptin receptor deficiency, proopiomelanocortin gene mutations, and melanocortin 4 receptor mutations (24), the latter being the most frequent monogenic disorder accounting for approximately 5% of morbid obesity in childhood (25). However, it is becoming increasingly evident that multiple genes influence the regulation of body weight and obesity is currently considered to be a polygenic disorder with many genes interacting at various levels.

## Environmental Factors Predisposing to the Development of Obesity

In addition to genetic factors, nongenetic environmental factors, such as an increasingly abundant calorie-dense, highly palatable diet and a technology-driven life of convenience and leisure at a time when physical activity is minimized, contribute to the current state of a rapidly increasing prevalence of obesity. These sedentary lifestyle changes play havoc with centuries of genetic selection that led to a "thrifty genotype," which may have conferred a survival benefit during times of sporadic food availability, but may be currently leading to the development of obesity (26). Physical exercise three or more times each week results in weight loss, in contrast to not exercising which may lead to weight gain (27). The net result of decreased energy expenditure combined with increased energy intake, even if only a small difference on a daily basis, has a profound effect on the long-term energy balance as measured by net weight gain over months or years. In contrast, it is now becoming evident that the relative stability of energy stores in nonobese subjects is due to the coordinate activity of a highly integrated complex system ranging from the hypothalamus to the adipocytes, which compensates for changes in daily energy intake and expenditure. Thus, it appears that there is a significant interplay between the centrally generated molecules, such as neuropeptide Y, melanocyte-concentrating hormone, galanin, and the peripherally generated molecules, such as insulin, leptin, ghrelin, and peptide YY with environmental factors in the regulation of the energy homeostasis, but this complex network of interactions is only now beginning to be deciphered (28,29).

## OBESITY AND INSULIN RESISTANCE

Insulin resistance is understood as an impaired biological response to the actions of insulin (30), where increasing amounts of insulin are needed to elicit a quantitatively normal response (31). Currently, there are several tests available to assess insulin resistance. Measuring insulin levels at baseline (fasting) or post–oral glucose tolerance testing (OGTT) is the easiest test to perform, but is a relatively less informative test (32). Measuring serial glucose levels after i.v. administration of insulin (insulin tolerance test) (32), performing the frequently sampled i.v. glucose tolerance test using the minimal model technique to estimate the index of insulin sensitivity (Si) (33), and measuring in vivo insulin-mediated glucose disposal (M) by the euglycemic hyper-insulinemic clamp (34) are more demanding tests, but provide a more detailed assessment of insulin sensitivity.

### Mechanism

Insulin is a hormone with pleiotropic effects and it mediates these effects by binding to a heterotetrameric glycoprotein insulin receptor that is expressed on the plasma membrane of almost all cells (35). Using both in vivo and in vitro techniques, insulin resistance has been described at the level of the muscle, where there is impaired insulin-stimulated glucose uptake, at the level of the liver, where there is impaired suppression of hepatic glucose production by insulin, and at the level of adipose tissue, where insulin becomes ineffective in suppressing lipolysis (36). Insulin resistance and hyperinsulinemia are closely associated with obesity and lead to the development of type 2 diabetes, hypertension, ischemic heart disease, and dyslipidemia; the coexistence of these disorders is called the metabolic syndrome (37,38).

## Genetics in the Etiology of Insulin Resistance

A significant body of evidence indicates that similar to obesity, insulin resistance is influenced by several genetic factors, each accounting for a relatively small percentage of its variability. The insulin receptor and the downstream signaling pathways have and are being investigated for potential genetic mechanisms of insulin resistance, with a specific focus on the insulin receptor, the insulin receptor substrates (IRS) and the phophatidylinositol 3-kinase (PI3-kinase) (39). More than 50 mutations of the insulin receptor gene have been identified (40), and have been associated with a number of rare clinical syndromes, the most common of which is type A insulin resistance, a syndrome characterized by insulin resistance, acanthosis nigricans, and hyperandrogenicity (41). In general, insulin receptor mutations are only rarely found in the garden variety type 2 diabetes, and are responsible for insulin resistance in only a few individuals (39). IRS-1 and IRS-2 mutations have also been described in humans, but these mutations are fairly common, occurring in 12% to 33% of nonobese healthy, as well as type 2 diabetic subjects (42). Because these mutations are found in such high percentages of normal healthy subjects the role of these mutations remains less clear. Mutations of PI3-kinase, a molecule playing a role in insulin-dependent glucose uptake, has not been associated with insulin resistance in a study in Pima Indians, but in contrast was associated with an increased insulin response after a glucose challenge test (43). Recently, loss-of-function mutations in the ligand-binding domain of peroxisome proliferator–activated receptor γ (PPAR γ), a nuclear receptor which plays a role in adipogenesis, insulin sensitivity, lipid metabolism, blood pressure regulation, and atherosclerosis (44), have been associated with the syndrome of familial partial lipodystrophy (45–47). This syndrome phenotypically manifests with loss of subcutaneous fat in the limbs, preserved subcutaneous and visceral abdominal fat depots, and severe insulin resistance (48). Although these loss-of-function mutations are rare and account for very few cases of insulin resistance, the PPAR γ genetic variant with a polymorphism replacing alanine for proline at codon 12 (Pro12Ala) is much more common, occurring in up to 15% of some Caucasian populations (49).

## Environmental Factors in the Etiology of Insulin Resistance

Obesity and lack of physical exercise are strongly associated with insulin resistance (50), whereas weight loss as well as exercise independent from weight loss have been shown to improve insulin sensitivity (39). The beneficial effects of exercise on insulin sensitivity are multiple—increased glucose uptake and glycogen synthesis (51), increased blood flow leading to improved insulin delivery to target tissues (52), and reduced hepatic glucose production (53). Weight reduction has also been shown to improve insulin sensitivity (50), and improvement in insulin sensitivity correlates with reduction in visceral fat (54). In addition, the role of diet has been investigated and it has been proposed that high carbohydrate diets reduce insulin sensitivity (55). High-fat diets lead to insulin resistance in the animal model (56), but this association remains to be fully elucidated in humans.

## Obesity, Insulin Resistance, Adipokines, and Inflammatory Markers

Adipose tissue is no longer considered to merely accrue fat, but rather is an active endocrine organ with adipocytes generating and secreting several inflammatory cytokines, including tumor necrosis factor $\alpha$ (TNF$\alpha$) (57), interleukin 6 (IL-6) (58), and adiponectin (59). Among the molecules that are generated from adipose tissue, free fatty acids (FFA) have traditionally been implicated in the pathogenesis of insulin resistance (60). FFA are taken up by the liver and skeletal muscle, and counteract the effects of insulin by increasing hepatic gluconeogenesis and by inhibiting glucose uptake and oxidation in skeletal muscle (61–63).

Recently the role of TNF$\alpha$ has been explored in association with obesity as related to insulin resistance. Several studies have demonstrated that TNF$\alpha$ is able to impair insulin signaling through serine kinase and tyrosine phosphatase–dependent modulation of the insulin signaling pathway in isolated cell systems (64,65). Clinical results from different insulin-resistant populations so far do not support a major role for circulating TNF$\alpha$ on the insulin resistance in humans (66), but this does not exclude a role for TNF$\alpha$ or other inflammatory mediators acting in a paracrine manner in the pathogenesis of insulin resistance.

Adiponectin, a recently discovered 244 amino acid adipose-specific protein (67), found in high concentrations in the peripheral circulation (68), is another adipokine implicated in insulin resistance and the metabolic syndrome. Adiponectin levels are more strongly associated with visceral obesity than with overall obesity, are correlated with hyperlipidemia and insulin resistance (69,70), and are decreased in obesity and type 2 diabetes mellitus (71–73). Resistin, another novel adipocyte-derived hormone, was initially thought to link obesity with insulin resistance and diabetes (74), but published data remain controversial. Obese mice were found to have markedly elevated resistin levels and these levels were decreased by insulin sensitizers such as rosiglitazone and other thiazolidinediones, and the administration of antiresistin antiserum neutralized the effect of resistin by leading to a significant decrease in blood glucose (74). These initial findings in mice were challenged by subsequent conflicting data demonstrating increased or decreased resistin levels in animal models of obesity and also variable responses of resistin expression to thiazolidinediones (70,75,76). Moreover, it has also been recently reported that circulating resistin is not associated with insulin resistance in humans (77,78). Thus, resistin levels may be associated with total and visceral obesity, but not with insulin resistance (70,77).

There is accumulating evidence that several adipokines respond to weight loss. Leptin and IL-6 levels decrease (78–82) and adiponectin levels increase (82,83) with weight loss, whereas the effect of weight loss on TNFα and C-reactive protein (CRP) remains controversial (80–82,84) and resistin levels do not change with weight loss (82).

Recent evidence implicates adipose tissue in general, and visceral adiposity in particular, as a key regulator of inflammation, coagulation, and fibrinolysis (85). Elevated levels of cytokines such as IL-6, fibrinogen, CRP, and TNFα have been associated not only with elevated body fat, but also with several CVD risk factors (86). Resistin has structural similarities to proteins involved with inflammatory processes (87), but has to be further studied in relation to inflammatory markers in humans. Adiponectin has also been associated with markers of inflammation, such as CRP and TNFα (88,89), but its association with inflammatory markers also needs to be investigated further.

## METABOLIC SYNDROME

### Defining the Metabolic Syndrome

The metabolic syndrome, as defined by the National Cholesterol Education Program (NCEP) expert panel, is the coexistence of three or more of the following conditions: waist circumference >102 cm in men and >88 cm in women, fasting plasma glucose of at least 110 mg/dL (6.1 mmol/L), serum triglycerides of at least 150 mg/dL (1.7 mmol/L), serum HDL less than 40 mg/dL (1.04 mmol/L) in men and less than 50 mg/dL (1.29 mmol/L) in women, and a blood pressure of at least 130/85 mmHg (90). Using the new NCEP definition, approximately 22% of U.S. adults (24% after age adjustment) have the metabolic syndrome and this increases to 43.5% in adults who are 60 years or older. African-American and Mexican-American women have significantly higher prevalence rates than do their male counterparts (91). A recent study reported a threefold increase in risk of coronary heart disease and stroke in subjects with the metabolic syndrome phenotype (92). Obesity has also been associated, through insulin resistance, with several malignancies such as breast, endometrial, and colon cancer (93–95). However, these cancers are not currently considered to be traditional components of the metabolic syndrome, and thus are not discussed here.

### Metabolic Syndrome and Glucose Intolerance/Diabetes

The pathogenesis of the syndrome is considered to be multifaceted, but obesity, especially central obesity, secondary to diet and a sedentary lifestyle appears to play a significant role. Increased visceral adiposity is associated with insulin resistance, hyperinsulinemia, glucose intolerance, and atherogenic lipoprotein profile (96). The relative contribution of beta cell dysfunction versus insulin resistance in the etiology of type 2 diabetes remains a contentious point of debate (31). Type 2 diabetes can be a smoldering disease for years, but the unknown hyperglycemia can cause macrovascular and microvascular disease years before the diagnosis is made (97). Persistent hyperglycemia can inhibit both insulin secretion and insulin gene expression (98), thereby further propagating hyperglycemia. In addition to the effects of "glucotoxicity," the metabolic syndrome is also characterized by chronically elevated levels of FFA generated by lipolysis of the abdominal visceral adipose depots, which leads to "lipotoxicity" that hinders glucose-induced insulin secretion and worsens insulin resistance at the level of the liver and skeletal muscle (60).

## Metabolic Syndrome and Hypertension

Hypertension associated with the metabolic syndrome is thought to be mediated by the combination of hyperinsulinemia with insulin resistance, which stimulates the sympathetic nervous system to release catecholamines, leading to vasoconstriction (99), increased cardiac output, and renal absorption of sodium. In addition, insulin either by direct action or in conjunction with other growth factors (100,101), may also promote the development of hypertension and atherosclerosis by stimulating the proliferation of vascular smooth muscle (102,103). Yet another possible explanation for the association of insulin resistance and hypertension is abnormal cellular ion fluxes involving increased intracellular calcium and decreased intracellular magnesium, which may lead to vascular dysfunction (104).

Studies show that approximately 50% of patients with hypertension have insulin resistance and hyperinsulinemia (96). Results from the European Group for the Study of Insulin Resistance indicate that blood pressure is directly related to both insulin resistance and insulin concentration; furthermore, these results were independent of differences in age, gender, and degree of obesity (105). Hyperinsulinemia alone, whether by insulin infusion or insulinoma-associated, does not cause hypertension in the absence of insulin resistance (106,107). Furthermore, not all patients with essential hypertension are insulin resistant or hyperinsulinemic, and this variability only further suggests the pleiotropic effects of insulin and the numerous other factors that interact to result in metabolic and cardiovascular consequences.

## Metabolic Syndrome and Lipid Profile

The lipid profile associated with the metabolic syndrome consists of the following: increased apolipoprotein B (apo B), plasma triglyceride, and intermediate density lipoprotein levels; reduced HDL; and smaller, dense LDL (96). In prospective studies, elevated levels of the small, dense LDL particles have been shown to be predictive of increased coronary artery disease (CAD) risk (108,109). The most frequent derangement of lipoproteins found in association with impaired carbohydrate metabolism is elevated triglycerides, which is attributed to an overproduction of very LDL (VLDL) in the liver and a slower clearance of lipoproteins (110,111). Additionally, the VLDL composition is altered; they are larger, more triglyceride rich, have less apo E and a decreased ratio of apo C-I or C-II to apo C-III, which decrease lipoprotein lipase activity (112,113).

In the setting of insulin resistance, the visceral adipocyte is more sensitive to the metabolic effects of the lipolytic hormones with glucocorticoids and catecholamines. This lipolytic activity results in an increased release of FFA in the portal system that serves as hepatic substrate for creating triglycerides and triglyceride-rich VLDLs (114). Patients with insulin resistance also have increased activity of the hepatic lipase that hydrolyzes HDL cholesterol, which leads to decreased levels of this antiatherogenic lipoprotein (115).

## CVD IN RELATION TO OBESITY, METABOLIC SYNDROME, AND INFLAMMATORY MARKERS

### Systolic and Diastolic Dysfunction

The effect of increased body weight on cardiovascular function results in increased blood volume, increased left ventricular preload, and increased resting cardiac output (116). The cardiac adaptation resulting in left ventricular remodeling is attributed to the increased intravascular volume, which eventually can result in systolic dysfunction due to dilation of the left ventricular cavity radius, and decreased contractility and diastolic dysfunction due to left ventricular hypertrophy. The combination of systolic and diastolic dysfunction may progress to clinically significant CHF (117), and body weight has been shown to be an independent risk factor for the development of CHF in the Framingham Heart Study (118). The association of increasing risk of heart failure across increasing categories of BMI, the temporal association of increased BMI before CHF, and support from experimental evidence suggest a causal relationship between increased BMI and CHF (119,120).

### CAD

Obesity is a major risk factor for CAD (121). Obese patients have increased oxidative stress and inflammation, as indicated by an increase in lipid peroxidation, protein carbonylation, and *ortho*-tyrosine and *meta*-tyrosine formation (122). Atherosclerosis is intimately linked with inflammation of the arterial wall (123), which starts with abnormalities in the endothelium, followed by adhesion of circulating monocytes and T cells that forms "foam cells" loaded with oxidized LDL. The foam cells release matrix metalloproteinases, which lyse the fibrous cap of the atherosclerotic plaque and contribute to plaque instability and ultimately thrombosis (124).

Adipose tissue generates and secretes inflammatory factors such as leptin, plasminogen activator inhibitor-1 (PAI-1), adiponectin, angiotensinogen, TNFα, and IL-6, which appear to have a significant impact on endothelial function (125), and induce endothelial expression of chemokines and adhesion molecules (126), which play a pivotal role in early atherogenesis (127,128). PAI-1 levels correlate with atherosclerotic burden and mortality, and there is data suggesting that PAI-1 may be an independent risk factor for CAD (129). PAI-1 contributes to atherosclerotic disease by inhibiting breakdown of fibrin clots and contributing to remodeling of vascular architecture (130). Angiotensinogen, via its cleaved product angiotensin II, contributes to foam cell formation, in addition to mediating vasoconstriction, by upregulating adhesion molecules, enhancing nitric oxide metabolism, and increasing macrophage accumulation at the cell wall (131–133). Both TNFα and IL-6 have proinflammatory activity that increases adhesion molecules, and IL-6 is associated with the generation of CRP, a strong predictor of atherosclerosis (134).

In addition to the inflammatory factors associated with obesity, there is also significant evidence that increased insulin levels (135) and hyperglycemia (136) may be directly associated with CVD. Thus, although hyperglycemia may be associated with deleterious effects through its association with the presence of other risk factors such as lipids and inflammatory markers, it may also have a direct effect on vascular disease by altering vascular wall matrix proteins, and by stimulating smooth muscle cells and/or endothelial cells to accelerate atherosclerosis (137). Clinically, a dose–response relationship between fasting and two-hour post-OGTT hyperglycemia and both CVD deaths and all-cause mortality independent of fasting insulin levels have been shown (136,137). Having a two-hour glucose level in the upper 20% was associated with a significantly higher risk of death when compared to those in the lower 80% among middle-aged nondiabetic men followed for over 20 years (136). Finally, the importance of glycemic control was also demonstrated in the United Kindgom Prospective Diabetes Study, where obese patients who were randomized to receive metformin had a significantly lower rate of myocardial infarction compared to those receiving conventional treatment (138).

## TREATMENT OPTIONS FOR OBESITY, METABOLIC SYNDROME, AND CVD AS ASSOCIATED TO OBESITY AND INFLAMMATION

In understanding and treating obesity it is critical to appreciate the redundancies in the various signaling pathways that make any single intervention unlikely to be successful. Although several treatment options are currently available, new more effective medications are urgently needed.

## Diet and Exercise

As with most diseases, the first line of treatment is lifestyle modification, which entails a diet and exercise program. Caloric restriction will lead to an initial weight loss; however, weight regain is a challenge for almost all patients. Over time, weight regain increases and virtually all patients in a moderate calorie-restricted diet regain all their pretreatment weight within five years (139). Very low calorie diets (<800 kcal/day) do not offer significant increases in weight loss in comparison to moderate low calorie diets (1200–1500 kcal/day), but do result in an increased risk of gallstones (140). Physical exercise is a key element in any weight-loss program, especially for maintaining the initial diet-induced weight loss (141). It is recommended to start slowly and gradually increase the duration of exercise as tolerated. The combination of caloric restriction and exercise usually results in a 5% to 10% of preintervention weight loss over four to six months (142), and though this may appear to be a small weight loss, it is significant in decreasing the risk of many obesity-related comorbidities (143). The Finnish Diabetes Prevention Study of 522 overweight subjects with impaired glucose tolerance demonstrated that lifestyle interventions of diet and exercise that resulted in weight loss decreased the risk of diabetes (144). Similar findings of decreased incidence of diabetes in the lifestyle-modification group of The Diabetes Prevention Program, a study of 3234 nondiabetics with elevated fasting glucose concentrations, further support the benefits associated with weight loss owing to diet and exercise programs (145). There are multiple benefits to increased physical activity, such as increased energy expenditure (146), decreased appetite, improved cardiovascular fitness (147), decreased intra-abdominal fat (148), and improved glycemic control. Reduction in body weight, particularly central adiposity, results in significant improvements in endothelial function, which correlates with reduction of cytokine and adhesion molecule levels (149).

## Medical Treatment

Medications that are currently used for weight loss fall into two categories—those that decrease food intake by reducing appetite or increasing satiety and those that decrease nutrient absorption. The class of medications that decrease food intake are appetite suppressants and work by increasing anorexigenic neurotransmitters such as norepinephrine, serotonin, and dopamine in certain nuclei of the central nervous system (150). Sibutramine (Meridia) is an inhibitor of both norepinephrine reuptake and serotonin reuptake that also weakly inhibits dopamine reuptake. Sibutramine is usually given in a dose of 10 to 15 mg once daily. Over a six-month period, subjects who adhere to a reduced-calorie diet and receive sibutramine typically lose 5% to 8% of their preintervention body weight, as compared with 1% to 4% among those treated with a placebo (151). Orlistat (Xenical), which decreases nutrient absorption, acts by binding to gastrointestinal lipases in the lumen of the gut, preventing hydrolysis of dietary fat (triglycerides) into absorbable FFA and monoacylglycerols (150). Ingestion of 120 mg of orlistat with or up to one hour after meals decreases absorption of ingested dietary fat by one-third. Subjects treated with orlistat for one year lost approximately 9% of their preintervention body weight, as compared to 5.8% among those treated with a placebo (152). A randomized, double-blind, placebo-controlled trial of orlistat or placebo combined with a reduced-calorie diet in overweight or obese adults with type 2 diabetes revealed a clinically significant decrease in fasting plasma glucose and HbA1c (153), suggesting orlistat may be useful as an antidiabetic agent as well as an antiobesity agent.

There is great anticipation for new medications that are currently in the development phase—Synthelabo in Paris has ongoing clinical trials for Rimonabant, which inhibits cannabinoid receptors in the brain; Regeneron is investigating a compound called ciliary neurotrophic factor (CNTF), which was originally conceived as a treatment for amyotrophic lateral sclerosis, but was found to induce significant weight loss. CNTF has been genetically modified to create Axokine, a less potent version of the original hormone; and, finally, melanocortins and agonists of their receptors have created excitement, with several pharmaceutical companies already initiating clinical trials (154).

## Surgical Treatment

Weight loss is usually not sustained because of the combined effects of multiple feedback loops from the level of the hypothalamus to the level of the adipocyte. These compensatory mechanisms attempt to maintain a stable energy homeostasis, which in the setting of intended weight loss leads inevitably to weight regain. Bariatric surgery, such as gastric bypass, can cause long-term weight loss, but is appropriate only for patients with a BMI of at least 40 or a BMI of at least 35 with obesity-related medical conditions (155). In addition to weight loss, bariatric surgery improves comorbidities as demonstrated in the Swedish Obese Subjects Study, where patients treated with bariatric surgery experienced a 47% resolution of diabetes in comparison to the 17% in the matched-control group and the two-year incidence of developing non–insulin dependent diabetes mellitus was decreased by 30-fold (156). Another study from Australia demonstrated a dramatic two-thirds of diabetic patients having resolution of their diabetes following laparoscopic gastric banding (157).

## Treatment of Insulin Resistance and the Metabolic Syndrome

As in the treatment of obesity, diet and exercise play a vital role in the treatment of insulin resistance. There are also many pharmacologic agents in the arsenal for treating insulin resistance: α-glucosidase inhibitors (such as acarbose), which delay the digestion of complex carbohydrates and disaccharides leading to decreased postprandial hyperglycemia, and this may improve insulin resistance by improving "glucotoxicity"; biguanides (such as metformin), a specific insulin sensitizer; thiazolidinediones (such as troglitazone or rosiglitazone), another insulin sensitizer that acts by activating the PPAR γ; sulfonylureas (such as glipizide or glimeperide), which mediates an antihyperglycemic effect by stimulating the pancreatic β-cell to secrete insulin; and finally insulin therapy per se, which also enhances peripheral insulin sensitivity and diminishes endogenous glucose production (39).

Several of the antidiabetic treatments listed above effect weight. Thiazolidinediones lead to increased body weight, which is associated with improved glycemic control (158), because treatment with thiazolidinedione reflects not only fluid retention, but also an increase of subcutaneous fat with a decrease in visceral fat resulting in fat redistribution (159). Acarbose and metformin in a randomized, placebo-controlled study led to modest weight loss of 3.5 and 1.0 kg, respectively (160). In addition to affecting weight, acarbose and metformin were also found to slow the progression of carotid intima-media thickness in subjects with impaired glucose tolerance and type 2 diabetes, respectively (161,162).

In addition to treating insulin resistance, a successful treatment of the metabolic syndrome should also target each component of the syndrome. Such a treatment will be needed to achieve the following goals: lower blood pressure to ideally <125/75 mmHg; LDL cholesterol <100 mg/dL; triglyceride level <150 mg/dL; and HDL cholesterol >40 mg/dL in men or >50 mg/dL in women (96). To that extent several antihypertensive and antihyperlipidemic medications are currently available, but a detailed discussion of each one is beyond the scope of this chapter.

## CONCLUSION

Obesity is a disease of rapidly increasing global prevalence. Obesity's multiple comorbidities and associated cost are the focus of attention of health care providers, researchers, and public policy makers. Importantly, in the past 10 years, basic and clinical researchers have made strides in improving our understanding of energy homeostasis, vascular function, and inflammation, and it is hoped that this new knowledge will soon lead to new and successful preventative and treatment options.

## ACKNOWLEDGMENT

Financial support (F32 DK64550–01A1) from the National Institutes of Health.

## REFERENCES

1. Kuczmarski RJ, Flegal KM, Campbell SM, Johnson CL. Increasing prevalence of overweight among US adults. JAMA 1994; 272:205–211.
2. Executive summary of the clinical guidelines on the identification, evaluation, and treatment of overweight and obesity in adults. Arch Intern Med 1998; 158:1855–1867.
3. Kraemer H, Berkowitz RI, Hammer LD. Methodological difficulties in studies of obesity. I: Measurement issues. Ann Behav Med 1990; 12:112–118.
4. Gallagher D, Visser M, Sepulveda D, Pierson RN, Harris T, Heymsfield SB. How useful is body mass index for comparison of body fatness across age, sex, and ethnic groups? Am J Epidemiol 1996; 143:228–239.
5. National task force on the prevention and treatment of obesity. Overweight, obesity and health risk. Arch Intern Med 2000; 160:898–904.
6. Manson JE, Stampfer MJ, Hennekens CH, Willett WC. Body weight and longevity. A reassessment. JAMA 1987; 257:353–358.
7. Colditz GA, Willett WC, Stampfer MJ, et al. Weight as a risk factor for clinical diabetes in women. Am J Epidemiol 1990; 132:501–513.
8. Lew EA. Mortality and weight: insured lives and the American Cancer Study. Ann Intern Med 1985; 103:1024–1029.
9. Kolterman OG, Insel J, Saekow M, Olefsky JM. Mechanisms of insulin resistance in human obesity. J Clin Invest 1980; 65:1272–1284.
10. Dyer AR, Elliot P. The INTERSALT study: relations in body mass index to blood pressure. INTERSALT Co-operative Research Group. J Hum Hypertens 1980; 3:299–308.
11. Anonymous: National Cholesterol Education Program. Second report of the expert panel on detection, evaluation, and treatment of high blood cholesterol in adults (adult treatment panel II). Circulation 1994; 89:1333–1445.
12. Kissebah AH, Krakower GR. Regional adiposity and morbidity. Physiol Rev 1994; 74:761–811.
13. Kissebah AH, Vydelingum N, Murray R, et al. Relation of body fat distribution to metabolic complications of obesity. J Clin Endocrinol Metab 1982; 54:254–260.
14. Despres JP, Moorjani S, Lupien PJ, Tremblay A, Nadeau A, Bouchard C. Regional distribution of body fat, plasma lipoproteins, and cardiovascular disease. Arteriosclerosis 1990; 10:497–511.
15. Carey VJ, Walters EE, Colditz GA, et al. Body fat distribution and risk of non-insulin dependent diabetes in women. Am J Epidemiol 1997; 145:614–619.

16. Folsom AR, Prineas RJ, Kaye SA, Munger RG. Incidence of hypertension and stroke in relation to body fat distribution and other risk factors in older women. Stroke 1990; 21:701–706.

17. Swanson CA, Potischman N, Wilbanks GD, et al. Relation of endometrial cancer risk to past and contemporary body size and body fat distribution. Cancer Epid Biomark Prev 1993; 2:321–327.

18. Ballard-Barbash R, Schatzkin A, Carter CL, et al. Body fat distribution and breast cancer in the Framingham Study. J Natl Cancer Inst 1990; 82:286–290.

19. Ducimetiere P, Richard JL. The relationship between subsets of anthropometric upper versus lower body measurements and coronary heart disease risk in middle-aged men. The Paris Prospective Study. I. Int J Obes 1989; 13:111–121.

20. Stunkard AJ, Foch TT, Hrubec Z. A twin study of human obesity. JAMA 1986; 256:51–54.

21. Stunkard AJ, Harris JR, Pedersen NL, McClearn GE. The body-mass index of twins who have been reared apart. N Engl J Med 1990; 322:1483–1487.

22. Bouchard C, Tremblay A, Despres JP, et al. The response to long term overfeeding in identical twins. N Engl J Med 1990; 322:1477–1482.

23. Zhang Y, Proenca R, Maffei M, Barone M, Leopold L, Friedman JM. Positional cloning of the mouse obese gene and its human homologue. Nature 1994; 372:425–432.

24. O'Rahilly S, Farooqi IS, Yeo GS, Challis BG. Minireview: human obesity lessons from monogenic disorders. Endocrinology 2003; 144:3757–3764.

25. Farooqi IS, Keogh JM, Yeo GS, Lank EJ, Cheetham T, O'Rahilly S. Clinical spectrum of obesity and mutations in the melanocortin 4 receptor gene. N Engl J Med 2003; 348:1085–1095.

26. Hales CN, Barker DJ. Type 2 (non-insulin-dependent) diabetes mellitus: the thrifty phenotype hypothesis. Diabetologia 1992; 35:595–601.

27. Rissanen AM, Heliovaara M, Knekt P, Reunanen A, Aromaa A. Determinants of weight gain and overweight in adult Finns. Eur J Clin Nutr 1991; 45:419–430.

28. Rosenbaum M, Leibel RL, Hirsch J. Obesity. NEJM 1997; 337:396–407.

29. Zigman JM, Elmquist JK. Minireview: from anorexia to obesity—the yin and yang of body weight control. Endocrinology 2003; 144:3749–3756.

30. American Diabetes Association. Consensus development conference on insulin resistance. Diabetes Care 1998; 21:310–314.

31. Mantzoros CS, Flier JS. Insulin resistance: the clinical spectrum. In: Mazzeferi E, ed. Advances in Endocrinology and Metabolism. 6. St. Louis: Mosby-Year Book, 1995:193–232.

32. Vidal-Puig A, Moller DE. Insulin resistance: classification, prevalence, clinical manifestations, and diagnosis. In: Azziz R, Nestler JE, Dewailly D, eds. Androgen Excess Disorders in Women. Philadelphia: Lippincott Raven, 1997:227–236.

33. Bergman RN. Toward physiological understanding of glucose tolerance: minimal model approach. Diabetes 1989; 38:1512–1527.

34. Bergman RN, Prager R, Volund A, Olefsky JM. Equivalence of the insulin sensitivity index in man derived by the minimal model method and the euglycemic glucose clamp. J Clin Invest 1987; 79:790–800.

35. Kahn CR. The molecular mechanism of insulin action. Annu Rev Med 1985; 36:429–451.

36. Chaiken RL. Insulin resistance and the metabolic syndrome. In: Poretsky L, ed. Principles of Diabetes Mellitus. Norwell: Kluwer Academic Publishers, 2002:723–737.
37. Reaven GM, Brand RJ, Chen YD, Mathur AK, Goldfine I. Insulin resistance and insulin secretion are determinants of oral glucose tolerance in normal individuals. Diabetes 1993; 42:1324–1332.
38. Kopp W. High-insulinogenic nutrition—an etiologic factor for obesity and the metabolic syndrome. Metabolism 2003; 52:840–844.
39. Matthaei S, Stumvoll M, Kellerer M, Haring HU. Pathophysiology and pharmacological treatment of insulin resistance. Endocrinol Rev 2000; 21:585–618.
40. Hone J, Accili D, al-Gazali LI, Lestringant G, Orban T, Taylor SI. Homozygosity for a new mutation (Ile$^{119}$ → Met) in the insulin receptor gene in 5 sibs with familial insulin resistance. J Med Genet 1994; 31:715–716.
41. Muller-Wieland D, Taub R, Tewari DS, et al. Insulin-receptor gene and its expression in patients with insulin resistance. Diabetes 1989; 38:31–38.
42. Almind K, Bjorbaek C, Vestergaard H, Hansen T, Echwald S, Pedersen O. Aminoacid polymorphisms of insulin receptors substrate-1 in non-insulin-dependent diabetes mellitus. Lancet 1993; 342:828–832.
43. Baier LJ, Wiedrich C, Hanson RL, Bogardus C. Variant in the regulatory subunit of phosphatidylinositol 3-kinase (p85alpha): preliminary evidence indicates a potential role of this variant in the acute insulin response and type 2 diabetes in Pima women. Diabetes 1998; 47:973–975.
44. Gurnell M, Savage DB, Chatterjee VK, O'Rahilly S. The metabolic syndrome: peroxisome proliferator-activated receptor γ and its therapeutic modulation. J Clin Endocrinol Metab 2003; 88:2412–2421.
45. Barroso I, Gurnell M, Crowley VE, et al. Dominant negative mutations in human PPAR γ are associated with severe insulin resistance, diabetes mellitus and hypertension. Nature 1999; 402:880–883.
46. Agarawal AK, Garg A. A novel heterozygous mutation in peroxisome-proliferator-activated receptor-gamma gene in a patient with familial partial lipodystrophy. J Clin Endocrinol Metab 2002; 87:408–411.
47. Hegele RA, Cao H, Frankowski C, Mathews ST, Leff T. PPARGF388L, a transactivation-deficient mutant, in familial partial lipodystrophy. Diabetes 2002; 51:3586–3590.
48. Reitman ML, Arioglu E, Gavrilova O, Taylor SI. Lipoatrophy revisited. Trends Endocrinol Metab 2000; 11:410–416.
49. Altshuler D, Hirschhorn JN, Klannemark M, et al. The common PPAR-gamma Pro12Ala polymorphism is associated with decreased risk of type 2 diabetes. Nat Genet 2000; 26:76–80.
50. Niskanen L, Uusitupa M, Sarlund H, Siitonen O, Paljarvi L, Laakso M. The effects of weight loss on insulin sensitivity, skeletal muscle composition, and capillary density in obese non-diabetic subjects. Int J Obes 1996; 20:154–160.
51. Perseghin G, Price TB, Petersen KF, et al. Increased glucose transport-phosphorylation and muscle glycogen synthesis after exercise training in insulin-resistant subjects. N Engl J Med 1996; 335:1357–1362.

52. Hespel P, Vergauwen L, Vandenberghe K, Richter EA. Important role of insulin and flow in stimulating glucose uptake in contracting skeletal muscle. Diabetes 1995; 44:210–215.
53. DeFronzo RA, Sherwin RS, Kraemer N. Effect of physical training on insulin action in obesity. Diabetes 1987; 36:1379–1385.
54. Goodpaster BH, Kelley DE, Wing RR, Meier A, Thaete FL. Effects of weight loss on regional fat distribution and insulin sensitivity in obesity. Diabetes 1999; 48:839–847.
55. Garg A, Grundy SM, Unger RH. Comparison of effects of high and low carbohydrate diets on plasma lipoproteins and insulin sensitivity in patients with mild NIDDM. Diabetes 1992; 41:1278–1285.
56. Storlien LH, Pan DA, Kriketos AD, Baur LA. High fat diet-induced insulin resistance. Lessons and implications from animal studies. Ann NY Acad Sci 1993; 683:82–90.
57. Hotamisligil GS, Shargill NS, Spiegelman BM. Adipose tissue expression of tumor necrosis factor α. Science 1993; 259:87–91.
58. Mohamed-Ali V, Goodrick S, Rawesh A, et al. Subcutaneous adipose tissue releases interleukin-6, but not tumor necrosis factor-α, in vivo. J Clin Endocrinol Metab 1997; 82:4196–4200.
59. Maeda K, Okubo K, Shimomura I, Funahashi T, Matsuzawa Y, Matsubara K. cDNA cloning and expression of a novel adipose specific collagen-like factor, apM1. Biochem Biophys Res Commun 1996; 221:286–289.
60. Boden G. Role of fatty acids in the pathogenesis of insulin resistance and NIDDM. Diabetes 1997; 46:3–10.
61. Randle PJ, Garland PB, Hales CN, Newsholme EA. The glucose fatty-acid cycle: its role in insulin sensitivity and the metabolic disturbances of diabetes mellitus. Lancet 1963; 1:785–789.
62. Gonzalez MC, Ayuso MS, Parrilla R. Control of hepatic gluconeogenesis: role of fatty acid oxidation. Arch Biochem Biophys 1989; 271:1–9.
63. Felley CP, Felley EM, van Melle GD, Frascarolo P, Jequier E, Felber JP. Impairment of glucose disposal by infusion of triglycerides in humans: role of glycemia. Am J Physiol 1989; 256:E747–E752.
64. Hotamisligil GS, Peraldi P, Budavari A, Ellis R, White MF, Spiegelman BM. IRS-1-mediated inhibition of insulin receptor tyrosine kinase activity in TNF-α- and obesity-induced insulin resistance. Science 1996; 271:665–668.
65. Kanety H, Hemi R, Papa MZ, Karasik A. Sphingomyelinase and ceramide suppress insulin-induced tyrosine phosphorylation of the insulin receptor substrated-1. J Biol Chem 1996; 271:9895–9897.
66. Kellerer M, Rett K, Renn W, Groop L, Haring HU. Circulating TNFα and leptin levels in offspring of NIDDM patients do not correlate to individual insulin sensitivity. Horm Metab Res 1996; 28:737–743.
67. Nakano Y, Tobe T, Choi-Miura NH, Mazda T, Tomita M. Isolation and characterization of GBP28, a novel gelatin-binding protein purified from human plasma. J Biochem (Tokyo) 1996; 120:803–812.
68. Tsao TS, Lodish HF, Fruebis J. ACRP30, a new hormone controlling fat and glucose metabolism. Eur J Pharmacol 2002; 440(2–3):213–221.

69. Yamamoto Y, Hirose H, Saito I, et al. Correlation of the adipocyte-derived protein adiponectin with insulin resistance index and serum high-density lipoprotein-cholesterol, independent of body mass index, in the Japanese population. Clin Sci (Lond) 2002; 103(2):137–142.

70. Matsubara M, Maruka S, Katayose S. Inverse relationship between plasma adiponectin and leptin concentrations in normal-weight and obese women. Eur J Endocrinol 2002; 147(2):173–180.

71. Arita Y, Kihara S, Ouchi N, et al. Paradoxical decrease of an adipose-specific protein, adiponectin, in obesity. Biochem Biophys Res Commun 1999; 257:79–83.

72. Yannakoulia M, Yiannakouris N, Bluher S, Matalas AL, Klimis-Zacas D, Mantzoros CS. Body fat mass and macronutrient intake in relation to circulating soluble leptin receptor, free leptin index, adiponectin, and resistin concentrations in healthy humans. J Clin Endocrinol Metab 2003; 88:1730–1736.

73. Gavrila A, Chan JL, Yiannakouris N, Kontogianni M, Miller LC, Orlova C, Mantzoros CS. Serum adiponectin levels are inversely associated with overall and central fat distribution but are not directly regulated by acute fasting or leptin administration in humans: cross-sectional and interventional studies. J Clin Endocrinol Metab 2003; 88:4823–4831.

74. Steppan CM, Bailey ST, Bhat S, et al. The hormone resistin links obesity to diabetes. Nature 2001; 409:307–312.

75. Steppan CM, Lazar MA. Resistin and obesity-associated insulin resistance. Trends Endocrinol Metab 2002; 13:18–23.

76. Way JM, Gorgun CZ, Tong Q, et al. Adipose tissue resistin expression is severely suppressed in obesity and stimulated by peroxisome proliferator-activator receptor gamma agonists. J Biol Chem 2001; 276:25651–25653.

77. Lee JH, Chan JL, Yiannakouris N, et al. Circulating resistin levels are not associated with obesity or insulin resistance in humans and are not regulated by fasting or leptin administration—cross-sectional and interventional studies in normal, insulin-resistant and diabetic subjects. J Clin Endocrinol Metab 2003; 88(10):4848–4856.

78. Silha JV, Krsek M, Hana V, et al. Perturbations in adiponectin, leptin and resistin levels in acromegaly: lack of correlation with insulin resistance. Clin Endocrinol 2003; 58(6):736–742.

79. Okazaki T, Himeno E, Nanri H, Ogata H, Ikeda M. Effects of mild aerobic exercise and a mild hypocaloric diet on plasma leptin in sedentary women. Clin Exp Pharmacol 1999; 26(5–6):415–420.

80. Xenachis C, Samojlik E, Raghuwanshi MP, Kirschner MA. Leptin, insulin and TNG-alpha in weight loss. J Endocrinol Invest 2001; 24(11):865–870.

81. Bastard JP, Jardel C, Bruckert E, et al. Elevated levels of interleukin 6 are reduced in serum and subcutaneous adipose tissue of obese women after weight loss. J Clin Endocrinol Metab 2000; 85(9):3338–3342.

82. Monzillo LU, Hamdy O, Horton ES, et al. Effect of lifestyle modification on adipokines in obese subjects with the insulin resistance syndrome. Obes Res 2003; 11:1048–1054.

83. Hotta K, Funahashi T, Arita Y, et al. Plasma concentration of a novel, adipose-specific protein, adiponectin, in type 2 diabetic patients. Arteriocler Thromb Vasc 2000; 20(6):1595–1599.

84. Heilbronn LK, Noakes M, Clifton PM. Energy restriction and weight loss on very-low-fat diets reduce C-reactive protein concentrations in obese, healthy women. Arterioscler Thromb Vasc Biol 2001; 21(6):968–970.

85. Yudkin JS. Abnormalities of coagulation and fibrinolysis in insulin resistance. evidence for a common antecedent? Diabetes Care 1999; 22(suppl 3):C25–C30.

86. Rosenson RS, Koenig W. Utility of inflammatory markers in the management of coronary artery disease. Am J Cardiol 2003; 92(suppl):10i–18i.

87. Holcomb IN, Kabakoff RC, Chan B, et al. FIZZ1, a novel cysteine-rich secreted protein associated with pulmonary inflammation, defines a new gene family. EMBO J 2000; 19:4046–4055.

88. Ouchi N, Kihara S, Funahashi T, et al. Reciprocal association of C-reactive protein with adiponectin in blood stream and adipose tissue. Circulation 2003; 107:671–674.

89. Krakoff J, Funahashi T, Stehouwer CD, et al. Inflammatory markers, adiponectin, and risk of type 2 diabetes in the Pima Indian. Diabetes Care 2003; 26:1745–1751.

90. Executive Summary of the Third Report of the National Cholesterol Education Program (NCEP) Expert Panel of Detection, Evaluation, and Treatment of High Blood Cholesterol in Adults (Adult Treatment Panel III). JAMA 2001; 285:2486–2497.

91. Ford ES, Giles WH, Dietz WH. Prevalence of the metabolic syndrome among US adults. Findings from the Third National Health and Nutrition Examination Survey. JAMA 2002; 287:356–359.

92. Isomaa B, Almgren P, Tuomi T, et al. Cardiovascular morbidity and mortality associated with the metabolic syndrome. Diabetes Care 2001; 24:683–689.

93. Petridou E, Mantzoros C, Dessypris N, et al. Plasma adiponectin concentrations in relation to endometrial cancer: a case-control study in Greece. J Clin Endocrinol Metab 2003; 88:993–997.

94. Deslypere JP. Obesity and cancer. Metabolism 1995; 44:24–27.

95. Carroll KK. Obesity as a risk factor for certain types of cancer. Lipids 1998; 33:1055–1059.

96. Scott CL. Diagnosis, prevention, and intervention for the metabolic syndrome. Am J Cardiol 2003; 92:35i–42i.

97. The Expert Committee on the Diagnosis and Classification of Diabetes Mellitus. American Diabetes Association. Clinical practice recommendations 2002. Diabetes Care 2002; 25:S1–S147.

98. Yki-Jarvinen H. Glucose toxicity. Endocrinol Rev 1992; 13:415–431.

99. Daly PA, Landsberg L. Pathogenesis of hypertension in NIDDM. Lessons from obesity. J Hum Hypertens 1991; 5:277–285.

100. Rocchini AP, Katch V, Kveselis D, et al. Insulin and renal sodium retention in obese adolescents. Hypertension 1989; 14:367–374.

101. Lever AF. Slow pressor mechanisms in hypertension. A role for hypertrophy of resistance vessels?. J Hypertens 1986; 4:515–524.

102. Sowers JR, Standley PR, Ram JL, Jacober S, Simpson L, Rose K. Hyperinsulinemia, insulin resistance and hyperglycemia: contributing factors in the pathogenesis of hypertension and atherosclerosis. Am J Hypertens 1993; 6(suppl):260–270.

103. Stout RW. Insulin and atheroma: 20 year perspective. Diabetes Care 1990; 13:631–654.
104. Resnick LM. Ionic basis of hypertension, insulin resistance, vascular disease and related disorders. Am J Hypertens 1993; 6(suppl):123–134.
105. Reaven GM. Insulin resistance/compensatory hyperinsulinemia, essential hypertension, and cardiovascular disease. J Clin Endocrinol Metab 2003; 88(6): 2399–2403.
106. Hall JE, Brands MW, Hildebrandt DA, Mizelle HL. Obesity associated hypertension. Hyperinsulinemia and renal mechanisms. Hypertension 1992; 19: I45–I55.
107. O'Brien T, Young WF Jr, Palumbo PJ, O'Brien PC, Service FJ. Hypertension and dyslipidemia in patients with insulinoma. Mayo Clin Proc 1993; 68: 141–146.
108. Stampfer MJ, Krauss RM, Ma J, et al. A prospective study of triglyceride level, low-density lipoprotein particle diameter, and risk of myocardial infarction. JAMA 1996; 276:882–888.
109. Gardner CD, Fortmann SP, Krauss RM. Association of small low-density lipoprotein particles with the incidence of coronary artery disease in men and women. JAMA 1996; 276:875–881.
110. Jones PH. A clinical overview of dyslipidemias: treatment strategies. Am J Med 1992; 93:187–198.
111. Howard BV, Howard WJ. Dyslipidemia in diabetes mellitus. Endocrinol Rev 1994; 15:263–274.
112. Mancini M, Steiner G, Betteridge DJ, Pometta D. Acquired (secondary) forms of hypertriglyceridemia. Am J Cardiol 1991; 68:17A–21A.
113. Pan XR, Cheung MC, Walden CE, Hu SX, Bierman EL, Albers JJ. Abnormal composition of apoproteins C-I, C-II and C-III in plasma and very-low-density lipoproteins of non-insulin-dependent diabetic Chinese. Clin Chem 1986; 32:1914–1920.
114. McFarlane SI, Banerji M, Sowers JR. Insulin resistance and cardiovascular disease. J Clin Endocrinol Metab 2001; 86:713–718.
115. Zambon A, Brown BG, Deeb SS, Brunzell JD. Hepatic lipase as a focal point for the development and treatment of coronary artery disease. J Invest Med 2001; 49:112–118.
116. de Divitiis O, Fazio S, Petitto M, Maddalena G, Contaldo F, Mancini M. Obesity and cardiac function. Circulation 1981; 64:477–482.
117. Kopelman PG. Obesity as a medical problem. Nature 2000; 404:635–643.
118. Hubert HB, Feinleib M, McNamara PM, Castelli WP. Obesity as an independent risk factor for cardiovascular disease: a 26-year follow-up of participants in the Framingham heart study. Circulation 1983; 67:968–977.
119. Kenchaiah S, Evans JC, Levy D, et al. Obesity and the risk of heart failure. N Engl J Med 2002; 347:305–313.
120. Cittadini A, Mantzoros CS, Hampton TG, et al. Cardiovascular abnormalities in transgenic mice with reduced brown fat: an animal model of human obesity. Circulation 1999; 100(21):2177–2183.
121. Barrett-Connor EL. Obesity, atherosclerosis and coronary artery disease. Ann Intern Med 1985; 103:1010–1019.

122. Dandona P, Alijada A. A rational approach to pathogenesis and treatment of type 2 diabetes mellitus, insulin resistance, inflammation, and atherosclerosis. Am J Cardiol 2002; 90(suppl):27g–33g.

123. Ross R. Atherosclerosis: an inflammatory disease. N Engl J Med 1999; 340: 115–126.

124. DiCorleto PE. Cellular mechanisms of atherogenesis. Am J Hypertens 1993; 6:314S–318S.

125. Bhagat K, Balance P. Inflammatory cytokines impair endothelium dependent dilatation in human veins in vivo. Circulation 1997; 96:3042–3047.

126. Romano M, Sironi M, Toniatti C, et al. Role of IL-6 and its soluble receptor in induction of chemokines and leukocyte recruitment. Immunity 1997; 6: 315–325.

127. Jang Y, Lincoff AM, Plow EF, Topol EJ. Cell adhesion molecules in coronary artery diseases. J Am Coll Cardiol 1994; 24:1591–1601.

128. Ahima RS, Flier JS. Adipose tissue as an endocrine organ. Trends Endocrinol Metab 2000; 11:327–332.

129. Thogersen AM, Jansson JH, Boman K, et al. High plasminogen activator inhibitor and tissue plasminogen activator levels in plasma precede a first acute myocardial infarction in both men and women: evidence for the fibrinolytic system as an independent primary risk factor. Circulation 1998; 98:2241–2247.

130. Sobel BE. Increased plasminogen activator inhibitor-1 and vasculopathy. A reconcilable paradox. Circulation 1999; 99:2496–2498.

131. Tham DM, Martin-McNulty B, Wang YX, et al. Angiotensin II is associated with activation of NF-κB-mediated genes and downregulation of PPARs. Physiol Genomics 2002; 11:21–30.

132. Wang YX, Martin-McNulty B, Freay AD, et al. Angiotensin II increases urokinase-type plasminogen activator expression and induces aneurysm in the abdominal aorta of apolipoprotein E-deficient mice. Am J Pathol 2001; 159:1455–1464.

133. Cai H, Li Z, Dikalov S, et al. NAD(P)H oxidase-derived hydrogen peroxide mediates endothelial nitric oxide production in response to angiotensin II. J Biol Chem 2002; 277:48311–48317.

134. Lyon CJ, Law RE, Hsueh WA. Minireview: adiposity, inflammation, and atherogenesis. Endocrinology 2003; 144:2195–2200.

135. Pyorala M, Miettinen H, Laakso M, Pyorala K. Hyperinsulinemia predicts coronary heart disease risk in healthy middle-aged men: the 22-year follow-up results of the Helsinki Policemen Study. Circulation 1998; 98:398–404.

136. Balkau B, Shipley M, Jarrett RJ, et al. High blood glucose concentration is a risk factor for mortality in middle-aged nondiabetic men. 20-year follow-up in the Whitehall Study, the Paris Prospective Study, and the Helsinki Policemen Study. Diabetes Care 1998; 21:360–367.

137. Wei M, Gaskill SP, Haffner SM, Stern MP. Effects of diabetes and level of glycemia on all-cause and cardiovascular mortality. The San Antonio Heart Study. Diabetes Care 1998; 21:1167–1172.

138. UK Prospective Diabetes Study (UKPDS) Group. Effect of intensive blood-glucose control with metformin on complications in overweight patients with type 2 diabetes (UKPDS 34). Lancet 1998; 352:854–865.

139. Kramer FM, Jeffery RW, Forster JL, Snell MK. Long-term follow-up of behavioral treatment for obesity: patterns of weight regain among men and women. Int J Obes 1989; 13:123–136.

140. Everhart JE. Contributions of obesity and weight loss to gallstone disease. Ann Intern Med 1993; 119:1029–1035.

141. McGuire MT, Wing RR, Klem ML, Hill JO. Behavioral strategies of individuals who have maintained long-term weight losses. Obes Res 1999; 7:334–341.

142. Wadden TA, Foster GD. Behavioral treatment of obesity. Med Clin North Am 2000; 84:441–461.

143. Blackburn G. Effect of degree of weight loss on health benefits. Obes Res 1995; 3(suppl 2):211s–216s.

144. Lindstrom J, Louheranta A, Mannelin M, et al. Finnish Diabetes Prevention Study Group. The Finnish Diabetes Prevention Study (DPS): Lifestyle intervention and 3-year results on diet and physical activity. Diabetes Care 2003; 26:3230–3236.

145. Knowler WC, Barrett-Connor E, Fowler SE, et al. Diabetes Prevention Program Research Group. Reduction in the incidence of type 2 diabetes with lifestyle intervention or metformin. N Engl J Med 2002; 346:393–403.

146. Frey-Hewitt B, Vranizan KM, Dreon DM, Wood PD. The effect of weight loss by dieting or exercise on resting metablolic rate in overweight men. Int J Obes 1990; 14:327–334.

147. Verit LS, Ismail AH. Effects of exercise on cardiovascular disease risk in women with NIDDM. Diabetes Res Clin Pract 1989; 6:27–35.

148. Centers for Disease Control, National Center for Chronic Disease Prevention and Health Promotion. Surgeon General's Report on Physical Activity and Health. Atlanta: Centers for Disease Control and Prevention, 1996.

149. Ziccardi P, Nappo F, Giugliano G, et al. Reduction of inflammatory cytokine concentrations and improvement of endothelial functions in obese women after weight loss over one year. Circulation 2002; 105:804–809.

150. Yanovski SZ, Yanovski JA. Obesity. N Engl J Med 2002; 346:591–602.

151. Fanghanel G, Cortinas L, Sanchez-Reyes L, Berber A. A clinical trial of the use of sibutramine for the treatment of patients suffering essential obesity. Int J Obes Relat Metab Disord 2000; 24:144–150.

152. Heck AM, Yanovski JA, Calis KA. Orlistat, a new lipase inhibitor for the management of obesity. Pharmacotherapy 2000; 20:270–279.

153. Kelley DE, Bray GA, Pi-Sunyer FX, et al. Clinical efficacy of orlistat therapy in overweight and obese patients with insulin-treated type 2 diabetes: a 1-year randomized controlled trial. Diabetes Care 2002; 25:1033–1041.

154. Gur T. Obesity drug pipeline not so fat. Science 2003; 299:849–852.

155. Clinical guidelines on the identification, evaluation, and treatment of overweight and obesity in adults—the Evidence Report. Obes Res 1998; 6(suppl 2): 51s–209s.

156. Sjostrom CD, Lissner L, Wedel H, Sjostrom L. Reduction in incidence of diabetes, hypertension and lipid disturbances after intentional weight loss induced by bariatric surgery: the SOS Intervention Study. Obes Res 1999; 7:477–484.

157. Dolan K, Bryant R, Fielding G. Treating diabetes in the morbidly obese by laparoscopic gastric banding. Obes Surg 2003; 13:439–443.

158. Patel J, Anderson RJ, Rappaport EB. Rosiglitazone monotherapy improves glycaemic control in patients with type 2 diabetes: a twelve-week, randomized, placebo-controlled study. Diabetes Obes Metab 1999; 1:165–172.
159. Nakamura T, Funahashi T, Yamashita S, et al. Thiazolidinedione derivative improves fat distribution and multiple risk factors in subjects with visceral fat accumulation—double-blind placebo-controlled trial. Diabetes Res Clin Pract 2001; 54:181–190.
160. Willms B, Ruge D. Comparison of acarbose and metformin in patients with Type 2 diabetes mellitus insufficiently controlled with diet and sulphonylureas: a randomized, placebo-controlled study. Diabet Med 1999; 16:755–761.
161. Hanefeld M, Chiasson JL, Koehler C, Henkel E, Schaper F, Temelkova-Kurktschiev T. Acarbose slows progression of intima-media thickness of the carotid arteries in subjects with impaired glucose tolerance. Stroke 2004; 35: 1073–1078.
162. Matsumoto K, Sera Y, Abe Y, Tominaga T, Yeki Y, Miyake S. Metformin attenuates progression of carotid arterial wall thickness in patients with type 2 diabetes. Diabetes Res Clin Pract 2004; 64:225–228.

# 4

# Obesity, Lipids, and Cardiovascular Disease

**Asha Thomas-Geevarghese**

*Columbia University, College of Physicians and Surgeons,
New York, New York, and Medstar Research Institute,
Washington, D.C., U.S.A.*

**Abraham Thomas**

*Division of Endocrinology, Diabetes, and Hypertension,
Brigham and Women's Hospital, Harvard Medical School, Boston,
Massachusetts, U.S.A.*

## INTRODUCTION

As the prevalence of obesity continues to increase in the United States, its role as a major public health issue grows. The effects of decreased physical activity and increased intake of calorie-dense foods have propelled the issue of obesity and its detrimental sequelae to the forefront of scientific thought. These detrimental effects are now manifested in younger and younger populations. The relationship between obesity and cardiovascular disease (CVD) is a complex one. It is mediated by a number of different factors including hypertension, diabetes, insulin resistance, and dyslipidemia, among others. Obesity in young men is associated with accelerated atherosclerosis (1). The progression from overweight to obesity to insulin resistance to glucose intolerance to type 2 diabetes and dyslipidemia is often a slow one. The role of the atherogenic dyslipidemic pattern [hypertriglyceridemia, low high-density lipoprotein cholesterol (HDL-C) and high low-density lipoprotein

(LDL-C) metabolism] has been well described. The role of weight loss and its beneficial impact on this dyslipidemic pattern make it a potent clinical target to reduce risk of CVD. Normal lipoprotein metabolism will be reviewed briefly followed by a review of the dyslipidemia of obesity.

## LIPOPROTEINS

Lipids and proteins that vary in composition, size, density, and function are carried by lipoproteins (2). The lipids are free and esterified cholesterol, triglycerides (TGs), and phospholipids. The hydrophobic TG and cholesteryl esters comprise the core (2). The lipid protein is covered by a surface containing both hydrophobic and hydrophilic phospholipids, and smaller amounts of free cholesterol and proteins (2). Apolipoproteins (Apos) are the proteins, which help to solubilize the core lipids and regulate plasma lipid and lipoprotein transport (Table 1). They are on the surface of the lipoproteins. Apo B100 is required for the secretion of hepatic-derived VLDL, intermediate-density lipoproteins (IDL), and low-density lipoproteins (LDLs) (2). Apo B48 is a form of Apo B100 that is required for secretion of chylomicrons from the small intestine. Apo A-I is the major structural protein in high-density lipoproteins (HDL). Apo A-I is also an important activator of the plasma enzyme, lecithin cholesteryl-acyl transferase, which plays a key role in reverse cholesterol transport (2,3).

TG and cholesterol are absorbed into the cells of the small intestine after food intake and are incorporated into the core of nascent chylomicrons that are secreted into the lymphatic system and enter the circulation via the superior vena cava (3). Chylomicrons acquire Apo C-II, Apo C-III, and Apo E in the blood stream. In adipose tissue and muscle, chylomicrons interact with the enzyme lipoprotein lipase (LPL), which is activated by Apo C-II, and the chylomicron core TG is hydrolyzed (2). The lipolytic products, free fatty acids, can be taken up by fat cells and reincorporated into TG, or into muscle cells where they can be used for energy. Chylomicron remnants, the product of this lipolytic process, are enriched in cholesterol esters and in Apo E (important for the interaction of chylomicron remnants with several pathways on hepatocytes that rapidly remove them from the circulation) (2). Uptake of chylomicron remnants involves binding to the LDL receptor, the LDL receptor–related protein, hepatic lipase, and cell-surface proteoglycans (4).

## RELATIONSHIP OF DYSLIPIDEMIA AND OBESITY

Obese individuals tend to be both insulin resistant and at increased risk to develop CVD. Obesity has also been shown to be associated with a clinically worsening lipid profile. The mechanisms are evolving, but the insulin resistance appears to be one of the central components. The Munster Heart

**Table 1** Apolipoprotein Characteristics

| Apolipoprotein | Lipoproteins | Metabolic functions |
|---|---|---|
| Apo A-I | HDL, chylomicrons | Structural component of HDL; LCAT activator |
| Apo B-48 | Chylomicrons | Necessary for assembly and secretion of chylomicrons from the small intestine |
| Apo B-100 | VLDL, IDL, LDL | Necessary for the assembly and secretion of VLDL from the liver; structural protein of VLDL, IDL and LDL; ligand for the LDL receptor |
| Apo C-1 | Chylomicrons, VLDL, IDL, HDL | May inhibit hepatic uptake of chylomicrons VLDL remnants |
| Apo C-II | Chylomicrons, VLDL, IDL, HDL | Activator of lipoprotein lipase |
| Apo C-III | Chylomicrons, VLDL, IDL, HDL | Inhibitor of lipoprotein lipase; inhibits hepatic uptake of chylomicron and VLDL remnants |
| Apo E | Chylomicrons, VLDL, IDL, HDL | Ligand for binding of several lipoproteins to the LDL receptor, LRP and proteoglycans |
| Apo(a) | Lp(a) | Composed of LDL Apo B linked covalently to Apo(a); an independent predictor of artery CAD |

*Abbreviations*: HDL, high-density lipoproteins; VLDL, very low-density lipoproteins; IDL, intermediate-density lipoproteins; LDL, low-density lipoproteins.
*Source*: From Ref. 3.

Study followed 16,288 men and 7325 women for up to seven years. There was a positive relationship between body mass index (BMI) and other coronary heart disease (CHD) risk factors including age, total serum cholesterol, LDL cholesterol, and systolic and diastolic blood pressure. The increase of CHD death associated with BMI was completely accounted for and mediated by these risk factors (5). HDL-C tended to increase with age, but decreased in graded fashion with increases in BMI in both sexes. TG increased with BMI in both sexes and with age in women, but decreased in the older age groups of overweight and obese men. Although fasting blood glucose increased with age and BMI in both sexes, the increase was more marked in women. Increased mortality was seen at a high BMI in both smokers and nonsmokers and was caused by CHD. Increased mortality at low BMI was seen in smokers but not in nonsmokers and was due to an increase in cancer deaths. The BMI-associated increase in CHD death was completely accounted for by the factors contained in the Munster Heart

Study risk algorithm, indicating that the effect of overweight and obesity on CHD is mediated via other risk factors (5).

Given the increased prevalence of obesity in the U.S. population, another study attempted to define the relationship between degree of obesity and insulin-mediated glucose disposal, as well as the relationship between obesity, insulin resistance, and CVD risk. The study evaluated the insulin-mediated glucose disposal in 465 healthy volunteers by determining the steady-state plasma glucose (SSPG) concentrations at the end of a 180-minute infusion of somatostatin, insulin, and glucose (6). A series of CVD risk factors were measured, including blood pressure, BMI and plasma glucose and insulin concentrations, before and after administration of 75 g of oral glucose, and fasting plasma lipid and lipoprotein concentrations. The SSPG concentration and BMI were significantly correlated, and 36% of the most insulin-resistant individuals were obese (BMI $\geq 30.0 \, \text{kg/m}^2$). However, 16% of those in the most insulin-resistant were of normal weight (BMI $<25.0 \, \text{kg/m}^2$). The higher the SSPG concentration, the greater the increase in plasma glucose, insulin, and TG concentrations, whereas the greater the BMI, the higher the LDL concentration (6). Significant differences in CVD risk were only apparent in the lowest BMI group, whereas CVD risk factors increased significantly with each tertile of insulin resistance. These results show that BMI and insulin resistance are related, but not synonymous, and that they make independent and different contributions to increasing CVD risk (6).

The insulin resistance of obesity is associated with hypertriglyceridemia (7). The risk of increased TG with increased body weight has been well described (8). The data have mainly been for studies conducted in whites, but the association has also been presented in black, Hispanic, and native American people (9–11). Studies of weight loss of greater than one year have shown significant reductions in TG (12).

Increased BMI has been associated with decreasing HDL levels in all ages, with the effects greater in women than in men (8,13). Weight loss has been shown to increase HDL (14), whereas an eight-year increase in BMI of 1 U was associated with a decrease in HDL of 3 mg/dL (12,15). These findings are similar in black, Hispanic, and native American populations (10,16,17).

The data on LDL is less clear. National Health and Nutrition Examination Surveys II data show an increase in LDL with increasing BMI in young men and women, but minimal differences in the older populations (8). The data regarding weight loss is conflicting, with only two showing a decrease in LDL with weight loss (18,19). In addition, the LDL trends in other groups are complex. In native Americans, the LDL increased until a BMI of 31.2 and then decreased with increasing BMI. Nonetheless, the LDL particles are smaller and more dense (12). The changes in lipoprotein patterns are similar in men and women, as BMI increases.

## INSULIN RESISTANCE

It is estimated that more than one-third of the U.S. population is insulin resistant (20). As part of the metabolic syndrome, these patients have glucose intolerance, type 2 diabetes, obesity, a prothrombotic state, CVD, hypertension, stroke, nonalcoholic fatty liver disease, polycystic ovary disease, and certain forms of cancer and dyslipidemia (21). The gold standard of diagnosis of insulin resistance is the euglycemic insulin clamp. Clinically, patients with central adiposity have an increased incidence of insulin resistance. In studies that have evaluated the effects of total versus central obesity, the data revealed that the central obesity was more closely associated with abnormal lipid profiles than total obesity in women, but both factors were equally important in men (12,22).

The ability of insulin to stimulate glucose disposal varies more than sixfold in apparently healthy individuals, and between 25% and 35% of the variability in insulin action is related to being overweight (23). Although the majority of individuals in the general population that can be considered insulin resistant are also overweight, not all overweight persons are insulin resistant and the abnormalities associated with insulin resistance are limited to the subset of overweight individuals that are also insulin resistant. Significant improvement in these metabolic abnormalities following weight loss is seen only in the subset of overweight/obese individuals that are also insulin resistant (23). Identifying these patients then becomes a key clinical goal.

The presence of increased visceral fat is predictive of the metabolic syndrome and an increased risk of CVD (24). The metabolic syndrome is associated with an increased risk of CVD. Visceral obesity is associated with low serum HDL, high serum TG, increased Apo B, small dense LDL particles, and insulin resistance. The hyperinsulinemia and central obesity of insulin resistance lead to VLDL overproduction. This is due to the increased free fatty acid and glucose levels that regulate hepatic VLDL output and the elevated TG levels in the liver, which inhibit Apo B degradation and result in an increased assembly and secretion of VLDL (25). There are decreased LPL levels that result in decreased VLDL clearance and increased serum TG–rich particles (Fig. 1) (25).

Visceral adiposity is correlated with larger very low-density lipoproteins (VLDL), smaller more dense LDL, and lower levels of $HDL_2$ (26), while obesity is related to decreased pre-beta-1-HDL (26,27). This pattern is seen in insulin-resistant lean subjects as well (28). Obese men have more LPL in visceral adipose tissue and plasma than lean subjects do. Owing to the fact that insulin resistance is often present, there are increased levels of TG-rich particles because the LPL is insulin sensitive (29,30).

Although obesity is defined by BMI, it does not take body fat distribution into consideration (31). The clinical criteria for the metabolic syndrome from the ATP guidelines include having three of the following

## Model of Insulin Resistance

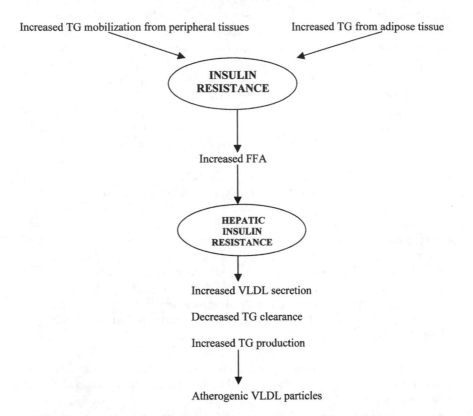

**Figure 1** Effect of insulin resistance on lipid metabolism. *Abbreviations*: TG, trigly-ceride; FFA, free fatty acids; VLDL, very low density lipoprotein.

components: abdominal obesity (waist circumference >40 in. in men, >35 in. in women), TG>150 mg/dL, blood pressure >130/≥80, fasting glucose ≥110 mg/dL, and HDL <40 mg/dL in men and <50 mg/dL in women (Table 2) (32). The characteristic findings of the dyslipidemic pattern are often found before any abnormality of glucose metabolism.

## THE LIPIDS

### Triglycerides

The effects of insulin resistance on liver, muscle, and fat are multifold. The persistent production of glucose by the liver, the decreased glucose uptake by muscle, and the continued fatty acid flux from fat all lead to the hyper-triglyceridemia of insulin resistance. The overproduction of VLDL, the pre-dominant TG-containing lipoprotein, by the liver is the culminating key

**Table 2**  Characteristics of the Metabolic Syndrome

| Risk factor | Definition |
|---|---|
| *Abdominal obesity (waist circumference):* | |
| Men | > 102 (cm) (> 40 in.) |
| Women | > 88 (cm) (> 35 in.) |
| Triglyceride level | > 150 (mg/dL) |
| *High density lipoprotein cholesterol:* | |
| Men | < 40 (mg/dL) |
| Women | < 50 (mg/dL) |
| Blood pressure | $\geq 130/\geq 85$ (mm Hg) |
| Fasting glucose | $\geq 110$ (mg/dL) |

Data taken from the National Cholesterol Education Program Adult Treatment Panel III.
Three of these characteristics are needed to diagnose the metabolic syndrome.
*Source*: From Ref. 32.

defect (12). VLDL is made in the liver and is stimulated by free fatty acids
(21). VLDL is cleared by the LDL receptor and LPL. In insulin resistance,
both of these mechanisms of clearance are decreased, contributing to the
hypertriglyceridemia found in this population. LPL activity is stimulated
by insulin. In insulin-resistant subjects, there is decreased LPL activity with
resulting decreased VLDL clearance (33,34).

## LDL

In insulin resistance, a change occurs to the LDL particle composition (which
is usually a cholesterol core with Apo B surrounding it). In part related to the
increased VLDL, there is increased transfer of TG into small, dense LDL
particles, which accumulate via the hepatic lipase conversion of VLDL
remnants. These particles have less cholesterol ester and more Apo B. With
increased VLDL, the protein cholesterol ester transfer protein (CETP) can
facilitate TG transfer into LDL and cholesterol transfer to VLDL. These
TG-enriched LDL particles undergo more oxidation and glycation (12).
Oxidated LDL binds to macrophages via scavenger receptors, which result
in foam cell formation (35). Hydrolysis of the TG-rich LDL results in small,
dense lipid-depleted particles. There is resultant decreased clearance of these
small LDL particles by the LDL receptor. The small dense LDL are associated with an increased risk of CVD in part due to their increased susceptibility to oxidation and increased uptake by macrophages (21).

Mamo et al. studied postprandial lipemia after an oral fat load in
middle-aged men with visceral obesity (36). The two groups had similar
plasma cholesterol levels, but obese subjects had higher levels of plasma TG
and reduced amounts of high-density cholesterol. Fasting plasma insulin
was fourfold greater in the obese subjects and the fasting concentration of

Apo B (37) was more than twofold greater. A delay in the conversion of chylomicrons to remnants probably contributed to postprandial dyslipidemia in viscerally obese subjects. The TG was greater in obese subjects and peak postprandial TG was delayed by approximately two hours in obese subjects. Postheparin plasma lipase rates were found to be similar for lean and obese subjects. In obese subjects, the binding of LDL was reduced by one-half compared with lean controls. Because the LDL receptor is involved in the removal of proatherogenic chylomicron remnants, the hepatic clearance of these particles might be decreased in insulin-resistant obese subjects. The authors hypothesized that atherogenesis in viscerally obese, insulin-resistant subjects may in part reflect delayed clearance of postprandial lipoprotein remnants.

## HDL

There are a number of factors that are likely to contribute to the HDL particles in obesity, which are smaller and fewer than in the nonobese population. With the impaired lipolysis of TG-rich particles, there is decreased transfer of lipoproteins and phospholipids to the HDL particle. In addition, there is an increased activity of hepatic lipase, which facilitates HDL clearance and decreased insulin stimulation of the hepatic HDL secretion and Apo A-1 production (12). This results in smaller HDL particles, which are cleared more quickly. With high levels of VLDL, CETP can exchange the TG of VLDL for the cholesterol of HDL, producing a highly atherogenic cholesterol-rich VLDL particle and a low cholesterol, TG-rich HDL particle (21). This ultimately results in a lower amount of effective circulating HDL.

Low plasma HDL cholesterol concentration has been associated with an increased risk of CHD, but is usually not observed as an isolated disorder. Pascot et al. assessed HDL particle size among 238 male subjects with visceral obesity and insulin resistance. HDL particle size was found to be significantly correlated with an increased plasma TG, decreased HDL cholesterol, high Apo B, elevated cholesterol/HDL cholesterol ratio, and small LDL particles as well as increased levels of visceral adipose tissue. Men with large HDL particles had a more favorable plasma lipoprotein–lipid profile compared with those with smaller HDL particles, reduced overall adiposity, and lower levels of visceral adipose. The authors concluded that small HDL particle size was a part of the dyslipidemia of obesity (38).

Reaven and Chen (39) showed an inverse relationship between HDL and insulin levels. In obese and nonobese patients who had elevated insulin levels, a lower HDL level was found than in those with insulin levels below the median.

## WEIGHT LOSS AND EFFECT ON LIPIDS

Several weight loss studies of one year duration show significant reductions in TG with weight loss (12,40), increases in HDL (14,18,40), and more inconsistent findings related to LDL. Only two (18,19) of five studies (14,18,40) have shown significant decreases in LDL with weight loss (12). A number of kinetic studies have been done to evaluate the metabolism of apoproteins and lipids in the obese state and in weight loss. These studies evaluate the production rate (PR) and the fractional catabolic rate (FCR).

In one study, Cummings et al. (41) measured the hepatic secretion of very-low-density lipoprotein apolipoprotein B-100 (VLDL Apo B) in six obese subjects and six lean control subjects. Plasma total cholesterol, triacylglycerol, and mevalonic acid (an index of cholesterol synthesis in vivo) concentrations were significantly higher in the obese subjects than in the control subjects. VLDL Apo B pool size and absolute secretion rate were significantly higher in the obese subjects than in the control subjects, but there was no significant difference in the FCR of VLDL Apo B (41).

In another study, Chan et al. (42) assessed the kinetics of hepatic Apo B-100 metabolism in men with visceral obesity to examine whether the kinetic defects are associated with elevated plasma concentration of Apo C-III VLDL, IDL, and LDL Apo B kinetics were measured in 48 viscerally obese men and 10 age-matched normolipidemic lean men using an intravenous bolus injection of D(3)-leucine. Apo B isotopic enrichment was measured. Compared with controls, obese subjects had significantly elevated plasma concentrations of plasma TG, cholesterol, LDL-cholesterol, VLDL-Apo B, IDL-Apo B, LDL-Apo B, Apo C-III, and insulin. The VLDL-Apo B secretion rate was significantly higher in obese than control subjects; the FCRs of IDL-Apo B and LDL-Apo B and percent conversion of VLDL-Apo B to LDL-Apo B were also significantly lower in obese subjects. The decreased VLDL-Apo B FCR, however, was not significantly different from the lean group. In the obese group, plasma concentration of Apo C-III was significantly and positively associated with VLDL-Apo B secretion rate and inversely with VLDL-Apo B FCR and percent conversion of VLDL to LDL. The authors suggested that plasma lipid and lipoprotein abnormalities in visceral obesity may be due to a combination of overproduction of VLDL-Apo B particles and decreased catabolism of Apo B–containing particles. Elevated plasma Apo C-III concentration is also a feature of dyslipidemia in obesity that contributes to the kinetic defects in Apo B metabolism (42).

Still other studies evaluating TG clearance using $^3H_2$-glycerol showed a 61% decrease in FCR in obese women compared to lean subjects, with no significant change in men (43). The obese men, however, had a 91% increase in PR compared to lean subjects, with no change found in the women. This reveals a gender difference in TG metabolism between men and women. The obese men had higher TG than lean controls secondary to increased production of TG, whereas obese women had a higher TG due to decreased clearance (28).

Other studies have looked at the effect of weight loss on a given subject (44). The effects of obesity and weight loss on lipoprotein kinetics were evaluated in six lean women [(BMI): $21 \pm 1 \, \text{kg/m}^2$] and seven women with abdominal obesity (BMI: $36 \pm 1 \, \text{kg/m}^2$). Stable isotope tracer techniques were used to determine VLDL-TG and Apo B-100 secretion rates in lean women and in obese women before and after 10% weight loss. VLDL-TG and VLDL-Apo B-100 secretion rates were similar in lean and obese women. Weight loss decreased the rate of VLDL-TG secretion by approximately 40%. The relative decline in VLDL-TG produced from nonsystemic fatty acids, derived from intraperitoneal and intrahepatic TG, was greater than the decline in VLDL-TG produced from systemic fatty acids, predominantly derived from subcutaneous TG. Weight loss did not affect VLDL-Apo B-100 secretion rate. The authors concluded that weight loss decreases the rate of VLDL-TG secretion in women with abdominal obesity, primarily by decreasing the availability of nonsystemic fatty acids. There is dissociation in the effect of weight loss on VLDL-TG and Apo B-100 metabolic pathways that may affect VLDL particle size (44).

Another study by Riches et al. also evaluated the effect of weight on the kinetics of Apo B metabolism in a dietary intervention study in 26 obese men (45). Hepatic secretion of VLDL Apo B was measured using an infusion of 1-[$^{13}$C] leucine. Subcutaneous and visceral adipose tissues were quantified by magnetic resonance imaging. With weight reduction, there was a significant decrease in BMI, waist circumference, and visceral adipose tissue. The plasma concentrations of total cholesterol, TG, and insulin also significantly decreased. Compared with weight maintenance, weight reduction significantly decreased the VLDL Apo B concentration, pool size, and hepatic secretion of VLDL Apo B, but did not significantly alter its fractional catabolism. Weight reduction was also associated with an increased FCR of LDL Apo B and conversion of VLDL to LDL Apo B. A change in hepatic VLDL Apo B secretion was significantly correlated with a change in visceral adipose tissue, but not plasma concentrations of insulin, or free fatty acids. The data support the hypothesis that a reduction in visceral adipose tissue is associated with a decrease in the hepatic secretion of VLDL Apo B, and this may be due to a decrease in portal lipid substrate supply. Weight reduction may also increase the fractional catabolism of LDL Apo B, but this requires further evaluation (45).

## TREATMENT

### Nonpharmacologic

Diet and exercise are the hallmark of therapy for lipid management in obese and insulin-resistant subjects. In overweight subjects, physical activity and weight control have been shown to be of benefit in the management of dyslipidemia (46). Exercise (47) and smoking cessation (48) can improve insulin sensitivity.

## Pharmacologic Treatment

### Lipid-Lowering Agents

**Statins:** The 3-hydroxy-3-methylgluatryl coenzyme A (HMG-CoA) reductase inhibitors have changed the course of lipid-lowering treatment. These agents decrease LDL, moderately decrease TG, and increase HDL. Lovastatin, pravastatin, fluvastatin, simvastatin, atorvastatin, and rosuvastatin are available in this category in the United States. They competitively inhibit HMG-CoA reductase, the rate-limiting enzyme in cholesterol synthesis, which results in both decreased hepatic production of Apo B–containing lipoproteins and upregulation of LDL receptors (3). The overall effect is a dramatic lowering of plasma levels of LDL cholesterol. VLDL TG concentrations are also reduced in many subjects with moderate hypertriglyceridemia (37). With decreased cholesterol synthesis, there is upregulation in the LDL receptors and resultant lower LDL (28,49). The reduction of TG is directly related to the reduction of LDL cholesterol achieved. These agents can lower LDL cholesterol by up to 45% to 60%, and decrease TG 20% to 45% (50). The reduction in TG achieved at these high levels of LDL cholesterol reduction depends on the starting TG level.

The main side effect associated with statin therapy is a myositis and elevated levels of creatine phosphokinase (usually greater than 1000 U). In severe cases, rhabdomyolysis and concomitant myoglobinemia can place the patients at risk for renal failure due to myoglobinuria. The incidence of myositis when statins are used as monotherapy is about 1 in 500 to 1000 patients. Statins can also cause nonclinically significant elevations in liver function tests in 1% to 2% of patients (3).

To determine the mechanisms whereby HMG-CoA reductase inhibitors lower the levels of LDL in patients with mixed hyperlipidemia, LDL turnover studies were conducted in 12 such patients during placebo treatment and then during treatment with lovastatin (49). Drug therapy reduced total cholesterol and TG concentrations by 33% and 32%, respectively. During lovastatin therapy, LDL-cholesterol levels fell by 37%, and LDL-Apo B concentrations decreased by an average of 29%. The decrease in LDL-Apo B concentrations on lovastatin therapy was largely due to an increase in FCRs for LDL Apo B (49). The average increase in FCRs was 34%, whereas transport rates (PRs) for LDL Apo B remained unchanged. These results strongly suggest that an increase in LDL-receptor activity is the major mechanism whereby LDL levels are lowered during lovastatin therapy (49). The data do not indicate that this drug inhibited the input of Apo B–containing lipoproteins, which would have been expected to result in a decrease in the rate of production of LDL. Interestingly, another study using deutroleucine in five lean hypertriglyceridemic male treated with lovastatin had no effect on LDL clearance but decreased the PR of Apo B-100 in IDL and LDL (28,51). This is an area of continued research.

**Niacin:**   Niacin, when used in pharmacologic doses (1–3 g/day), has the ability to potently lower TG (25–40%), lower LDL cholesterol (15–20%), and raise HDL cholesterol (10–25%) (3). The mechanism of action is thought to be through lowering hepatic VLDL Apo B production and increasing the synthesis of Apo A-I. Niacin unfortunately has several side effects that often limit its use. It produces a prostaglandin-mediated flush that occurs about 30 minutes after ingestion and can last as long as one hour. Niacin can cause gastric irritation, exacerbate peptic ulcer disease, dry skin, and hyperuricemia, and precipitate gouty attacks. Its use is associated with elevations of hepatic transaminases in about 5% of patients and rarely can also cause hepatitis. Some studies have demonstrated that niacin therapy worsens diabetic control, likely by inducing insulin resistance (52). Yet more recent studies have demonstrated that glycemic control could be maintained with intensive glucose management during niacin therapy (53).

**Fibric acid derivatives:**   This class of drugs lowers TG and raises HDL levels. The effects on LDL are more variable. Fenofibrate and gemfibrozil, the agents available in the United States at present, result in lowering of TG from 20% to 35% and increases in HDL cholesterol from 10% to 20% (54). These agents appear to work by both decreasing hepatic VLDL production, as well as increasing the activity of LPL. Fibrates are peroxisome proliferator–activated receptor $\alpha$ agonists, which activate genes involved in TG and HDL metabolism (21). Fibrates have modest and variable effects on LDL cholesterol in most patients and may even raise LDL levels in patients who present with more significant hypertriglyceridemia and lower LDL cholesterol levels pretreatment (3). The usual dose is 600 mg twice daily of gemfibrozil and 160 mg once daily for micronized fenofibrate. These agents are contraindicated in patients with gallstones, and because they are tightly bound to plasma proteins, levels of other drugs (e.g., Coumadin) should be monitored carefully. Fibrates do not significantly affect glycemic control.

**Orlistat:**   Orlistat inhibits pancreatic and gastric lipases, thereby inhibiting absorption of ingested fat. Weight loss is maximal after treatment for six months (55). This agent has shown some promise in decreasing cholesterol and LDL, independent of weight loss. In a 57-week randomized double-blind placebo-controlled study of 391 obese patients with type 2 diabetes, 120 mg orlistat or placebo was administered orally three times a day with a mildly hypocaloric diet. The orlistat group lost 6% of body weight while the placebo group lost 4% ($p$ <0.001) (56). The orlistat group had significantly greater decreases in total cholesterol and LDL cholesterol than placebo, independent of the degree of weight loss (56). The HbA1c values decreased in both groups, correlating with the weight loss (56).

In another study, Erdmann et al. evaluated the cholesterol-lowering effect of orlistat treatment, independent of its weight-reducing efficacy (57).

Three hundred eighty-four patients with elevated cholesterol were assigned to double-blind treatment with orlistat ($3 \times 120$ mg/day) or placebo for six months with a hypocaloric diet. The weight loss in the orlistat group was 7.4 kg versus 4.9 kg compared with the placebo group (57). Total and LDL cholesterol decreased by 25 to 30 mg/dL versus 10 to 15 mg/dL with placebo (57). Reduction of cholesterol with orlistat was significantly greater than anticipated from weight loss alone. The authors concluded that orlistat has a cholesterol-lowering efficacy independent of its weight-reducing effect (57).

**Sibutramine:** Sibutramine inhibits norepinephrine and serotonin reuptake. It reduces food intake by causing early satiety and may increase thermogenesis in humans (58,59). Among obese subjects treated with sibutramine, weight loss is associated with a decrease in serum TG and LDL cholesterol concentrations (60). Dujovne et al., as part of the Sibutramine Study Group, studied the effects of sibutramine on body weight and serum lipids in a double-blind, randomized, placebo-controlled trial (61). Three hundred twenty-two obese patients with dyslipidemia and TG $\geq 250$ and $\leq 1000$ mg/dL and HDL $\leq 45$ mg/dL (women) and $\leq 40$ mg/dL (men) were placed on a step I American Heart Association diet and randomized to sibutramine 20 mg or placebo once daily for six months (62). Patients taking sibutramine had greater weight loss than those receiving placebo ($-4.9$ kg vs. $-0.6$ kg, $p \leq 0.05$) (61). TG levels decreased among 5% and 10% weight-loss responders in the sibutramine group to 33.4 and 72.3 mg/dL, respectively, compared with an increase of 31.7 mg/dL among all patients receiving placebo ($p \leq 0.05$) (61). Mean increases in HDL levels for 5% and 10% weight-loss responders in the sibutramine group were 4.9 and 6.7 mg/dL, respectively, compared with an increase of 1.7 mg/dL among all patients in the placebo group ($p \leq 0.05$) (61). The authors concluded that in overweight and obese patients with elevated TG levels and low serum HDL levels, treatment with sibutramine was associated with significant improvements in body weight and TG and HDL levels (61).

Sabuncu et al. evaluated the effect of sibutramine treatment on glucose tolerance, insulin sensitivity, and serum lipid profiles in obese subjects (62). Seventy-two obese subjects were given sibutramine at a dose of 10 mg/day and a 1200-calorie diet for 12 months. Nine patients were withdrawn from the study (five because of side effects, two because of ineffective therapy, and two for unknown reasons). Sixty-three (6 male, 57 female) patients completed the study (62). At one year, obese subjects had lower body weights, waist-to-hip ratios, serum TG levels, and areas under the curve for glucose and insulin (all $p < 0.001$) (62). Serum HDL cholesterol levels and the insulin sensitivity index were higher after treatment (both $p < 0.001$). Serum total and LDL cholesterol levels did not change significantly during the study (62).

## CONCLUSION

The effect of obesity on lipids and CVD is an intricate one. The underlying role of insulin resistance is clear, but its complexities continue to evolve. Increased TG, decreased HDL levels, and small dense atherogenic LDL describe the dyslipidemia of obesity. Continued research is necessary to better describe the relationship between obesity and insulin resistance and the impact of each of these factors individually and together on their effect on CVD. Diet modification, exercise, weight loss, and lipid-lowering therapy can improve the obesity-related dyslipidemia and decrease cardiovascular risk.

## REFERENCES

1. McGill HC Jr, McMahan CA, Herderick EE, et al. Obesity accelerates the progression of coronary atherosclerosis in young men. Circulation 2002:2712–2718.
2. Ginsberg HN. Lipoprotein physiology. Endocrinol Metab Clin North Am 1998; 27(3):503–519.
3. Thomas-Geevarghese ATC, Ginsberg HN. Diabetes and dyslipidemia. In: Johnstone MT, Veves A, eds. Diabetes and Cardiovascular Disease. Towata, NJ: Humana Press. In press.
4. Cooper AD. Hepatic uptake of chylomicron remnants. J Lipid Res 1997; 38(11):2173–2192.
5. Schulte H, Cullen P, Assmann G. Obesity, mortality and cardiovascular disease in the Munster Heart Study (PROCAM). Atherosclerosis 1999; 144(1):199–209.
6. McLaughlin T, Allison G, Abbasi F, Lamendola C, Reaven G. Prevalence of insulin resistance and associated cardiovascular disease risk factors among normal weight, overweight, and obese individuals. Metabolism 2004:495–499.
7. Moro E, Gallina P, Pais M, Cazzolato G, Alessandrini P, Bittolo-Bon G. Hypertriglyceridemia is associated with increased insulin resistance in subjects with normal glucose tolerance: evaluation in a large cohort of subjects assessed with the 1999 World Health Organization criteria for the classification of diabetes. Metabolism 2003:616–619.
8. Denke MA, Sempos CT, Grundy SM. Excess body weight. An underrecognized contributor to high blood cholesterol levels in white American men. Arch Intern Med 1993; 153(9):1093–1103.
9. Folsom AR, Burke GL, Ballew C, et al. Relation of body fatness and its distribution to cardiovascular risk factors in young blacks and whites. The role of insulin. Am J Epidemiol 1989:911–924.
10. Haffner SM, Stern MP, Hazuda HP, Pugh J, Patterson JK. Do upper-body and centralized adiposity measure different aspects of regional body-fat distribution? Relationship to non-insulin-dependent diabetes mellitus, lipids, and lipoproteins. Diabetes 1987:43–51.
11. Howard BV, Bogardus C, Ravussin E, et al. Studies of the etiology of obesity in Pima Indians. Am J Clin Nutr 1991:1577S–1585S.
12. Howard BV, Ruotolo G, Robbins DC. Obesity and dyslipidemia. Endocrinol Metab Clin North Am 2003:855–867.

13. Denke MA, Sempos CT, Grundy SM. Excess body weight. An under-recognized contributor to dyslipidemia in white American women. Arch Intern Med 1994; 154(4):401–410.

14. Karvetti RL, Hakala P. A seven-year follow-up of a weight reduction programme in Finnish primary health care. Eur J Clin Nutr 1992; 46(10):743–752.

15. Anderson KM, Wilson PW, Garrison RJ, Castelli WP, eds. Longitudinal and secular trends in lipoprotein cholesterol measurements in a general population sample. The Framingham Offspring Study. Atherosclerosis 1987; 68(1–2): 59–66.

16. Burke GL, Bild DE, Hilner JE, Folsom AR, Wagenknecht LE, Sidney S. Differences in weight gain in relation to race, gender, age and education in young adults: the CARDIA Study. Coronary Artery Risk Development in Young Adults. Ethn Health 1996; 1(4):327–335.

17. Howard BV, Davis MP, Pettitt DJ, Knowler WC, Bennett PH. Plasma and lipoprotein cholesterol and triglyceride concentrations in the Pima Indians: distributions differing from those of Caucasians. Circulation 1983; 68(4):714–724.

18. Wood PD, Stefanick ML, Williams PT, Haskell WL. The effects on plasma lipoproteins of a prudent weight-reducing diet, with or without exercise, in overweight men and women. N Engl J Med 1991:461–466.

19. Wood PD, Stefanick ML, Dreon DM, et al. Changes in plasma lipids and lipoproteins in overweight men during weight loss through dieting as compared with exercise. N Engl J Med 1988:1173–1179.

20. Ford ES, Giles WH, Dietz WH. Prevalence of the metabolic syndrome among US adults: findings from the third National Health and Nutrition Examination Survey. JAMA 2002:356–359.

21. Watson KE, Horowitz BN, Matson G. Lipid abnormalities in insulin resistant states. Rev Cardiovasc Med 2003; 4:228–236.

22. Hu D, Hannah J, Gray RS, et al. Effects of obesity and body fat distribution on lipids and lipoproteins in nondiabetic American Indians: The Strong Heart Study. Obes Res 2000:411–421.

23. Reaven G, Abbasi F, McLaughlin T. Obesity, insulin resistance, and cardiovascular disease. Recent Prog Horm Res 2004:207–223.

24. Sowers JR. Obesity as a cardiovascular risk factor. Am J Med 2003; 115(suppl 8A):37S–41S.

25. Howard BV. Insulin resistance and lipid metabolism. Am J Cardiol 1999: 28J–32J.

26. Nieves DJ, Cnop M, Retzlaff B, et al. The atherogenic lipoprotein profile associated with obesity and insulin resistance is largely attributable to intra-abdominal fat. Diabetes 2003:172–179.

27. Sasahara T, Yamashita T, Sviridov D, Fidge N, Nestel P. Altered properties of high density lipoprotein subfractions in obese subjects. J Lipid Res 1997: 600–611.

28. Marsh JB. Lipoprotein metabolism in obesity and diabetes: insights from stable isotope kinetic studies in humans. Nutr Rev 2003:363–375.

29. Jeppesen J, Hollenbeck CB, Zhou MY, et al. Relation between insulin resistance, hyperinsulinemia, postheparin plasma lipoprotein lipase activity, and postprandial lipemia. Arterioscler Thromb Vasc Biol 1995:320–324.

30. Cominacini L, Garbin U, Davoli A, et al. High-density lipoprotein cholesterol concentrations and postheparin hepatic and lipoprotein lipases in obesity: relationships with plasma insulin levels. Ann Nutr Metab 1993:175–184.
31. Sowers JR. Obesity as a cardiovascular risk factor. Am J Med 2003:37S–41S.
32. Executive Summary of The Third Report of The National Cholesterol Education Program (NCEP) Expert Panel on Detection, Evaluation, and Treatment of High Blood Cholesterol in Adults (Adult Treatment Panel III). JAMA 2001:2486–2497.
33. Miyashita Y, Shirai K, Itoh Y, et al. Low lipoprotein lipase mass in preheparin serum of type 2 diabetes mellitus patients and its recovery with insulin therapy. Diabetes Res Clin Pract 2002:181–187.
34. Taskinen MR. Lipoprotein lipase in diabetes. Diabetes Metab Rev 1987: 551–570.
35. Schunkert H. Obesity and target organ damage: the heart. Int J Obes Relat Metab Disord 2002:S15–S20.
36. Mamo JC, Watts GF, Barrett PH, Smith D, James AP, Pal S. Postprandial dyslipidemia in men with visceral obesity: an effect of reduced LDL receptor expression? Am J Physiol Endocrinol Metab 2001:E626–E632.
37. Ginsberg HN. Effects of statins on triglyceride metabolism. Am J Cardiol 1998:32B–35B.
38. Pascot A, Lemieux I, Prud'homme D, et al. Reduced HDL particle size as an additional feature of the atherogenic dyslipidemia of abdominal obesity. J Lipid Res 2001:2007–2014.
39. Reaven GM, Chen YD. Insulin resistance, its consequences, and coronary heart disease. Must we choose one culprit? Circulation 1996:1780–1783.
40. Jalkanen L. The effect of a weight reduction program on cardiovascular risk factors among overweight hypertensives in primary health care. Scand J Soc Med; 1991:66–71.
41. Cummings MH, Watts GF, Pal C, et al. Increased hepatic secretion of very-low-density lipoprotein apolipoprotein B-100 in obesity: a stable isotope study. Clin Sci (Lond) 1995:225–233.
42. Chan DC, Watts GF, Redgrave TG, Mori TA, Barrett PH. Apolipoprotein B-100 kinetics in visceral obesity: associations with plasma apolipoprotein C-III concentration. I. Metabolism 2002:1041–1046.
43. Mittendorfer B, Patterson BW, Klein S. Effect of sex and obesity on basal VLDL-triacylglycerol kinetics. Am J Clin Nutr 2003:573–579.
44. Mittendorfer B, Patterson BW, Klein S. Effect of weight loss on VLDL-triglyceride and apoB-100 kinetics in women with abdominal obesity. Am J Physiol Endocrinol Metab 2003:E549–E556.
45. Riches FM, Watts GF, Hua J, Stewart GR, Naoumova RP, Barrett PH. Reduction in visceral adipose tissue is associated with improvement in apolipoprotein B-100 metabolism in obese men. J Clin Endocrinol Metab 1999: 2854–2861.
46. Grundy SM. Hypertriglyceridemia, insulin resistance, and the metabolic syndrome. Am J Cardiol 1999:25F–29F.
47. Knowler WC, Narayan KM, Hanson RL, et al. Preventing non-insulin-dependent diabetes. Diabetes 1995:483–488.

48. Eliasson BSU. Insulin resistance. In: Reaven GMLA, ed. Insulin Resistance: The Metabolic Syndrome X. Totowa, NJ: Humana Press, 1999:121–136.
49. Vega GL, Grundy SM. Influence of lovastatin therapy on metabolism of low density lipoproteins in mixed hyperlipidaemia. J Intern Med 1991:341–350.
50. Stein EA, Lane M, Laskarzewski P. Comparison of statins in hypertriglyceridemia. Am J Cardiol 1998:66B–69B.
51. Cuchel M, Schaefer EJ, Millar JS, et al. Lovastatin decreases de novo cholesterol synthesis and LDL Apo B-100 production rates in combined-hyperlipidemic males. Arterioscler Thromb Vasc Biol 1997:1910–1917.
52. Garg A, Grundy SM. Nicotinic acid as therapy for dyslipidemia in non-insulin-dependent diabetes mellitus. JAMA 1990:723–726.
53. Elam MB, Hunninghake DB, Davis KB, et al. Effect of niacin on lipid and lipoprotein levels and glycemic control in patients with diabetes and peripheral arterial disease: the ADMIT study: a randomized trial. Arterial Disease Multiple Intervention Trial. JAMA 2000:1263–1270.
54. Steiner G. Effects of various lipid-lowering treatments in diabetics. J Cardiovasc Pharmacol 1990:S35–S39.
55. Davidson MH, Hauptman J, DiGirolamo M, et al. Weight control and risk factor reduction in obese subjects treated for 2 years with orlistat: a randomized controlled trial. JAMA 1999; 281(3):235–242.
56. Hollander PA, Elbein SC, Hirsch IB, et al. Role of orlistat in the treatment of obese patients with type 2 diabetes. A 1-year randomized double-blind study. Diabetes Care 1998; 21(8):1288–1294.
57. Erdmann J, Lippl F, Klose G, Schusdziarra V. Cholesterol lowering effect of dietary weight loss and orlistat treatment—efficacy and limitations. Aliment Pharmacol Ther 2004; 19(11):1173–1179.
58. Seagle HM, Bessesen DH, Hill JO. Effects of sibutramine on resting metabolic rate and weight loss in overweight women. Obes Res 1998; 6(2):115–121.
59. Hansen DL, Toubro S, Stock MJ, Macdonald IA, Astrup A. Thermogenic effects of sibutramine in humans. Am J Clin Nutr 1998; 68(6):1180–1186.
60. Bray GA, Blackburn GL, Ferguson JM, et al. Sibutramine produces dose-related weight loss. Obes Res 1999; 7(2):189–198.
61. Dujovne CA, Zavoral JH, Rowe E, Mendel CM. Effects of sibutramine on body weight and serum lipids: a double-blind, randomized, placebo-controlled study in 322 overweight and obese patients with dyslipidemia. Am Heart J 2001; 142(3):489–497.
62. Sabuncu T, Ucar E, Birden F, Yasar O. The effect of 1-yr sibutramine treatment on glucose tolerance, insulin sensitivity and serum lipid profiles in obese subjects. Diabetes Nutr Metab 2004; 17(2):103–107.

# 5

# Vascular Dysfunction and Obesity

**Kieren J. Mather**

*Indiana University School of Medicine, Indianapolis, Indiana, U.S.A.*

**Alain D. Baron**

*Indiana University School of Medicine, Indianapolis, Indiana, and
Amylin Pharmaceuticals, Inc., San Diego, California, U.S.A.*

## INTRODUCTION: OBESITY AND CV RISK

The obesity epidemic has resulted in increased interest in the health consequences of obesity. Obesity is associated with a number of adverse health outcomes. Among these are an increased risk of subsequent development of type 2 diabetes mellitus (DM2) and an increased risk for cardiovascular (CV) disease. Together, these conditions already account for the majority of morbidity and mortality in industrialized nations, and the prospect of a ballooning population with augmented disease susceptibility threatens to undo the significant advances in the prevention of CV disease we have seen in the last few decades.

The pathogenesis of vascular disease is meaningfully linked to changes in vascular function. Investigations of vascular function both in animal models and in humans have provided valuable insights into the mechanisms of disease, the relative importance of various pathogenic factors, and the utility of various therapeutic interventions. Importantly, in vivo measurements of vascular function, in particular, measurements of endothelium-dependent vasodilation, have been shown to predict the occurrence of CV events in high-risk populations (1–3). Impairments of endothelium-dependent vasodilation are a feature of obesity (discussed in detail in section "OB/IR and Endothelial

Dysfunction"), and it seems likely that the pathogenesis of vascular dysfunction and CV disease are linked in obese subjects as in other populations.

## Metabolic Syndrome and CV Risk

There are a number of candidate pathophysiologic mechanisms that account for increased CV risk and impairments in vascular function in obesity. Perhaps most obviously, the prevalence of diabetes and prediabetic dysglycemia is increased in obesity, and these factors alone are recognized to increase the risk of CV disease. Obesity is also associated with increased rates of hypertension, another well-recognized CV risk factor.

An association between hypertension, hyperglycemia, and obesity has been recognized for decades. In 1988, Reaven reintroduced and refined this concept and referred to the clustering of hypertension, glucose intolerance, high triglycerides, and low high-density lipoprotein cholesterol as "Syndrome X" (4). This syndrome has been variably labeled over the years as the insulin resistance syndrome, the dysmetabolic syndrome, and the metabolic syndrome. More recently, the World Health Organization proposed a formal definition for the metabolic syndrome (5). In its most recent guidelines for the treatment and management of CV risk factors, the National Institutes of Health expert panel has also provided a formal definition for the syndrome and settled on the label of "metabolic syndrome" (6).

The presence of this clustering of risk factors is associated with increased CV risk, over and above the risk conferred by the individual component risk factors. A number of epidemiologic studies have been reanalyzed to assess the relationships between the various metabolic syndrome components and vascular outcomes (7,8). A striking finding from these studies is that the presence of multiple components results in synergism in the relationship between the components and CV disease outcomes. In other words, the clustering of components is itself an independent risk factor for adverse outcomes, beyond the contributions of the individual components (8,9). Therefore, the increased prevalence of the metabolic syndrome in obesity is an important contributor to overall CV risk in obesity.

## Insulin Resistance and CV Risk

Insulin resistance is a common feature in obesity, conferring an increased risk for diabetes and likely contributing to derangements in the metabolic syndrome components. The potential impact of insulin resistance per se on vascular risk has been of interest for decades, and a number of large clinical trials have evaluated the relationship between fasting or postprandial insulin levels (as an index of insulin resistance) and incident CV disease. Many large longitudinal studies, including the Paris prospective study (10), the Quebec CV study (11), the Helsinki policemen study (12), and the Bogalusa heart study (13), have shown an increased risk of CV events in subjects with higher insulin levels compared to subjects with lower levels. Ruige et al. undertook a meta-analysis addressing this question (14), and examined 17 prospective studies evaluating insulin levels (fasting and non-fasting) in relation to CV outcomes (death for coronary heart disease, myocardial infarction, or electrocardiogram changes) with follow-up periods ranging from 5 to 11.5 years. In this analysis, insulin concentrations correlated significantly with the incidence of CV events [relative risk 1.18 (1.08–1.29)]. These association studies do not provide information regarding the mechanisms underlying the relationships. However, it is clear that insulin resistance per se is associated with increased CV risk.

Overall, the human literature equates obesity with insulin resistance, although gradations of insulin resistance within a given body mass index (BMI) range can clearly be discerned using detailed, formal measurements of insulin sensitivity. The natural variation in human biology is such that some lean individuals are objectively insulin resistant, and conversely, not all obese individuals are insulin resistant.

Recently, investigations of the contributions of specific fat depots to metabolic status have suggested different contributions from intra-abdominal versus subcutaneous fat to insulin resistance (15–18). These findings suggest that the biology of adipocytes from these different fat depots differs, and this suggests an opportunity to explore different possible underlying mechanisms linking adipocyte stores to insulin resistance. For example, it has been hypothesized that free fatty acid (FFA) production, specifically by intraperitoneal fat depots, produces a high concentration of FFA in the liver directly via the portal vein. This in turn may directly affect the metabolic balance in the liver, and either initiate or perpetuate the whole-body changes in metabolic balance, which results in insulin resistance. Therefore, not all versions of excess body fat are equal. These factors may underlie some of the observed variability in the relationship between obesity and insulin sensitivity.

Nonetheless, the association between obesity and insulin resistance is strong, and many studies in the literature equate obesity with insulin resistance. Also, the intrinsic association between obesity and insulin resistance makes it difficult to distinguish their separate contributions to a given physiologic state or therapeutic response. For this reason we will use the categorical description of obesity/insulin resistance (OB/IR) to describe these obese, insulin-resistant subjects, as a reminder that both features are generally present.

## OB/IR AND ENDOTHELIAL DYSFUNCTION

### Associations

Endothelial dysfunction, manifest either as abnormal circulating products of endothelial cells (ECs) or more rigorously as impaired physiologic responses to endothelium-dependent vasodilator stimuli, is readily demonstrated both in animal models of obesity (19,20) and in studies of human obesity (21–24). A number of metabolic features of obesity have been invoked as potential causes of endothelial dysfunction in obesity, including increased levels of circulating FFAs, an increased prevalence of hypertension, insulin resistance, and (independent of insulin resistance) hyperinsulinemia. Perhaps the most extensively investigated has been the relationship between insulin resistance and endothelial dysfunction.

Impaired endothelial function has been observed in most studies of nondiabetic states of insulin resistance, including obesity and hypertension (25,26), normotensive relatives of subjects with DM2 (27), women with prior gestational diabetes (28,29), and women with polycystic ovary syndrome (30). In many studies, the natural gradations of insulin sensitivity across the study groups were significantly correlated with the impairment in endothelium-dependent vascular responses (31–35). Together, these studies suggest not only that the presence of insulin resistance relate to the endothelial dysfunction, but also that a strong linear relationship links these phenomena. An interesting situation has been reported where this linkage was not evident in lean subjects. Utriainen et al. (36) studied lean, healthy subjects (BMI 23.6 kg/m$^2$ and ~14.2% body fat) who were divided into insulin-sensitive and insulin-resistant subgroups according to their responses to hyperinsulinemic euglycemic clamps. The insulin-resistant subgroup was statistically more obese (BMI 24.7 vs. 22.5) and fatter (percent fat 16.1 vs. 12.2), although both groups were evidently lean. Neither group exhibited impaired endothelium-dependent vasodilation. In this analysis, in the absence of obesity, there was no measured effect of increasing degrees of insulin resistance on impaired endothelium-dependent vasodilation. The authors interpreted this finding as evidence against a relationship between insulin resistance and endothelial function, perhaps suggesting that the effect of obesity on the endothelium was independent of insulin sensitivity. To our knowledge this finding has not been replicated using similar or complementary techniques. Overall, there is a strong association of the presence of obesity and insulin resistance with impaired endothelium-dependent vasodilation.

In endogenous states of insulin resistance, it is unclear what role each of the diverse metabolic aberrations plays in observed impairments of endothelial function. If these associations reflect a direct effect of insulin resistance and/or hyperinsulinemia on vascular biology, then we might predict that the imposition of insulin resistance should reproduce these same changes. This has been explored in a number of complementary ways, for example using diverse metabolic stimuli to impair insulin's actions or using genetic manipulations to induce an inability to respond to insulin.

### Inducing Insulin Resistance

The fructose-fed rat (37,38) and the glucosamine infusions in rats (39–42) are both models where the experimental induction of insulin resistance is associated with the induction of endothelial dysfunction. The effects of targeted disruptions of the insulin signaling system on vascular function have also been studied; these studies further support the close connection between insulin resistance and vascular dysfunction. The insulin receptor (IR) substrate-1 knockout mouse, a nonobese model of insulin resistance, exhibits a spectrum of metabolic abnormalities parallel to those seen in the insulin-resistance syndrome including endothelial dysfunction (43). IR knockout mice develop a severe form of diabetes associated with high triglycerides and FFAs. The Cre-LoxP targeted gene insertion approach has been used to target specific tissues for disruption of the IR. For example, muscle-specific IR knockout mice maintain normoglycemia, but exhibit features of the metabolic syndrome, with impaired insulin-mediated glucose uptake and elevated fat mass, triglycerides and FFAs (44). The initial studies of the vascular endothelium–specific targeted IR knockout have revealed surprisingly little effect on either vascular function or glucose homeostasis (45), although detailed studies of vascular function have not yet been reported. To date, studies of vascular function in these animals or in animals with targeted disruption of the IRs in other tissues have not been published, but are eagerly awaited.

A significant recent advance has been the discovery of adiponectin, a multimeric peptide secreted by adipocyte, which functions as an adipocytokine (46). A role for adiponectin in the integrated regulation of insulin sensitivity is suggested by the observation of insulin resistance in the adiponectin knockout mouse (47). OB/IR is associated with reduced circulating levels of adiponectin (48–50). Adiponectin knockout mice exhibit endothelial dysfunction (51), and human endothelial dysfunction is associated with reduced adiponectin levels (49) (adiponectin is discussed in further detail in section "Adipocytokines"). These developments raise the possibility that adiponectin deficiency, rather than insulin resistance, plays a role in the endothelial dysfunction observed in OB/IR.

Increased circulating FFAs, a product of adipocyte fat store turnover, are a typical metabolic feature of human obesity. Elevated FFA concentrations have been suggested as a proximate cause of both hepatic and peripheral resistance to the actions of insulin. Insulin resistance can be reliably induced by acute exposure to FFA, evident as an inhibition of insulin-stimulated peripheral glucose uptake. This can be demonstrated both in animals (52,53) and in humans (54,55). Physiological elevations in plasma FFA concentrations also induce vascular dysfunction (55–57). Interestingly, the induction of endothelial dysfunction by FFA appears to precede the effects of FFA on skeletal muscle insulin resistance (55,57). This is notable in light of the presumed association between vascular and tissue insulin resistance: The underlying assumption here is that insulin-mediated vasodilation is an important component of insulin's net metabolic effect, and this action of insulin is lost along with its classical tissue effects in states of insulin resistance. In other words, the same mechanism for insulin resistance is thought to act at both the endothelial level and the tissue level. However, the demonstration of FFA-induced vascular dysfunction prior to tissue dysfunction perhaps suggests different mechanisms for insulin resistance at each site and calls into question this presumed mechanistic connection between vascular and tissue insulin resistance.

Tumor necrosis factor alpha (TNFα) is another adipocyte product that has been proposed as a mediator of fat-related insulin resistance. In vivo, in humans and in rats, circulating levels of TNFα are increased in subjects with obesity and impaired glucose tolerance (58–60). TNFα mRNA and protein levels in human adipocytes correlate with the degree of obesity or hyperinsulinemia (61). TNFα protein and TNFα-receptor knockout mice generally exhibit some amelioration of metabolic parameters with a resistance to obesity-induced insulin resistance [reviewed in detail in Ref. (62)]. Studies in rats have suggested an acute effect of TNFα on vascular function as well (63,64), and the effect appears to be mediated by the endothelium rather than being a direct effect on vascular smooth muscle cells (VSMCs) (63). In human obesity, neutralization of TNFα with monoclonal antibodies had no apparent effect on insulin sensitivity (65). No studies of vascular function with neutralizing antibodies have been reported in rodents or in humans.

## Reducing Insulin Resistance

Concurrent improvement of endothelial function and metabolism with interventions improving insulin sensitivity has been reported. Physical exercise, independent of weight loss, improves insulin resistance and vascular function in obesity (66,67) and diabetes (68,69). Weight loss, with or without exercise, clearly has significant effects on insulin sensitivity but the reports to date have been inconsistent regarding demonstrable improvements in endothelial function. In one recent publication (70), weight-loss diet plus Orlistat, but not weight-loss diet alone, was associated with improved endothelium-dependent vasodilation and appeared to be related more strongly to associated changes in low-density lipoprotein (LDL) cholesterol than to the reduction in obesity. A comparable reduction in circulating insulin levels (the only index of insulin sensitivity assessed) was seen in both groups. Other published studies of weight loss include a beneficial effect of two weeks of exposure to a very low calorie diet (71), and an improved profile of circulating markers of endothelial activation in obese subjects following 12 weeks of caloric restriction (800 kcal/day), achieving ~9% weight loss (72). Circulating levels of inflammatory cytokines were similarly reduced in obese women following a one-year multidisciplinary weight-loss program, which achieved at least 10% reduction in weight (73). This literature suggests beneficial effects of both exercise and weight loss on a number of axes related to vascular function, perhaps mediated by reductions in insulin resistance.

Pharmacologic therapies that improve insulin sensitivity exist, and their effects on vascular function in states of insulin resistance have been assessed. The biguanide metformin improves whole-body insulin sensitivity, primarily through effects on hepatic metabolism (74,75) that involve stimulation of glucose transport via adenosine monophosphate kinase (76–79). In rats, metformin has been found to block the development of fructose-induced hypertension, hyperinsulinemia, and endothelial dysfunction (80). In humans, we and others have shown a concurrent improvement in insulin sensitivity and endothelium-dependent vascular responses in subjects with DM2 treated with metformin (81,82). The newest class of insulin-sensitizing drugs, the peroxizome-proliferator activator receptor (PPAR)-gamma agonists, have widespread metabolic effects. These effects include alterations in adipocyte biology, including changes in the pattern of secreted proteins, as well as improvements in tissue responsiveness to insulin (including both vascular ECs and more classical insulin targets such as skeletal muscle cells) (83). Interestingly, improvements in insulin sensitivity with PPAR-gamma agonists are seen even in the absence of weight loss, and can be seen despite weight gain associated with the therapy (84). Beneficial effects of PPAR-gamma agonists on vascular function in animal models and in human obesity have been reported with troglitazone (84–87). Data suggesting similar benefits of the currently available members of this class, rosiglitazone and pioglitazone, are becoming available (88–93). Not all studies, however, are able to demonstrate beneficial vascular effects with PPAR-gamma agonists (23,94,95), and different agents within the class are not necessarily equivalent in this regard (96).

Together, these findings point to a tight association between OB/IR and endothelial dysfunction. But what is the mechanism of this association? In the remainder of this manuscript we will explore this question in the context of the current understanding of the molecular mechanisms of endothelial function in general. The concepts explored are presented diagrammatically in Figure 1.

## DETERMINANTS OF VASCULAR FUNCTION

### The Balance of Regulators in Vascular Biology

Nitric oxide (NO) production, both from constitutively active NO synthase present in the endothelial layer (eNOS, endothelial NO synthase) and from augmented eNOS activity under stimulated conditions, is an important contributor to overall vascular health (97). This is manifested as acute vasodilatory and antithrombotic effects, and longer-term antiatherosclerotic effects including impaired smooth muscle cell migration and proliferation

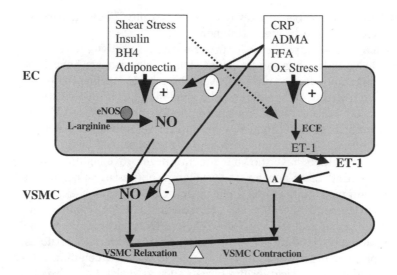

**Figure 1** Conceptual diagram of the sites of interaction between components of the metabolic syndrome and the principal determinants of vascular tone. Plus signs represent actions to augment the indicated function; minus signs represent actions that reduce the indicated function. The *dashed line* represents a possible stimulation of ET-1 by insulin. Glucose acts principally via oxidative stress in this paradigm. Not depicted are direct interactions of NO and ET-1 to limit each other's actions. *Abbreviations*: ADMA, asymmetric dimethylarginine; BH4, tetrahydropiopterin; CRP, C-reactive protein, EC, endothelial cell; ECE, endothelin converting enzyme; eNOS, endothelial nitric oxide synthase; ET-1, endothelin-1; FFA, free fatty acids; NO, nitric oxide; Ox stress, oxidative stress; VSMC, vascular smooth muscle cell.

(97). In the current paradigm, NO is viewed as the principal vasodilatory/ antiatherosclerotic agent. The main counterbalancing vasoconstrictor is endothelin-1 (ET-1), which, in addition to acute effects on vasomotion, has chronic proatherogenic effects (98). In many diseases endothelial dysfunction results in impaired production or action of NO, and therefore the balance of acute and chronic effects is less favorable. In addition to the loss of beneficial effects from NO, the actions of constrictor agents such as ET-1 are relatively unopposed in states of impaired endothelial function (Fig. 1). In this section we will explore the data documenting diminished NO action and increased ET-1 action in states of obesity and insulin resistance.

### Reduced NO Bioactivity

There is considerable debate whether states of insulin resistance are associated with reduced absolute production of NO. The literature on this point is inconsistent, and no consensus has been reached. Some studies suggest increased or normal total NO production (99,100) (measured as urinary or systemic total nitrates, $NO_x$, or by the total capacity of platelets to produce NO when stimulated). Others find frankly reduced indices of NO production (101–103). Increased consumption could be reflected in normal to elevated total $NO_x$ levels, whereas reduced production should result in reduced $NO_x$. Recently, a kinetic modeling approach has been developed and applied to diabetic humans, showing a reduction in the rate of NO synthesis from L-arginine (104); this approach has not yet been extended to subjects with obesity. It is not yet clear why some studies suggest changes in production while others point to increased consumption.

eNOS produces NO from the precursor L-arginine, along with molecular oxygen and electrons derived from nicotinamide adenine dinucleotide phosphate. eNOS is regulated by a number of factors, including the availability of the redox cofactor tetrahydrobiopterin (BH4) and the endogenous inhibitor asymmetric dimethylarginine (ADMA), and direct activation by regulatory factors including insulin. We will next explore the evidence for alterations in these regulators of eNOS in OB/IR.

Oxidative stress has been implicated in atherogenesis. Oxidative stress may impair NO bioactivity through the direct consumption of NO (contributing to reduced bioavailability) or through decreased availability of BH4 (105) as discussed below. Fructose-fed rats were found to develop insulin resistance and decreased expression of antioxidant enzymes (106). Concurrently treatment with metformin improved antioxidant enzyme activity in these rats (107), but metformin also had the same effect in normally fed control rats. In human studies, oxidative stress is linked to impaired endothelial function in insulin resistance (108) and treatment with vitamin C improved endothelial function in obese insulin-resistant subjects (21). Troglitazone therapy inhibited LDL oxidation and reduced reactive oxygen species in obese subjects (109), but it is again uncertain whether this effect is mediated directly through improvement of insulin resistance. Also, neither self-reported intake of vitamins E and/or C nor the circulating levels of these antioxidants track with whole-body insulin sensitivity (110,111), perhaps suggesting a mechanistic or temporal disconnect between the direct vascular effects of these antioxidants and any metabolic effects. A considerable body of evidence has been produced disproving the notion that antioxidant therapy with vitamins E and/or C is of overall benefit regarding CV events (112,113). This does not discount the importance of oxidative stress in the molecular events in the vessel wall, and this parameter of vessel wall biology is clearly adversely affected by states of insulin resistance.

The role of BH4 in the vascular pathogenesis of OB/IR is unclear. BH4 functions as a redox cofactor for NO synthase, but the metabolic pathways, which reduce dihydrobiopterin to BH4 (recycling), are themselves subject to the oxidative environment of the cell. Therefore, states of increased oxidative stress are expected to result in impairment in the available supply of BH4. A recent report describes a phosphatidyl inositol-3 kinase–dependent effect of insulin to stimulate BH4 production (114), although it is uncertain if this effect is impaired in states of insulin resistance. No published data, to our knowledge, address the question of possible effects of hyperinsulinemia or dyslipidemia on the production or recycling of BH4. Glucose, through well-described pathways involving protein kinase C, functions as a stimulus to the production of oxidant species (115–117).

The importance of cellular redox state in the normal functioning of eNOS, and the capacity of nonspecific antioxidant therapies to correct endothelial dysfunction in both type 1 (118) and type 2 diabetes (119) raise the possibility that the mechanism of these beneficial effects is mediated by restoration of BH4 availability. In a rat model of obesity, BH4 treatment improved vascular and cardiac function (120). Parallel benefits were seen with specifically replacing BH4 in type 1 (121) and type 2 diabetes (122). Unfortunately, these important findings do not aid in addressing the question of the mechanistic connection between the metabolic syndrome and BH4 availability. No studies of possible associations between insulin sensitizing medications and alterations in BH4 availability have been published.

ADMA is endogenously produced and functions as an endogenous competitive inhibitor of eNOS. Elevated levels of ADMA have been found in association with the various components of the metabolic syndrome (123–127) and, furthermore, appear to be increased in direct proportion to the degree of insulin resistance (128). The mechanism that mediates this association is less clear. No published data describe effect of either hyperinsulinemia or hyperlipidemia to stimulate the production of ADMA or to alter the levels or activity of enzymes responsible for the production or destruction of ADMA. A recent report, however, did find that hyperglycemia reduced the levels of dimethylarginine dimethylaminohydrolase, the enzyme that catalyzes the destruction of ADMA, thereby causing increases in ADMA levels (129). In hyperglycemic insulin deficient rats without other components of the metabolic syndrome, insulin therapy to reduce glucose levels normalized ADMA levels (130). In humans with type 2 diabetes, angiotensin converting enzyme inhibition, rosiglitazone, and metformin have all been found to reduce ADMA levels (128,131,132). Notably, in a recent report, the 3-hydroxy-3-methylglutaryl coenzyme A–reductase antagonist pravastatin failed to reduce ADMA levels in young hypercholesterolemic subjects (125), suggesting that the above relationships and responses to therapy reflect a specific effect of the metabolic syndrome rather than the accompanying vasculopathy.

Increased Endothelin Activity

ET-1, produced directly by vascular ECs, is the most important local vasoconstrictor, acting principally through endothelin type A ($ET_A$) receptors on VSMCs (133). A number of studies point to a significant effect of insulin to directly stimulate the production and release of ET-1 from ECs in culture (134,135). Elevated circulating levels of ET-1 have been reported in most (136–142), but not all (143,144) studies of human insulin resistance. The ET-1 elevation has been reported to be proportional to the hyperinsulinemia (141,145,146), and a dietary weight loss can reduce both serum insulin and ET-1 concentrations (141). Furthermore, acute endogenous and exogenous elevations in circulating insulin levels in normal controls and in insulin-resistant subjects have been shown to acutely elevate circulating ET-1 (137,147,148), although again, opposing findings exist (127,149,150).

Experiments to delineate the effect of these changes on vascular biology in states of insulin resistance are beginning to appear in the literature. Fructose-induced insulin resistance is associated with augmented vascular ET-1 sensitivity (38,151) and with beneficial effects of endothelin receptor blockade on vascular function (152). In insulin-resistant galactose-fed rats, augmented extracellular matrix production was partially prevented by endothelin receptor blockade (153). Similarly, in mesenteric artery and thoracic aorta from spontaneously insulin-resistant obese Zucker rats, increased endothelin receptor mRNA expression and receptor levels were noted (154). Most recently, an in vitro effect of resistin, a hormone secreted by adipocytes in proportion to adipocyte mass to activate ECs including augmenting endothelin production, has been reported (155). This raises the possibility that adipocytes act directly in the genesis of endothelial dysfunction, which will be addressed in detail below.

Literature addressing the role of ET-1 in the vascular dysfunction of human OB/IR and diabetes is sparse. Conflicting reports of normal (156) and impaired (157) constrictor responses to ET-1 in human type 2 diabetes (studying different vascular beds) have been published. A recent report found no vasodilator effect of $ET_A$ blockade in subjects with type 2 diabetes (158), but $ET_A$ blockade has been reported to normalize endothelium-dependent vascular responses in human subjects with type 2 diabetes (159,160). To date, only data from our laboratory has specifically addressed the separate question of obesity-associated endothelial dysfunction, independent of the added metabolic aberrations of frank diabetes. We found that the response to the $ET_A$ antagonist BQ123 was greater in obese subjects than in lean controls, and in fact indistinguishable from the response of a similarly obese group of diabetic subjects (Fig. 2) (160). We interpret these findings as evidence for increased endogenous activity of the endothelin system in obesity and diabetes. Of note, the impaired vasodilation apparent in obese subjects at baseline was essentially corrected by acute $ET_A$ antagonism, suggesting an important contribution of ET-1 to the pathogenesis of endothelial dysfunction in obesity. Clearly the biology of ET-1 in states of obesity, hyperinsulinemia, and insulin resistance needs to be further explored.

These findings suggest a dual pathogenesis of endothelial dysfunction in obesity, namely a concurrent impairment in NO bioavailability and

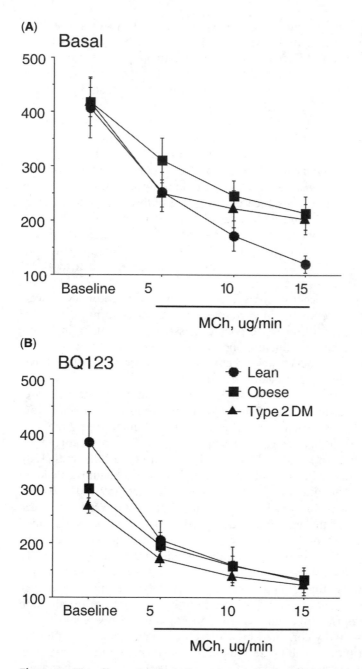

**Figure 2** The effects of endothelin antagonism using BQ123, a specific antagonist of type A endothelin receptors, on impaired endothelium-dependent vasodilation in obese subjects with and without DM2, compared to lean healthy controls. (*Top*) Basal untreated state; (*bottom*) following 90-minute exposure to BQ123 0.6 mg/hr. *Abbreviation*: DM2, type 2 diabetes mellitus. *Source*: From Ref. 161.

augmented endothelin activity. Interestingly, a number of interactions between NO and endothelin have been described, which might contribute to this imbalance. In particular, NO and ET-1 appear to act to limit one another at multiple levels, including reciprocal gene downregulation (162–164), changes in cell surface receptors (165), and cross-talk in post-receptor signaling (166,167). Furthermore, ET-1, acting through EC $ET_B$ receptors, can produce an NO-dependent vasodilator response (151,168), which can partially counteract the constrictor actions through $ET_A$ receptors in health. These interactions suggest mechanisms whereby perturbations in the balance between NO and ET-1 would serve to amplify the imbalance. This may contribute to the pathogenesis of vascular disease, but also provides an opportunity for augmented effectiveness of therapeutic interventions, adding to the support for novel therapeutic approaches using endothelin blockade in states of insulin resistance.

## Novel Determinants of Vascular Health

### Adipocytokines

An exciting development in obesity research was the discovery that adipose tissue is a source of regulatory and communication molecules, rather than simply serving as location for fat storage. A recently described adipocyte-derived hormone, resistin, was found to induce insulin resistance in rodents (169). As discussed above, in vitro resistin has recently been shown to activate ECs, markedly altering the various proteins produced including upregulating endothelin production (155). Leptin, the first adipocyte product described with clear links to body weight regulation, has been found to have direct effects on vascular cells in vitro through both NO-dependent and NO-independent mechanisms (170–172). Interestingly, leptin also can induce ET-1 production by ECs (173), but conversely ET-1 affects leptin, resistin, and adiponectin production in vitro (174–176). In vivo in humans, intracoronary arterial infusion of leptin induced NO-independent vasodilation (177). Perhaps more promising still is adiponectin, which is also produced by adipocytes but in inverse relation to obesity and insulin resistance (46). A role for adiponectin in the maintenance of insulin sensitivity has been described (47), and therapies that alter insulin sensitivity also change adiponectin production from adipocytes in vitro (178) as well as in vivo in humans (50). A direct correlation between endothelial function and adiponectin levels has been described in animals (47) and in humans (49,51), and adiponectin appears to directly stimulate the production of NO by ECs (179,180). These novel proteins provide a new set of potential connections between the metabolic syndrome and vascular dysfunction, and suggest that adipocyte–endothelium cross-talk may be an important mechanism of CV disease in the metabolic syndrome.

Inflammation

A central role of inflammation in atherogenesis is increasingly recognized (181). The association of C-reactive protein (CRP) levels with CV outcome has been convincingly established in recent years, using stored samples from previous prospective studies as well as using CRP as a defined endpoint in ongoing prospective studies (182–188). Obesity and insulin resistance are associated with a host of inflammatory marker abnormalities. In a study involving nondiabetic subjects, CRP was related to insulin resistance measured by the homeostasis model and to circulating markers of endothelial dysfunction (plasma levels of von Willebrand factor, tissue plasminogen activator, and cellular fibronectin) (189). In the nondiabetic subpopulation free of coronary disease in the Insulin Resistance and Atherosclerosis Study, CRP, fibrinogen, and white blood cell correlated with insulin levels and insulin sensitivity (190). Similarly, in the Rotterdam study, insulin resistance as measured by postload insulin was significantly associated with CRP, interleukin-6 (IL-6), and soluble intercellular adhesion molecule after adjustment for age and gender (191). It is therefore evident that insulin-resistant states are associated with increases in inflammatory markers. Furthermore, CRP levels are independently predictive of CV outcomes above and beyond the risk assessment provided by accounting for the metabolic syndrome (186,192).

A relationship between obesity per se and increased CRP levels is well described (189,193–195), and predicts a variety of adverse outcomes of obesity (8,182,186,192,196). One proposed mechanism for the association is via adipocyte secretion of IL-6 (197), which in turn stimulates CRP production by the liver, and possibly also directly within the vascular wall (198). This may be independent of insulin resistance: No reports in the literature connect the pharmacologic or dietary induction of insulin resistance in rats with changes in markers of inflammation. Similarly, no effects of hyperinsulinemia, hyperglycemia, or hyperlipidemia on CRP levels have been reported in in vivo animal models or in cell studies.

The treatment of insulin resistance is associated with improvements in inflammatory marker profiles. Diabetic patients treated with troglitazone or metformin showed decreased markers of inflammation such as CRP (199), although not all investigators have reported this effect (71). Recently, in a large cohort of diabetic subjects, treatment with the insulin sensitizer rosiglitazone decreased markers of inflammation such as CRP, proportional to improvements in insulin resistance (200). Again, these beneficial effects are not limited to pharmacologic agents: Lifestyle interventions, which reduce obesity and improve the metabolic syndrome, also reduce CRP (201,202).

## SUMMARY

Endothelial dysfunction is a feature of human obesity. In obese humans, there appears to be a strong association between insulin resistance and endothelial dysfunction. This is seen both in association studies and in experimental study designs, which induce or reduce insulin resistance, with concordant effects on vascular function.

The presence of vascular dysfunction reflects some combination of reduced vasodilator action (largely NO bioactivity) and increased vasoconstrictor action (largely ET-1 activity through $ET_A$ receptors). There is reason to believe that NO bioactivity is reduced in human obesity due to some combination of increased oxidative stress, reduced BH4 availability and increased levels of ADMA. The precise contributions of these factors and the reasons for alterations in their status in obesity remain to be clarified. Preclinical work suggests that increased action of ET-1 is an important component of vascular dysfunction associated with obesity and insulin resistance, and the early human literature suggests this is true in human obesity as well.

A number of novel contributors to the regulation of vascular function are also abnormal in obesity, including reduced levels of adiponectin and increased levels of CRP. The relative contributions of these factors to overall vascular health remains to be worked out, but these promising fields are providing new insights into the physiology and pathophysiology of the vascular wall in health and disease.

In summary, despite many steps forward, much remains to be done to better understand the pathogenesis of vascular dysfunction in obesity. A better understanding of these processes will ultimately allow better targeting of therapies to reduce obesity-associated CV disease.

## REFERENCES

1. Halcox JP, Schenke WH, Zalos G, et al. Prognostic value of coronary vascular endothelial dysfunction. Circulation 2002; 106:653–658.
2. Heitzer T, Schlinzig T, Krohn K, Meinertz T, Munzel T. Endothelial dysfunction, oxidative stress, and risk of cardiovascular events in patients with coronary artery disease. Circulation 2001; 104:2673–2678.
3. Schachinger V, Britten MB, Zeiher AM. Prognostic impact of coronary vasodilator dysfunction on adverse long-term outcome of coronary heart disease. Circulation 2000; 101:1899–1906.
4. Reaven GM. Role of insulin resistance in human disease. Diabetes 1988; 37:1595–1607.
5. Alberti KG, Zimmet PZ. Definition, diagnosis and classification of diabetes mellitus and its complications. Part 1: Diagnosis and classification of diabetes mellitus provisional report of a WHO consultation. Diabet Med 1998; 15:539–553.
6. Executive Summary of the Third Report of the National Cholesterol Education Program (NCEP) Expert Panel on Detection, Evaluation, and Treatment of High Blood Cholesterol in Adults (Adult Treatment Panel III). JAMA 2001; 285:2486–2497.

7.  Meigs JB, Wilson PW, Nathan DM, D'Agostino RB Sr, Williams K, Haffner SM. Prevalence and characteristics of the metabolic syndrome in the San Antonio Heart and Framingham Offspring Studies. Diabetes 2003; 52:2160–2167.
8.  Sattar N, Gaw A, Scherbakova O, et al. Metabolic syndrome with and without C-reactive protein as a predictor of coronary heart disease and diabetes in the West of Scotland Coronary Prevention Study. Circulation 2003; 108:414–419.
9.  Kannel WB. Risk stratification in hypertension: new insights from the Framingham Study. Am J Hypertens 2000; 13:3S–10S.
10. Balkau B, Bertrais S, Ducimetiere P, Eschwege E. Is there a glycemic threshold for mortality risk? Diabetes Care 1999; 22:696–699.
11. Despres JP, Lamarche B, Mauriege P, et al. Hyperinsulinemia as an independent risk factor for ischemic heart disease. N Engl J Med 1996; 334: 952–957.
12. Pyorala M, Miettinen H, Halonen P, Laakso M, Pyorala K. Insulin resistance syndrome predicts the risk of coronary heart disease and stroke in healthy middle-aged men: the 22-year follow-up results of the Helsinki Policemen Study. Arterioscler Thromb Vasc Biol 2000; 20:538–544.
13. Bao W, Srinivasan SR, Berenson GS. Persistent elevation of plasma insulin levels is associated with increased cardiovascular risk in children and young adults. The Bogalusa Heart Study. Circulation 1996; 93:54–59.
14. Ruige JB, Assendelft WJJ, Dekker JM, Kostense PJ, Heine RJ, Bouter LM. Insulin and risk of cardiovascular disease—a meta-analysis. Circulation 1998; 97:996–1001.
15. Cruz ML, Bergman RN, Goran MI. Unique effect of visceral fat on insulin sensitivity in obese Hispanic children with a family history of type 2 diabetes. Diabetes Care 2002; 25:1631–1636.
16. Goran MI, Bergman RN, Gower BA. Influence of total vs. visceral fat on insulin action and secretion in African American and white children. Obes Res 2001; 9:423–431.
17. Mittelman SD, Van Citters GW, Kirkman EL, Bergman RN. Extreme insulin resistance of the central adipose depot in vivo. Diabetes 2002; 51:755–761.
18. Wagenknecht LE, Langefeld CD, Scherzinger AL, et al. Insulin sensitivity, insulin secretion, and abdominal fat: the Insulin Resistance Atherosclerosis Study (IRAS) Family Study. Diabetes 2003; 52:2490–2496.
19. Laight DW, Desai KM, Anggard EE, Carrier MJ. Endothelial dysfunction accompanies a pro-oxidant, pro-diabetic challenge in the insulin resistant, obese Zucker rat in vivo. Eur J Pharmacol 2000; 402:95–99.
20. McNamee CJ, Kappagoda CT, Kunjara R, Russell JC. Defective endothelium-dependent relaxation in the JCR:LA-corpulent rat. Circ Res 1994; 74: 1126–1132.
21. Perticone F, Ceravolo R, Candigliota M, et al. Obesity and body fat distribution induce endothelial dysfunction by oxidative stress: protective effect of vitamin C. Diabetes 2001; 50:159–165.
22. Steinberg HO, Chaker H, Leaming R, Johnson A, Brechtel G, Baron AD. Obesity/insulin resistance is associated with endothelial dysfunction. Implications for the syndrome of insulin resistance. J Clin Invest 1996; 97:2601–2610.

23. Tack CJJ, Ong MKE, Lutterman JA, Smits P. Insulin-induced vasodilatation and endothelial function in obesity/insulin resistance. Effects of troglitazone. Diabetologia 1998; 41:569–576.
24. Vigili de Kreutzenberg S, Kiwanuka E, Tiengo A, Avogaro A. Visceral obesity is characterized by impaired nitric oxide-independent vasodilation. Eur Heart J 2003; 24:1210–1215.
25. Higashi Y, Oshima T, Sasaki N, et al. Relationship between insulin resistance and endothelium-dependent vascular relaxation in patients with essential hypertension. Hypertension 1997; 29:280–285.
26. Panza JA, Quyyumi AA, Brush JE, Epstein SE. Abnormal endothelium-dependent vascular relaxation in patients with essential hypertension. N Engl J Med 1990; 323:22–27.
27. Balletshofer BM, Rittig K, Enderle MD, et al. Endothelial dysfunction is detectable in young normotensive first-degree relatives of subjects with type 2 diabetes in association with insulin resistance. Circulation 2000; 101: 1780–1784.
28. Anastasiou E, Lekakis JP, Alevizaki M, et al. Impaired endothelium-dependent vasodilatation in women with previous gestational diabetes. Diabetes Care 1998; 21:2111–2115.
29. Knock GA, McCarthy AL, Lowy C, Poston L. Association of gestational diabetes with abnormal maternal vascular endothelial function. Br J Obstet Gynaecol 1997; 104:229–234.
30. Paradisi G, Steinberg HO, Hempfling A, et al. Polycystic ovary syndrome is associated with endothelial dysfunction. Circulation 2001; 103:1410–1415.
31. Baron AD, Steinberg HO, Chaker H, Leaming R, Johnson A, Brechtel G. Insulin-mediated skeletal muscle vasodilation contributes to both insulin sensitivity and responsiveness in lean humans. J Clin Invest 1995; 96:786–792.
32. Cleland SJ, Petrie JR, Small M, Elliott HL, Connell JM. Insulin action is associated with endothelial function in hypertension and type 2 diabetes. Hypertension 2000; 35:507–511.
33. Olsen MH, Andersen UB, Wachtell K, Ibsen H, Dige-Petersen H. A possible link between endothelial dysfunction and insulin resistance in hypertension. A LIFE substudy. Losartan Intervention For Endpoint-Reduction in Hypertension. Blood Press 2000; 9:132–139.
34. Petrie JR, Ueda S, Webb DJ, Elliott HL, Connell JM. Endothelial nitric oxide production and insulin sensitivity. A physiological link with implications for pathogenesis of cardiovascular disease. Circulation 1996; 93:1331–1333.
35. Serne EH, Stehouwer CD, ter Maaten JC, et al. Microvascular function relates to insulin sensitivity and blood pressure in normal subjects. Circulation 1999; 99:896–902.
36. Utriainen T, Makimattila S, Virkamaki A, Bergholm R, Yki-Jarvinen H. Dissociation between insulin sensitivity of glucose uptake and endothelial function in normal subjects. Diabetologia 1996; 39:1477–1482.
37. Verma S, Bhanot S, Yao L, McNeill JH. Defective endothelium-dependent relaxation in fructose-hypertensive rats. Am J Hypertens 1996; 9:370–376.
38. Verma S, Bhanot S, Yao L, McNeill JH. Vascular insulin resistance in fructose-hypertensive rats. Eur J Pharmacol 1997; 322:R1–R2.

39. Baron AD, Zhu JS, Zhu JH, Weldon H, Maianu L, Garvey WT. Glucosamine induces insulin resistance in vivo by affecting GLUT 4 translocation in skeletal muscle. Implications for glucose toxicity. J Clin Invest 1995; 96: 2792–2801.

40. Gabriely I, Yang XM, Cases JA, Ma XH, Rossetti L, Barzilai N. Hyperglycemia induces PAI-1 gene expression in adipose tissue by activation of the hexosamine biosynthetic pathway. Atherosclerosis 2002; 160:115–122.

41. Holmang A, Nilsson C, Niklasson B, Lonroth P. Induction of insulin resistance by glucosamine reduces blood flow but not interstitial levels of either glucose or insulin. Diabetes 1999; 48:106–111.

42. Patti ME, Virkamaki A, Landaker EJ, Kahn CR, Yki-Jarvinen H. Activation of the hexosamine pathway by glucosamine in vivo induces insulin resistance of early postreceptor insulin signaling events in skeletal muscle. Diabetes 1999; 48:1562–1571.

43. Abe H, Yamada N, Kamata K, et al. Hypertension, hypertriglyceridemia, and impaired endothelium-dependent vascular relaxation in mice lacking insulin receptor substrate-1. J Clin Invest 1998; 101:1784–1788.

44. Bruning JC, Michael MD, Winnay JN, et al. A muscle-specific insulin receptor knockout exhibits features of the metabolic syndrome of NIDDM without altering glucose tolerance. Mol Cell 1998; 2:559–569.

45. Vicent D, Ilany J, Kondo T, et al. The role of endothelial insulin signaling in the regulation of vascular tone and insulin resistance. J Clin Invest 2003; 111: 1373–1380.

46. Yamauchi T, Kamon J, Waki H, et al. The fat-derived hormone adiponectin reverses insulin resistance associated with both lipoatrophy and obesity. Nat Med 2001; 7:941–946.

47. Kubota N, Terauchi Y, Yamauchi T, et al. Disruption of adiponectin causes insulin resistance and neointimal formation. J Biol Chem 2002; 277:25863–25866.

48. Matsuzawa Y, Funahashi T, Nakamura T. Molecular mechanism of metabolic syndrome X: contribution of adipocytokines adipocyte-derived bioactive substances. Ann NY Acad Sci 1999; 892:146–154.

49. Shimabukuro M, Higa N, Asahi T, et al. Hypoadiponectinemia is closely linked to endothelial dysfunction in man. J Clin Endocrinol Metab 2003; 88: 3236–3240.

50. Yang WS, Lee WJ, Funahashi T, et al. Weight reduction increases plasma levels of an adipose-derived anti-inflammatory protein, adiponectin. J Clin Endocrinol Metab 2001; 86:3815–3819.

51. Ouchi N, Ohishi M, Kihara S, et al. Association of hypoadiponectinemia with impaired vasoreactivity. Hypertension 2003; 42:231–234.

52. Clerk LH, Rattigan S, Clark MG. Lipid infusion impairs physiologic insulin-mediated capillary recruitment and muscle glucose uptake in vivo. Diabetes 2002; 51:1138–1145.

53. Mason TM, Goh T, Tchipashvili V, et al. Prolonged elevation of plasma free fatty acids desensitizes the insulin secretory response to glucose in vivo in rats. Diabetes 1999; 48:524–530.

54. de Kreutzenberg SV, Crepaldi C, Marchetto S, et al. Plasma free fatty acids and endothelium-dependent vasodilation: effect of chain-length and cyclooxygenase inhibition. J Clin Endocrinol Metab 2000; 85:793–798.
55. Steinberg HO, Tarshoby M, Monestel R, et al. Elevated circulating free fatty acid levels impair endothelium-dependent vasodilation. J Clin Invest 1997; 100:1230–1239.
56. Egan BM, Lu G, Greene EL. Vascular effects of non-esterified fatty acids: implications for the cardiovascular risk factor cluster. Prostaglandins Leukot Essent Fatty Acids 1999; 60:411–420.
57. Steinberg HO, Paradisi G, Hook G, Crowder K, Cronin J, Baron AD. Free fatty acid elevation impairs insulin-mediated vasodilation and nitric oxide production. Diabetes 2000; 49:1231–1238.
58. Hotamisligil GS, Shargill NS, Spiegelman BM. Adipose expression of tumor necrosis factor-alpha: direct role in obesity-linked insulin resistance. Science 1993; 259:87–91.
59. Sewter CP, Digby JE, Blows F, Prins J, O'Rahilly S. Regulation of tumour necrosis factor-alpha release from human adipose tissue in vitro. J Endocrinol 1999; 163:33–38.
60. Zinman B, Hanley AJ, Harris SB, Kwan J, Fantus IG. Circulating tumor necrosis factor-alpha concentrations in a native Canadian population with high rates of type 2 diabetes mellitus. J Clin Endocrinol Metab 1999; 84: 272–278.
61. Hotamisligil GS, Arner P, Caro JF, Atkinson RL, Spiegelman BM. Increased adipose tissue expression of tumor necrosis factor-alpha in human obesity and insulin resistance. J Clin Invest 1995; 95:2409–2415.
62. Moller DE. Potential role of TNF-alpha in the pathogenesis of insulin resistance and type 2 diabetes. Trends Endocrinol Metab 2000; 11:212–217.
63. Hollenberg SM, Cunnion RE, Parrillo JE. The effect of tumor necrosis factor on vascular smooth muscle. In vitro studies using rat aortic rings. Chest 1991; 100:1133–1137.
64. Wang P, Ba ZF, Chaudry IH. Administration of tumor necrosis factor-alpha in vivo depresses endothelium-dependent relaxation. Am J Physiol 1994; 266: H2535–H2541.
65. Paquot N, Castillo MJ, Lefebvre PJ, Scheen AJ. No increased insulin sensitivity after a single intravenous administration of a recombinant human tumor necrosis factor receptor: Fc fusion protein in obese insulin-resistant patients. J Clin Endocrinol Metab 2000; 85:1316–1319.
66. Arvola P, Wu X, Kahonen M, et al. Exercise enhances vasorelaxation in experimental obesity associated hypertension. Cardiovasc Res 1999; 43: 992–1002.
67. Lavrencic A, Salobir BG, Keber I. Physical training improves flow-mediated dilation in patients with the polymetabolic syndrome. Arterioscler Thromb Vasc Biol 2000; 20:551–555.
68. Fuchsjager-Mayrl G, Pleiner J, Wiesinger GF, et al. Exercise training improves vascular endothelial function in patients with type 1 diabetes. Diabetes Care 2002; 25:1795–1801.

69. Maiorana A, O'Driscoll G, Cheetham C, et al. The effect of combined aerobic and resistance exercise training on vascular function in type 2 diabetes. J Am Coll Cardiol 2001; 38:860–866.

70. Bergholm R, Tiikkainen M, Vehkavaara S, et al. Lowering of LDL cholesterol rather than moderate weight loss improves endothelium-dependent vasodilatation in obese women with previous gestational diabetes. Diabetes Care 2003; 26:1667–1672.

71. Ebeling P, Teppo AM, Koistinen HA, et al. Troglitazone reduces hyperglycaemia and selectively acute-phase serum proteins in patients with Type II diabetes. Diabetologia 1999; 42:1433–1438.

72. Ferri C, Desideri G, Valenti M, et al. Early upregulation of endothelial adhesion molecules in obese hypertensive men. Hypertension 1999; 34:568–573.

73. Ziccardi P, Nappo F, Giugliano G, et al. Reduction of inflammatory cytokine concentrations and improvement of endothelial functions in obese women after weight loss over one year. Circulation 2002; 105:804–809.

74. Bailey CJ, Path MRC, Turner RC. Metformin. N Engl J Med 1996; 334: 574–579.

75. Kirpichnikov D, McFarlane SI, Sowers JR. Metformin: an update. Ann Intern Med 2002; 137:25–33.

76. Hawley SA, Gadalla AE, Olsen GS, Hardie DG. The antidiabetic drug metformin activates the AMP-activated protein kinase cascade via an adenine nucleotide-independent mechanism. Diabetes 2002; 51:2420–2425.

77. Musi N, Hirshman MF, Nygren J, et al. Metformin increases AMP-activated protein kinase activity in skeletal muscle of subjects with type 2 diabetes. Diabetes 2002; 51:2074–2081.

78. Ruderman NB, Cacicedo JM, Itani S, et al. Malonyl-CoA and AMP-activated protein kinase (AMPK): possible links between insulin resistance in muscle and early endothelial cell damage in diabetes. Biochem Soc Trans 2003; 31: 202–206.

79. Zhou G, Myers R, Li Y, et al. Role of AMP-activated protein kinase in mechanism of metformin action. J Clin Invest 2001; 108:1167–1174.

80. Verma S, Yao L, Dumont AS, McNeill JH. Metformin treatment corrects vascular insulin resistance in hypertension. J Hypertens 2000; 18:1445–1450.

81. Abbink EJ, Pickkers P, Jansen van Rosendaal A, et al. Vascular effects of glibenclamide vs. glimepiride and metformin in Type 2 diabetic patients. Diabet Med 2002; 19:136–143.

82. Mather K, Verma S, Anderson T. Effect of modulating insulin resistance on endothelial function in type 2 diabetes mellitus [abstr]. Circulation 1999; 100:I-832.

83. Plutzky J. Peroxisome proliferator-activated receptors in endothelial cell biology. Curr Opin Lipidol 2001; 12:511–518.

84. Paradisi G, Steinberg HO, Shepard MK, Hook G, Baron AD. Troglitazone therapy improves endothelial function to near normal levels in women with polycystic ovary syndrome. J Clin Endocrinol Metab 2003; 88:576–580.

85. Caballero AE, Saouaf R, Lim SC, et al. The effects of troglitazone, an insulin-sensitizing agent, on the endothelial function in early and late type 2 diabetes: a placebo-controlled randomized clinical trial. Metabolism 2003; 52:173–180.

86. Watanabe Y, Sunayama S, Shimada K, et al. Troglitazone improves endothelial dysfunction in patients with insulin resistance. J Atheroscler Thromb 2000; 7:159–163.

87. Yamagishi T, Saito Y, Nakamura T, et al. Troglitazone improves endothelial function and augments renal klotho mRNA expression in Otsuka Long-Evans Tokushima Fatty (OLETF) rats with multiple atherogenic risk factors. Hypertens Res 2001; 24:705–709.

88. Martin-Nizard F, Furman C, Delerive P, et al. Peroxisome proliferator-activated receptor activators inhibit oxidized low-density lipoprotein-induced endothelin-1 secretion in endothelial cells. J Cardiovasc Pharmacol 2002; 40: 822–831.

89. Phillips JW, Barringhaus KG, Sanders JM, et al. Rosiglitazone reduces the accelerated neointima formation after arterial injury in a mouse injury model of type 2 diabetes. Circulation 2003; 108:1994–1999.

90. Tao L, Liu HR, Gao E, et al. Antioxidative, antinitrative, and vasculoprotective effects of a peroxisome proliferator-activated receptor-{gamma} agonist in hypercholesterolemia. Circulation 2003; 108:2805–2811.

91. Toriumi Y, Hiraoka M, Watanabe M, Yoshida M. Pioglitazone reduces monocyte adhesion to vascular endothelium under flow by modulating RhoA GTPase and focal adhesion kinase. FEBS Lett 2003; 553:419–422.

92. Walker AB, Chattington PD, Buckingham RE, Williams G. The thiazolidinedione rosiglitazone (BRL-49653) lowers blood pressure and protects against impairment of endothelial function in Zucker fatty rats. Diabetes 1999; 48:1448–1453.

93. Yoshimoto T, Naruse M, Shizume H, et al. Vasculo-protective effects of insulin sensitizing agent pioglitazone in neointimal thickening and hypertensive vascular hypertrophy. Atherosclerosis 1999; 145:333–340.

94. Naderali EK, Pickavance LC, Wilding JP, Doyle PJ, Williams G. Troglitazone corrects metabolic changes but not vascular dysfunction in dietary-obese rats. Eur J Pharmacol 2001; 416:133–139.

95. Takase H, Hakamata M, Toriyama T, et al. Effect of troglitazone on endothelial function in type 2 diabetic patients. Arzneimittelforschung 2002; 52:34–38.

96. Walker AB, Naderali EK, Chattington PD, Buckingham RE, Williams G. Differential vasoactive effects of the insulin sensitizers rosiglitazone (BRL 49653) and troglitazone on human small arteries in vitro. Diabetes 1998; 47:810–814.

97. Cooke JP, Dzau VJ. Nitric oxide synthase: role in the genesis of vascular disease. Ann Rev Med 1997; 48:489–509.

98. Schiffrin EL. The endothelium and control of blood vessel function in health and disease. Clin Invest Med 1994; 17:602–620.

99. Catalano M, Carzaniga G, Perilli E, et al. Basal nitric oxide production is not reduced in patients with noninsulin-dependent diabetes mellitus. Vasc Med 1997; 2:302–305.

100. Sharma AC, Fogelson BG, Nawas SI, et al. Elevated coronary endothelin-1 but not nitric oxide in diabetics during CABG. Ann Thorac Surg 1999; 67: 1659–1663.

101. Honing ML, Morrison PJ, Banga JD, Stroes ES, Rabelink TJ. Nitric oxide availability in diabetes mellitus. Diabetes Metab Rev 1998; 14:241–249.

102. Kurioka S, Koshimura K, Murakami Y, Nishiki M, Kato Y. Reverse correlation between urine nitric oxide metabolites and insulin resistance in patients with type 2 diabetes mellitus. Endocr J 2000; 47:77–81.

103. Martina V, Bruno GA, Trucco F, et al. Platelet cNOS activity is reduced in patients with IDDM and NIDDM. Thromb Haemost 1998; 79:520–522.

104. Avogaro A, Toffolo G, Kiwanuka E, de Kreutzenberg SV, Tessari P, Cobelli C. L-Arginine-nitric oxide kinetics in normal and type 2 diabetic subjects: a stable-labelled 15N arginine approach. Diabetes 2003; 52:795–802.

105. Shinozaki K, Nishio Y, Okamura T, et al. Oral administration of tetrahydrobiopterin prevents endothelial dysfunction and vascular oxidative stress in the aortas of insulin-resistant rats. Circ Res 2000; 87:566–573.

106. Cavarape A, Feletto F, Mercuri F, Quagliaro L, Daman G, Ceriello A. High-fructose diet decreases catalase mRNA levels in rat tissues. J Endocrinol Invest 2001; 24:838–845.

107. Faure P, Rossini E, Wiernsperger N, Richard MJ, Favier A, Halimi S. An insulin sensitizer improves the free radical defense system potential and insulin sensitivity in high fructose-fed rats. Diabetes 1999; 48:353–357.

108. Shinozaki K, Hirayama A, Nishio Y, et al. Coronary endothelial dysfunction in the insulin-resistant state is linked to abnormal pteridine metabolism and vascular oxidative stress. J Am Coll Cardiol 2001; 38:1821–1828.

109. Garg R, Kumbkarni Y, Aljada A, et al. Troglitazone reduces reactive oxygen species generation by leukocytes and lipid peroxidation and improves flow-mediated vasodilatation in obese subjects. Hypertension 2000; 36:430–435.

110. Facchini F, Coulston AM, Reaven GM. Relation between dietary vitamin intake and resistance to insulin-mediated glucose disposal in healthy volunteers. Am J Clin Nutr 1996; 63:946–949.

111. Facchini FS, Humphreys MH, DoNascimento CA, Abbasi F, Reaven GM. Relation between insulin resistance and plasma concentrations of lipid hydroperoxides, carotenoids, and tocopherols. Am J Clin Nutr 2000; 72:776–779.

112. Dagenais GR, Yusuf S, Bourassa MG, et al. Effects of ramipril on coronary events in high-risk persons: results of the Heart Outcomes Prevention Evaluation Study. Circulation 2001; 104:522–526.

113. Yusuf S, Dagenais G, Pogue J, Bosch J, Sleight P. Vitamin E supplementation and cardiovascular events in high-risk patients. The Heart Outcomes Prevention Evaluation Study Investigators. N Engl J Med 2000; 342:154–160.

114. Ishii M, Shimizu S, Nagai T, Shiota K, Kiuchi Y, Yamamoto T. Stimulation of tetrahydrobiopterin synthesis induced by insulin: possible involvement of phosphatidylinositol 3-kinase. Int J Biochem Cell Biol 2001; 33:65–73.

115. Ceolotto G, Gallo A, Miola M, et al. Protein kinase C activity is acutely regulated by plasma glucose concentration in human monocytes in vivo. Diabetes 1999; 48:1316–1322.

116. Esberg LB, Ren J. Role of nitric oxide, tetrahydrobiopterin and peroxynitrite in glucose toxicity-associated contractile dysfunction in ventricular myocytes. Diabetologia 2003.

117. Tesfamariam B, Brown ML, Cohen RA. Elevated glucose impairs endothelium-dependent relaxation by activating protein kinase C. J Clin Invest 1991; 87: 1643–1648.

118. Timimi FK, Ting HH, Haley EA, Roddy MA, Ganz P, Creager MA. Vitamin C improves endothelium-dependent vasodilation in patients with insulin-dependent diabetes mellitus. J Am Coll Cardiol 1998; 31:552–557.

119. Ting HH, Timimi FK, Boles KS, Creager SJ, Ganz P, Creager MA. Vitamin C improves endothelium-dependent vasodilation in patients with non-insulin-dependent diabetes mellitus. J Clin Invest 1996; 97:22–28.

120. Brunner F, Wolkart G, Pfeiffer S, Russell JC, Wascher TC. Vascular dysfunction and myocardial contractility in the JCR:LA-corpulent rat. Cardiovasc Res 2000; 47:150–158.

121. Bagi Z, Koller A. Lack of nitric oxide mediation of flow-dependent arteriolar dilation in type I diabetes is restored by sepiapterin. J Vasc Res 2003; 40: 47–57.

122. Heitzer T, Krohn K, Albers S, Meinertz T. Tetrahydrobiopterin improves endothelium-dependent vasodilation by increasing nitric oxide activity in patients with Type II diabetes mellitus. Diabetologia 2000; 43:1435–1438.

123. Boger RH, Bode-Boger SM. Asymmetric dimethylarginine, derangements of the endothelial nitric oxide synthase pathway, and cardiovascular diseases. Semin Thromb Hemost 2000; 26:539–545.

124. Chan NN, Chan JC. Asymmetric dimethylarginine (ADMA): a potential link between endothelial dysfunction and cardiovascular diseases in insulin resistance syndrome? Diabetologia 2002; 45:1609–1616.

125. Eid HM, Eritsland J, Larsen J, Arnesen H, Seljeflot I. Increased levels of asymmetric dimethylarginine in populations at risk for atherosclerotic disease. Effects of pravastatin. Atherosclerosis 2003; 166:279–284.

126. Paiva H, Laakso J, Lehtimaki T, Isomustajarvi M, Ruokonen I, Laaksonen R. Effect of high-dose statin treatment on plasma concentrations of endogenous nitric oxide synthase inhibitors. J Cardiovasc Pharmacol 2003; 41:219–222.

127. Surdacki A, Nowicki M, Sandmann J, et al. Effects of acute euglycemic hyperinsulinemia on urinary nitrite/nitrate excretion and plasma endothelin-1 levels in men with essential hypertension and normotensive controls. Metabolism 1999; 48:887–891.

128. Stuhlinger MC, Abbasi F, Chu JW, et al. Relationship between insulin resistance and an endogenous nitric oxide synthase inhibitor. JAMA 2002; 287:1420–1426.

129. Lin KY, Ito A, Asagami T, et al. Impaired nitric oxide synthase pathway in diabetes mellitus: role of asymmetric dimethylarginine and dimethylarginine dimethylaminohydrolase. Circulation 2002; 106:987–992.

130. Xiong Y, Fu YF, Fu SH, Zhou HH. Elevated levels of the serum endogenous inhibitor of nitric oxide synthase and metabolic control in rats with streptozotocin-induced diabetes. J Cardiovasc Pharmacol 2003; 42:191–196.

131. Asagami T, Abbasi F, Stuelinger M, et al. Metformin treatment lowers asymmetric dimethylarginine concentrations in patients with type 2 diabetes. Metabolism 2002; 51:843–846.

132. Ito A, Egashira K, Narishige T, Muramatsu K, Takeshita A. Angiotensin-converting enzyme activity is involved in the mechanism of increased endogenous nitric oxide synthase inhibitor in patients with type 2 diabetes mellitus. Circ J 2002; 66:811–815.

133. Levin ER. Endothelins. N Engl J Med 1995; 333:356–363.
134. Anfossi G, Cavalot F, Massucco P, et al. Insulin influences immunoreactive endothelin release by human vascular smooth muscle cells. Metabolism 1993; 42:1081–1083.
135. Hu RM, Levin ER, Pedram A, Frank HJ. Insulin stimulates production and secretion of endothelin from bovine endothelial cells. Diabetes 1993; 42: 351–358.
136. Caballero AE, Arora S, Saouaf R, et al. Microvascular and macrovascular reactivity is reduced in subjects at risk for type 2 diabetes. Diabetes 1999; 48: 1856–1862.
137. Cardillo C, Nambi SS, Kilcoyne CM, et al. Insulin stimulates both endothelin and nitric oxide activity in the human forearm. Circulation 1999; 100:820–825.
138. Donatelli M, Colletti I, Bucalo ML, Russo V, Verga S. Plasma endothelin levels in NIDDM patients with macroangiopathy. Diabetes Res 1994; 25:159–164.
139. Donatelli M, Hoffmann E, Colletti I, et al. Circulating endothelin-1 levels in type 2 diabetic patients with ischaemic heart disease. Acta Diabetol 1996; 33:246–248.
140. Ferri C, Bellini C, Desideri G, et al. Circulating endothelin-1 levels in obese patients with the metabolic syndrome. Exp Clin Endocrinol Diabetes 1997; 105:38–40.
141. Ferri C, Bellini C, Desideri G, et al. Plasma endothelin-1 levels in obese hypertensive and normotensive men. Diabetes 1995; 44:431–436.
142. Juan CC, Fang VS, Kwok CF, Perng JC, Chou YC, Ho LT. Exogenous hyperinsulinemia causes insulin resistance, hyperendothelinemia, and subsequent hypertension in rats. Metabolism 1999; 48:465–471.
143. Bertello P, Veglio F, Pinna G, et al. Plasma endothelin in NIDDM patients with and without complications. Diabetes Care 1994; 17:574–577.
144. Kanno K, Hirata Y, Shichiri M, Marumo F. Plasma endothelin-1 levels in patients with diabetes mellitus with or without vascular complication. J Cardiovasc Pharmacol 1991; 17:S475–S476.
145. Mangiafico RA, Malatino LS, Santonocito M, Spada RS. Plasma endothelin-1 concentrations in non-insulin-dependent diabetes mellitus and nondiabetic patients with chronic arterial obstructive disease of the lower limbs. Int Angiol 1998; 17:97–102.
146. Piatti PM, Monti LD, Galli L, et al. Relationship between endothelin-1 concentration and metabolic alterations typical of the insulin resistance syndrome. Metabolism 2000; 49:748–752.
147. Ferri C, Bellini C, Desideri G, De Mattia G, Santucci A. Endogenous insulin modulates circulating endothelin-1 concentrations in humans. Diabetes Care 1996; 19:504–506.
148. Ferri C, Carlomagno A, Coassin S, et al. Circulating endothelin-1 levels increase during euglycemic hyperinsulinemic clamp in lean NIDDM men. Diabetes Care 1995; 18:226–233.
149. Gottsater A, Rendell M, Anwaar I, Lindgarde F, Hulthen UL, Mattiasson I. Increasing neopterin and decreasing endothelin-1 in plasma during insulin infusion in women. Scand J Clin Lab Invest 1999; 59:417–424.

150. Katsumori K, Wasada T, Saeki A, Naruse M, Omori Y. Lack of acute insulin effect on plasma endothelin-1 levels in humans. Diabetes Res Clin Pract 1996; 32:187–189.
151. Katakam PV, Pollock JS, Pollock DM, Ujhelyi MR, Miller AW. Enhanced endothelin-1 response and receptor expression in small mesenteric arteries of insulin-resistant rats. Am J Physiol Heart Circ Physiol 2001; 280:H522–H527.
152. Verma S, Skarsgard P, Bhanot S, Yao L, Laher I, McNeill JH. Reactivity of mesenteric arteries from fructose hypertensive rats to endothelin-1. Am J Hypertens 1997; 10:1010–1019.
153. Evans T, Deng DX, Chen S, Chakrabarti S. Endothelin receptor blockade prevents augmented extracellular matrix component mRNA expression and capillary basement membrane thickening in the retina of diabetic and galactose-fed rats. Diabetes 2000; 49:662–666.
154. Wu SQ, Hopfner RL, McNeill JR, Wilson TW, Gopalakrishnan V. Altered paracrine effect of endothelin in blood vessels of the hyperinsulinemic, insulin resistant obese Zucker rat. Cardiovasc Res 2000; 45:994–1000.
155. Verma S, Li SH, Wang CH, et al. Resistin promotes endothelial cell activation: further evidence of adipokine-endothelial interaction. Circulation 2003; 108: 736–740.
156. Blochl-Daum B, Vierhapper H, Eichler HG, Waldhausl W. Endothelin-induced venoconstriction is unaffected by type 2-diabetes: in vivo effect of histamine on the endothelin action on veins. Arch Int Pharmacodyn Ther 1992; 316:90–96.
157. McAuley DF, McGurk C, Nugent AG, Hanratty C, Hayes JR, Johnston GD. Vasoconstriction to endothelin-1 is blunted in non-insulin-dependent diabetes: a dose-response study. J Cardiovasc Pharmacol 2000; 36:203–208.
158. McAuley DF, Nugent AG, McGurk C, Maguire S, Hayes JR, Johnston GD. Vasoconstriction to endogenous endothelin-1 is impaired in patients with Type II diabetes mellitus. Clin Sci (Colch) 2000; 99:175–179.
159. Cardillo C, Campia U, Bryant MB, Panza JA. Increased activity of endogenous endothelin in patients with type II diabetes mellitus. Circulation 2002; 106:1783–1787.
160. Mather K, Steinberg H, Mirzamohammadi B, Hook G, Baron A. ET-1A receptor blockade improves endothelium-dependent vasodilation in insulin resistant obese and Type 2 diabetic patients [abstr]. Diabetes 2000; 49(suppl 1):A143.
161. Mather K, Mirzamohammadi B, Lteif A, Steinberg H, Baron A. Endothelin contributes to basal vascular tone and endothelial dysfunction in human obesity and Type 2 diabetes mellitus. Diabetes 2002; 51:3517–3523.
162. Flowers MA, Wang Y, Stewart RJ, Patel B, Marsden PA. Reciprocal regulation of endothelin-1 and endothelial constitutive NOS in proliferating endothelial cells. Am J Physiol 1995; 269:H1988–H1997.
163. Marsen TA, Egink G, Suckau G, Baldamus CA. Tyrosine-kinase-dependent regulation of the nitric oxide synthase gene by endothelin-1 in human endothelial cells. Pflugers Arch 1999; 438:538–544.
164. Schena M, Mulatero P, Schiavone D, et al. Vasoactive hormones induce nitric oxide synthase mRNA expression and nitric oxide production in human endothelial cells and monocytes. Am J Hypertens 1999; 12:388–397.

165. Hopfner RL, Hasnadka RV, Wilson TW, McNeill JR, Gopalakrishnan V. Insulin increases endothelin-1-evoked intracellular free calcium responses by increased ET(A) receptor expression in rat aortic smooth muscle cells. Diabetes 1998; 47:937–944.

166. Goligorsky MS, Tsukahara H, Magazine H, Andersen TT, Malik AB, Bahou WF. Termination of endothelin signaling: role of nitric oxide. J Cell Physiol 1994; 158:485–494.

167. Jiang ZY, Zhou QL, Chatterjee A, et al. Endothelin-1 modulates insulin signaling through phosphatidylinositol 3-kinase pathway in vascular smooth muscle cells. Diabetes 1999; 48:1120–1130.

168. Verhaar MC, Strachan FE, Newby DE, et al. Endothelin-A receptor antagonist-mediated vasodilation is attenuated by inhibition of nitric oxide synthesis and by endothelin-B receptor blockade. Circulation 1998; 97:752–756.

169. Steppan CM, Bailey ST, Bhat S, et al. The hormone resistin links obesity to diabetes. Nature 2001; 409:307–312.

170. Kimura K, Tsuda K, Baba A, et al. Involvement of nitric oxide in endothelium-dependent arterial relaxation by leptin. Biochem Biophys Res Commun 2000; 273:745–749.

171. Lembo G, Vecchione C, Fratta L, et al. Leptin induces direct vasodilation through distinct endothelial mechanisms. Diabetes 2000; 49:293–297.

172. Vecchione C, Maffei A, Colella S, et al. Leptin effect on endothelial nitric oxide is mediated through Akt-endothelial nitric oxide synthase phosphorylation pathway. Diabetes 2002; 51:168–173.

173. Quehenberger P, Exner M, Sunder-Plassmann R, et al. Leptin induces endothelin-1 in endothelial cells in vitro. Circ Res 2002; 90:711–718.

174. Clarke KJ, Zhong Q, Schwartz DD, Coleman ES, Kemppainen RJ, Judd RL. Regulation of adiponectin secretion by endothelin-1. Biochem Biophys Res Commun 2003; 312:945–949.

175. Xiong Y, Tanaka H, Richardson JA, et al. Endothelin-1 stimulates leptin production in adipocytes. J Biol Chem 2001; 276:28471–28477.

176. Zhong Q, Lin CY, Clarke KJ, Kemppainen RJ, Schwartz DD, Judd RL. Endothelin-1 inhibits resistin secretion in 3T3-L1 adipocytes. Biochem Biophys Res Commun 2002; 296:383–387.

177. Matsuda K, Teragawa H, Fukuda Y, Nakagawa K, Higashi Y, Chayama K. Leptin causes nitric-oxide independent coronary artery vasodilation in humans. Hypertens Res 2003; 26:147–152.

178. Yamauchi T, Kamon J, Waki H, et al. The mechanisms by which both heterozygous peroxisome proliferator-activated receptor gamma (PPARgamma) deficiency and PPARgamma agonist improve insulin resistance. J Biol Chem 2001; 276:41245–41254.

179. Chen H, Montagnani M, Funahashi T, Shimomura I, Quon MJ. Adiponectin stimulates production of nitric oxide in vascular endothelial cells. J Biol Chem 2003; 278:45021–45026.

180. Hattori Y, Suzuki M, Hattori S, Kasai K. Globular adiponectin upregulates nitric oxide production in vascular endothelial cells. Diabetologia 2003; 46:1543–1549.

181. Ross R. Atherosclerosis is an inflammatory disease. Am Heart J 1999; 138:S419–S420.

182. Chambers JC, Eda S, Bassett P, et al. C-reactive protein, insulin resistance, central obesity, and coronary heart disease risk in Indian Asians from the United Kingdom compared with European whites. Circulation 2001; 104:145–150.

183. Danesh J, Collins R, Appleby P, Peto R. Association of fibrinogen, C-reactive protein, albumin, or leukocyte count with coronary heart disease: meta-analyses of prospective studies. JAMA 1998; 279:1477–1482.

184. Folsom AR, Aleksic N, Catellier D, Juneja HS, Wu KK. C-reactive protein and incident coronary heart disease in the Atherosclerosis Risk In Communities (ARIC) study. Am Heart J 2002; 144:233–238.

185. Retterstol L, Eikvar L, Berg K. A twin study of C-Reactive Protein compared to other risk factors for coronary heart disease. Atherosclerosis 2003; 169:279–282.

186. Ridker PM, Buring JE, Cook NR, Rifai N. C-reactive protein, the metabolic syndrome, and risk of incident cardiovascular events: an 8-year follow-up of 14 719 initially healthy American women. Circulation 2003; 107:391–397.

187. Ridker PM, Hennekens CH, Buring JE, Rifai N. C-reactive protein and other markers of inflammation in the prediction of cardiovascular disease in women. N Engl J Med 2000; 342:836–843.

188. van der Meer IM, de Maat MP, Kiliaan AJ, van der Kuip DA, Hofman A, Witteman JC. The value of C-reactive protein in cardiovascular risk prediction: the Rotterdam Study. Arch Intern Med 2003; 163:1323–1328.

189. Yudkin JS, Stehouwer CD, Emeis JJ, Coppack SW. C-reactive protein in healthy subjects: associations with obesity, insulin resistance, and endothelial dysfunction: a potential role for cytokines originating from adipose tissue? Arterioscler Thromb Vasc Biol 1999; 19:972–978.

190. Festa A, D'Agostino R Jr, Howard G, Mykkanen L, Tracy RP, Haffner SM. Chronic subclinical inflammation as part of the insulin resistance syndrome: the Insulin Resistance Atherosclerosis Study (IRAS). Circulation 2000; 102:42–47.

191. Hak AE, Pols HA, Stehouwer CD, et al. Markers of inflammation and cellular adhesion molecules in relation to insulin resistance in nondiabetic elderly: the Rotterdam study. J Clin Endocrinol Metab 2001; 86:4398–4405.

192. Han TS, Sattar N, Williams K, Gonzalez-Villalpando C, Lean ME, Haffner SM. Prospective study of C-reactive protein in relation to the development of diabetes and metabolic syndrome in the Mexico City Diabetes Study. Diabetes Care 2002; 25:2016–2021.

193. Ford ES. Body mass index, diabetes, and C-reactive protein among U.S. adults. Diabetes Care 1999; 22:1971–1977.

194. Hak AE, Stehouwer CD, Bots ML, et al. Associations of C-reactive protein with measures of obesity, insulin resistance, and subclinical atherosclerosis in healthy, middle-aged women. Arterioscler Thromb Vasc Biol 1999; 19:1986–1991.

195. Visser M, Bouter LM, McQuillan GM, Wener MH, Harris TB. Elevated C-reactive protein levels in overweight and obese adults. JAMA 1999; 282:2131–2135.

196. Spranger J, Kroke A, Mohlig M, et al. Inflammatory cytokines and the risk to develop type 2 diabetes: results of the prospective population-based European

Prospective Investigation into Cancer and Nutrition (EPIC)-Potsdam Study. Diabetes 2003; 52:812–817.

197. Yudkin JS, Kumari M, Humphries SE, Mohamed-Ali V. Inflammation, obesity, stress and coronary heart disease: is interleukin-6 the link? Atherosclerosis 2000; 148:209–214.

198. Calabro P, Willerson JT, Yeh ET. Inflammatory cytokines stimulated C-reactive protein production by human coronary artery smooth muscle cells. Circulation 2003; 108:1930–1932.

199. Chu NV, Kong AP, Kim DD, et al. Differential effects of metformin and troglitazone on cardiovascular risk factors in patients with type 2 diabetes. Diabetes Care 2002; 25:542–549.

200. Haffner SM, Greenberg AS, Weston WM, Chen H, Williams K, Freed MI. Effect of rosiglitazone treatment on nontraditional markers of cardiovascular disease in patients with type 2 diabetes mellitus. Circulation 2002; 106: 679–684.

201. Esposito K, Pontillo A, Di Palo C, et al. Effect of weight loss and lifestyle changes on vascular inflammatory markers in obese women: a randomized trial. JAMA 2003; 289:1799–1804.

202. Sasaki S, Higashi Y, Nakagawa K, et al. A low-calorie diet improves endothelium-dependent vasodilation in obese patients with essential hypertension. Am J Hypertens 2002; 15:302–309.

# 6

# Obesity and Inflammatory and Thrombotic Factors

**Vincent Ricchiuti**

*Division of Endocrinology, Diabetes and Hypertension, Department of Medicine, Brigham and Women's Hospital, Harvard Medical School, Boston, Massachusetts, U.S.A.*

## INTRODUCTION

The prevalence of obesity has escalated dramatically in the United States (1). This has led to a marked increase in the metabolic syndrome, a clustering of atherosclerotic cardiovascular disease (CVD) risk factors characterized by visceral adiposity, hypertension, diabetes, insulin resistance, low high-density lipoprotein (HDL) cholesterol, and a systemic proinflammatory state (2). Although obesity is a powerful risk factor for type 2 diabetes mellitus (DM-2) and CVDs across populations, considerable heterogeneity exists in the relationship between metabolic and cardiovascular abnormalities and the degree of obesity (3). Significant subgroups of subjects who are defined as obese by current guidelines do not develop insulin resistance; conversely, insulin resistance can be present in lean individuals (4). Genetic and environmental factors may have a major impact on the metabolic and cardiovascular consequences of obesity, although the mechanisms by which genetic factors modify the effects of obesity are largely unknown.

Waist circumference reflects abdominal subcutaneous as well as visceral adipose tissue and is a general index of central (trunk) fat mass. Visceral adipose tissue has been proposed as the major determinant of metabolic and cardiovascular complications of obesity (5). However, this remains controversial, and it is unclear whether more accurate measures of total body fat, trunk fat mass, or specific abdominal subcutaneous adipose tissue or visceral adipose tissue compartments provide superior information regarding obesity complications (6). Alternatively, the use of novel biochemical measures of adipose mass and function may be a more practical way to incorporate additional adipose readouts into large epidemiological studies and clinical practice.

Adipose tissue is an active secretory organ that elaborates a variety of molecules known as "adipokines," including tumor necrosis factor alpha (TNFα), interleukin-6 (IL-6), leptin, adiponectin, and resistin, which may mediate many of the metabolic changes seen in the metabolic syndrome (7). Some of these fat-derived factors may be directly atherogenic. Plasma leptin, which is largely derived from adipose tissue, increases in obesity and insulin-resistant states. Leptin deficiency in mice protects against atherosclerosis despite causing massive obesity (8), and plasma leptin levels were found to be predictive of cardiovascular events, independent of traditional risk factors, body mass index (BMI), and C-reactive protein (CRP) levels (9). In contrast, plasma levels of adiponectin are reduced in obesity and DM-2, and early evidence suggests that this molecule may have antiatherosclerotic properties in murine models and in humans (10,11). Whether these measures of adipose tissue hormonal activity will be superior markers of cardiovascular risk over anatomic measures of obesity, such as waist/hip ratio (WHR), remains to be determined. The connection between obesity and disordered hemostasis is well established, but not completely understood. In this chapter, the relationship between inflammatory and thrombotic factors that lead to CVD risk in obesity will be discussed.

## ADIPOKINES: INFLAMMATION AND ROLE OF WHITE ADIPOSE TISSUE

### Definition of Adipokines

As the number of protein signals recognized to be secreted from adipose tissue rapidly increased, it became helpful to agree on a collective name. The term introduced by Funahashi et al. (12) at first was "adipocytokines" and was used widely by others. This term is confusing because there is an inference that the adipocyte-secreted proteins are cytokines, or cytokine-like. While this is the case for some such as TNFα and IL-6, it is obviously not so with the majority of proteins. An alternative name that has been suggested was "adipokines," which may be more appropriate because it does not imply that the proteins belong to a particular functional group. However, this term should be only used to describe those proteins that are released by adipocytes themselves. Macrophages, which also secrete protein signals such as TNFα and IL-6 are found in a number of organs as well as being present in adipose tissue. The number of macrophages in adipose tissue increases in obesity and these macrophages participate in inflammatory pathways that are activated in adipose tissues of obese individuals (13). There is also an uncertainty of whether the term adipokine should be restricted to proteins released from white adipocytes or also include proteins secreted from brown adipocytes. White and brown adipocytes are functionally different and do not produce the same proteins. In contrast to other cells, including white adipocytes, brown adipocytes express mitochondrial-uncoupling protein, which gives the cell's mitochondria an ability to uncouple oxidative phosphorylation and utilize substrates to generate heat rather than adenosine triphosphate.

## Inflammation and Obesity

An essential advance in the understanding of obesity is the emergence of the paradigm of low-grade inflammation (14). The basis for this observation is that increased signaling levels of several inflammatory markers, both pro-inflammatory cytokines and acute phase proteins are elevated in obesity. These markers include IL-6, TNFα, CRP, and haptoglobin (15,16). The implications in terms of the site of inflammation itself, whether systemic or local, are unclear. Nevertheless, it is increasingly evident that the inflammatory state may contribute to the development of insulin resistance and other disorders associated with obesity, such as hyperlipidemia and metabolic syndrome (17,18).

There are three different origins for inflammatory markers in obesity: (i) production and release from organs other than adipose tissue, primarily the liver and immune cells; (ii) secretion of factors from white adipose tissue (WAT) that stimulate the production of inflammatory factors from the liver and other organs (such a marker could be CRP); and (iii) production of inflammatory markers directly from adipocytes themselves. In obesity, the rise in the circulating levels of inflammatory markers may reflect the production from an increased WAT mass. It is not completely understood whether adipose tissue directly contributes to the raised circulating levels of specific inflammatory markers and to what limit.

## Cytokines

### TNFα and IL-6

Numerous inflammatory cytokines are expressed in, and secreted by, white adipocytes. The first to be identified was TNFα (17). TNFα expression in WAT was initially demonstrated in rodents, and was found to be clearly increased in obese animal models (17). Furthermore, it was proposed that TNFα is linked to the development of insulin resistance. This cytokine has been extensively examined in relation to insulin action, and multiple effects have been described, including the inhibition of the insulin receptor–signaling pathway (17,19). In humans, the secretion of TNFα was reported to be mainly from the cells of the stromal vascular matrix fractions, which include the macrophages, regardless of the fact that most of the mRNA for TNFα was thought to be found within the adipocytes themselves (13,20). In recent reports by Fain et al. (20,21), an apparent disparity between mRNA and protein secretion in human WAT is evident for several adipokines and requires further assessment.

TNFα within adipose tissue acts in both an autocrine and a paracrine manner to influence a range of processes, including apoptosis (19,22). There appears to be a hierarchy of cytokines within WAT, with TNFα playing a pivotal role in relation to the production of several cytokines and other adipokines (19). Thus, TNFα is a key regulator of the synthesis of IL-6, of the acute-phase protein, haptoglobin (23), and of neurotrophin [nerve growth factor (NGF)] (24). The extent to which TNFα is formed in WAT and released into the circulation has been a matter of debate, but an association between the plasma TNFα system (including the soluble receptors) and indices of obesity has been reported (15).

The other cytokine that has been the subject of major interest in WAT is IL-6. It is expressed in, and secreted by, adipocytes and has local actions within the tissue and after it is released into the circulation (25). Plasma levels of IL-6 as well as expression in WAT are elevated in obesity and insulin resistance (25–27). It has been proposed that IL-6 has direct central nervous system actions, because IL-6 receptors are found in the hypothalamus of mice (25,28). Furthermore, IL-6 is a candidate molecule for conveying information from adipocytes to the hypothalamus in the regulation of energy balance, in addition to leptin.

### Other Cytokines

Although there has been considerable focus on TNFα and IL-6 as described above, several other cytokines and related factors are synthesized within adipose tissue, including IL-1-β, transforming growth factor-β (TGF-β), and leptin. Recent reports have also included IL-8, IL-10, and IL-17-D. The IL-8 gene is expressed in human adipocytes and the protein released from both fat cells and adipose tissue fragments (29,30). IL-1-β and TNFα stimulate IL-8 release, while dexamethasone is inhibitory (30). As with IL-6, the plasma level of IL-8 is increased in obesity (31). The levels of IL-10, an anti-inflammatory cytokine, are also raised in the obese (32); the secretion of IL-10 from human adipocytes as well as from the stromal vascular fraction and tissue matrix of human fat deposits have been documented (21).

The expression of IL-17-D, believed to be the last member of the IL-17 family to be identified, has recently been described in adipocytes (33). This cytokine stimulates the production of IL-6 and IL-8 from endothelial cells

(33). However, its release from adipocytes has not been documented, and so at present it can only be considered as a putative adipokine.

## Acute-Phase Proteins

There are a number of acute-phase proteins whose plasma concentrations increase substantially during the early stages of the inflammatory response, and a small number where the levels decrease (34). Several of these proteins are now recognized as adipokines, with adipose tissue being a potential contributor to the raised circulating levels in obesity. These proteins are discussed in detail below.

### CRP

The circulating level of CRP rises with obesity as well as diabetes. Elevated levels of CRP have been associated with increased BMI (15,35,36), and levels fall with weight loss (37). There is evidence from a study using real-time polymerase chain reaction that the mRNA coding for CRP is expressed in adipose tissue. It was shown that an inverse correlation between the levels of the mRNA for CRP and adiponectin exists (38). This raises the possibility that adipose tissue contributes directly to the circulating levels of CRP.

IL-6 is secreted by adipose tissue in increased amounts in obesity. IL-6 is the major cytokine regulating the hepatic production of CRP (39,40). Thus WAT may be a major player in the raised circulating levels of CRP in obesity, but through the indirect route of adipocyte-derived IL-6.

### PAI-1

Plasminogen activator inhibitor-1 (PAI-1) is an essential factor in the maintenance of vascular hemostasis, inhibiting the activation of plasminogen, the precursor of plasmin, which is involved in the breakdown of fibrin (41). The expression and secretion of PAI-1 by adipocytes, both rodent and human, is well documented (41–44). The circulating level of PAI-1 is increased in obesity and synthesis in WAT is also raised (45). This has led to the view that adipose tissue is the major source of the elevated PAI-1 levels in the obese (42,45,46). In addition to its role in hemostasis, PAI-1 is also an acute-phase response protein as PAI-1 levels increase in an inflammatory response (34). Because the risk of atherothrombotic disease is increased in obesity, this is a potent example of how the comorbidities, such as diabetes and cardiovascular risk, associated with an increase in adipocity can be directly linked to alterations in the production of specific adipokines. The role of PAI-1 and fibrinolysis will be discussed later in this chapter.

### Haptoglobin

Levy et al. recently demonstrated in multiple independent population-based longitudinal and cross-sectional analyses that the haptoglobin 2–2 genotype is associated with an increased risk for diabetic CVD (47,48). The chief function of haptoglobin is to bind to hemoglobin and thereby prevent hemoglobin-induced oxidative tissue damage. This antioxidant function of haptoglobin is mediated in part by the ability of haptoglobin to prevent the release of iron from hemoglobin on its binding. Several studies have now reported that the haptoglobin gene is expressed in murine adipose tissue (16,23,49). Similarly, gene expression has also been shown in human WAT (16). A very recent study has reported that haptoglobin was released directly from human adipose tissue explants (20). Release of haptoglobin into the medium has been observed in 3T3-L1 adipocytes by a proteomic approach (50). Both transgenic studies and studies in 3T3-L1 adipocytes indicate that TNFα is a key factor in the stimulation of haptoglobin expression (23,51). IL-6 also was stimulatory for haptoglobin expression.

Stimulation of the peroxisome proliferator–activated receptor-gamma (PPAR-γ) nuclear receptor through administration of the thiazolidinedione, rosiglitazone, strongly inhibits haptoglobin gene expression. This is consistent with the emerging view that PPARs have substantial anti-inflammatory actions (52). Indeed, several other adipokines are downregulated by PPAR-γ ligands, including TNFα, leptin, and NGF, while adiponectin is upregulated (52).

### SAA

Serum amyloid A (SAA) is the precursor to amyloid A protein and is found in secondary amyloid plaques and consists of a family of apolipoproteins that bind to, and substitute for, apo A-I in HDL. These apolipoproteins are expressed as either major acute-phase reactants SAA, or constitutive SAA, the functions of which are largely unknown. However, a few clinically important functions have been suggested that include proinflammatory and anti-inflammatory roles. A number of genes have now been identified in man and mouse that share very similar sequence identities and genomic organization (53). These genes are upregulated by proinflammatory cytokines such as TNFα and IL-6, as well as by glucocorticoids. The expression of SAA is predominantly in the liver as with other acute-phase reactants. However, extrahepatic expression of SAA has been reported in adipocytes. The expression and release of SAA3 occurs in murine adipocytes, and this is upregulated under hyperglycemic conditions (54).

### Additional Inflammation-Related Proteins: Leptin, Adiponectin, and Resistin

#### Leptin

Leptin is an adipocyte-derived polypeptide hormone that controls body weight through central regulation of food intake and energy expenditure (55). Large quantities of leptin mRNA were found in adipose tissue and concentrations of leptin in the circulation are strongly and positively correlated with body weight and adiposity in man. Most, but not all, human obesity is characterized by elevated circulating leptin levels (56). Both leptin and its receptor share structural and functional similarities with the IL-6 family of cytokines (57), and leptin appears to play a critical role in the inflammatory response. Defective immune responses are present in both leptin-deficient mice (58) and infants (59) as well as during starvation and malnutrition, two conditions characterized by low levels of circulating leptin (58). CD34+ hemopoietic stem cells (57) and most leukocytes express the leptin receptor (58), and the stimulating effects of leptin on leukocyte proliferation have been well established in vitro (57). Further evidence from in vitro and animal studies suggests that leptin is also involved in regulation of the humoral inflammatory response through its direct effects on T cells (57), monocytes (57,60), neutrophils (61), and endothelial cells (62,63).

Weight loss reduces circulating leptin levels and concurrently lowers the plasma levels of inflammation markers associated with obesity (64). The question of whether leptin levels underlie the proinflammatory state in human obesity was investigated a decade ago (65). Hukshorn et al. sought evidence for a proinflammatory role of leptin in obesity by maintaining elevated plasma leptin levels during weight loss (66). Moderately obese men who had profound weight loss induced by a very low calorie diet, received weekly injections of long-acting pegylated human recombinant leptin (PEG-OB) or placebo (67). Treatment with PEG-OB protein modified subjective appetite at a dosage that produced no changes in body composition, energy expenditure, or body mass loss relative to placebo treatment, suggesting that PEG-OB protein has central rather than peripheral biological activity in obese men (67). It was clear that if elevated leptin levels were an important factor in inducing an inflammatory state in obese humans, exogenous leptin administration during weight loss would counteract the concurrent beneficial effects of weight loss on the proinflammatory state.

### Adiponectin

The recently identified hydrophilic protein adiponectin (also known as Acrp30, AdipQ, apM1, and GBP28) is exclusively produced by adipocytes and has high homology to complement factor C1q (68). Plasma adiponectin levels are decreased in obesity (69), insulin resistance (70), DM 2 (71), and dyslipidemia (72), and particularly low in patients with coronary artery disease (73). Weight loss and pharmacological improvement of insulin sensitivity by thiazolidinediones (74,75) are associated with increased adiponectin levels. Lack of adiponectin resulted in increased susceptibility to diet-induced insulin resistance, and treatment of animals with adiponectin improved insulin resistance and other metabolic abnormalities associated with obesity and lipoatrophy (76,77). In vitro, adiponectin suppressed adhesion molecule expression in endothelial cells (11), reduced vascular inflammatory responses by inhibition of endothelial cell nuclear factor-(kappa) B signaling (78), and suppressed macrophage function (79). In vivo, adiponectin adhered to endothelial lesions (80) and prevented neointimal formation (81) and athero-sclerosis in mice (10). In contrast to other adipokine molecules, adiponectin thus seems to have protective metabolic and anti-inflammatory properties. Much remains to be learned about adiponectin regulation; however, it is known that adiponectin mRNA levels in adipose tissue decrease in patients with obesity. Engeli et al. examined the relationship between decreased adiponectin levels and IL-6, TNFα, and high-sensitive CRP as mediators of inflammation and markers of cardiovascular risk in nondiabetic postmenopausal women. The authors demonstrated that low levels of adiponectin in obese women are associated with higher levels of CRP and IL-6 (82).

### Resistin

Resistin is a 10-kDa protein secreted by the adipocytes and has been claimed to represent an important link between obesity and insulin resistance. Originally, resistin administration was reported to cause glucose intolerance and insulin resistance in mouse. However, resistin antibody administration improved glucose intolerance. Moreover, serum levels of resistin were higher in mouse models of obesity and decreased after PPAR-γ agonist (e.g., thiazolidinedione) treatment. WAT resistin mRNA and serum protein levels dropped during fasting and increased during refeeding (83). Other groups confirmed resistin's existence by using different experimental approaches (84,85). Resistin has a rapid effect on hepatic, but not peripheral, insulin sensitivity (84). Mouse lacking resistin show evidence of low blood glucose levels after fasting owing to reduced hepatic glucose production. This is in part mediated by 5'-adenosine monophosphate–activated protein kinase C activation and decreased expression of gluconeogenic enzymes in the liver (86). The original concept is still open to discussion following major controversial results concerning resistin expression in obese rodents and thiazolidinedione effects. Identification of the receptor and signaling pathways and analysis of the phenotypes resulting from deletion or overexpression of resistin in transgenic mice will help to further define the biological roles of this adipokine. Finally, the role of resistin in human insulin resistance remains quite controversial. A human homolog of murine resistin has been identified. However, because its sequence and expression in WAT are quite different from that in rodents, it is not yet clear whether this protein plays a significant role in the development of insulin resistance in humans (87).

## COAGULATION AND ABNORMAL FIBRINOLYSIS IN OBESITY

### Obesity and Prothrombotic Factors

Studies performed in obese and normal weight patients have shown that obese patients have elevated plasma concentrations of all prothrombotic factors—fibrinogen, von Willebrand factor (vWF) antigen and activity, and factor VII (FVII)—as compared to nonobese controls. In particular, plasma levels of the vWF antigen have been shown to be directly associated with central fat (as measured by waist circumference) independently of other metabolic and nonmetabolic variables (88).

A study performed in men has shown that obesity per se may account for higher concentrations of fibrinogen and vWF, with plasma levels of fibrinogen correlating with central fat (as measured by WHR) independently of metabolic factors (88). A further study conducted in men has shown that men with more visceral fat have significantly higher plasma fibrinogen and factor VIII clotting activity (89). However, in this study, fibrinogen and factor VIII clotting were not associated with abdominal visceral fat areas after controlling for plasma insulin levels, thus suggesting that hyperinsulinemia may be responsible for higher fibrinogen and factor VIII activity in patients with visceral obesity (89). In a recent epidemiological study, fibrinogen clustered with the inflammation factor rather than with procoagulant activity, supporting the position that fibrinogen principally reflects underlying inflammation rather than procoagulant potential (90). A number of clinical studies have shown that obese patients have an increase in coagulation mediated by a tissue factor that serves as a cell surface receptor for the activation of FVII and may be the major cellular initiator of the coagulation cascade (91). A recent study has demonstrated higher D-dimer levels in obese children and adolescents. In addition, cholesterol was found to be significantly associated with D-dimer, thus suggesting an unfavorable correlation between metabolic and hemostatic risk factors (92).

### Fibrinolysis and PAI-1

PAI-1 is the primary physiological inhibitor of plasminogen activation in vivo. Circulating PAI-1 levels are elevated in patients with coronary heart disease and may play an important role in the development of atherothrombosis by decreasing fibrin degradation. Increased PAI-1 expression can also directly influence vessel wall remodeling. Prospective cohort studies have underlined the association between increased plasma PAI-1 levels and the risk of coronary events.

In studies performed in obese and normal weight subjects (men and women), obese patients had higher plasma concentrations of PAI-1 (antigen and activity) as compared to nonobese controls, with plasma concentrations of PAI-1 antigen directly correlating with visceral fat independently of metabolic and nonmetabolic variables (89). Interestingly, it appears that all of the genetic influences for PAI-1 are more or less shared with those for triglycerides and BMI. These correlations could reflect genetic and/or environmental factors in common to PAI-1, triglycerides, and BMI (93).

PAI-1 4G/5G Gene Polymorphism and Obesity

PAI-1, a cardiovascular risk factor linked to insulin resistance, may be influenced by a 4G/5G gene polymorphism in disease states. A recent study performed in obese patients and lean normal subjects has shown that 4G/5G polymorphism is a determinant of PAI-1 antigen levels, which were highest in 4G/4G, intermediate in 4G/5G, and lowest in 5G/5G wild type genotype carriers. PAI-1 antigen levels were significantly associated with most of anthropometric and endocrine-metabolic parameters only in 4G allele obese carriers (94). In each genotype subset of patients with central, but not peripheral, obesity, PAI-1 antigen levels were significantly increased compared to their lean counterparts. Therefore, 4G/5G polymorphism may influence PAI-1 expression in obesity, with a crucial role in central but not peripheral adiposity (94). Because subjects with central obesity are at a high risk for CVD, the effects of the 4G/5G polymorphism on PAI-1 concentration may further enhance this risk.

## Obesity and Antithrombotic and Profibrinolytic Factors

Obese women are also characterized by higher plasma concentrations of antithrombotic factors such as tissue-type plasminogen activator (t-PA) antigen and protein C as compared to nonobese controls, although these factors are not independently correlated with the waist circumference or the WHR (88). Men with more visceral fat also have significantly higher plasma t-PA antigen (89). Moreover, plasma levels of inhibitors of the tissue factor pathway are higher in obese patients (95). The increase in all these antithrombotic factors may represent a protective response partly counteracting the increase in prothrombotic factors in these individuals. However, even though plasma t-PA antigen levels are higher in men with more visceral fat, t-PA activity is lower in these subjects (89). Concerning this point, obesity is also characterized by resistance to activated protein C, a protein with antithrombotic activity (96). Family history of DM-2 is an additional factor for a lower sensitivity to activated protein C due to obesity (97). Antithrombin III plasma levels are not different between obese and normal weight men and women (88). Therefore, all the described abnormalities in antithrombotic factors have an unfavorable global impact on coagulation balance.

## Role of Adipose Tissue in the Production of Prothrombotic Factors

Adipose tissue has the capacity to synthesize PAI-1, and both plasma and abdominal subcutaneous fat PAI-1 values are reduced significantly after weight reduction (98). Regarding fat distribution, subcutaneous adipose tissue has been shown to secrete greater amounts of PAI-1 and to have higher PAI-1 gene expression than visceral adipose tissue from the same obese individuals (99,100). Bearing in mind that subcutaneous adipose tissue is the largest fat depot, these findings may be important for coagulation abnormalities associated with obesity. Moreover, only the abdominal, but not the femoral, subcutaneous fat PAI-1 expression is a potential contributor to increased plasma PAI-1 in obesity (99,100). Noteworthy, within human adipose tissue, stromal cells appear to be the main cells involved in PAI-1 synthesis (99).

Adipose tissue produces elevated levels of cytokines such as TNFα and TGF-β; these cytokines may act in an autocrine and paracrine manner to alter gene expression in adipose tissue and to increase PAI-1 and tissue factor (101). The issue of whether adipose tissue directly contributes to plasma PAI-1 is still not resolved.

t-PA is the major plasminogen activator (PA) in preadipocytes (i.e., mouse 3T3-L1 preadipocytes), but it dramatically decreases with cell differentiation. On the other hand, urinary-type PA (u-PA) and PAI-1 increase with adipocyte differentiation (102). In particular, u-PA has been considered as a differentiation marker in 3T3-L1 cells.

## Insulin Resistance and Changes in Hemostatic Factors in Central Obesity

The insulin resistance syndrome, which is characterized by central obesity with visceral fat accumulation, is commonly considered as a major regulation of PAI-1 expression (94). Prospective studies demonstrating an association between increased plasma PAI-1 levels and the risk of coronary events have shown that the predictive capacity of PAI-1 disappears after adjustment for markers of insulin resistance. Moreover, amelioration for insulin resistance and reduction of insulin levels obtained by troglitzone enhance the activity of the fibrinolytic system in insulin-resistant DM-2 patients (103).

Both insulin and proinsulin increase the expression of PAI-1 in intra-abdominal adipose tissue 2.5-fold and 5.3-fold, respectively (104). Insulin continues to stimulate PAI-1 gene expression in insulin-resistant mice and adipocytes (105), thus explaining high PAI-1 levels in patients with visceral obesity and insulin resistance. However, insulin significantly decreases both u-PA and t-PA production (102).

Concentrations of the endothelial cell protein vWF are elevated in insulin-resistant states as well (106). Levels of a third coagulation factor, fibrinogen, are elevated in insulin-resistant subjects, an association that suggests a possible role for acute-phase cytokines in the abnormalities of coagulation and endothelial function (106). The plasma levels of IL-6 and TNFα, cytokines produced by adipose tissue, are higher in obese patients; because these substances induce insulin resistance, it has been proposed that IL-6 and TNFα may indirectly induce coagulopathy, endothelial dysfunction, and coronary heart disease (106).

Regarding platelet activity, recent data demonstrate that normal in vivo insulin action inhibits platelet interaction with collagen under conditions mimicking thrombus formation and decreases aggregation to several agonists (107). These platelet-inhibitory actions of insulin are absent or blunted in obese subjects. This provides a potential mechanism linking insulin resistance to atherothrombotic disease (107).

Hypertriglyceridemia is a further typical feature of the insulin resistance syndrome and upper body obesity. A pronounced increase in triglycerides may be associated with a hypercoagulable state, mainly due to significant elevation of factors VIII, VII, and PAI-1 (108). In experimental systems, increased expression and secretion of PAI-1 by hepatocytes and endothelial cell lines can be induced by insulin, proinsulin-like molecules, triglyceride-rich lipoproteins, and oxidized low-density lipoproteins, as well as by inducing insulin resistance in isolated hepatocytes (106).

## Endocrine Changes in Obesity and Thrombotic Risk

Cortisol secretion is, in general, higher in patients with central obesity. Moreover, experiments performed in human adipose tissue have demonstrated that dexamethasone induces PAI-1 activity and enhances PAI-1 stimulation by IL-1$\beta$ (109), thus suggesting that glucocorticoids may be involved in higher PAI-1 levels in patients with central obesity. Interestingly, dexamethasone significantly decreases both u-PA and t-PA production (102).

Excess adipose tissue is responsible for higher estrogen production. The induction of PAI-1 activity and PAI-1 mRNA expression by IL-1$\beta$ is attenuated by estrogens (109).

Hypertensive obese patients are characterized by higher levels of catecholamines and angiotensin II. Exposure of differentiated human adipocytes in primary culture to angiotensin II is associated to a dose- and time-dependent induction of PAI-1 release into the culture medium, and this stimulation is preceded by an augmentation in specific PAI-1 mRNA copies (110). This effect is mediated by Angiotensin II type 1 (AT$_1$) receptors. However, catecholamines have a negative effect on PAI-1 synthesis in cultured human adipose tissue (111).

In summary, these results indicate that multiple cytokines and hormones may be involved in the regulation of PAI-1 biosynthesis in human adipose tissue and suggest that there is a relationship between cytokines and these hormones. The association between these hormones may be of importance regarding the levels of PAI-1 observed in obesity and associated states.

Obese men have lower androgenicity that amplifies the cardiovascular risk in these patients. A decrease of testosterone levels is associated with higher plasma levels of prothrombotic factors such as fibrinogen and FVII plasma concentrations, irrespective of age, obesity, body fat distribution, and related metabolic parameters in men (109). However, obese women have higher androgenicity that also amplifies the cardiovascular risk in these patients. An elevation of testosterone levels in women is associated with higher plasma levels of PAI-1 antigen plasma levels, independent of age, obesity, body fat distribution, and related metabolic parameters. The paradigm that testosterone may directly influence PAI-1 production has never been tested in vitro. However, these results seem to suggest that this may be the case with different effects of this androgen, depending on the genes, sex, and/or the counteracting influence of estrogens.

### Leptin and Hemostasis

Human obesity is associated with elevated leptin concentrations in the circulation. Recent reports suggest that high leptin levels may directly promote arterial thrombosis in vivo and raise the possibility that elevated plasma levels of leptin may contribute to the risk of atherothrombotic complications in human obesity. Konstantinides et al. found that leptin-deficient ob/ob mice had prolonged times to thrombosis after arterial injury and that exogenously administered leptin corrected their phenotype in a dose-dependent manner (112). These effects appear to result from a direct, receptor-mediated effect of leptin on platelets because leptin stimulates the aggregation of murine (wild type and ob/ob) and human platelets, but it has no effect on platelets from leptin receptor-deficient db/db mice (112). Moreover, it has been shown that leptin concentrations that correspond to those in the circulation of obese individuals induce thrombotic tendency by acting on both platelet and endothelial cells (113). However, other authors have cast doubts on the role of leptin in platelet aggregation in human obesity and leptin deficiency (114). Finally, it has been suggested that leptin may have an autocrine direct effect on PAI-1 production in adipose tissue.

A very low caloric diet has been shown to significantly decrease plasma PAI-1 concentrations, but surprisingly to increase PAI-1 mRNA and protein abundance in subcutaneous adipose tissue, thus indicating that changes in subcutaneous adipose tissue PAI-1 expression are not involved in the decrease of plasma PAI-1 levels during very low calorie diets in obese subjects (115).

Concerning the quality of food, the optimal antithrombotic diet is a low-fat diet with a high content of foods rich in complex carbohydrates and dietary fiber. The dietary fatty acid composition has a profound effect on blood lipids, but seems of minor importance in the hemostatic system (116). However, dietary fish-oil supplementation (n-3) of polyunsaturated fatty acid led to the normalization of the hypercoagulable state in nondiabetic subjects with obesity, hypertension, and dyslipidemia (117).

### CONCLUSION

Accumulating evidence shows that the adipokines (such as IL-6 or TNFα), inflammatory markers (such as CRP), coagulation factors (such as fibrinogen,

FVII, FVIII, and vWF) and the fibrinolytic systems (such as PAI-1 and t-PA) are involved in the CVD process. However, the extreme complexity of all these systems, and the fact that factors sometimes correlate with each other, make it difficult to study the effects and determinants of each separate factor. Also, changes in levels of these proinflammatory, acute-phase molecules, adipocyte-derived molecules (such as leptin, adiponectin, or resistin) and procoagulants such as hemostatic and fibrinolytic factors were found to be involved to various degrees with obesity. The biological mechanism underlying these associations is not yet completely understood. Factors of the proinflammatory, acute-phase molecules and procoagulant systems could be directly linked to the insulin resistance syndrome or be a reflection of a larger underlying disease such as endothelial cell activation or chronic low-grade inflammation, both of which are associated with the atherosclerotic process and CVDs.

## REFERENCES

1. Flegal KM, Carroll MD, Ogden CL, Johnson CL. Prevalence and trends in obesity among US adults, 1999–2000. Jama 2002; 288(14):1723–1727.
2. Ford ES, Giles WH, Dietz WH. Prevalence of the metabolic syndrome among US adults: findings from the third National Health and Nutrition Examination Survey. Jama 2002; 287(3):356–359.
3. Kissebah AH, Vydelingum N, Murray R, et al. Relation of body fat distribution to metabolic complications of obesity. J Clin Endocrinol Metab 1982; 54(2):254–260.
4. Reaven GM. Banting lecture 1988. Role of insulin resistance in human disease. Diabetes 1988; 37(12):1595–1607.
5. Nieves DJ, Cnop M, Retzlaff B, et al. The atherogenic lipoprotein profile associated with obesity and insulin resistance is largely attributable to intra-abdominal fat. Diabetes 2003; 52(1):172–179.
6. Smith SR, Lovejoy JC, Greenway F, et al. Contributions of total body fat, abdominal subcutaneous adipose tissue compartments, and visceral adipose tissue to the metabolic complications of obesity. Metabolism 2001; 50(4):425–435.
7. Steppan CM, Lazar MA. Resistin and obesity-associated insulin resistance. Trends Endocrinol Metab 2002; 13(1):18–23.
8. Hasty AH, Shimano H, Osuga J, et al. Severe hypercholesterolemia, hypertriglyceridemia, and atherosclerosis in mice lacking both leptin and the low density lipoprotein receptor. J Biol Chem 2001; 276(40):37402–37408.
9. Wallace AM, McMahon AD, Packard CJ, et al. Plasma leptin and the risk of cardiovascular disease in the west of Scotland coronary prevention study (WOSCOPS). Circulation 2001; 104(25):3052–3056.
10. Okamoto Y, Kihara S, Ouchi N, et al. Adiponectin reduces atherosclerosis in apolipoprotein E-deficient mice. Circulation 2002; 106(22):2767–2770.
11. Ouchi N, Kihara S, Arita Y, et al. Novel modulator for endothelial adhesion molecules: adipocyte-derived plasma protein adiponectin. Circulation 1999; 100(25):2473–2476.

12. Funahashi T, Nakamura T, Shimomura I, et al. Role of adipocytokines on the pathogenesis of atherosclerosis in visceral obesity. Intern Med 1999; 38(2):202–206.
13. Weisberg SP, McCann D, Desai M, Rosenbaum M, Leibel RL, Ferrante AW, Jr. Obesity is associated with macrophage accumulation in adipose tissue. J Clin Invest 2003; 112(12):1796–1808.
14. Maachi M, Pieroni L, Bruckert E, et al. Systemic low-grade inflammation is related to both circulating and adipose tissue TNFalpha, leptin and IL-6 levels in obese women. Int J Obes Relat Metab Disord 2004; 28(8):993–997.
15. Bullo M, Garcia-Lorda P, Megias I, Salas-Salvado J. Systemic inflammation, adipose tissue tumor necrosis factor, and leptin expression. Obes Res 2003; 11(4):525–531.
16. Chiellini C, Santini F, Marsili A, et al. Serum haptoglobin: a novel marker of adiposity in humans. J Clin Endocrinol Metab 2004; 89(6):2678–2683.
17. Hotamisligil GS, Shargill NS, Spiegelman BM. Adipose expression of tumor necrosis factor-alpha: direct role in obesity-linked insulin resistance. Science 1993; 259(5091):87–91.
18. Yudkin JS. Adipose tissue, insulin action and vascular disease: inflammatory signals. Int J Obes Relat Metab Disord 2003; 27(Suppl 3):S25–S28.
19. Coppack SW. Pro-inflammatory cytokines and adipose tissue. Proc Nutr Soc 2001; 60(3):349–356.
20. Fain JN, Bahouth SW, Madan AK. Haptoglobin release by human adipose tissue in primary culture. J Lipid Res 2004; 45(3):536–542.
21. Fain JN, Madan AK, Hiler ML, Cheema P, Bahouth SW. Comparison of the release of adipokines by adipose tissue, adipose tissue matrix, and adipocytes from visceral and subcutaneous abdominal adipose tissues of obese humans. Endocrinology 2004; 145(5):2273–2282.
22. Prins JB, Niesler CU, Winterford CM, et al. Tumor necrosis factor-alpha induces apoptosis of human adipose cells. Diabetes 1997; 46(12):1939–1944.
23. Chiellini C, Bertacca A, Novelli SE, et al. Obesity modulates the expression of haptoglobin in the white adipose tissue via TNFalpha. J Cell Physiol 2002; 190(2):251–258.
24. Peeraully MR, Jenkins JR, Trayhurn P. NGF gene expression and secretion in white adipose tissue: regulation in 3T3-L1 adipocytes by hormones and inflammatory cytokines. Am J Physiol Endocrinol Metab 2004; 287(2):E331–E339.
25. Mohamed-Ali V, Goodrick S, Rawesh A, et al. Subcutaneous adipose tissue releases interleukin-6, but not tumor necrosis factor-alpha, in vivo. J Clin Endocrinol Metab 1997; 82(12):4196–4200.
26. Bastard JP, Jardel C, Bruckert E, et al. Elevated levels of interleukin 6 are reduced in serum and subcutaneous adipose tissue of obese women after weight loss. J Clin Endocrinol Metab 2000; 85(9):3338–3342.
27. Vozarova B, Weyer C, Hanson K, Tataranni PA, Bogardus C, Pratley RE. Circulating interleukin-6 in relation to adiposity, insulin action, and insulin secretion. Obes Res 2001; 9(7):414–417.
28. Wallenius K, Wallenius V, Sunter D, Dickson SL, Jansson JO. Intracerebroventricular interleukin-6 treatment decreases body fat in rats. Biochem Biophys Res Commun 2002; 293(1):560–565.

29. Bruun JM, Pedersen SB, Richelsen B. Interleukin-8 production in human adipose tissue. inhibitory effects of anti-diabetic compounds, the thiazolidinedione ciglitazone and the biguanide metformin. Horm Metab Res 2000; 32(11–12):537–541.
30. Bruun JM, Pedersen SB, Richelsen B. Regulation of interleukin 8 production and gene expression in human adipose tissue in vitro. J Clin Endocrinol Metab 2001; 86(3):1267–1273.
31. Straczkowski M, Dzienis-Straczkowska S, Stepien A, Kowalska I, Szelachowska M, Kinalska I. Plasma interleukin-8 concentrations are increased in obese subjects and related to fat mass and tumor necrosis factor-alpha system. J Clin Endocrinol Metab 2002; 87(10):4602–4606.
32. Esposito K, Pontillo A, Giugliano F, et al. Association of low interleukin-10 levels with the metabolic syndrome in obese women. J Clin Endocrinol Metab 2003; 88(3):1055–1058.
33. Starnes T, Broxmeyer HE, Robertson MJ, Hromas R. Cutting edge: IL-17D, a novel member of the IL-17 family, stimulates cytokine production and inhibits hemopoiesis. J Immunol 2002; 169(2):642–646.
34. Gabay C, Kushner I. Acute-phase proteins and other systemic responses to inflammation. N Engl J Med 1999; 340(6):448–454.
35. Visser M, Bouter LM, McQuillan GM, Wener MH, Harris TB. Elevated C-reactive protein levels in overweight and obese adults. Jama 1999; 282(22):2131–2135.
36. Pannacciulli N, Cantatore FP, Minenna A, Bellacicco M, Giorgino R, De Pergola G. C-reactive protein is independently associated with total body fat, central fat, and insulin resistance in adult women. Int J Obes Relat Metab Disord 2001; 25(10):1416–1420.
37. Tchernof A, Nolan A, Sites CK, Ades PA, Poehlman ET. Weight loss reduces C-reactive protein levels in obese postmenopausal women. Circulation 2002; 105(5):564–569.
38. Ouchi N, Kihara S, Funahashi T, et al. Reciprocal association of C-reactive protein with adiponectin in blood stream and adipose tissue. Circulation 2003; 107(5):671–674.
39. Heinrich PC, Castell JV, Andus T. Interleukin-6 and the acute phase response. Biochem J 1990; 265(3):621–636.
40. Yudkin JS, Kumari M, Humphries SE, Mohamed-Ali V. Inflammation, obesity, stress and coronary heart disease: is interleukin-6 the link? Atherosclerosis 2000; 148(2):209–214.
41. Mutch NJ, Wilson HM, Booth NA. Plasminogen activator inhibitor-1 and haemostasis in obesity. Proc Nutr Soc 2001; 60(3):341–347.
42. Lundgren CH, Brown SL, Nordt TK, Sobel BE, Fujii S. Elaboration of type-1 plasminogen activator inhibitor from adipocytes. A potential pathogenetic link between obesity and cardiovascular disease. Circulation 1996; 93(1):106–110.
43. Eriksson P, Reynisdottir S, Lonnqvist F, Stemme V, Hamsten A, Arner P. Adipose tissue secretion of plasminogen activator inhibitor-1 in non-obese and obese individuals. Diabetologia 1998; 41(1):65–71.
44. Cigolini M, Tonoli M, Borgato L, et al. Expression of plasminogen activator inhibitor-1 in human adipose tissue: a role for TNF-alpha? Atherosclerosis 1999; 143(1):81–90.

45. Alessi MC, Bastelica D, Morange P, et al. Plasminogen activator inhibitor 1, transforming growth factor-beta1, and BMI are closely associated in human adipose tissue during morbid obesity. Diabetes 2000; 49(8):1374–1380.
46. Samad F, Yamamoto K, Loskutoff DJ. Distribution and regulation of plasminogen activator inhibitor-1 in murine adipose tissue in vivo. Induction by tumor necrosis factor-alpha and lipopolysaccharide. J Clin Invest 1996; 97(1):37–46.
47. Asleh R, Guetta J, Kalet-Litman S, Miller-Lotan R, Levy AP. Haptoglobin genotype- and diabetes-dependent differences in iron-mediated oxidative stress in vitro and in vivo. Circ Res 2005; 96(4):435–441.
48. Levy AP, Roguin A, Hochberg I, et al. Haptoglobin phenotype and vascular complications in patients with diabetes. N Engl J Med 2000; 343(13):969–970.
49. Friedrichs WE, Navarijo-Ashbaugh AL, Bowman BH, Yang F. Expression and inflammatory regulation of haptoglobin gene in adipocytes. Biochem Biophys Res Commun 1995; 209(1):250–256.
50. Kratchmarova I, Kalume DE, Blagoev B, et al. A proteomic approach for identification of secreted proteins during the differentiation of 3T3-L1 preadipocytes to adipocytes. Mol Cell Proteomics 2002; 1(3):213–222.
51. Chinetti G, Fruchart JC, Staels B. Peroxisome proliferator-activated receptors and inflammation: from basic science to clinical applications. Int J Obes Relat Metab Disord 2003; 27(Suppl 3):S41–S45.
52. Moller DE, Berger JP. Role of PPARs in the regulation of obesity-related insulin sensitivity and inflammation. Int J Obes Relat Metab Disord 2003; 27(Suppl 3):S17–S21.
53. Uhlar CM, Whitehead AS. Serum amyloid A, the major vertebrate acute-phase reactant. Eur J Biochem 1999; 265(2):501–523.
54. Lin Y, Rajala MW, Berger JP, Moller DE, Barzilai N, Scherer PE. Hyperglycemia-induced production of acute phase reactants in adipose tissue. J Biol Chem 2001; 276(45):42077–42083.
55. Ahima RS, Flier JS. Leptin. Annu Rev Physiol 2000; 62:413–437.
56. Considine RV, Sinha MK, Heiman ML, et al. Serum immunoreactive-leptin concentrations in normal-weight and obese humans. N Engl J Med 1996; 334(5):292–295.
57. Fantuzzi G, Faggioni R. Leptin in the regulation of immunity, inflammation, and hematopoiesis. J Leukoc Biol 2000; 68(4):437–446.
58. Lord GM, Matarese G, Howard JK, Baker RJ, Bloom SR, Lechler RI. Leptin modulates the T-cell immune response and reverses starvation-induced immunosuppression. Nature 1998; 394(6696):897–901.
59. Farooqi IS, Matarese G, Lord GM, et al. Beneficial effects of leptin on obesity, T cell hyporesponsiveness, and neuroendocrine/metabolic dysfunction of human congenital leptin deficiency. J Clin Invest 2002; 110(8):1093–1103.
60. Zarkesh-Esfahani H, Pockley G, Metcalfe RA, et al. High-dose leptin activates human leukocytes via receptor expression on monocytes. J Immunol 2001; 167(8):4593–4599.
61. Caldefie-Chezet F, Poulin A, Tridon A, Sion B, Vasson MP. Leptin: a potential regulator of polymorphonuclear neutrophil bactericidal action? J Leukoc Biol 2001; 69(3):414–418.

62. Yamagishi SI, Edelstein D, Du XL, Kaneda Y, Guzman M, Brownlee M. Leptin induces mitochondrial superoxide production and monocyte chemoattractant protein-1 expression in aortic endothelial cells by increasing fatty acid oxidation via protein kinase A. J Biol Chem 2001; 276(27):25096–25100.
63. Bouloumie A, Marumo T, Lafontan M, Busse R. Leptin induces oxidative stress in human endothelial cells. Faseb J 1999; 13(10):1231–1238.
64. Ziccardi P, Nappo F, Giugliano G, et al. Reduction of inflammatory cytokine concentrations and improvement of endothelial functions in obese women after weight loss over one year. Circulation 2002; 105(7):804–809.
65. Loffreda S, Yang SQ, Lin HZ, et al. Leptin regulates proinflammatory immune responses. Faseb J 1998; 12(1):57–65.
66. Hukshorn CJ, Lindeman JH, Toet KH, et al. Leptin and the proinflammatory state associated with human obesity. J Clin Endocrinol Metab 2004; 89(4):1773–1778.
67. Westerterp-Plantenga MS, Saris WH, Hukshorn CJ, Campfield LA. Effects of weekly administration of pegylated recombinant human OB protein on appetite profile and energy metabolism in obese men. Am J Clin Nutr 2001; 74(4):426–434.
68. Berg AH, Combs TP, Scherer PE. ACRP30/adiponectin: an adipokine regulating glucose and lipid metabolism. Trends Endocrinol Metab 2002; 13(2):84–89.
69. Arita Y, Kihara S, Ouchi N, et al. Paradoxical decrease of an adipose-specific protein, adiponectin, in obesity. Biochem Biophys Res Commun 1999; 257(1):79–83.
70. Weyer C, Funahashi T, Tanaka S, et al. Hypoadiponectinemia in obesity and type 2 diabetes: close association with insulin resistance and hyperinsulinemia. J Clin Endocrinol Metab 2001; 86(5):1930–1935.
71. Hotta K, Funahashi T, Bodkin NL, et al. Circulating concentrations of the adipocyte protein adiponectin are decreased in parallel with reduced insulin sensitivity during the progression to type 2 diabetes in rhesus monkeys. Diabetes 2001; 50(5):1126–1133.
72. Matsubara M, Maruoka S, Katayose S. Decreased plasma adiponectin concentrations in women with dyslipidemia. J Clin Endocrinol Metab 2002; 87(6):2764–2769.
73. Zoccali C, Mallamaci F, Tripepi G, et al. Adiponectin, metabolic risk factors, and cardiovascular events among patients with end-stage renal disease. J Am Soc Nephrol 2002; 13(1):134–141.
74. Maeda N, Takahashi M, Funahashi T, et al. PPARgamma ligands increase expression and plasma concentrations of adiponectin, an adipose-derived protein. Diabetes 2001; 50(9):2094–2099.
75. Yang WS, Jeng CY, Wu TJ, et al. Synthetic peroxisome proliferator-activated receptor-gamma agonist, rosiglitazone, increases plasma levels of adiponectin in type 2 diabetic patients. Diabetes Care 2002; 25(2):376–380.
76. Yamauchi T, Kamon J, Waki H, et al. The fat-derived hormone adiponectin reverses insulin resistance associated with both lipoatrophy and obesity. Nat Med 2001; 7(8):941–946.
77. Combs TP, Berg AH, Obici S, Scherer PE, Rossetti L. Endogenous glucose production is inhibited by the adipose-derived protein Acrp30. J Clin Invest 2001; 108(12):1875–1881.

78. Ouchi N, Kihara S, Arita Y, et al. Adiponectin, an adipocyte-derived plasma protein, inhibits endothelial NF-kappaB signaling through a cAMP-dependent pathway. Circulation 2000; 102(11):1296–1301.
79. Ouchi N, Kihara S, Arita Y, et al. Adipocyte-derived plasma protein, adiponectin, suppresses lipid accumulation and class A scavenger receptor expression in human monocyte-derived macrophages. Circulation 2001; 103(8):1057–1063.
80. Okamoto Y, Arita Y, Nishida M, et al. An adipocyte-derived plasma protein, adiponectin, adheres to injured vascular walls. Horm Metab Res 2000; 32(2): 47–50.
81. Matsuda M, Shimomura I, Sata M, et al. Role of adiponectin in preventing vascular stenosis. The missing link of adipo-vascular axis. J Biol Chem 2002; 277(40):37487–37491.
82. Engeli S, Feldpausch M, Gorzelniak K, et al. Association between adiponectin and mediators of inflammation in obese women. Diabetes 2003; 52(4):942–927.
83. Steppan CM, Bailey ST, Bhat S, et al. The hormone resistin links obesity to diabetes. Nature 2001; 409(6818):307–312.
84. Rajala MW, Lin Y, Ranalletta M, et al. Cell type-specific expression and coregulation of murine resistin and resistin-like molecule-alpha in adipose tissue. Mol Endocrinol 2002; 16(8):1920–1930.
85. Kim KH, Lee K, Moon YS, Sul HS. A cysteine-rich adipose tissue-specific secretory factor inhibits adipocyte differentiation. J Biol Chem 2001; 276(14):11252–11256.
86. Banerjee RR, Rangwala SM, Shapiro JS, et al. Regulation of fasted blood glucose by resistin. Science 2004; 303(5661):1195–1198.
87. Savage DB, Sewter CP, Klenk ES, et al. Resistin / Fizz3 expression in relation to obesity and peroxisome proliferator-activated receptor-gamma action in humans. Diabetes 2001; 50(10):2199–2202.
88. Mertens I, Van Gaal LF. Obesity, haemostasis and the fibrinolytic system. Obes Rev 2002; 3(2):85–101.
89. Cigolini M, Targher G, Bergamo Andreis IA, Tonoli M, Agostino G, De Sandre G. Visceral fat accumulation and its relation to plasma hemostatic factors in healthy men. Arterioscler Thromb Vasc Biol 1996; 16(3):368–374.
90. Sakkinen PA, Wahl P, Cushman M, Lewis MR, Tracy RP. Clustering of procoagulation, inflammation, and fibrinolysis variables with metabolic factors in insulin resistance syndrome. Am J Epidemiol 2000; 152(10):897–907.
91. Kario K, Matsuo T, Kobayashi H, Matsuo M, Sakata T, Miyata T. Activation of tissue factor-induced coagulation and endothelial cell dysfunction in non-insulin-dependent diabetic patients with microalbuminuria. Arterioscler Thromb Vasc Biol 1995; 15(8):1114–1120.
92. Gallistl S, Sudi KM, Borkenstein M, Weinhandl G, Zotter H, Muntean W. Correlation between cholesterol, soluble P-selectin, and D-dimer in obese children and adolescents. Blood Coagul Fibrinolysis 2000; 11(8):755–760.
93. Hong Y, Pedersen NL, Egberg N, de Faire U. Moderate genetic influences on plasma levels of plasminogen activator inhibitor-1 and evidence of genetic and environmental influences shared by plasminogen activator inhibitor-1, triglycerides, and body mass index. Arterioscler Thromb Vasc Biol 1997; 17(11):2776–2782.

94. Sartori MT, Vettor R, De Pergola G, et al. Role of the 4G/5G polymorphism of PaI-1 gene promoter on PaI-1 levels in obese patients: influence of fat distribution and insulin-resistance. Thromb Haemost 2001; 86(5):1161–1169.

95. Vambergue A, Rugeri L, Gaveriaux V, et al. Factor VII, tissue factor pathway inhibitor, and monocyte tissue factor in diabetes mellitus: influence of type of diabetes, obesity index, and age. Thromb Res 2001; 101(5):367–375.

96. Lowe GD, Rumley A, Woodward M, Reid E, Rumley J. Activated protein C resistance and the FV:R506Q mutation in a random population sample–associations with cardiovascular risk factors and coagulation variables. Thromb Haemost 1999; 81(6):918–924.

97. Pannacciulli N, De Mitrio V, Sciaraffia M, Giorgino R, De Pergola G. A family history of type 2 diabetes is associated with lower sensitivity to activated protein C in overweight and obese premenopausal women. Thromb Haemost 2001; 86(6):1593–1594.

98. Mavri A, Alessi MC, Bastelica D, et al. Subcutaneous abdominal, but not femoral fat expression of plasminogen activator inhibitor-1 (PAI-1) is related to plasma PAI-1 levels and insulin resistance and decreases after weight loss. Diabetologia 2001; 44(11):2025–2031.

99. Alessi MC, Morange P, Juhan-Vague I. Fat cell function and fibrinolysis. Horm Metab Res 2000; 32(11–12):504–508.

100. Eriksson P, Van Harmelen V, Hoffstedt J, et al. Regional variation in plasminogen activator inhibitor-1 expression in adipose tissue from obese individuals. Thromb Haemost 2000; 83(4):545–548.

101. Loskutoff DJ, Fujisawa K, Samad F. The fat mouse. A powerful genetic model to study hemostatic gene expression in obesity/NIDDM. Ann N Y Acad Sci 2000; 902:272–81; discussion 81–82.

102. Seki T, Miyasu T, Noguchi T, et al. Reciprocal regulation of tissue-type and urokinase-type plasminogen activators in the differentiation of murine preadipocyte line 3T3-L1 and the hormonal regulation of fibrinolytic factors in the mature adipocytes. J Cell Physiol 2001; 189(1):72–78.

103. Kruszynska YT, Yu JG, Olefsky JM, Sobel BE. Effects of troglitazone on blood concentrations of plasminogen activator inhibitor 1 in patients with type 2 diabetes and in lean and obese normal subjects. Diabetes 2000; 49(4):633–639.

104. Nordt TK, Bode C, Sobel BE. Stimulation in vivo of expression of intra-abdominal adipose tissue plasminogen activator inhibitor Type I by proinsulin. Diabetologia 2001; 44(9):1121–1124.

105. Samad F, Pandey M, Bell PA, Loskutoff DJ. Insulin continues to induce plasminogen activator inhibitor 1 gene expression in insulin-resistant mice and adipocytes. Mol Med 2000; 6(8):680–692.

106. Yudkin JS. Abnormalities of coagulation and fibrinolysis in insulin resistance. Evidence for a common antecedent? Diabetes Care 1999; 22(Suppl 3): C25–C30.

107. Westerbacka J, Yki-Jarvinen H, Turpeinen A, et al. Inhibition of platelet-collagen interaction: an in vivo action of insulin abolished by insulin resistance in obesity. Arterioscler Thromb Vasc Biol 2002; 22(1):167–172.

108. Chan P, Huang TY, Shieh SM, Lin TS, Tsai CW. Thrombophilia in Patients with Hypertriglyceridemia. J Thromb Thrombolysis 1997; 4(3/4):425–429.

109. He G, Pedersen SB, Bruun JM, Richelsen B. Regulation of plasminogen activitor inhibitor-1 in human adipose tissue: interaction between cytokines, cortisol and estrogen. Horm Metab Res 2000; 32(11–12):515–520.
110. Skurk T, Lee YM, Hauner H. Angiotensin II and its metabolites stimulate PAI-1 protein release from human adipocytes in primary culture. Hypertension 2001; 37(5):1336–1340.
111. Halleux CM, Declerck PJ, Tran SL, Detry R, Brichard SM. Hormonal control of plasminogen activator inhibitor-1 gene expression and production in human adipose tissue: stimulation by glucocorticoids and inhibition by catecholamines. J Clin Endocrinol Metab 1999; 84(11):4097–4105.
112. Konstantinides S, Schafer K, Loskutoff DJ. The prothrombotic effects of leptin possible implications for the risk of cardiovascular disease in obesity. Ann N Y Acad Sci 2001; 947:134–41; discussion 41–42.
113. Maruyama I, Nakata M, Yamaji K. Effect of leptin in platelet and endothelial cells. Obesity and arterial thrombosis. Ann N Y Acad Sci 2000; 902:315–319.
114. Ozata M, Avcu F, Durmus O, Yilmaz I, Ozdemir IC, Yalcin A. Leptin does not play a major role in platelet aggregation in obesity and leptin deficiency. Obes Res 2001; 9(10):627–630.
115. Bastard JP, Vidal H, Jardel C, et al. Subcutaneous adipose tissue expression of plasminogen activator inhibitor-1 gene during very low calorie diet in obese subjects. Int J Obes Relat Metab Disord 2000; 24(1):70–74.
116. Marckmann P. Dietary treatment of thrombogenic disorders related to the metabolic syndrome. Br J Nutr 2000; 83(Suppl 1):S121–S126.
117. Yosefy C, Viskoper JR, Laszt A, et al. The effect of fish oil on hypertension, plasma lipids and hemostasis in hypertensive, obese, dyslipidemic patients with and without diabetes mellitus. Prostaglandins Leukot Essent Fatty Acids 1999; 61(2):83–87.

# 7

# Obstructive Sleep Apnea

## Sanjay R. Patel

*Case Western Reserve University,
Cleveland, Ohio, U.S.A.*

## Robert B. Fogel

*Division of Sleep Medicine, Brigham and Women's Hospital,
Boston, Massachusetts, U.S.A.*

## INTRODUCTION

### Definition of Obstructive Sleep Apnea

Over the last 20 years, there has been increasing recognition by the medical community of obstructive sleep apnea (OSA) as a relatively common disorder, with important clinical consequences for afflicted individuals. In this chapter, we will review the pathophysiology of OSA, along with its clinical consequences and appropriate treatment. We will then discuss the relationship between obesity and sleep apnea. Finally, we will conclude with an in-depth discussion of the potential mechanisms by which OSA may contribute to cardiovascular disease, including mechanisms by which it may overlap, or interact directly, with the effects of obesity.

The International Classification of Sleep Disorders Manual describes OSA syndrome as a disorder " .... characterized by repetitive episodes of upper airway obstruction that occur during sleep, usually associated with a reduction in blood oxygen saturation. Associated features include loud snoring, fragmented sleep (because repetitive airway obstruction, hypoxia, and hypercapnia lead to recurrent arousal from sleep to open the upper

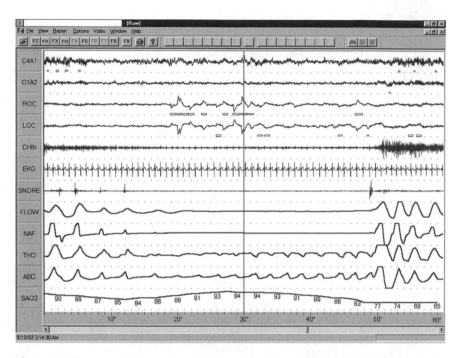

**Figure 1** Two epochs (one minute) of an overnight polysomnogram demonstrating OSA. Note the reduction in airflow followed by complete cessation of flow (apnea). Respiratory effort continues as demonstrated by movement of the thorax and abdomen although this movement becomes paradoxical (out of phase) due to the obstructed airway. The apnea is followed by oxygen desaturation and is terminated by cortical arousal (increased high frequency activity in EEG and EMG leads) at 48 seconds. With arousal, airflow is restored and thoracic and abdominal movement become in-phase again. C4A1, O1A2: EEG. *Abbreviations*: EEG, electroencephalography; ROC, LOC: right and left electro-oculography; CHIN, chin EMG; EKG, electrocardiography; EMG, electromyography; SNORE, microphone to detect snoring; FLOW, airflow measured by oronasal thermistor; NAF, nasal pressure tracing; THO, thoracic movement; ABD, abdominal movement; SAO$_2$, oxygen saturation; OSA, obstructive sleep apnea.

airway) and daytime sleepiness." The diagnosis is typically confirmed by overnight polysomnography during which sleep is recorded while breathing, respiratory effort, oxygen saturation, and the electrocardiogram are simultaneously monitored (Fig. 1). Upper airway obstruction can be complete, in which case there is no airflow (obstructive apnea), or partial, during which there is a substantial reduction in, but not a complete cessation of, airflow (obstructive hypopnea). Patients with sleep apnea are typically characterized by an apnea–hypopnea index (AHI) or respiratory disturbance index (RDI), which is the average number of apneas plus hypopneas per hour of sleep.

## Pathophysiology and Treatment

The principal event in OSA is recurrent collapse of the pharyngeal airway, which characteristically occurs at sleep onset and during rapid eye movement (REM) sleep (1). Although there is continued respiratory effort, this pharyngeal closure prevents effective ventilation. Both apneas and hypopneas lead to substantial hypoxia and hypercapnia with arousal from sleep generally being required to reestablish airway patency and resumption of ventilation. This cycle of recurrent pharyngeal collapse with subsequent arousal from sleep leads to the primary symptom of OSA—daytime somnolence.

Collapse of the pharyngeal airway occurs between the choanae (back of the nasal septum) and the epiglottis, typically behind the soft palate, the tongue, or a combination of the two (2,3). This event is likely a product of deficient pharyngeal anatomy and state-related influences on pharyngeal muscle function. The human pharyngeal airway is relatively unique in that it lacks the rigid bony support found in most other mammals. Therefore, patency of the upper airway depends on a balance of forces between the upper airway muscles dilating the pharynx and the negative intraluminal airway pressure generated by the respiratory pump muscles during inspiration tending to collapse it. In addition, an individual's dependence on pharyngeal dilator muscle activity is likely a product of the intrinsic anatomy and collapsibility of their airway. Individuals with an anatomically large airway may be less dependent on muscles to maintain airway patency than someone with an anatomically small airway.

There is abundant evidence to suggest anatomical differences in the pharyngeal airway between patients with OSA and controls. Cephalometric X rays were among the earliest techniques used to image the pharyngeal airway and showed OSA patients to have a reduction in the length of the mandible, an inferiorly positioned hyoid bone, and a retroposition of the maxilla (4). Using more sophisticated imaging techniques including computed tomography (CT) scanning, acoustic reflection, and, most recently, magnetic resonance imaging, a number of investigators have shown apnea patients to have a smaller airway lumen than controls (5–9). Recent studies by Schwab et al. have also demonstrated a number of soft-tissue abnormalities in apnea patients, including an increase in the volume of the tongue, soft-palate, parapharyngeal fat pads, and the lateral walls surrounding the pharynx (9). The observed variability in airway size is likely determined by genetic influences on bony structure, tongue size, tonsillar tissue, etc. as well as acquired factors such as obesity. Obesity may affect pharyngeal size by direct deposition of fat around the airway or by altering muscle orientation and function.

Although the muscles responsible for maintaining upper airway patency and the mechanisms controlling their function are at best incompletely understood, certain generalizations can be made. The muscles of primary importance fall into three groups: (a) the muscles influencing hyoid bone position (geniohyoid, sternohyoid, etc.), (b) the muscle of the tongue (genioglossus), and (c) the muscles of the palate (tensor palatini, levator palatini, etc.). The activity of many of these muscles is increased during inspiration thus stiffening and dilating the upper airway and acting to counteract the collapsing influence of negative airway pressure. These are referred to as inspiratory phasic upper airway muscles with the genioglossus being the best studied such muscle. The activity of these muscles is substantially reduced (although not eliminated) during expiration (tonic activation) when pressure inside the airway becomes positive, and there is lesser tendency for collapse. Other muscles, such as tensor palatini, do not consistently demonstrate inspiratory phasic activity but instead maintain a relatively constant level of activity throughout the respiratory cycle. These are called tonic or postural muscles and are also thought to play a role in the maintenance of airway patency. The activity of the pharyngeal dilator muscles can be influenced by a number of physiological stimuli. Chemical stimulation [rising partial pressure of carbon dioxide ($PaCO_2$) or falling partial pressure of oxygen ($PaO_2$)] can substantially augment the activity of these muscles. Perhaps more importantly, negative pressure in the pharynx (which would tend to collapse the airway) markedly activates these muscles, which in turn counteract this collapsing influence (10–12). This response to negative pressure is likely driven by pressure or stretch-sensitive receptors because it can be substantially attenuated by the application of topical anesthesia (13). It is this receptor mechanism that is likely activated in an individual with an anatomically small airway in response to greater negative pressure, airway stretch, or collapse itself.

In the apnea patient with an anatomically small airway, there is evidence that this negative pressure reflex is activated, leading to augmented dilator muscle activity as a neuromuscular compensatory mechanism. This has been shown for genioglossus, which in apnea patients functions at nearly 40% of its maximal capacity during wakefulness, while in control subjects the muscle functions at only about 12% of maximum (14,15). Thus, were it not for this increased activity of the pharyngeal dilator muscles, the airway of the apnea patient would substantially narrow or collapse even during wakefulness. Sleep has a measurable effect on airway patency in everyone. In the apnea patient, as stated, there is a reflex-driven augmentation of dilator muscle activity compensating for deficient anatomy during wakefulness. Several studies indicate a marked attenuation or loss of this reflex mechanism even in normal subjects during sleep (16,17). With the loss of this reflex, the neuromuscular compensatory mechanism of the apnea patient is lost leading to falling dilator muscle activity and airway collapse. In normal individuals, who are not dependent on this reflex-driven dilator muscle activity, this loss may be associated with a rise in upper airway resistance, but patency is maintained.

Current therapeutic strategies for OSA are aimed at either enlarging the pharyngeal airway, and thereby rendering it less susceptible to collapse, or using positive airway pressure to pneumatically splint the airway during sleep. Although effective therapy along these lines does exist, patient acceptance of such therapy is often less than optimal, and new therapeutic approaches are continually being sought. Because obesity is the single most important predictor of apnea, weight loss would be expected to lead to an increase in upper airway dimensions and an improvement in sleep-disordered breathing. Indeed, it has been shown that weight loss can lead to a decrease in the RDI, reduced blood pressure, improved sleep efficiency, decreased snoring, improved oxygenation, and a decreased requirement for continuous positive airway pressure (CPAP) (18). The most dramatic results have been reported with surgical weight loss, with the largest series reported by Sugerman et al. who evaluated 36 patients following gastric reduction surgery (either banding or stapling) with a typical weight loss of between 40 and 50 kg. Sleep apnea was improved in all subjects and was cured (AHI<10) in many (19,20). Less dramatic weight loss by medical means has also been shown to be beneficial. With moderate weight loss (10 kg or 10% of the body weight), the AHI decreased by approximately 50% in one series of 15 patients (21,22).

Since its initial description in 1981, CPAP, applied via a nasal mask, has been the primary therapy for patients with OSA (23,24). The device consists of a mask attached to a blower unit that maintains positive airway pressure at designated levels by alterations in flow, acting as a pneumatic splint on the pharyngeal airway (25,26). The prescribed CPAP pressure is typically determined in the sleep laboratory as the pressure that is required to eliminate all snoring and sleep-disordered breathing, during all sleep stages, in all body positions. There is strong evidence supporting improvements in measures of both daytime sleepiness and neurocognitive function with nasal CPAP. In the largest randomized, placebo-controlled trial, Jenkinson et al. found that nasal CPAP led to greater improvements in sleepiness and quality-of-life measurements (27). (Effects of CPAP on cardiovascular/metabolic outcomes are discussed below.) Despite CPAP's near-universal effectiveness in treating sleep apnea, it suffers from major compliance limitations. These problems primarily relate to the facial interface (mask) and pressure required to prevent airway collapse, with many patients being intolerant of therapy (28). When assessed objectively, compliance with CPAP ranges from 50% to 70%, with the most important predictor of compliance being the patient's perception of improvement with CPAP (29,30).

## Epidemiology

Recent research has demonstrated how common sleep-disordered breathing truly is. In a survey of Wisconsin State employees less than 65 years of age,

Young et al. found a prevalence of sleep-disordered breathing (RDI > 5) of 9% in women and 24% in men. Defining the OSA syndrome as an RDI > 5 plus a complaint of daytime somnolence, Young observed a prevalence of 2% and 4% in middle-aged women and men, respectively (31). Other epidemiological studies have provided widely varying estimates, revealing the importance of the RDI cutoff used to define the syndrome in estimating prevalence (32,33). The above data suggest that OSA is quite common in middle-aged adults with a likely prevalence of 2% to 4%, which is similar to asthma or diabetes mellitus.

Male gender is an important risk factor for the development of sleep-disordered breathing. In studies of sleep clinic populations, the ratio of men to women is as high as 10:1 (34). However, in community-based samples, this ratio seems to be closer to 2–3:1 (35). This difference may in part be due to referral bias because women are less likely to report snoring, a cardinal symptom in OSA (36). This gender difference in the incidence of apnea is most noticeable between the ages of 25 and 55, and becomes less evident after menopause (35). As well, studies have reported that women typically need to become much more obese than men to develop clinically important sleep apnea (37). The reasons for this gender effect remain poorly understood but could result from differences in body fat distribution (or other influences on upper airway anatomy), the control of ventilation, and/or the physiology of the pharyngeal airway dilator muscles.

Increasing age appears to be an independent risk factor for the development of apnea in the majority of the epidemiological studies described above. As with gender, the explanation for this aging effect remains unknown. Other risk factors for OSA are likely less prominent but do exist. Although uncommon, craniofacial abnormalities such as retrognathia, micrognathia, and macroglossia all predispose to the development of sleep apnea (38,39).

## OSA AND OBESITY

### Obesity as a Risk Factor for OSA

OSA and obesity commonly occur together, with some studies suggesting that 25% to 75% of obese subjects suffer from OSA. Furthermore, those obese individuals with the greatest cardiovascular risk, those with *Syndrome X* (the combination of visceral obesity, insulin resistance, hypertension, and dyslipidemia), are those most likely to suffer from sleep-disordered breathing as well. The prevalence of sleep apnea in the syndrome mentioned above is so common that one group has termed this combination *Syndrome Z* (40). Numerous studies have also confirmed that obesity is the strongest risk factor for the development of OSA. A body mass index (BMI) greater than 28 kg/m$^2$ is found in 60% to 90% of patients diagnosed with apnea (41), and the relative risk of sleep apnea from obesity (BMI>29 kg/m$^2$) is as great as 10 to

14 (42,43). In the Wisconsin Sleep Study, a 1 standard deviation increase in BMI was associated with a 4.5-fold increased risk of OSA (31). Furthermore, in a prospective study of community dwelling individuals, Redline found that those in the highest BMI quartile had a much greater increase in their AHI over five years than did those in the lowest quartile (44).

However, the relationship between measures of obesity and severity of OSA is only moderate and not linear. In fact, several studies of obese subjects have shown that the severity of apnea varies widely in these subjects. In a group of 250 morbidly obese men and women (mean BMI 45 kg/m$^2$), Vgontzas et al. found that only 50% of the men and 8.5% of the women had more than 30 epsiodes of apneas + hypopneas over the course of the night (an AHI>5). There was no difference in mean BMI in the group with and without apnea (45). Similarly, Rajala et al. found no difference in mean BMI or neck circumference in a group of morbidly obese subjects (BMI = 50 kg/m$^2$) with and without sleep-disordered breathing (46). Finally, in a large population of patients referred to a sleep laboratory in Israel, the correlation between BMI and AHI, while significant, was found to be only moderate ($r^2 = 0.23$) and weakened when the group was restricted to individuals who were overweight ($r^2 = 0.17$) (47). Taken together, these data suggest that other factors must interact with obesity in the development of OSA. Such features might include variability in upper airway anatomy (fat deposition), specific tissue characteristics of the upper airway, neuromuscular control of pharyngeal dilator muscles, lung volume, or ventilatory control mechanisms.

### Central Obesity

Several investigators have also suggested that upper body or truncal obesity may be a better predictor of sleep apnea than BMI, perhaps by signifying greater fat deposition in the pharynx (48). More recently, neck circumference and waist-to-hip ratio (WHR) have been recognized as better predictors of sleep apnea than previous measures and may be especially useful in predicting risk in thin subjects (49). In a study of obese women with polycystic ovarian syndrome and age/BMI matched controls, we found WHR to be a much better predictor of AHI than BMI (50). Although the mechanism(s) by which central obesity may affect upper airway patency is not well understood, a number of possibilities exist. There may be direct effects on the pharyngeal airway, such as increased neck circumference and pharyngeal fat altering collapsibility of the airway. Alternatively, upper body obesity may indirectly affect the upper airway by lowering lung volume (which increases airway collapsibility) or by increasing total respiratory system resistance.

### Pharyngeal Abnormalities in Obesity

Obesity may predispose to OSA by leading to abnormalities in upper airway anatomy or pharyngeal muscle function. As stated previously, numerous studies have shown the pharyngeal airway of the apnea patient to be smaller than that of controls, although these studies did not typically include weight-matched controls. Several studies have suggested that increased fat deposition around the airway, and/or total fat deposition in the neck is greater in apnea patients (7,48). In a study of morbidly obese subjects being evaluated for gastric bypass surgery, we found that while airway size (area or volume) was not different between those with and without OSA, the shape of the airway in those with OSA was oriented with its major axis in the A–P dimension rather than horizontally, which may predispose to collapse (51). Furthermore, we found that those with OSA had greater airway collapse during voluntary changes in resting lung volume. By measuring genioglossal muscle function, we found no evidence that obesity impaired pharyngeal dilator muscle activity or its response to negative pressure. With weight loss, we found a decrease in resting genioglossal muscle activity as apnea improved, suggesting less need for neuromuscular compensation. Taken together, these data strongly suggest that the primary effect of obesity on the upper airway is anatomical in nature and that local effects may be more important than global measures of obesity.

## OSA as a Risk Factor for Obesity

While obesity is clearly a strong risk factor for OSA, there is some evidence to suggest that OSA may predispose to obesity as well. Individuals with sleep apnea have serum leptin levels elevated beyond that expected for their level of obesity (52–54). Leptin, a hormone produced by adipocytes, is an important regulator of long-term weight, by stimulating satiety centers in the hypothalamus. Obesity in humans is associated with elevated levels of leptin suggesting that there may be resistance to its effects in the central nervous system (CNS) (55). The heightened level of leptin found in OSA has been postulated to represent a further resistance to the anorexic effects of leptin and thus a predilection for further weight gain. The mechanism for leptin resistance in OSA is unclear but appears to be reversible, because treatment with CPAP results in reductions to a level comparable to that in BMI-matched controls (54,56,57). Besides potentially leading to increased weight, elevated leptin levels may also have adverse cardiovascular effects. Leptin is known to produce sympathetic activation, and chronic leptin infusion has been associated with elevations in both sympathetic activity and blood pressure (58,59).

Besides these metabolic effects, OSA has neuropsychological effects that may predispose to weight gain. The sleep fragmentation and hypoxia caused by OSA lead to increases in symptoms of daytime sleepiness and fatigue as well as loss of energy and vitality (60). Depressive symptoms including a loss of motivation are another effect. Treatment with CPAP improves these neurocognitive and quality-of-life measures (27,61). Although not well studied, these symptoms may result in reductions in physical activity and poor eating habits. In support of this theory, sleep deprivation has been found to increase symptoms of hunger and consumption of high-fat and high-carbohydrate foods (62). Several studies have reported that patients with OSA had greater weight gain in the year prior to diagnosis than weight-matched controls (53,63). However, these retrospective findings may be the result of selection bias in that the rapid weight gain may have been responsible for the presentation of the OSA patients to medical attention.

Despite these data supporting a role for OSA in worsening obesity, treatment of OSA has not been found to reduce weight. This may be because

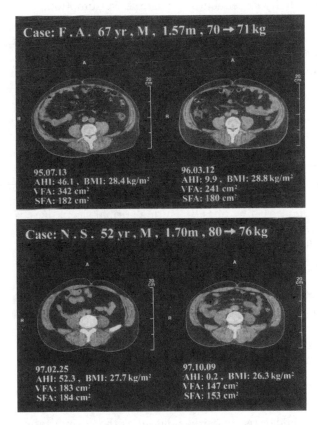

**Figure 2** The effect of CPAP on visceral fat. CT scans at the level of the umbilicus taken before and after more than six months of CPAP therapy in two patients with severe OSA demonstrate a large reduction in the amount of visceral fat with treatment. While the second patient had a slight reduction in weight during this time (80–76 kg), the first patient lost visceral fat despite no loss in overall weight. *Abbreviations*: CPAP, continuous positive airway pressure; CT, computed tomography; OSA, obstructive sleep apnea. *Source*: From Ref. 56.

the weight-promoting effects of OSA are counterbalanced by anorectic effects. The appetite-stimulating hormone, ghrelin, is elevated in patients with sleep apnea, and CPAP therapy leads to a reduction in the levels (57). In addition, energy expenditure during sleep is markedly elevated in OSA (64). This may be a result of the elevated sympathetic tone or the frequent arousals from sleep characteristic of sleep apnea. In addition, the work of breathing in sleep apneics becomes markedly elevated during sleep because the respiratory muscles generate massive amounts of negative intrathoracic pressure in attempting to overcome the occluded airway. Treatment with CPAP results in a normalization of nocturnal energy expenditure that may actually lead to further weight gain if not compensated for by daytime increases in activity or reductions in caloric consumption.

Although there is typically no overall change in weight with OSA treatment, CPAP may reduce levels of visceral fat (Fig. 2) (56). Because visceral fat appears to be more strongly implicated in the development of insulin resistance and cardiovascular disease (65,66), this effect may have important clinical consequences.

## OSA AND CARDIOVASCULAR/METABOLIC DYSFUNCTION

### Autonomic Dysfunction

Obesity is clearly a strong risk factor for the development of cardiovascular dysfunction and disease. OSA further disrupts normal cardiovascular function above and beyond that posed by obesity. During normal sleep, there is a marked reduction in sympathetic activity accompanied by a drop in blood pressure (67). In OSA, this withdrawal of sympathetic activity is lost. Peroneal nerve recordings demonstrate that muscle sympathetic activity slowly rises over the course of each obstructive event peaking right before apnea termination (Fig. 3) (68). This is thought to be mediated through the hypoxia and hypercapnia produced by apnea. In addition, apnea eliminates the sympathoinhibitory effect of pulmonary afferents (the diving reflex) leading to a further increase in sympathetic output. At resumption of breathing, there is an abrupt fall in sympathetic nerve activity. Concurrent with rising sympathetic activity, blood pressure also slowly increases over the course of an apnea. At apnea termination, however, there is a sharp surge in blood pressure before a decline to baseline levels (68). This surge is thought to be due to a sudden rise in cardiac output as the normalization of intrathoracic pressure allows venous blood to return to the heart. Over the course of the night, sympathetic activity is markedly elevated in OSA whether measured by muscle sympathetic nerve activity or by norepinephrine levels (68,69).

OSA is also associated with daytime elevations in sympathetic activity. Both muscle sympathetic burst frequency and plasma norepinephrine

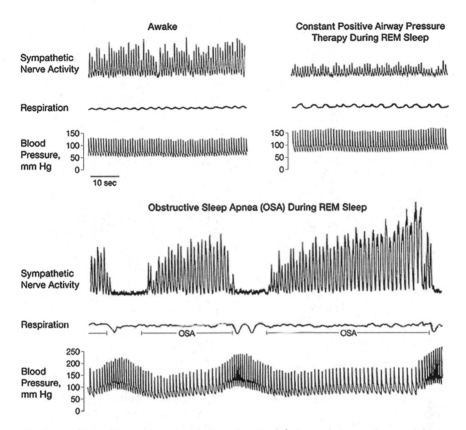

**Figure 3** Recordings of sympathetic nerve activity, respiratory rate, and intra-arterial blood pressure in the same individual with OSA while awake, during REM sleep, and during REM sleep with CPAP treatment to eliminate OSA. Sympathetic activity is elevated during wakefulness and rises even further during apneic episodes. Blood pressure rises substantially at the end of each apnea. Elimination of apnea with CPAP results in reduced sympathetic activity and prevents blood pressure surges. *Abbreviations*: CPAP, continuous positive airway pressure; OSA, obstructive sleep apnea; REM, rapid eye movement. *Source*: From Ref. 68.

levels are elevated during wakefulness (68,70). Treatment with CPAP reduces the elevated sympathetic activity both while asleep and while awake (68,69,71).

Other abnormalities noted in OSA include an increased variability in blood pressure and a reduced variability in heart rate (72). Increased blood pressure variability is an independent risk factor for end organ hypertensive injury (73,74), while reduced heart rate variability has been associated with increased mortality in several disease states (75,76). Again, treatment with CPAP appears to reduce these abnormalities (77).

## Baroreceptor Dysfunction

The cause of the elevated daytime sympathetic levels is unclear. One hypothesis is that the repeated nocturnal surges in blood pressure over time lead to a blunting in the sensitivity of the baroreflex, the feedback system linking the baroreceptors in the carotid bulb to sympathetic tone via synapses in the medulla, which is important in maintaining an appropriate perfusion pressure. Decreases in blood pressure are sensed by baroreceptor afferents and result in increases in sympathetic efferent activity. Several studies have found that the sensitivity of this reflex arc as measured by the change in muscle sympathetic burst frequency in response to an induced drop in blood pressure is reduced in OSA (78,79). This loss of sensitivity may lead to the heightened daytime sympathetic activity observed. Studies on the effect of CPAP on restoring the baroreceptor control of muscle sympathetic neural activity have not been performed. However, baroreceptor sensitivity as measured by changes in heart rate does appear to normalize with CPAP (77,80). Whether this reduced sensitivity occurs at the level of the baroreceptor or the medulla is unknown.

## Insulin Resistance

In addition to autonomic effects, OSA has been shown to have important metabolic effects. Several epidemiologic studies have investigated the relationship between OSA and insulin resistance as a potential pathway by which OSA may contribute to cardiovascular disease. Observational studies of this relationship have been difficult to perform because of the common underlying risk factor of obesity and specifically, central obesity, making adjustment or matching for obesity measures critical for any meaningful interpretation of associations. Two cross-sectional studies have attempted to study the association between OSA severity and glucose metabolism independent of obesity. Both studies used the homeostasis model adjustment (HOMA) index to quantify insulin resistance. The HOMA index is simply the product of fasting insulin and glucose normalized by a constant and has been shown to correlate reasonably well with insulin resistance measures determined by clamp techniques (81). Both studies found that AHI was an independent predictor of the HOMA index after controlling for obesity measures including BMI, WHR, and percent body fat (Fig. 4) (82,83). One study also found a correlation between OSA severity as measured by hypoxemia and insulin resistance (83). Despite these findings, the relationship between OSA and insulin resistance is not completely clear. The possibility of residual confounding by obesity or fat distribution pattern remains a possibility.

Interventional studies aimed at better understanding the causal relationship between OSA and insulin resistance have revealed mixed find-

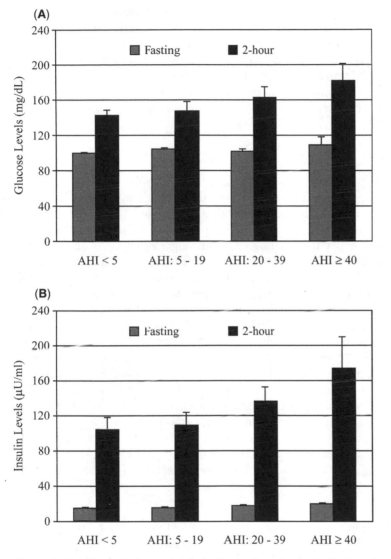

**Figure 4** Insulin and glucose levels in the fasting state and after two-hour oral glucose tolerance testing by AHI. Values represent means ± SE. Significant trends ($P<0.05$) across AHI severity were found for fasting insulin and two-hour glucose and insulin levels. *Abbreviations*: AHI, apnea–hypopnea index; SE, standard error. *Source*: From Ref. 83.

ings. Four studies have evaluated the effect of treating OSA with CPAP on insulin sensitivity measured using euglycemic clamp methods. While two studies found no effect of therapy (84,85), two others found a 30% to 40% improvement in insulin sensitivity with CPAP (86,87).

There are several biologically plausible mechanisms whereby OSA may lead to insulin resistance. The increased sympathetic tone in OSA, by stimulating glycogenolysis and lipolysis, may promote insulin resistance. Intermittent hypoxia may also play a role because it disrupts glucose control in mouse models of obesity (88). Finally, given recent findings suggesting sleep deprivation impairs glucose regulation, the sleep disruption and chronic sleep debt of OSA may be another pathway leading to insulin resistance (89).

## Dyslipidemia

Dyslipidemia is another manifestation of the metabolic syndrome that has been variably associated with OSA in the literature. The prevalence of lipid abnormalities in OSA has been reported to be over 60%, but again this is in large part due to the common underlying risk factor of obesity and in particular, central obesity (90). A large epidemiologic study using self-reported history of snoring and breathing pauses as a measure of OSA reported elevated triglycerides in OSA independent of fat deposition and fat distribution but only in women (91). The Sleep Heart Health Study, the largest study to perform sleep studies in order to quantify OSA severity, found an association between OSA severity and lipid abnormalities (92). Independent of obesity, this group found elevations in total cholesterol in men and reductions in high-density lipoprotein (HDL) in women that correlated with increasing AHI. Ip et al. matching on BMI, waist, and neck circumference, found that apneics had a 33% greater fasting triglyceride level than controls and that CPAP treatment eliminated this difference (54). No differences were observed in low-density lipoprotein (LDL) or HDL levels. Chin et al. however, have reported in multiple experiments that CPAP does not affect triglycerides but does improve LDL and HDL levels (56,93,94). Thus the association between OSA and lipid abnormalities is still unclear.

## Endothelial Dysfunction

The endothelium performs many vital roles including controlling vascular tone. Endothelial-dependent vasodilation induced by either reactive hyperemia or acetylcholine infusion is impaired in OSA, and treatment with CPAP results in normalization of this important function (95,96).

In addition, circulating levels of endothelial adhesion molecules such as intercellular adhesion molecule-1 (ICAM-1) and E-selectin have been reported to be elevated in OSA with normalization following treatment (93,97). The increase in ICAM-1 is thought to be secondary to hypoxic stimulation of nuclear transcription factor (NF-κB).

Circulating levels of vascular endothelial growth factor (VEGF) are also increased in OSA and thought to be secondary to hypoxic activation of the transcription factor hypoxia inducible factor-1. Again, treatment with

CPAP reduces plasma VEGF levels (98). The significance of these findings is unclear. VEGF is associated with angiogenesis, and so increased levels may represent an adaptive response to hypoxia promoting the development of collateral circulation (99,100). However, by inducing monocyte migration and activation and modulating smooth muscle growth, VEGF may also contribute to the development of atherosclerosis (101).

## Inflammation

Many cytokines including tumor necrosis factor (TNF) alpha and interleukin (IL)-6 are produced by adipocytes, and obesity has been identified as a proinflammatory state. Whether OSA further increases inflammation has been the subject of much research. Although TNF levels have been reported to be elevated in OSA, the higher BMI in apneics compared to controls in these studies makes it difficult to separate out the effects of obesity from sleep apnea (102,103). In addition, CPAP therapy has not been found to affect TNF levels suggesting that OSA does not have a direct effect on this cytokine (104). Studies of C-reactive peptide (CRP) and IL-6, on the other hand, do appear to show a clear association with OSA independent of obesity (Fig. 5) (105,106). Yokoe et al. found that individuals with an AHI > 20 had a nearly fourfold elevation in serum CRP and twice the

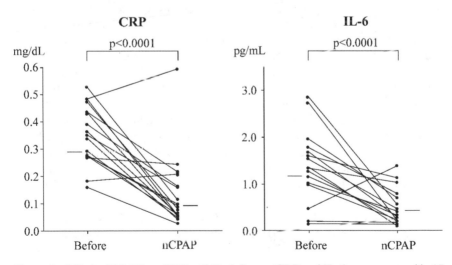

**Figure 5** Effect of CPAP on CRP and IL-6. Serum CRP and IL-6 was measured in 17 patients with moderate to severe OSA (AHI > 20 events/hr) before and after one month of nCPAP therapy. Significant reductions in both cytokines were demonstrated. *Abbreviations*: IL-6, interleukin-6; CPAP, continuous positive airway pressure; CRP, C-reactive peptide; nCPAP, nasal CPAP; OSA, obstructive sleep apnea; AHI, apnea–hypopnea index. *Source*: From Ref. 106.

level of IL-6 (106). One month of treatment with CPAP resulted in a normalization of both cytokines. The increased IL-6 levels may also be secondary to hypoxic activation of NF-κB. Carpagnano et al. found exhaled levels of IL-6 correlated with OSA severity independent of obesity suggesting that OSA may also cause localized inflammation in the upper airway through repetitive occlusion and reopening (107). Another cytokine whose expression is regulated by NF-κB is IL-8. Ohga et al. have reported a correlation between IL-8 and OSA severity and normalization of levels with CPAP therapy (108). Monocyte chemoattractant protein-1 has also been reported to be elevated in OSA (108). On the other hand, no association has been found between IL-1 or transforming growth factor-beta and OSA (102,103).

Sleep apnea also appears to have an effect on leukocyte function. Neutrophil and monocyte production of oxygen radicals is elevated in OSA and falls with CPAP use (109,110). In addition, the expression of adhesion molecules, adhesion to endothelial cells in vitro, and production of proinflammatory cytokines including TNF, IL-6, and IL-8 is increased in both monocytes and $\gamma\delta-$T cells in OSA (106,111).

## Coagulation Abnormalities

Sleep apnea has also been associated with a prothrombotic state. As with many other studies on the effects of OSA, the literature on the hemostatic effects of OSA has been limited by the ability to control for the confounding effects of obesity, smoking, and related disorders. All studies in this area have thus far been small further limiting the ability to draw conclusions. The most consistent coagulation abnormality reported has been an increased fibrinogen level in apneics relative to controls with a dose–response relationship between levels and OSA severity (112). In addition, a drop in fibrinogen levels has been reported with CPAP therapy (113). OSA has also been associated with increased clotting activity of factor VII, which normalized with CPAP (114). Plasminogen activator inhibitor-1 has been reported to be elevated in apneics, but this difference was not significant after adjusting for BMI (115). Elevations in homocysteine levels among subjects with OSA appear to be due to comorbid hypertension and heart disease rather than OSA itself (116). Studies of D-dimer, von Willebrand factor, and thrombin–antithrombin III complex have found no association with OSA (117).

Because epinephrine is an activator of platelet activity, several investigators have studied platelet function in sleep apnea postulating that the sympathetic activation of OSA may lead to platelet activation. The results have been mixed. Rangemark et al. have reported no difference in platelet aggregation in vitro between apneics and controls (115). Although Sanner et al. could find no difference in aggregation parameters between those with and without OSA, they did find a significant decrease in epinephrine-induced platelet aggregation measured overnight with six months of CPAP use (118). A study by Bokinsky et al. has suggested that though awake measures of platelet function are unaffected, CPAP does reduce both platelet activation and aggregation while asleep (119).

The clinical significance of these laboratory abnormalities is unclear. The only study examining the association between OSA and venous thromboembolic events has been small and lacking control groups (120,121). The prothrombotic association may be more important in the development of atherosclerotic vascular disease for which there is more evidence implicating OSA.

## OSA AND CARDIOVASCULAR/METABOLIC DISEASE

### Hypertension

As described previously, blood pressure normally falls during non-REM stages of sleep (67). Overnight studies on OSA, however, have clearly demonstrated that blood pressure rises with each obstructive event peaking just after resumption of breathing (68). In addition, mean nocturnal blood pressure is elevated, likely a result of both the brief spikes occurring with each apneic event as well as the elevated nocturnal sympathetic tone. Thus blood pressure when asleep is often equal to if not higher than blood pressure when awake. This type of 24-hour blood pressure pattern has been referred to as "nondipping" and is associated with an increased risk of cardiovascular events independent of daytime blood pressure (73,122). CPAP appears effective in converting "nondippers" to "dippers" (123).

In addition, OSA has been implicated in the development of daytime hypertension. Brooks et al. have created an animal model of OSA that has provided insight on this issue (Fig. 6) (124). This group tracheotomized dogs and inserted a computer-controlled occlusion valve that was triggered whenever continuous electroencephalography (EEG) monitoring revealed the dog was asleep. The valve would open again once the dog awoke, thereby simulating the obstructive episodes of sleep apnea. Nocturnal blood pressure in these dogs rose once the occluding mechanism was activated and remained elevated over a month. Blood pressure returned to normal on the first night that the valve was left open. More importantly, the "apneic" dogs also had a significant increase in daytime blood pressure. Daytime mean arterial pressure rose 15 mmHg, and this was again reversible with cessation of the nocturnal occlusions. A control group of dogs were aroused from sleep by an acoustic alarm so that the degree of sleep fragmentation was similar to that of the apneic dogs. These dogs were found to have a similar rise in nocturnal blood pressure but no rise in daytime pressures. Thus recurrent arousal and sleep fragmentation alone were not

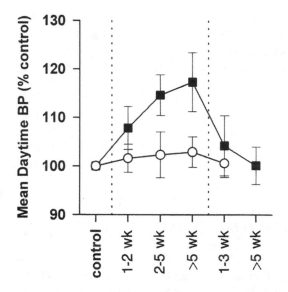

**Figure 6** Mean daytime blood pressure in dogs during OSA (*filled squares*) and sleep fragmentation (*open circles*). Error bars represent the standard error of the mean. The dashed lines represent the beginning and end of the OSA or sleep fragmentation phase. *Abbreviation*: OSA, obstructive sleep apnea. *Source*: From Ref. 124.

sufficient to produce sustained hypertension in this model, suggesting a role for recurrent hypoxemia.

Human data also support a role for sleep apnea in the development of hypertension. Several large cross-sectional studies of patients referred to a sleep clinic have reported the odds of hypertension increasing 11% to 13% for every 10-unit increase in AHI (125,126). Prospectively studying a middle-aged cohort over four years, Peppard et al. found AHI to be an independent risk factor for the development of hypertension (Fig. 7) (127). A clear dose–response relationship existed between OSA severity and hypertension risk such that mild OSA (AHI between 5 and 15) was associated with twice the risk and moderate to severe OSA (AHI > 15) was associated with nearly triple the risk.

Several interventional trials have assessed the relationship between OSA and hypertension with mixed results. Barbe et al. studying asymptomatic sleep apneics randomized to either CPAP or a sham-CPAP treatment found no significant change in blood pressure in either arm (128). Faccenda et al. performed a crossover study comparing CPAP with oral placebo in a group of normotensive apneics (129). With four weeks of therapy, they found a small (1.4 mmHg) but statistically significant reduction in diastolic blood pressure with CPAP. The effect was greatest in those with the most

ADJUSTED ODDS RATIOS FOR HYPERTENSION AT A FOLLOW-UP SLEEP STUDY,
ACCORDING TO THE APNEA–HYPOPNEA INDEX AT BASE LINE

| BASE-LINE APNEA-HYPOPNEA INDEX | ODDS RATIO, ADJUSTED FOR BASE-LINE HYPERTENSION STATUS | ODDS RATIO, ADJUSTED FOR BASE-LINE HYPERTENSION STATUS AND NONMODIFIABLE RISK FACTORS (AGE AND SEX) | ODDS RATIO, ADJUSTED FOR BASE-LINE HYPERTENSION STATUS, NON-MODIFIABLE RISK FACTORS, AND HABITUS (BMI AND WAIST AND NECK CIRCUMFERENCE) | ODDS RATIO, ADJUSTED FOR BASE-LINE HYPERTENSION STATUS, NON-MODIFIABLE RISK FACTORS, HABITUS, AND WEEKLY ALCOHOL AND CIGARETTE USE |
|---|---|---|---|---|
| | | odds ratio (95% confidence interval) | | |
| 0 events/hr | 1.0 | 1.0 | 1.0 | 1.0 |
| 0.1–4.9 events/hr | 1.66 (1.35–2.03) | 1.65 (1.33–2.04) | 1.42 (1.14–1.78) | 1.42 (1.13–1.78) |
| 5.0–14.9 events/hr | 2.74 (1.82–4.12) | 2.71 (1.78–4.14) | 2.03 (1.29–3.19) | 2.03 (1.29–3.17) |
| >15.0 events/hr | 4.54 (2.46–8.36) | 4.47 (2.37–8.43) | 2.89 (1.47–5.69) | 2.89 (1.46–5.64) |
| P for trend | <0.001 | <0.001 | 0.002 | 0.002 |

**Figure 7** The odds ratio of developing hypertension as a function of OSA severity as assessed by the AHI. An AHI of 0 is used as the reference group. *p*-Values are for a linear trend in the logistic regression coefficients across AHI categories. *Abbreviations*: OSA, obstructive sleep apnea; AHI, apnea–hypopnea index. *Source*: From Ref. 127.

severe apnea and those most compliant with therapy. It has been suggested that the small effect size in this study may have been due to the fact that the population was normotensive at baseline.

Pepperell et al. found that CPAP reduced mean ambulatory blood pressure 3.3 mmHg more than sham therapy after four weeks of treatment (130). Similar reductions were observed in both daytime and nighttime pressures. Again, the blood pressure reduction was greatest in patients with more severe OSA and more compliant with treatment.

Most recently, Becker et al. randomized 32 patients with severe OSA to nine weeks of treatment with either CPAP or sham therapy (131). Nearly two-third of the population was hypertensive at baseline. Both systolic and diastolic blood pressure dropped by about 10 mmHg in the treated group relative to placebo with reductions noted in both the daytime and nighttime (Fig. 8). Overall, these studies suggest that CPAP therapy is effective in reducing blood pressure but that the effect is most evident in patients with severe OSA, with elevated blood pressure, and who are adherent to therapy. It should be noted that all of these intervention studies were of short duration (30 days), and thus the long-term benefit of treating OSA in terms of blood pressure reduction may be even greater.

Thus there is now strong evidence from animal models, longitudinal cohort studies, and interventional trials demonstrating that OSA is an independent risk factor for hypertension and that treatment of OSA can help treat high blood pressure. Sleep apnea should be considered in the

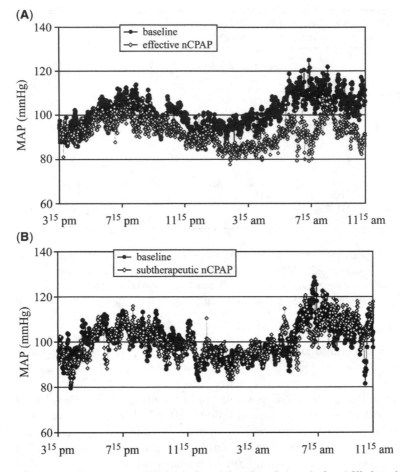

**Figure 8** Time course of MAP before (*closed circles*) and after (*filled circles*) randomization to treatment of OSA with either effective nasal CPAP (*Panel A*) or subtherapeutic CPAP (*Panel B*). While subtherapeutic CPAP had no effect on blood pressure, therapeutic levels of CPAP significantly reduced mean arterial pressure, and this reduction was found both at nighttime and during the day. *Abbreviations*: MAP, mean arterial blood pressure; CPAP, continuous positive airway pressure; OSA, obstructive sleep apnea. *Source*: From Ref. 131.

evaluation of patients with high blood pressure. A recent study found that 83% of patients with resistant hypertension had OSA on overnight polysomnography (132). The most recent guidelines set out by the Joint National Committee on Prevention, Detection, Evaluation and Treatment of High Blood Pressure (JNC 7) list OSA first among the causes of secondary hypertension and recommend that patients with resistant hypertension be screened for OSA (133).

## Coronary Artery Disease

The data implicating OSA as a causative factor for coronary artery disease are not as compelling. Clearly, the acute effects of sleep apnea such as hypoxemia, hypercapnia, and sympathetic activation can predispose to myocardial ischemia. In addition, the negative intrathoracic pressures generated when an individual attempts to breathe against the occluded airway result in elevations in ventricular afterload and thus wall stress, the primary determinant of myocardial oxygen consumption. ST-segment depression on overnight electrocardiography (EKG) monitoring has been reported to occur with OSA and has been correlated with both oxygen desaturation and the postapneic surges in heart rate and blood pressure. Among those with coexisting coronary disease and OSA, the prevalence of nocturnal ischemic EKG changes has been reported to range from 20% to 90% (134–136). In addition, nocturnal ST-segment depression has been reported in as many as 30% of OSA patients without coronary disease (137). The chronic consequences of OSA including insulin resistance, activation of inflammatory and prothrombotic pathways as well as hypertension may also contribute to the development of atherosclerotic heart disease.

Case–control studies have suggested a high prevalence of OSA in patients surviving myocardial infarction. Peker et al. found an odds ratio of 3.1 for OSA in patients with myocardial infarction or unstable angina when compared to controls after adjusting for obesity and conventional cardiac risk factors (138). Only smoking and diabetes were stronger risk factors in this analysis. Other studies have found odds ratios as high as 23 associated with OSA (139). Because of the retrospective nature of these studies, it is not clear if some part of this association is due to postinfarct changes in cardiac or neurologic function that predispose coronary heart disease patients to develop OSA.

The Sleep Heart Health Study found a strong relationship between prevalent coronary heart disease and AHI with a relative risk for coronary disease of 1.27 comparing top and bottom quartiles of AHI (140). A trend for association persisted after adjustment for blood pressure supporting the notion that hypertension is not the only mechanism by which OSA affects coronary disease risk.

Prospective studies have typically used snoring as a surrogate for sleep apnea. The Nurses Health Study found a history of regular snoring to be associated with a 33% excess risk of incident coronary heart disease over eight years after controlling for obesity and conventional cardiac risk factors. In those with coronary artery disease, OSA appears to have an important effect on prognosis. A five-year prospective study of patients with established heart disease found mortality to be fourfold greater in those with OSA (38% vs. 9%) (141). Prospective data on OSA as a risk factor for incident heart disease are currently being collected within the Sleep Heart

Health Study and should hopefully be able to better define this relationship in the near future.

No controlled trials have been performed assessing the effect of treating OSA on coronary artery disease. However, uncontrolled studies of patients with OSA and nocturnal angina have found a reduced frequency of ischemic EKG changes and resolution of anginal symptoms with positive pressure therapy (135,136,142).

## Cerebrovascular Disease

A strong association between stroke and OSA has been known for some time. The prevalence of OSA among acute stroke survivors has been reported to be as high as 70% to 95% (143,144). This may be in part because of the large number of common underlying risk factors such as obesity, smoking, and alcohol use. In addition, acute stroke likely increases the risk of sleep apnea by affecting pharyngeal muscle tone and ventilatory control. In support of this hypothesis is the finding that the AHI falls in the weeks following a stroke as the brain regains function (145). Whether OSA is a risk factor for stroke is still a matter of much debate. To reduce concerns about reverse causation, a recent study recruited patients suffering a transient ischemic attack instead of stroke. Because of the lack of a permanent neurologic deficit, it was thought unlikely that the neurologic event would produce OSA. In this study, no difference in AHI was found between patients and matched controls (146).

The Sleep Heart Health investigators found a clear dose–response relationship between severity of OSA and stroke, similar to heart disease, with stroke nearly 60% more prevalent in the highest quartile of AHI when compared to the lowest. Again a trend for association persisted after adjusting for hypertension suggesting that other mechanisms contribute to this association (140). Because this study was also cross-sectional, the potential for this association to be due to an effect of stroke on OSA cannot be ruled out however.

The only prospective studies to be performed in this arena have used snoring as a surrogate for OSA. The largest of these was conducted by the Nurses Health Study (147). Following over 71,000 women for eight years, this group found a 60% to 88% excess risk of stroke associated with snoring. After controlling for BMI, smoking, alcohol consumption, and other potential confounders, an excess risk of 35% to 42% remained apparent.

The same pathways implicated in the pathogenesis of coronary artery disease likely also play a role in predisposing those with OSA to stroke. These include the acute effects of hypoxemia and catecholamine surges as well as the chronic effects of hypertension, insulin resistance, and upregulation of prothrombotic factors such as fibrinogen and platelet activation. In addition, Doppler ultrasound imaging of the middle cerebral artery has found that obstructive apneas and hypopneas are associated with acute marked reductions in cerebral blood flow (148).

## Congestive Heart Failure

Sleep apnea is extremely common in those with heart failure and can be obstructive or central (Cheyne–Stokes respirations) in nature. While the close relationship between heart failure and Cheyne–Stokes breathing has been known for some time, the association between heart failure and OSA has only recently become apparent. Although early studies reported a high prevalence of close to 40% of OSA among patients with left ventricular systolic dysfunction, these studies were biased by recruiting patients referred to a sleep clinic. Prospective studies based on recruitment from heart failure clinics or transplant waiting lists have reported that the prevalence of sleep-disordered breathing in patients with systolic dysfunction has ranged from 45% to 82%, but the majority of these patients have Cheyne–Stokes respirations (149–152). The prevalence of OSA in these studies has ranged from 5% to 20%. Among those with diastolic dysfunction on the other hand, OSA appears to be the most common manifestation of sleep-disordered breathing, present in up to 35% (153).

Hypoxemia, sympathetic activation, and increases in blood pressure all may contribute to hypertensive heart disease, which can lead to both systolic and diastolic dysfunction. The extreme negative intrathoracic pressure generated during an obstruction, by rapidly changing transmural cardiac pressures, increases myocardial wall stress and left ventricular afterload. Furthermore, the inflammatory changes associated with OSA may lead to reductions in myocardial contractility, and the induced endothelial dysfunction may lead to maladaptive ventricular remodeling.

Heart failure may in turn predispose to OSA. Heart failure is a known risk factor for periodic breathing. During the nadirs in ventilation, not only does the diaphragm relax but neurologic input to genioglossus and other upper airway muscles also decreases (154). This combined with reduced lung volumes predisposes the upper airway to collapse. In fact, many heart failure patients have a combination of central and obstructive respiratory events.

Few population-based studies have assessed the relationship between OSA and heart failure. The largest, the Sleep Heart Health Study, found a strong relationship between increasing OSA severity and presence of heart failure. The odds of heart failure for individuals in the top quartile of AHI (AHI>11.0) was 2.2 times greater than that in the lowest quartile after controlling for major cardiac risk factors (140). As with myocardial infarction and stroke, longitudinal follow-up of the Sleep Heart Health cohort is eagerly awaited to assess the association between OSA and incident cases of heart failure.

In the meantime, interventional studies have supported the notion that treatment of sleep-disordered breathing can improve ventricular function. A recent randomized trial evaluated the efficacy of treating OSA as an adjunctive therapy for heart failure. Kaneko et al. randomized 24 patients with left ventricular systolic dysfunction to receive either maximal medical therapy or medical therapy plus CPAP (155). Patients were evenly divided between ischemic and nonischemic etiologies of their cardiomyopathy. After one month of treatment, the group assigned to CPAP had a 10 mmHg reduction in systolic blood pressure. More importantly, the left ventricular ejection fraction increased from 25% to 34%.

## Diabetes

While several studies have found an independent association between OSA and insulin resistance, the data implicating OSA as a risk factor for the development of overt diabetes are not as clear. As with many of the other conditions described, it is difficult to separate the association between OSA and diabetes with the common risk factor of obesity. The potential for confounding exists in observational studies even after controlling for overall obesity because certain fat distribution patterns are more important in the development of both OSA and diabetes. An android fat deposition pattern and increased visceral fat are both more important for the development of sleep-disordered breathing, glucose dysregulation, and cardiovascular disease.

Several prospective epidemiologic studies have used self-reported snoring as a surrogate marker for sleep apnea in investigating the relationship between OSA and diabetes. A 10-year study of 2668 middle-aged Swedish men found that the odds ratio for incident diabetes was 1.4 times greater in obese snorers when compared to obese nonsnorers (156). Relative to never snorers, the Nurses Health Study found that women who were occasional snorers and regular snorers had 1.5- and 2.3-fold greater odds, respectively, of developing diabetes over 10 years after adjusting for age and BMI (157). Due to concerns regarding residual confounding by fat deposition patterns, the relative risks were adjusted for WHR in the subset of women for whom this measure was available. The adjusted odds ratios for occasional and regular snoring in this subgroup were 1.2 and 1.6, respectively. Using a more restrictive definition for OSA (self-reported snoring plus breathing pauses), the Swedish Obese Subjects study also found an association between OSA and diabetes with an odds ratio of 1.8 (91).

Prospective studies on new onset diabetes using polysomnography to define sleep apnea severity have not been done. The largest cross-sectional study using polysomnography, the Sleep Heart Health Study found no relationship between prevalent diabetes and AHI after adjusting for obesity and other potential confounders (158). They did, however, find an association between diabetes and periodic breathing suggesting that diabetes may have effects on central regulation of breathing. A recent study of nonobese patients with diabetes found a significant association between OSA and the presence of autonomic neuropathy suggesting that diabetes may be a risk factor for OSA by causing neuropathic effects on ventilatory control mechanisms (159).

Only one intervention study has assessed the effect of treating OSA in diabetics. Brooks et al. recruited 10 type 2 diabetics with severe OSA (86). Hyperinsulinemic euglycemic clamping was performed before and after four months of CPAP therapy. The authors found a 32% improvement in insulin responsiveness with CPAP. Unfortunately, no control group was included for comparison.

## SUMMARY

In summary, OSA is an extremely common complication of obesity. This disorder exposes the patient to recurrent hypoxia and hypercapnia, large intrathoracic pressure swings, and sleep fragmentation. These nocturnal disturbances lead to disruptions in the normal functioning of a whole host of physiologic pathways affecting neurologic, metabolic, inflammatory, and hemostatic systems. The end result of these abnormalities in terms of clinical disease is only now being fully understood. The data that exist implicate OSA as an independent risk factor for hypertension. While OSA is clearly associated with other cardiovascular diseases as well as obesity and diabetes, further research is needed to better elucidate the causal relationships responsible for this association. OSA may be a cause of these diseases, but many of these disorders may predispose to OSA. In addition, these disorders may share common risk factors in addition to obesity and fat distribution patterns. It is likely that several, if not all, of these types of causal relationships exist making longitudinal and interventional studies vital to understanding the importance of OSA in cardiovascular disease better. In the meantime, given the high prevalence of OSA in these disease states, all patients with obesity, diabetes, and cardiovascular disease should be questioned for symptoms attributable to OSA and formal diagnostic studies conducted if the history is suggestive.

## REFERENCES

1. Remmers JE et al. Pathogenesis of upper airway occlusion during sleep. J Appl Physiol 1978; 44(6):931–938.
2. Shepard JW Jr, Thawley SE. Localization of upper airway collapse during sleep in patients with obstructive sleep apnea. Am Rev Respir Dis 1990; 141(5 Pt 1):1350–1355.

3. Hudgel DW. Variable site of airway narrowing among obstructive sleep apnea patients. J Appl Physiol 1986; 61(4):1403–1409.
4. Lowe AA et al. Cephalometric and computed tomographic predictors of obstructive sleep apnea severity [see comments]. Am J Orthodont Dentofacial Orthop 1995; 107(6):589–595.
5. Bradley TD et al. Pharyngeal size in snorers, nonsnorers, and patients with obstructive sleep apnea. N Engl J Med 1986; 315(21):1327–1331.
6. Haponik E et al. Computerized tomography in obstructive sleep apnea: correlation of airway size with physiology during sleep and wakefulness. Am Rev Respir Dis 1983; 127:221–226.
7. Horner RL et al. Sites and sizes of fat deposits around the pharynx in obese patients with obstructive sleep apnoea and weight matched controls. Eur Respir J 1989; 2(7):613–622.
8. Schwab R et al. Dynamic upper airway imaging during awake respiration in normal subjects and patients with sleep disordered breathing. Am Rev Respir Dis 1993; 148:1375–1400.
9. Schwab RJ et al. Upper airway and soft tissue anatomy in normal subjects and patients with sleep-disordered breathing. Significance of the lateral pharyngeal walls. Am J Respir Crit Care Med 1995; 152(5 Pt 1):1673–1689.
10. Horner RL, Innes JA, Murphy K, Guz A. Evidence for reflex upper airway dilator muscle activation by sudden negative airway pressure in man. J Physiol (Lond) 1991; 436:15–29.
11. Mathew OP. Upper airway negative pressure effects on respiratory activity of upper airway muscles. J Appl Physiol 1984; 56:500.
12. Wheatley J, White D. The influence of sleep on pharyngeal reflexes. Sleep 1993; 16(8 suppl):S87–S89.
13. Fogel RB et al. Reduced genioglossal activity with upper airway anesthesia in awake patients with OSA. J Appl Physiol 2000; 88(4):1346–1354.
14. Fogel R et al. Genioglossal activation in patients with obstructive sleep apnea versus control subjects. Mechanisms of muscle control. Am J Respir Crit Care Med 2001; 164:2025–2030.
15. Mezzanotte WS, Tangel DJ, White DP. Waking genioglossal EMG in sleep apnea patients versus normal controls (a neuromuscular compensatory mechanism). J Clin Invest 1992; 89:1571–1579.
16. Wheatley J et al. Influence of sleep on genioglossus muscle activation by negative pressure in normal men. Am Rev Respir Dis 1993; 148(3):597–605.
17. Fogel R et al. Within-breath control of genioglossal muscle activation in humans: effect of sleep-wake state. J Physiol 2003; 550:899–910.
18. Harman EM, Wynne JW, Block AJ. The effect of weight loss on sleep-disordered breathing and oxygen desaturation in morbidly obese men. Chest 1982; 82(3):291–294.
19. Sugerman HJ et al. Gastric surgery for respiratory insufficiency of obesity. Chest 1986; 90(1):81–86.
20. Sugerman HJ et al. Long-term effects of gastric surgery for treating respiratory insufficiency of obesity. Am J Clin Nutr 1992; 55(2 suppl):597S–601S.
21. Strobel RJ, Rosen RC. Obesity and weight loss in obstructive sleep apnea: a critical review. Sleep 1996; 19(2):104–115.

22. Smith PL et al. Weight loss in mildly to moderately obese patients with obstructive sleep apnea. Ann Intern Med 1985; 103(6 Pt 1):850–855.
23. Sullivan CE et al. Reversal of obstructive sleep apnoea by continuous positive airway pressure applied through the nares. Lancet 1981; 1(8225):862–865.
24. Sullivan CE, Berthon-Jones M, Issa FG. Remission of severe obesity-hypoventilation syndrome after short-term treatment during sleep with nasal continuous positive airway pressure. Am Rev Respir Dis 1983; 128(1):177–181.
25. Sanders MH, Moore SE, Eveslage J. CPAP via nasal mask: a treatment for occlusive sleep apnea. Chest 1983; 83(1):144–145.
26. Sanders MH. Nasal CPAP effect on patterns of sleep apnea. Chest 1984; 86(6):839–844.
27. Jenkinson C et al. Comparison of therapeutic and subtherapeutic nasal continuous positive airway pressure for obstructive sleep apnoea: a randomised prospective parallel trial. Lancet 1999; 353(9170):2100–2105.
28. Hoffstein V et al. Treatment of obstructive sleep apnea with nasal continuous positive airway pressure. Patient compliance, perception of benefits, and side effects. Am Rev Respir Dis 1992; 145(4 Pt 1):841–845.
29. McArdle N et al. Long-term use of CPAP therapy for sleep apnea/hypopnea syndrome. Am J Respir Crit Care Med 1999; 159(4 Pt 1):1108–1114.
30. Engleman HM, Martin SE, Douglas NJ. Compliance with CPAP therapy in patients with the sleep apnoea/hypopnoea syndrome. Thorax 1994; 49(3):263–266.
31. Young T et al. The occurrence of sleep-disordered breathing among middle-aged adults. N Engl J Med 1993; 328(17):1230–1235.
32. Olson LG et al. A community study of snoring and sleep-disordered breathing. Symptoms. Am J Respir Crit Care Med 1995; 152(2):707–710.
33. Redline S et al. Racial differences in sleep-disordered breathing in African-Americans and Caucasians. Am J Respir Crit Care Med 1997; 155(1):186–192.
34. Guilleminault C et al. Women and the obstructive sleep apnea syndrome. Chest 1988; 93(1):104–109.
35. Redline S et al. Gender differences in sleep disordered breathing in a community-based sample. Am J Respir Crit Care Med 1994; 149(3 Pt 1):722–726.
36. Ambrogetti A, Olson LG, Saunders NA. Differences in the symptoms of men and women with obstructive sleep apnoea. Aust N Z J Med 1991; 21(6):863–866.
37. Block AJ et al. Sleep apnea, hypopnea and oxygen desaturation in normal subjects. A strong male predominance. N Engl J Med 1979; 300(10):513–517.
38. Lowe AA et al. Cephalometric and demographic characteristics of obstructive sleep apnea: an evaluation with partial least squares analysis. Angle Orthodontist 1997; 67(2):143–153.
39. Bacon WH et al. Craniofacial characteristics in patients with obstructive sleep apneas syndrome. Cleft Palate J 1988; 25(4):374–378.
40. Wilcox I et al. "Syndrome Z": the interaction of sleep apnoea, vascular risk factors and heart disease. Thorax 1998; 53:S25–S28.
41. Wilhoit SC, Suratt PM. Obstructive sleep apnea in premenopausal women. A comparison with men and with postmenopausal women. Chest 1987; 91(5):654–8.

42. Dealberto MJ et al. Factors related to sleep apnea syndrome in sleep clinic patients. Chest 1994; 105(6):1753–1758.
43. Grunstein R et al. Snoring and sleep apnoea in men: association with central obesity and hypertension. Int J Obes 1993; 17(9):533–540.
44. Redline S et al. Predictors of longitudinal change in sleep-disordered breathing in a nonclinic population. Sleep 2003; 26(6):703–709.
45. Vgontzas AN, et al. Sleep apnea and sleep disruption in obese patients. Arch Intern Med 1994; 154(15):1705–1711.
46. Rajala R et al. Obstructive sleep apnoea syndrome in morbidly obese patients. J Intern Med 1991; 230(2):125–129.
47. Pillar G et al. Predictive value of specific risk factors, symptoms and signs, in diagnosing obstructive sleep apnoea and its severity. J Sleep Res 1994; 3(4): 241–244.
48. Mortimore IL et al. Neck and total body fat deposition in nonobese and obese patients with sleep apnea compared with that in control subjects. Am J Respir Crit Care Med 1998; 157(1):280–283.
49. Millman RP et al. Body fat distribution and sleep apnea severity in women. Chest 1995; 107(2):362–366.
50. Fogel RB et al. Increased prevalence of obstructive sleep apnea syndrome in obese women with polycystic ovary syndrome. J Clin Endocrinol Metab 2001; 86(3):1175–1180.
51. Fogel R. Anatomic and physiologic predictors of apnea severity in morbidly obese subjects. Sleep 2003; 6(2):150–155.
52. Vgontzas AN et al. Sleep apnea and daytime sleepiness and fatigue: relation to visceral obesity, insulin resistance, and hypercytokinemia. J Clin Endocrinol Metab 2000; 85(3):1151–1158.
53. Phillips BG et al. Increases in leptin levels, sympathetic drive, and weight gain in obstructive sleep apnea. Am J Physiol Heart Circ Physiol 2000; 279(1): H234–H237.
54. Ip MS et al. Serum leptin and vascular risk factors in obstructive sleep apnea. Chest 2000; 118(3):580–586.
55. Considine RV et al. Serum immunoreactive-leptin concentrations in normal-weight and obese humans. N Engl J Med 1996; 334(5):292–295.
56. Chin K et al. Changes in intra-abdominal visceral fat and serum leptin levels in patients with obstructive sleep apnea syndrome following nasal continuous positive airway pressure therapy. Circulation 1999; 100(7):706–712.
57. Harsch IA et al. Leptin and ghrelin levels in patients with obstructive sleep apnoea: effect of CPAP treatment. Eur Respir J 2003; 22(2):251–257.
58. Haynes WG et al. Receptor-mediated regional sympathetic nerve activation by leptin. J Clin Invest 1997; 100(2):270–278.
59. Shek EW, Brands MW, Hall JE. Chronic leptin infusion increases arterial pressure. Hypertension 1998; 31(1 Pt 2):409–414.
60. Sateia MJ. Neuropsychological impairment and quality of life in obstructive sleep apnea. Clin Chest Med 2003; 24(2):249–259.
61. Douglas NJ, Engleman HM. Effects of CPAP on vigilance and related functions in patients with the sleep apnea/hypopnea syndrome. Sleep 2000; 23(suppl 4):S147–S149.

62. Spiegel K et al. Sleep curtailment results in decreased leptin levels and increased hunger and appetite [abstr.]. Sleep 2003; 26:A174.
63. Phillips BG et al. Recent weight gain in patients with newly diagnosed obstructive sleep apnea. J Hypertens 1999; 17(9):1297–1300.
64. Stenlof K et al. Energy expenditure in obstructive sleep apnea: effects of treatment with continuous positive airway pressure. Am J Physiol 1996; 271(6 Pt 1):E1036–E1043.
65. Zamboni M et al. Relation of body fat distribution in men and degree of coronary narrowings in coronary artery disease. Am J Cardiol 1992; 70(13): 1135–1138.
66. Ross R et al. Abdominal obesity, muscle composition, and insulin resistance in premenopausal women. J Clin Endocrinol Metab 2002; 87(11):5044–5051.
67. Somers VK et al. Sympathetic-nerve activity during sleep in normal subjects. N Engl J Med 1993; 328(5):303–307.
68. Somers VK et al. Sympathetic neural mechanisms in obstructive sleep apnea. J Clin Invest 1995; 96(4):1897–1904.
69. Hedner J et al. Reduction in sympathetic activity after long-term CPAP treatment in sleep apnoea: cardiovascular implications. Eur Respir J 1995; 8(2): 222–229.
70. Carlson JT et al. Augmented resting sympathetic activity in awake patients with obstructive sleep apnea. Chest 1993; 103(6):1763–1768.
71. Narkiewicz K et al. Nocturnal continuous positive airway pressure decreases daytime sympathetic traffic in obstructive sleep apnea. Circulation 1999; 100(23):2332–2335.
72. Narkiewicz K et al. Altered cardiovascular variability in obstructive sleep apnea. Circulation 1998; 98(11):1071–1077.
73. Palatini P et al. Clinical relevance of nighttime blood pressure and of daytime blood pressure variability. Arch Intern Med 1992; 152(9):1855–1860.
74. Sega R et al. Blood pressure variability and organ damage in a general population: results from the PAMELA study (Pressioni Arteriose Monitorate E Loro Associazioni). Hypertension 2002; 39(2 Pt 2):710–714.
75. La Rovere MT et al. Short-term heart rate variability strongly predicts sudden cardiac death in chronic heart failure patients. Circulation 2003; 107(4): 565–570.
76. Filipovic M et al. Heart rate variability and cardiac troponin I are incremental and independent predictors of one-year all-cause mortality after major noncardiac surgery in patients at risk of coronary artery disease. J Am Coll Cardiol 2003; 42(10):1767–1776.
77. Belozeroff V et al. Effects of CPAP therapy on cardiovascular variability in obstructive sleep apnea: a closed-loop analysis. Am J Physiol Heart Circ Physiol 2002; 282(1): H110–H121.
78. Carlson JT et al. Depressed baroreflex sensitivity in patients with obstructive sleep apnea. Am J Respir Crit Care Med 1996; 154(5):1490–1496.
79. Narkiewicz K et al. Baroreflex control of sympathetic nerve activity and heart rate in obstructive sleep apnea. Hypertension 1998; 32(6):1039–1043.

80. Bonsignore MR et al. Continuous positive airway pressure treatment improves baroreflex control of heart rate during sleep in severe obstructive sleep apnea syndrome. Am J Respir Crit Care Med 2002; 166(3):279–286.

81. Bonora E et al. Homeostasis model assessment closely mirrors the glucose clamp technique in the assessment of insulin sensitivity: studies in subjects with various degrees of glucose tolerance and insulin sensitivity. Diabetes Care 2000; 23(1):57–63.

82. Ip MS et al. Obstructive sleep apnea is independently associated with insulin resistance. Am J Respir Crit Care Med 2002; 165(5):670–676.

83. Punjabi NM et al. Sleep-disordered breathing and insulin resistance in middle-aged and overweight men. Am J Respir Crit Care Med 2002; 165(5):677–682.

84. Saarelainen S, Lahtela J, Kallonen E. Effect of nasal CPAP treatment on insulin sensitivity and plasma leptin. J Sleep Res 1997; 6(2):146–147.

85. Smurra M et al. CPAP treatment does not affect glucose-insulin metabolism in sleep apneic patients. Sleep Med 2001; 2(3):207–213.

86. Brooks B et al. Obstructive sleep apnea in obese noninsulin-dependent diabetic patients: effect of continuous positive airway pressure treatment on insulin responsiveness. J Clin Endocrinol Metab 1994; 79(6):1681–1685.

87. Harsch IA et al. CPAP treatment rapidly improves insulin sensitivity in patients with OSAS. Am J Respir Crit Care Med 2004; 169(2):15–62.

88. Polotsky VY et al. Intermittent hypoxia increases insulin resistance in genetically obese mice. J Physiol 2003; 552(Pt 1):253–264.

89. Spiegel K, Leproult R, Van Cauter E. Impact of sleep debt on metabolic and endocrine function. Lancet 1999; 354(9188):1435–1439.

90. Kiely JL, McNicholas WT. Cardiovascular risk factors in patients with obstructive sleep apnoea syndrome. Eur Respir J 2000; 16(1):128–133.

91. Grunstein RR et al. Impact of obstructive sleep apnea and sleepiness on metabolic and cardiovascular risk factors in the Swedish Obese Subjects (SOS) Study. Int J Obes Relat Metab Disord 1995; 19(6):410–418.

92. Newman AB et al. Relation of sleep-disordered breathing to cardiovascular disease risk factors: the Sleep Heart Health Study. Am J Epidemiol 2001; 154(1):50–59.

93. Chin K et al. Effects of nasal continuous positive airway pressure on soluble cell adhesion molecules in patients with obstructive sleep apnea syndrome. Am J Med 2000; 109(7):562–567.

94. Chin K et al. Effects of obstructive sleep apnea syndrome on serum aminotransferase levels in obese patients. Am J Med 2003; 114(5):370–376.

95. Kato M et al. Impairment of endothelium-dependent vasodilation of resistance vessels in patients with obstructive sleep apnea. Circulation 2000; 102(21):2607–2610.

96. Ip MS et al. Endothelial function in obstructive sleep apnea and response to treatment. Am J Respir Crit Care Med 2004; 169(3):348–353.

97. Ohga E et al. Increased levels of circulating ICAM-1, VCAM-1, and L-selectin in obstructive sleep apnea syndrome. J Appl Physiol 1999; 87(1):10–14.

98. Lavie L et al. Plasma vascular endothelial growth factor in sleep apnea syndrome: effects of nasal continuous positive air pressure treatment. Am J Respir Crit Care Med 2002; 165(12):1624–1628.

99. Baumgartner I et al. Constitutive expression of phVEGF165 after intramuscular gene transfer promotes collateral vessel development in patients with critical limb ischemia. Circulation 1998; 97(12):1114–1123.

100. Losordo DW et al. Gene therapy for myocardial angiogenesis: initial clinical results with direct myocardial injection of phVEGF165 as sole therapy for myocardial ischemia. Circulation 1998; 98(25):2800–2804.

101. Inoue M et al. Vascular endothelial growth factor (VEGF) expression in human coronary atherosclerotic lesions: possible pathophysiological significance of VEGF in progression of atherosclerosis. Circulation 1998; 98(20): 2108–2116.

102. Vgontzas AN et al. Elevation of plasma cytokines in disorders of excessive daytime sleepiness: role of sleep disturbance and obesity. J Clin Endocrinol Metab 1997; 82(5):1313–1316.

103. Alberti A et al. Plasma cytokine levels in patients with obstructive sleep apnea syndrome: a preliminary study. J Sleep Res 2003; 12(4):305–311.

104. Entzian P et al. Obstructive sleep apnea syndrome and circadian rhythms of hormones and cytokines. Am J Respir Crit Care Med 1996; 153(3):1080–1086.

105. Shamsuzzaman AS et al. Elevated C-reactive protein in patients with obstructive sleep apnea. Circulation 2002; 105(21):2462–2464.

106. Yokoe T et al. Elevated levels of C-reactive protein and interleukin-6 in patients with obstructive sleep apnea syndrome are decreased by nasal continuous positive airway pressure. Circulation 2003; 107(8):1129–1134.

107. Carpagnano GE et al. Increased 8-isoprostane and interleukin-6 in breath condensate of obstructive sleep apnea patients. Chest 2002; 122(4):1162–1167.

108. Ohga E et al. Effects of obstructive sleep apnea on circulating ICAM-1, IL-8, and MCP-1. J Appl Physiol 2003; 94(1):179–184.

109. Schulz R et al. Enhanced release of superoxide from polymorphonuclear neutrophils in obstructive sleep apnea. Impact of continuous positive airway pressure therapy. Am J Respir Crit Care Med 2000; 162(2 Pt 1):566–570.

110. Dyugovskaya L, Lavie P, Lavie L. Increased adhesion molecules expression and production of reactive oxygen species in leukocytes of sleep apnea patients. Am J Respir Crit Care Med 2002; 165(7):934–939.

111. Dyugovskaya L, Lavie P, Lavie L. Phenotypic and functional characterization of blood gammadelta T cells in sleep apnea. Am J Respir Crit Care Med 2003; 168(2):242–249.

112. Schafer H et al. Body fat distribution, serum leptin, and cardiovascular risk factors in men with obstructive sleep apnea. Chest 2002; 122(3):829–839.

113. Chin K et al. Effects of NCPAP therapy on fibrinogen levels in obstructive sleep apnea syndrome. Am J Respir Crit Care Med 1996; 153(6 Pt 1): 1972–1976.

114. Chin K et al. Improvement of factor VII clotting activity following long-term NCPAP treatment in obstructive sleep apnoea syndrome. QJM 1998; 91(9): 627–633.

115. Rangemark C et al. Platelet function and fibrinolytic activity in hypertensive and normotensive sleep apnea patients. Sleep 1995; 18(3):188–194.

116. Lavie L, Perelman A, Lavie P. Plasma homocysteine levels in obstructive sleep apnea: association with cardiovascular morbidity. Chest 2001; 120(3):900–908.

117. von Kanel R et al. The hypercoagulable state in sleep apnea is related to comorbid hypertension. J Hypertens 2001; 19(8):1445–1451.
118. Sanner BM et al. Platelet function in patients with obstructive sleep apnoea syndrome. Eur Respir J 2000; 16(4):648–652.
119. Bokinsky G et al. Spontaneous platelet activation and aggregation during obstructive sleep apnea and its response to therapy with nasal continuous positive airway pressure. A preliminary investigation. Chest 1995; 108(3):625–630.
120. Arnulf I et al. Obstructive sleep apnea and venous thromboembolism. JAMA 2002; 287(20):2655–2656.
121. Hasegawa R et al. Sleep apnea syndrome in patients with pulmonary thromboembolism. Psychiat Clin Neurosci 2000; 54(3):342–343.
122. Ko GT, Chan HC. Restoration of nocturnal dip in blood pressure is associated with improvement in left ventricular ejection fraction. A 1-year clinical study comparing the effects of amlodipine and nifedipine retard on ambulatory blood pressure and left ventricular systolic function in Chinese hypertensive type 2 diabetic patients. Int J Cardiol 2003; 89(2/3):159–166.
123. Akashiba T et al. Nasal continuous positive airway pressure changes blood pressure "non-dippers" to "dippers" in patients with obstructive sleep apnea. Sleep 1999; 22(7):849–853.
124. Brooks D et al. Obstructive sleep apnea as a cause of systemic hypertension. Evidence from a canine model. J Clin Invest 1997; 99(1):106–109.
125. Grote L et al. Sleep-related breathing disorder is an independent risk factor for systemic hypertension. Am J Respir Crit Care Med 1999; 160(6):1875–1882.
126. Lavie P, Herer P, Hoffstein V. Obstructive sleep apnoea syndrome as a risk factor for hypertension: population study. BMJ 2000; 320(7233):479–482.
127. Peppard PE et al. Prospective study of the association between sleep-disordered breathing and hypertension. N Engl J Med 2000; 342(19):1378–1384.
128. Barbe F et al. Treatment with continuous positive airway pressure is not effective in patients with sleep apnea but no daytime sleepiness. A randomized, controlled trial. Ann Intern Med 2001; 134(11):1015–1023.
129. Faccenda JF et al. Randomized placebo-controlled trial of continuous positive airway pressure on blood pressure in the sleep apnea-hypopnea syndrome. Am J Respir Crit Care Med 2001; 163(2):344–348.
130. Pepperell JC et al. Ambulatory blood pressure after therapeutic and subtherapeutic nasal continuous positive airway pressure for obstructive sleep apnoea: a randomised parallel trial. Lancet 2002; 359(9302):204–210.
131. Becker HF et al. Effect of nasal continuous positive airway pressure treatment on blood pressure in patients with obstructive sleep apnea. Circulation 2003; 107(1):68–73.
132. Logan AG et al. High prevalence of unrecognized sleep apnoea in drug-resistant hypertension. J Hypertens 2001; 19(12):2271–2277.
133. Chobanian AV et al. The Seventh Report of the Joint National Committee on Prevention, Detection, Evaluation, and Treatment of High Blood Pressure: the JNC 7 report. JAMA 2003; 289(19):2560–2572.
134. Mooe T et al. Sleep-disordered breathing and myocardial ischemia in patients with coronary artery disease. Chest 2000; 117(6):1597–1602.

135. Peled N et al. Nocturnal ischemic events in patients with obstructive sleep apnea syndrome and ischemic heart disease: effects of continuous positive air pressure treatment. J Am Coll Cardiol 1999; 34(6):1744–1749.
136. Franklin KA et al. Sleep apnoea and nocturnal angina. Lancet 1995; 345(8957):1085–1087.
137. Hanly P et al. ST-segment depression during sleep in obstructive sleep apnea. Am J Cardiol 1993; 71(15):1341–1345.
138. Peker Y et al. An independent association between obstructive sleep apnoea and coronary artery disease. Eur Respir J 1999; 14(1):179–184.
139. Hung J et al. Association of sleep apnoea with myocardial infarction in men. Lancet 1990; 336(8710):261–264.
140. Shahar E et al. Sleep-disordered breathing and cardiovascular disease: cross-sectional results of the Sleep Heart Health Study. Am J Respir Crit Care Med 2001; 163(1):19–25.
141. Peker Y et al. Respiratory disturbance index: an independent predictor of mortality in coronary artery disease. Am J Respir Crit Care Med 2000; 162(1): 81–86.
142. Philip P, Guilleminault C. ST segment abnormality, angina during sleep and obstructive sleep apnea. Sleep 1993; 16(6):558–559.
143. Good DC et al. Sleep-disordered breathing and poor functional outcome after stroke. Stroke 1996; 27(2):252–259.
144. Dyken ME et al. Investigating the relationship between stroke and obstructive sleep apnea. Stroke 1996; 27(3):401–407.
145. Parra O et al. Time course of sleep-related breathing disorders in first-ever stroke or transient ischemic attack. Am J Respir Crit Care Med 2000; 161(2 Pt 1):375–380.
146. McArdle N et al. Sleep-disordered breathing as a risk factor for cerebrovascular disease: a case-control study in patients with transient ischemic attacks. Stroke 2003; 34(12):2916–2921.
147. Hu FB et al. Snoring and risk of cardiovascular disease in women. J Am Coll Cardiol 2000; 35(2):308–313.
148. Netzer N et al. Blood flow of the middle cerebral artery with sleep-disordered breathing: correlation with obstructive hypopneas. Stroke 1998; 29(1):87–93.
149. Lofaso F et al. Prevalence of sleep-disordered breathing in patients on a heart transplant waiting list. Chest 1994; 106(6):1689–1694.
150. Javaheri S et al. Sleep apnea in 81 ambulatory male patients with stable heart failure. Types and their prevalences, consequences, and presentations. Circulation 1998; 97(21):2154–2159.
151. Tremel F et al. High prevalence and persistence of sleep apnoea in patients referred for acute left ventricular failure and medically treated over 2 months. Eur Heart J 1999; 20(16):1201–1209.
152. Lanfranchi PA et al. Prognostic value of nocturnal Cheyne-Stokes respiration in chronic heart failure. Circulation 1999; 99(11):1435–1440.
153. Chan J et al. Prevalence of sleep-disordered breathing in diastolic heart failure. Chest 1997; 111(6):1488–1493.
154. Alex CG, Onal E, Lopata M. Upper airway occlusion during sleep in patients with Cheyne-Stokes respiration. Am Rev Respir Dis 1986; 133(1):42–45.

155. Kaneko Y et al. Cardiovascular effects of continuous positive airway pressure in patients with heart failure and obstructive sleep apnea. N Engl J Med 2003; 348(13):1233–1241.

156. Elmasry A et al. The role of habitual snoring and obesity in the development of diabetes: a 10-year follow-up study in a male population. J Intern Med 2000; 248(1):13–20.

157. Al-Delaimy WK et al. Snoring as a risk factor for type II diabetes mellitus: a prospective study. Am J Epidemiol 2002; 155(5):387–393.

158. Resnick HE et al. Diabetes and sleep disturbances: findings from the Sleep Heart Health Study. Diabetes Care 2003; 26(3):702–709.

159. Bottini P et al. Sleep-disordered breathing in nonobese diabetic subjects with autonomic neuropathy. Eur Respir J 2003; 22(4):654–660.

# 8

# Molecular Genetics of Obesity and Cardiovascular Diseases

Yvon C. Chagnon

*Psychiatric Genetic Unit, Laval University Robert-Giffard Research Center, Beauport, Québec, Canada*

## INTRODUCTION

Metabolic syndrome or syndrome X was defined initially according to the presence of atherogenic risk factors combined with underlying insulin resistance (1). This definition now includes insulin resistance, impaired glucose tolerance, presence or absence of type 2 diabetes mellitus, and any two of the following: hypertension, obesity, dyslipidemia, and microalbumineria (2). Dyslipidemia [low high-density lipoprotein cholesterol (HDL-C), high triglycerides (TGs)] and insulin resistance predict risk for atherosclerotic cardiovascular disease (CVD) even in healthy individuals. Three times more coronary heart diseases and strokes are observed in subjects with metabolic syndrome, while central obesity is a key etiological factor for underlying insulin resistance (3).

Both obesity and CVD are complex traits showing multiple environmental and polygenic influences in their expression. This chapter will review some of the genes and their variations involved in obesity-related phenotypes and in cardiovascular risk factors, highlighting those genes shared by both pathologies. Obesity and CVD show numerous candidate genes from various metabolic pathways, and trying to combine and synthesize all known results and studies for both traits is outside the capacity and the goal of the actual chapter. To focus on the most sustainable results, different independent lines of evidence will be used to narrow the possible candidates to those showing the strongest evidence. Among these lines, studies reporting statistically strong results will be included to produce a sharper image of the possible molecular genetic links between obesity and CVD. The author apologizes for the numerous and very valuable studies that will be set aside in the present work because of these guidelines.

## LINES OF EVIDENCE

### Genome Scans

The first line of evidence will be quantitative trait loci or QTLs identified by linkage analysis following human genome scans. In a genome scan, highly variable genetic markers, usually di, tri or tetra repeat microsatellites, located regularly at each 5 to 10 centimorgans (cM) on all the 22 autosomal and the sexual pairs of chromosomes are amplified by the polymerase chain reaction in informative family members. Because the entire genome represents some 4 Morgans, about 400 markers are needed to cover the genome at a 10 cM spacing. The number of subjects to be analyzed can be as low as 10 to 20 in an informative multigenerational pedigree, to as high as 1000 and more subjects from hundreds of smaller nuclear families. Following genotyping of all the subjects, linkage analysis is done to detect chromosomal regions sharing genetic characteristics or QTL among affected subjects. One major advantage of the genome scan approach is that all the genome is investigated simultaneously. A second advantage is that there is no a priori hypothesis on which chromosomal regions should show linkages with the trait under study. This unbiased non–hypothesis-driven approach, when used and interpreted correctly, allows prioritizing known candidate genes located in detected linked regions among those candidates defined according to their biochemical functions in relevant metabolic pathways. But more importantly, the genome scan approach allows the identification of unsuspected new candidate genes. This is an important issue since we learned from the Human Genome Sequencing Project that fewer genes than expected (about 30,000 genes in contrast to the 100,000 expected initially) are encoded in the genome. This implies more forms, functions, and interactions of these genes to fulfill all the needed biological processes, and consequently, more unsuspected functions for our genes. The new candidate genes that will be detected by the genome scan are those genes located in the linked region but that did not show functions obviously related to the trait under study. They also could be expressed transcripts or ESTs with no known function or metabolic pathway.

To associate formally these candidate genes and ESTs to the trait under study, a search for genetic variants within these genes and ESTs, usually single nucleotide polymorphism, is done. The detected variants are then characterized among cases and controls by association studies with trait-related phenotypes. Alternatively, or complementarily, gene invalidation (KO, knockout) and/or overexpression (Tg, transgenic) of the candidate genes and ESTs could be done to evaluate the effects of a perturbed expression of these new candidate genes on the trait of interest.

## Association Studies

Association studies represent an independent line of evidence from the genome scan when candidate genes are defined a priori according to their biological functions and metabolic pathways potentially related to the trait under study. For example, the uncoupling protein genes have been targeted as candidate genes for obesity because of their potential role in energy expenditure (EE). Similarly, the apolipoprotein (APO) genes are candidates for atherosclerosis because of their role in cholesterol transport. The nomenclature of the variations observed in genes is problematic because the same terminology is used for different phenomena. A strict molecular definition of a variation observed at any frequency in a gene is a mutation. However, clinically, a variation in a gene would be called a mutation when this genetic variation produced a deleterious effect on the function of the product encoded by this gene. A variation in a gene that is associated with obesity or CVD-related phenotypes, but showing no obvious deleterious effect on product activity, should be named a variant or a polymorphism. In this case, it is postulated that the variant or polymorphism studied is in linkage disequilibrium with the true variant at the origin of the effect within the gene or in a physically close gene. The deleterious effects of a mutation could come from some change either in the expression of the mutated gene, or in the processing and the translation of its primary RNA, or in the structure or the cellular localization of the encoded product, all resulting in an altered activity. For example, a variation in the promoter of a gene can reduce or stop its expression, whereas a variation in the coding region could produce a reduction or a loss of activity of the gene encoded product. The strict molecular definition of a mutation should not be used when reporting genetic association results for gene variations with unknown effects.

In association studies, the frequency of the different forms or alleles of a gene, or the distribution of the genotypes produced by the combination of these alleles, are compared between cases and controls. If the effect of the gene is relatively strong in the population studied, a difference in the frequency of the alleles or of the genotypes should be observed between cases and controls. Alternatively, mean values of continuous trait-related phenotypes such as body mass index (BMI) in obesity or lipid levels in CVD could be tested among genotypes by variance analysis or by regression. Candidate genes defined because of their location within linked regions of genome scans are tested for association in the same way, but these candidate genes do not represent an independent line of evidence from that of genome scans.

Another way of defining candidate genes independently of their metabolic roles or of their location in linked regions is to analyze their differential expression between case and control subjects. For example, the melanin-concentrating hormone, or MCH, encoded by the pro-MCH gene located on chromosome 12q23-q24, was detected initially as a transcript overexpressed in the hypothalamus of the obese ob/ob mouse mutated in the leptin gene (4). MCH proved to be an orexigenic peptide stimulating food intake (FI) in rats (4), while its receptor is becoming a target for drug control of FI and obesity (5). Similarly, Eurlings et al. (6) investigated adipose tissue for differential gene expression in subjects with familial combined hyperlipidemia matched for BMI with controls. Twenty-two genes with a greater expression and three with a lower expression were identified, including the tumor necrosis factor alpha, the interleukin 6, and the intracellular adhesion molecule 1 (6). However, very few of these differential expression studies are actually available, and few of the detected genes or ESTs over- or underexpressed have been sufficiently characterized to be included in the actual lines of evidence.

## KO and Tg Rodent Models

KO and Tg rodent models also represent an independent line of evidence for obesity or CVD when genes have been selected according to other traits and metabolic functions. For example, metallothionein (MT) has several alleged roles in metal detoxification, in Zn and Cu homeostasis, in scavenging free radicals, and in the acute phase response that does not obviously target MT as a significant factor in obesity or CVD. However, KO mice for both MT-I and MT-II genes are more sensitive to toxic metals and oxidative stress, but also showed moderate obesity from a higher fat accretion, indicating a link between MT and the regulation of energy balance (7). More recently, a higher expression of MT-I in adipose tissue of human obese subjects has also been reported (8), supporting earlier observations in KO mice. Such KO and Tg genes including unsuspected obesity-related phenotypes have been reviewed recently (9), whereas some reviews are available for CVD candidate genes per se (10,11). Unfortunately, KO and Tg models are not evaluated systematically for obesity or CVD-related phenotypes when there are no obvious indications present to indicate that these phenotypes have been perturbed. Moreover, obesity and CVD phenotypes are not necessarily of obvious interest to the investigators developing these Tg models. The consequences are that besides evident exterior characteristics such as obesity and greatly increased FI, for example, weaker but significant effects on body weight, fat distribution, or lipids profile will not be detected or reported at all if outside the scope of published research papers.

When both KO and Tg are available for a same gene, it is expected that they will produce opposite metabolic perturbations: KO will suppress the gene product whereas Tg will enhance its expression. However, it appears that this occurrence is not always the case, probably because of the multiple mechanisms involved in complex traits such as obesity and CVD showing redundant and compensatory pathways. This absence of occurrence could also come from the use of different mouse strains in KO and Tg, which carry different genetic backgrounds. For example, it has been shown that the ob mutation when expressed on different genetic backgrounds will or will not induce insulin resistance (12). But most often, KO and Tg models are not available for a same gene; yet its occurrence does reflect to some extent how long this gene has been recognized as a candidate for obesity or CVD. For example, numerous Tg models are available for the former candidate APO genes family that is reflected by the numerous combined KO/Tg or Tg/Tg models. Nevertheless, because different genome sequencing projects have led to an easier access to gene structure information, and thanks to new Tg facilities that are now provided in most research centers, KO and Tg models are now being developed rapidly and simultaneously for most new candidate genes.

## GENETIC EPIDEMIOLOGY OF OBESITY AND CVD

### Phenotypes

Obesity-related phenotypes include weight, FI, BMI, fatness, skinfold thickness, abdominal fat and waist circumference, fat-free mass, and some plasma hormone levels such as those of leptin and adiponectin. CVD-related phenotypes include alterations in glucose and insulin levels, insulin resistance/sensitivity, changes in lipid profile including cholesterol, TG, HDL, low density lipoprotein (LDL), very LDL (VLDL), atheroschlerosis, and some familial dyslipidemias.

### Heritability

Heritability estimates for obesity and CVD are relatively high for both traits. Estimates varied according to the obesity- or CVD-related phenotypes analyzed. For obesity-related phenotypes, heritability estimate values ranged between 0.32 and 0.59 for BMI (13–16), between 0.48 and 0.80 for fat percentage (13,14,17), between 0.65 and 0.76 for fat-free mass (13,14), and between as low as 0.06 and as high as 0.86 for waist-to-hip ratio (14,18–20). For LDL, heritabilities between 0.34 and 0.50 (20,21) up to 0.90 in Hutterites (14) have been reported, whereas estimates for HDL heritabilities ranged between 0.42 and 0.83 (14,20–23). TGs showed slightly lower values ranging between 0.19 and 0.55 (14,20–24), whereas lipoprotein (a) [Lp(a)] presented a heritability similar to that of LDL [0.51–0.90 (20,25–27)].

## GENOME SCAN RESULTS FOR OBESITY AND CVD

### Linkages for Obesity or CVD

In the last 10 years, results from 35 genome scans for obesity-related phenotypes have been reported (9): for CVD, 15 on HDL-C genetics (28), 16 for
TG, 10 for cholesterol, 11 for LDL-cholesterol (LDL-C), and close to 40
additional for other CVD-related phenotypes including various lipid trans-
porters ratio and familial lipid perturbations (29). Among these studies,
only those reporting results with Lod scores of 3.0 and higher will be
retained (Table 1).

This is usually the significant Lod score at the genome-wide level,
while it corresponds to a lower threshold level according to Lander and
Kruglyak (73) guidelines recommending a minimum Lod score of 3.5 and of
2.5 for a significant or a suggestive linkage result, respectively (73). Based on
a minimum Lod score of 3.0, results from 23 genome scans for obesity and
20 for CVD have been retained (Table 1). At this Lod score threshold, some
valuably informative results may be lost. This selection, however, will help
to focus on the more consistent results across studies that should be
supported by our other independent lines of evidence, namely association
studies and Tg rodent models. For comparison purposes, markers and genes
in the positive-linked regions have all been relocated according to the same
genetic map (LDB, genetic location database; http://cedar.genetics.soton.
ac.uk/public_html/). In Table 1, it can be seen that almost all chromosomes
except chromosomes 21, 22, and Y harbored QTLs related to obesity, CVD,
or to both traits. This is a larger coverage of the human genome than those
observed in other combined complex traits. For example, schizophrenia (SZ)
and bipolar disorder (BP) are two complex traits for which specific and
shared genes between both traits are expected (74,75). A review of linkage
findings in SZ and BP showed that 15 out of the 23 chromosome pairs harbored linkages with a Lod score over 3.0 (75–77). For diabetes, another individual complex trait similar to obesity or CVD because it is also involved in
the metabolic disorder syndrome, replicated linkage signals have been
observed in 10 out of the 23 human chromosomes (78,79). In a similar
undertaking, Goldin et al. (80) have also analyzed different metabolic syndrome phenotypes in the Framingham Heart Study families in an attempt to
map underlying genes. They observed consistent linkage in regions of chromosomes 2, 11, 16, 19, and 22, only the latter not being in the present results
(Table 1). The lower number of genome scans included in the analysis could
explain the lower number of linked regions detected by Goldin et al. (80).

### Linked Regions Shared by Obesity and CVD

From Table 1, it can also be seen that 11 out of the 32 chromosomal regions
showing linkages with either obesity or CVD showed linkages with both traits.

**Table 1** Significant (Lod Score > 3.0) Linkages with Obesity-Related or CVD-Related Phenotypes

| Chr | Location | cM | Obesity | CVD | References |
|-----|----------|-----|---------|-----|------------|
| 1 | 1p36.32-p34.2 | 3–56 | | FH | (30–33) |
| | **1p31.1-p22.3** | **74–91** | **Leptin** | **TGs** | (34,35) |
| | 1q24.1 | 182 | | Chol | (35) |
| 2 | **2p25.2-p21** | **10–49** | **Leptin, fat** | **HDL-C** | (36–38) |
| | 2q14.2 | 125 | | TGs | (14,39) |
| 3 | **3p22.1-p21.2** | **40–62** | **BMI** | **FHBL** | (40,41) |
| | 3q22.1 | 150 | BMI | | (42) |
| | **3q26.32-q29** | **192–213** | **BMI** | **LDL-3** | (42,43) |
| 4 | 4p15.1 | 34 | BMI | | (44) |
| | 4q22.1-q28.2 | 98–143 | | LDL-3 | (45) |
| 5 | **5p15.2-p12** | **15–46** | **Adiponectin** | **HDL-C** | (46,47) |
| 6 | **6q23.1-q27** | **142–180** | **BMI, leptin** | **Lp(a)** | (14,48,49) |
| 7 | 7q31.33-q35 | 134–156 | BMI, skinfolds, fat, WC | | (50–52) |
| 8 | 8p12 | 37 | BMI | | (53) |
| | 8q23.3-q24.3 | 124–145 | | HDL-C | (38,54) |
| 9 | 9p22.3-p22.2 | 16–17 | | HDL-C, TGs | (39,55) |
| 10 | **10p12.33** | **20–49** | **Obesity** | **TGs** | (56–58) |
| 11 | 11p12 | 44 | | LDL-C | (59) |
| | **11q14.3-q24.3** | **100–138** | **BMI** | **LDL-C** | (60,61) |
| 12 | 12q14.3 | 75 | | HDL-C | (61) |
| | 12q24.11-q24.31 | 115–134 | | TGs | (35) |
| 13 | 13q11-q14 | 16–21 | BMI | | (40,50) |
| | 13q21.33-q32.3 | 73–101 | | Chol, FH | (30,62) |
| 14 | 14q13.1-q21.1 | 32–41 | Adiponectin | | (46) |
| 15 | 15q11.1-q21.3 | 19–60 | | TGs, HDL-C | (54,63) |
| | **15q26.1-q26.3** | **97–105** | **FFM** | **FH, LDL-C** | (61,64,65) |
| 16 | 16q22.1–24.1 | 78–95 | | HDL-C | (57,56) |
| 17 | **17p12-q21.33** | **16–56** | **Leptin** | **LPL-PPD** | (43,61) |
| 18 | **18p11.23-q12.3** | **8–45** | **FFM** | **Lp(a)** | (14,64) |
| 19 | 19p13.3-q13.43 | 6–64 | | Chol, LDL-C, ApoE, TGs | (14,61,67–69) |
| 20 | 20q13.12-q13.31 | 48–64 | BMI, fat | | (32,70,71) |
| X | Xq23 | 113 | Obesity | | (72) |

Linkage regions shared between obesity and CVD are indicated in bold.
*Abbreviations*: BMI, body mass index; WC, waist circumference; FFM, fat-free mass; Chol, cholesterol; LDL-C, low-density lipoprotein-cholesterol; ApoE, apolipoprotein E; TGs, triglycerides; Lp(a), lipoprotein (a); LPL-PPD, lipoprotein lipase-luminogen PPD; HDL-C, high-density lipoprotein-cholesterol; FH, familial hypercholesteronemia; FHBL, familial hyper-betalipoproteinemia; CVD, cardiovascular disease.

For example, at chromosome 1p32.1-p22.3, in two independent genome scans, one showed linkages with leptin (34), the other with TGs (35). A second linkage with cholesterol at 1q24, outside the shared region for leptin and TGs, was also observed (35). Chromosomal region 1p32.1-p22.3 covered 17 cM (74–91 cM according to the LDB genetic map), a large chromosomal region, when trying to identify positional candidate genes. Different hypothesis on the genetic origin of these common linkages could be drawn. A first possibility is that the common region of linkage at 1p32.1-p22.3 comes from a gene located in this region, involved in the control of both leptin and TGs. A second is that a gene located within 1p32.1-p22.3 is responsible for the linkage with leptin, while a different gene also located within 1p32.1-p22.3 is responsible for the linkage with TGs. A third is that one gene is responsible for either the linkage with leptin or TGs, while another gene is involved in the control of both leptin and TGs levels. These three hypotheses do not cover all the combinations possible with two or more genes, but such combinations are less likely. In any case, if we consider at this point the possibility of one common gene, it has to be stressed that the leptin receptor (LEPR) gene is located at 1p31 within the linked region. Mutations in LEPR have shown to be associated with obesity or body composition changes, but have not, up to now, been reported to be associated with CVD risk factors (Table 2 A–D). However, mice KO in fat for LEPR have shown higher TG levels (Table 2 A–D), underlying the possibilities that known or new mutations in LEPR could be associated with lipid levels in humans. This should be investigated in future studies in humans. In fact, mutations in the leptin gene, located at 7q31.1, have been shown to be associated not only with obesity but also with TGs levels (Table 2 A–D).

Other linked chromosomal regions shared by obesity and CVD are also observed at 6q23.1-q27 (38 cM) or 17p12-q21.33 (40 cM). These represent fairly large chromosomal regions similar to those reported in the study of Goldin et al. (80), but where many hundreds of genes are encoded. Usually, one should proceed to a fine mapping at a 1 cM interval within these regions before beginning a systematic candidate genes analysis. However, using independent lines of evidence could accelerate the identification and the choice of positional candidate genes from the linked regions to be further tested.

## RESULTS OF ASSOCIATION STUDIES FOR OBESITY AND CVD

Table 2 A–D summarizes results from association studies for obesity or CVD-related phenotypes. For association studies, those with $P$ values of 0.005 and less were retained when available. Our annual compilation of the obesity gene map (9) and the review of Ordovas (28) for CVD were used as a starting point to select relevant genes and association studies. These were completed by a PubMed electronic search for additional relevant

*(Text continues on p. 197.)*

**Table 2** Polymorphisms, Mutations, or KO in Human (Uppercase in Bold) and Rodent (Lowercase) Genes and Tg in Rodent Models of Obesity and CVD

| Genes | Chr | Variations | Obesity | CVD | References |
|---|---|---|---|---|---|
| *(A) Genes showing greater weight and food intake in KO mice or mutated gene, or lower weight and food intake in Tg mice* | | | | | |
| **LEP** | 7q31.3 | GGTΔ133ΔG398 (KO) | Weight >, FI >, no leptin | Insulin > (age) | (81) |
| Lep | 6 | Arg35**Trp** (KO) | Weight >, FI >, no leptin Leptin (corrected) | Insulin >, TG >, Chol= Dyslipidemia: no | (82) (83) |
| | | ob/ob (KO) | **Weight >, FI >**, fat cell # & size > | **Lipogenesis >**, insulin≫, glucose > (transient) | (12) |
| | | Tg | Weight <, FI <, fat < | PLIN <, PKA <, lipolysis < | (84) |
| | | Tg (A-ZIP/F-1) | ΔWeight < | TG <, FFA < (VLDL-TG, LPL >) | (85) |
| **LEPR** | 1p31 | IV18G/A (KO) Gln223**Arg** | Weight >, FI >, leptin > BMI >, fat >, FFM > in males | Insulin=, TG=, Chol= TG <, HDLC < | (86) (87–89) |
| Lepr | 4 | db/db (KO) | **Weight >, FI >**, fat cell size > | Insulin >, glucose > | (12) |
| | | Antisense (fat) KO | FI=, fat > | | (90) |
| **MC4R** | 18q22 | Lys211**del**CTCT (KO) | Weight >, FI >, | **TG >**, IR, glucose > | (91) |
| | | Tyr35**X** (KO) | Weight >, leptin > | Lipids=, glucose= | (92) |
| | | N62**Ser**, Cys279**Ins**GT | Weight >, FI >, fat >, leptin > | Insulin > | (93) |
| | | NcoI+ | Fat > | Insulin=, glucose= | (94) |
| Mc4r | 18 | KO | **Weight >, FI >** | Insulin > | (95) |

*(Continued)*

**Table 2** Polymorphisms, Mutations, or KO in Human (Uppercase in Bold) and Rodent (Lowercase) Genes and Tg in Rodent Models of Obesity and CVD (*Continued*)

| Genes | Chr | Variations | Obesity | CVD | References |
|---|---|---|---|---|---|
| **CCKAR** | 4p15.2 | −128G/T | Fat >, leptin > | Insulin > | (96) |
| Cckar | 5 | 5′_exons1,2 **del** (KO) | **Weight** >, **FI** > | Glucose > (half of rats) | (97) |
| **APM1** (adiponectin) | 3q27 | Gly15(45T/G)_IVS2+276G/T | Weight >, WC > | Insulin >, IR >, Tot/**HDL** >, TG=, Chol=, HDL-C= | (98) |
| | | Gly15 (45T/G) | BMI=, leptin= | LDL >, insulin=, TG=, Chol= | (99) |
| Acrp30 | 16 | Tg (adenovirus) | **Weight** <, **FI** < | TG <, **lipogenesis** <, IS >, glucose > | (100) |
| **GAD2** | 10p12 | −243 A/**G** +61450**C**/ T_+83897T/A | **Weight** >, **FI** >, RNA > Weight < | | (101) |
| Gad2 | 2 | KO | | Fear <, anxiety >, corticosterone= | (102,103) |
| **HSD11B1** | 1q32-q41 | 4436**ins**A | BMI > | Insulin >, lipid= | (104) |
| Hsd11b1 | 1 | KO | | **TG** <, HDL-Chol >, ApoA1 >, IS > | (105) |
| **POMC** | 2p23.3 | Tg Glu79X_Ala131X (KO) E2 3804C/A (KO) RsaI++_C7556T | **Fat** > (visceral) HFD, **FI** > Weight > | **Lipid** >, IR (diabetes) | (106) (107) |
| Pomc | 12 | KO | Leptin > **weight** > | | (37) |
| **AGRP** | 16q22.1 | **Thr67Ala** | Fat > | Insulin= | (108) |
| | | **Thr67**Ala | > in anorexia | | (109) |
| Agrp | 8 | Tg | **Weight** >, fat >, fat cell # & size > | Insulin >, glucose > (late onset) | (110) (111) |

| Gene | Locus | Variant | Phenotype | | Ref |
|---|---|---|---|---|---|
| **FABP2** | 4q26 | Ala54Thr | BMI >, fat > | IR > (not in FH), HDL-TG >, LDL-TG > | (112,113) |
| Fabp2 | 3 | KO | **Weight** > males, weight < females HFD | **Triacylglycerols** > males, insulin > | (114) |
| **FABP4** | 8q21 | | | IS, lipids, lipolysis , atherosclerosis | (115) |
| Fabp4 (aP2) | 3 | KO | **Weight** > HFD | No IR HFD, glucose < | (116,117) |
| **CYP19A1** | 15q21 | IVS4 TCTdelTTTA(n) **168** | Obesity abdominal | | (118) |
| | | IVS4 TCTdelTTTA(n) **187** | Leanness | | (119) |
| Cyp19 | 9 | KO | **Weight** > (females), **FI**=, fat > (abdominal), FFM <, activity <, fat cell # & size > | **Chol** >, HDL >, insulin > | (120,121) |
| **PPARG** | 3p25 | Phe388Leu | No fat (FPLD2) | | (122) |
| | | Pro115Gln | BMI > 35, fat cell # > | TG >, insulin <, diabetes | (123) |
| | | C161T | Leptin > | TG=, Chol=, insulin= | (124) |
| | | Pro12Ala | Weight > | LDL-Chol >, Chol >, ApoB > | (125) |
| | | | WC > (overweight) | Insulin <, IR <, TG= (normal weight) | (126) |
| | | | ASF > | Insulin= | (127) |
| | | | ΔBMI > in obese & < in lean | | (128) |
| Pparg | 6 | KO (muscle) | **Weight** >, **FI** < HFD; fat pads > CD | **TG (fat)** >, insulin >, Glucose > HFD; IR, glucose = CD | (129) |

*(Continued)*

**Table 2** Polymorphisms, Mutations, or KO in Human (Uppercase in Bold) and Rodent (Lowercase) Genes and Tg in Rodent Models of Obesity and CVD (*Continued*)

| Genes | Chr | Variations | Obesity | CVD | References |
|---|---|---|---|---|---|
| *(B) Genes showing no change in weight (obesity resistant) and a higher or equal* | | | | | |
| **PLIN** | 15q26 | IVS6 rs894160 A/G | BMI= | Lipolysis >, perilipin < (obese women), TG=, insulin=, glucose= | (130) |
| Plin | 7 | KO | **Weight= HFD, FI >**, lean, fat cell size < | **Lipolysis (constitutive)**, FFA < | (131,132) |
| NCOA2 (TIF2) | 8q13.2 | KO-Lepr$^{db/db}$ KO | Weight normal, EE > | | (133) |
| Ncoa2 | 1 | KO | **Weight= HFD, FI >**, EE >, fat cell # >, size < | Lipolysis >, FFA storage <, IS > | (134) |
| **LIPE (HSL)** | 19q13.2 | −60C/**G** | Fat < (white women) BMI > & SF > (black women) | Insulin=, FFA= | (135) |
| | | −60C/G | BMI=, RNA < | Insulin <, HOMAB >, Chol=, TG= | (136) |
| Lipe | 7 | KO Tg | **Weight= HFD, FI >**, EE > | **FFA** < CD, insulin > CD **Atherosclerosis** > HFD, cholesteryl ester > | (137) (138) |
| | | Tg-ApoA IV Tg | | HDL >, atherosclerosis > HFD < | (138) |
| **MCHR-1 (GPR24)** | 22q13.2 | | | | |
| Mchr-1 | 15 | KO | **Weight= HFD, FI >**, fat <, EE >, activity > | | (139) |

| Gene | Location | Model | Phenotype | Metabolic | Ref. |
|---|---|---|---|---|---|
| **DGAT1** Dgat1 | 8q24.3 / 15 | KO | **Weight= HFD, FI=**, lean, EE >, activity > Fat >, Δweight > HFD, | **TG <, IS >** (GTT), FFA=, glucose=, insulin= TG=, glucose=, insulin= | (140,141) |
| **PKARIIβ** PkarIIβ | | Tg (fat) | **Weight= HFD, FI=**, lean, fat cell # = | **Lipolysis >** | (142) (142,143) |
| **HMGIC** Hmgic | | KO | **Weight= HFD, FI=** | | (145) |
| | | KO-Lep$^{ob/ob}$ KO | Obesity <, fat <, fat cell # < | Insulin=, glucose= | (145) |
| **PTPN1 (PTP-1B)** Ptpn1 | 20q13.1 / 2 | KO | **Weight= HFD, FI=** | Insulin <, glucose < | (146) |
| **PLA2G1B (PLA2)** Pla2g1b | 12q24.3 / 5 | KO | **Weight= HFD, FI=**, fat < | **TG <**, insulin < HFD, (TG > in stool) | (147) |
| **SCD** Scd1 | 10q24.3 / 19 | KO | **Weight= HFD**, fat <: EE > | IS > | (148) |
| | | ab$^J$/ab$^J$ (KO) | | **TG <** (liver) (VLDL, LDL), CE < | (149) |
| | | ab$^J$/ab$^J$ KO-Lep$^{ob/ob}$ KO | Obesity <, FI >, EE= | TG normal, VLDL < | (150) |
| **ATRN** Atrn | 20p13 / 2 | Mahogany (KO) | **Weight= HFD** | | (151,152) |

*(Continued)*

**Table 2** Polymorphisms, Mutations, or KO in Human (Uppercase in Bold) and Rodent (Lowercase) Genes and Tg in Rodent Models of Obesity and CVD (*Continued*)

| Genes | Chr | Variations | Obesity | CVD | References |
|---|---|---|---|---|---|
| **ESR1** | 6q25.1 | XbaI ++ | > Obesity (android), C-peptide < | | (153) |
| Esr1 | 10 | KO | **Weight**=, **FI**= (resistant) | Lipids= | (154) |
| **RETN** | 19p13.3 | g.-537A/C | BMI > | | (155) |
| | | 3'UTR +62G/A | BMI= | | (156) |
| Retn | 8 | Tg (fat) | **Weight**=, fat= | < in diabetes, TG=, Chol=, glucose = | (157) |
| **MC3R** | 20q13.2 | +2138**Ins**CAGACC | Fat > (normal weight), fat < (overweight), FI= | **FFA** >, **TG** > (muscle), insulin=, glucose =, glucose tolerance < | (158) |
| Mc3r | 2 | KO | **Weight**=, **FI** <, fat >, FFM <, activity < | na | (159,160) |
| | | | | Insulin > (males), glucose= | |

*(C) Genes showing lower weight or no fat when invalidated or overexpressed*

| Genes | Chr | Variations | Obesity | CVD | References |
|---|---|---|---|---|---|
| **PMCH** | 12q24.2 | | | | |
| Mch | 10 | KO | **Weight** <, **FI** <, lean, EE > | | (161) |
| | | KO-Lep[ob/ob] KO | Fat <, FI >, EE > | | (162) |
| | | Tg | **Weight** >, **FI** > | IR | (163) |
| **PRKCQ** | 10p15.1 | | | | |
| Prkcq | 2 | **Tg** | **Weight** > | Insulin >, glucose > | (164) |
| **EIF4EBP1** | 8p12 | | | | |
| Eif4ebp1 | 8 | KO | **Weight** <, **FI**=, fat≪, EE > (males) | Insulin=, glucose >, TG= | (165) |

| Gene (Location) | Variant/Model | Obesity phenotype | Metabolic phenotype | Ref. |
|---|---|---|---|---|
| CD36 (7q11.2) | HaeIII+−150delCCCCGCC-GT | BMI < (females) | >CAD, HDL-C, ApoA1 | (166) |
|  |  | RNA < | HDL-C> | (167) |
| Cd36 (5) | IVS5 C/T_E8 C/T |  | HDL> | (168) |
|  | KO |  | Chol> (HDL), TG > (VLDL), FA >, Gluc <, IS > (muscle), IR > (liver) | (169,170) |
| LPIN1 (2p25.1) |  |  |  |  |
| Lpin1 (12) | Tg (muscle) | Weight <, fat < | Chol <, TG < (VLDL), FA <, Gluc >, insulin= | (171) |
| B-ZIP | Fld (KO) | No fat (lipodystrophy) | TG>, IR | (172) |
| B-ZIP (1q21.3) | KO (A-ZIP/F-1) | No fat, liver fat >, FI > | FFA>, TG >, IR, glucose > | (173) |
| LMNA | Arg482Gln | No fat (FPLD2) | TG >, insulin >, HDL-Chol < | (174,175) |
|  | 1908T/C | BMI>, fat>, WHR > |  | (176,177) |
| Lmna (3) |  |  |  |  |
| SREBF1 (17p11.2) | SMS del (17) (p11.2p11.2) | BMI= | Chol> | (178) |
| Srebf1 (8) | Tg | No fat (lipodystrophy) | Lipids > (liver) | (179,180) |
| BATF (14q24.3) |  |  |  |  |
| Batf (12) | Tg | No fat, weight > (females) |  | (173) |
| GPD1 (12q13.2) | IVS3+18T/A_+26 delTTTTAA |  | Diabetes | (181) |
|  | His264Arg |  | FFA>, glycerol > in non-diabetics | (182) |
| Gpd1 (15) | Tg | No fat |  | (183) |

(D) Other genes

*(Continued)*

**Table 2** Polymorphisms, Mutations, or KO in Human (Uppercase in Bold) and Rodent (Lowercase) Genes and Tg in Rodent Models of Obesity and CVD (*Continued*)

| Genes | Chr | Variations | Obesity | CVD | References |
|---|---|---|---|---|---|
| **APOC1** | 19q13.2 | −317**InsCGTT** (HpaI) | RNA < | TG < in African-Americans | (184) |
| Apoc1 | 7 | Tg | | TG >, Chol > (VLDL clearance <), ApoB > | (185,186) |
| | | Tg-ApoE KO | | Chol > (IDL+LDL), TG > | (187) |
| | | Tg-Ldlr KO | | Chol >, TG > | (187) |
| | | Tg-Lepob/ob KO | Weight <, fat <, fat cell size= | FFA >, TG >, IS > | (188) |
| **APOC2** | 19q13.2 | Tyr63X (KO) | FI < | TG >, hyperchylomicronemia | (189) |
| | | Trp26**Arg** (KO) | | TG > | (190) |
| Apoc2 | 7 | KO | | TG≫ (VLDL >), apoC/apoE ratio > | (191) |
| **APOC3** | 11q23.1 | 3′UTR +C3238**G** | | LDL-C > | (192) |
| | | 3′UTR +C3238**G** (SstI) | | TG > | (193) |
| | | −455**T**/C_−625**T**/del | | | |
| Apoc3 | 9 | KO | | Chol >, LDL-C > | (194) |
| | | KO-ApoE KO | | TG <, Chol < | (195) |
| | | Tg-Ldlr KO | | TG <, VLDL-C < Chol of HDL, IDL-LDL→VLDL | (196) |
| | | | | TG of VLDL→ HDL, IDL-LDL LDL | (197) |
| **APOC4** | 19q13.2 | **Leu36Pro, Leu96Arg** | | TG > in women | (198) |
| Apoc4 | | Tg | | TG > in VLDL, Chol= (> in VLDL) | (199) |

| Gene | Locus | Variant | Phenotype | Ref. |
|---|---|---|---|---|
| **APOE** | 19q13.2 | E1/E3/**E4** | Chol>, LDL-C>, CHD risk>, ApoB> in men | (200–202) |
| | | Lys146**Gln**, Arg158**Cys** | FHBL | (203) |
| | | E1/E3/**E4**, −219G/T | CHD risk>, ApoE<, glucose> (OGTT) | (204,205) |
| ApoE | 7 | SHL (KO) | Chol≫, atherosclerosis (<KO) | (206) |
| | | KO | Chol> (VLDL,chylomicron), atherosclerosis | (207,208) |
| | | KO-IL10 Tg (muscle) | Chol>, no atherosclerosis | (209) |
| | | KO-FABP2 KO  Weight> | Chol=, TG=, FFA=, insulin=, atherosclerosis< | (210) |
| **APOB** | 2p22.3 | KO-Cav1 KO | Non-HDL Chol> (2x) | (211) |
| | | KO-Ldlr KO | ApoB-48>, apoB-100> | (212) |
| | | 5564**InsC**, 11040T/G, 1018_1025**del**, 3600T/A, 82+1G/A | FHBL (LDL-C<, ApoB<), atherosclerosis< | (228) |
| | | Arg463**Trp** | FHBL (LDL-C<, ApoB<) | (213) |
| | | Thr2488 (XbaI+) | LDL-C>, ApoB>, IHD risk< | (214) |
| | | E1 **del** Leu-Ala-Leu | LDL-C>, ApoB>, IHD risk> | (215) |
| | | Lys4154Lys (EcoRI-) | LDL-C>, ApoB>, IHD risk> | (215) |
| | | PvuII/Thr2488 (XbaI)  BMI> | LDL-C<, Chol<, IHD risk= | (216) |
| | | Arg3611Gln/ Glu4154Lys | Chol> | (216) |
| ApoB | 12 | Thr2488/Arg3611Gln | CHD risk> | (216) |
| | | Tg | LDL> CD, TG> | (217) |
| | | | Atherosclerosis HFD (VLDL+LDL-Chol>) | (218,219) |
| | | Tg-Cetp Tg | Lipids= | (220) |

*(Continued)*

**Table 2** Polymorphisms, Mutations, or KO in Human (Uppercase in Bold) and Rodent (Lowercase) Genes and Tg in Rodent Models of Obesity and CVD (*Continued*)

| Genes | Chr | Variations | Obesity | CVD | References |
|---|---|---|---|---|---|
| **APOA1** | 11q23 | −75G/A, 83C/T | BMI < (in diabetics) | HDL-C > (males) | (221) |
| Apoa1 | 9 | Tg | | Atherosclerosis: LP(a) > | (217,222) |
| **APOA4** | 11q23 | Xbal∗**2**, Thr347**Ser** | BMI > (in smokers) | | (223) |
| | | Gln360**His** | WC > (in nonsmokers), BMI <, fat < | | (223,224) |
| Apoa4 | 9 | Thr347Ser | BMI >, WHR >, BMI >, fat > | TG > | (224,225) |
| | | KO | FI= | Chol <, TG <, (HDL <, VLDL <), ApoCIII < | (226) |
| **CETP** | 16q21 | Taq1**B1B2**(−) | | HDL-C >, CETP < | (227,228) |
| | | IVS14Δ (KO) | | Atherosclerosis, hyperalphalipoproteinemia | (229) |
| Cetp | 8 | Tg | | Atherosclerosis: VLDL+LDL/ HDL ratio > (VLDL+LDL-Chol, ApoB >; HDL-Chol <) | (230) |
| | | Tg-ApoA1 KO | | HDL-C <: CETP= | (231) |
| | | Tg-ApoC-III KO | | HDL-C <; ApoA1, HDL size < | (232) |
| | | Tg-Lcat KO | | CETP < | (233) |
| | | Tg-ApoC1 KO | | Chol <; CE > in VLDL | (42) |
| | | Tg-Pltp KO | | HDL-PL <, HDL-CE <, HDL-APOAI < | (234) |
| | | Tg-ApoE KO | | HDL-C < | (235) |
| | | Tg-Ldlr KO | | Atherosclerosis | (236) |
| **LCAT** | 16q22.1 | PvuII +− | | HDL-C << (in baboons) | (237,238) |
| Lcat | 8 | Tg | | Atherosclerosis > in spite of HDL-Chol > | (239) |
| | | Tg-Cetp Tg | | Atherosclerosis <: HDL-CE > (liver) | (240) |

| Gene | Locus | Variant | Phenotype | Ref. |
|---|---|---|---|---|
| **LPL** | 8p22 | Asp9Asn | TG >, HDL-C <, CHD risk > | (241–243) |
| | | N291S | HDL-C < | (243,244) |
| | | Ser447X | TG <, VLDL-TG < in obese | (245,246) |
| | | | ΔBMI <, Δfat < (white women; training) | (247) |
| | | Gly188Glu_Asp250Asn (KO) | HDL-C>, VLDL-C <, VLDL-TG <, TG <, CHD risk < | (242,244) |
| | | Arg243His_Asp250Asn (KO) | Familial hyperchylomicronemia | (248) |
| Lpl | 8 | Tg-ApoE KO | Atherosclerosis < | (249) |
| | | Tg-Ldlr KO | No atherosclerosis HFD | (250) |
| **ENPP1** | 6q23.1 | Lys121Gln | Leptin >, TG > | (251) |
| Enpp1 | 10 | KO | Bone hypermineralization | (252) |
| **SLC6A3** | 5p15.33 | E15 VNTR 9/10 | Risk obesity > (in smokers) | (253) |
| Slc6a3 | 13 | KO | Activity > | (254) |
| **ADRB1** | 10q25.2 | Gly389Arg | Weight >, fat >, FI= | (255) |
| Adrb1 | 19 | KO | | (256) |
| **ADRB2** | 5q32 | Gln27Glu | BMI >, ASF >, > in obese / HR >, BP <, catecholamines / Chol>, TG > (both in VLDL), > in diabetes | (257–259) |
| | | **Gln27Glu_Arg16Gly** | BMI <, fat < in obese | (260) |
| | | | Weight >, BMI >, WC >, WHR > in men | (261) |
| | | Arg16Gly | BMI > | (257) |
| | | | BMI <, fat < in obese white women | (260) |
| Adrb2 | 18 | KO | | (262) |
| | | KO-Adrb1 KO | | (263) |

*(Continued)*

**Table 2** Polymorphisms, Mutations, or KO in Human (Uppercase in Bold) and Rodent (Lowercase) Genes and Tg in Rodent Models of Obesity and CVD (*Continued*)

| Genes | Chr | Variations | Obesity | CVD | References |
|---|---|---|---|---|---|
| **ADRB3** | 8p11.2 | Trp64Arg | Δweight > in morbid obese<br>BMI > | Insulin > (OGTT) | (264)<br>(265) |
| Adrb3 | 8 | KO<br>KO-Adrb1,2 KO | Fat > (mild in females)<br>FI=, cold intolerant | FFA >, glycerol >, lipolysis > | (266)<br>(267) |

Variations associated with effects are in bold.

*Abbreviations:* LEP, leptin; LEPR, leptin receptor; GPD1, α-glycerol phosphate dehydrogenase; BATF, regulator of transcription factor B-ZIP; SREBF1, sterol regulatory element binding protein 1; DGAT1, Acyl CoA: diacylglycerol transferase; LDLR, low density lipoprotein receptor; CETP, cholesteryl ester transfer protein; FABP4 (AP2), fatty acid binding protein 4; ATRN, attractin; CCKAR, cholecystokinin receptor A; LCAT, lecithin:cholesterol acyl-transferase; LPIN1, lipin; HSD11B1, 11-beta-hydroxysteroid dehydrogenase type 1; LPL, lipoprotein lipase; RETN (FIZZ3), resistin; SCD, stearoyl-CoA desaturase (delta-9-desaturase); GPR24 (MCHR1), G protein-coupled receptor 24; NCOA2 (TIF2), nuclear receptor coactivator 2; PLIN, perilipin; APM1 (Acrp30, adiponectin), adipocyte complement related protein; B-ZIP, transcription factors of the C/EBP and Jun families; Eif4ebp1, eukaryotic translation initiation factor 4E binding protein 1; PTPN1 (PTP-1B), protein tyrosine phosphatase, non-receptor type 1; PLA2G1B (PLA2), group 1B phospholipase A2; PKARIIβ, protein kinase A RIIβ; LIPE (HSL), lipase, hormone-sensitive; Cav-1, caveolin-1; PON, paraoxonase; PPARG, peroxisome proliferator receptor gamma; SLC6A3 (DAT), dopamine transporter; ESR1, estrogen receptor 1; PRKCQ, protein kinase C, theta; ENPP1(PC-1), plasma cell membrane glycoprotein; GAD2, glutamic acid decarboxylase; CYP19A1, cytochrome P450 aromatase; FFA, free fatty acids; TG, triglycerides; CE, cholesteryl ester; HDL-C, high density lipoprotein-cholesterol; LDL-C, low density lipoprotein-cholesterol; CD, chow diet; HFD, high fat diet; FI, food intake; GH, growth hormone; GTT, glucose tolerance test; IS, insulin sensitivity; IR, insulin resistant; AVF, abdominal visceral fat; lean, weight normal with less fat; FPLD2, familial partial lypodystrophy 2; FD, familial dysbetalipoproteinemia; IHD, ischemic heart disease; FHBL, familial hypobetalipo-proteinemia; OGTT, oral glucose tolerance test; HOMA-B, homeostatic assessment of β-cells function; Tgly, triacylglycerol; fld, fatty liver dystrophy; SMS, Smith-Magenis syndrome; FFM, fat-free mass.

publications. Gene symbols were those from the National Center for Biotechnology Information Locus Link website (http://www.ncbi.nlm.nih. gov/LocusLink). Mutations and polymorphisms within genes are presented with the allele or haplotype producing the phenotypic changes highlighted in bold. For example, in the naturally occurring mutation Arg35Trp in the leptin gene producing an inactive leptin i.e., a natural KO, the tryptophane or Trp is highlighted in bold (Arg35**Trp**) because it is in the presence of this allele that leptin was shown to be inactive. Similarly, the arginine allele of the Gln223**Arg** variant in LEPR is responsible for greater BMI, fat amount, and fat-free mass in males carrying this allele. In other instances, the highlighted allele showed a greater frequency in cases than in controls. For example, the threonine allele of the **Thr**67Ala variant in the agouti-related peptide (AGRP) showed a higher frequency in patients of *Anorexia nervosa* for which FI is largely reduced. Interestingly, carriers of the alternative alanine allele of this AGRP variant (Thr67**Ala**) showed higher amounts of fat in contrast to excessive leanness in anorexia patients. Compound heterozygotes and haplotypes are indicated by linking the two mutations by means of a lower dash, as for Glu79**X**_Ala131**X** in the pro-opiomelanocortin (POMC) gene.

Not all studies related to the genes presented in Table 2 A–D will be reported in the actual compilation, nor will all the genes that have been analyzed by association studies with obesity- or CVD-related phenotypes be considered. As stated earlier, this comes from the exclusion of statistically weaker results that have been observed in these studies. The author acknowledges that these results remain valuable and could become variations for the genes involved in further studies focusing on a more subtle control of obesity or CVD. Similarly, published and unpublished negative result reports are not included. For instance, negative association results can be observed between studies involving the same gene and variation within this gene, and the same phenotype that previously showed a positive association in other studies. These results are not necessarily contradictory because they can arise from differences in the genetic structure of the populations from which the subjects have been sampled. For example, racial and ethnic origins of subjects are important factors contributing to variations in association or linkage results. This is particularly expected for complex traits such as obesity and CVD arising from the combined effects of different genes and environmental factors such as one's diet and way of life (schooling, physical activity, habits, etc.). Gene pools are different among different races and ethnic groups because of the previous historic separation of these groups. Different combinations of the variations within the obesity- or CVD-related genes would produce the same obesity or CVD phenotypes. The same holds true for gender differences, more particularly for phenotypes such as fat mass and leptin for which a well-known sexual dimorphism is observed with women showing higher levels of both fat and leptin.

## KO AND Tg RODENT MODELS

Ko and Tg mouse models are presented together with association results in Table 2 A–D. This should facilitate comparisons of their effects on obesity- and CVD-related phenotypes with those observed for human gene mutations and variants. Genes have been roughly grouped according to the effects of mutations on weight and FI. According to these criteria, a first group of genes showed a greater weight in KO than in control mice, and conversely, a lower weight in Tg mice (Table 2 A). Generally, they also showed a greater FI except for the peroxisome proliferative activated receptor, gamma (PPARG) gene where a lower FI was observed in KO mice. The genes of this group could be considered as the actual "classical" candidate genes for obesity, including the adipose tissue–specific hormones leptin gene, its receptor LEPR, and the new adipose-specific hormone adiponectin (APM1). In the same group are also present some of the genes of the melanocortin system, including the melanocortin receptor 4 (MC4R), the POMC gene encoding, among other peptides, the MC4R agonist α-melanocyte–stimulating hormone (α-MSH), and the AGRP gene encoding the natural antagonist of MC4R. In this group of genes are also found the fatty acid–binding protein 2 (FABP2) and 4 (FABP4) genes encoding, respectively, the intestinal and the adipose tissue form of the protein, and the PPARG gene as well, all three being strong candidates for CVD. In this group, KO mice [LEP, FABP2, cytochrome P450 aromatase (CYP19A1), and PPARG] showed a higher level of lipids and a greater lipogenesis. In Tg mice (LEPR and APM1), the inverse was observed i.e., a lower level of lipids and of lipogenesis. Tg mice for 11-beta-hydroxysteroid dehydrogenase type 1 escaped the rule for this group of genes with lipid levels being lower in KO and higher in Tg mice.

The second group of genes are those genes showing no significant changes in weight under normal chow diet (CD) or high-fat diet (HFD) (Table 2 B). Additionally, some of the genes within this group did not show significant differences in FI, such as diacylglycerol transferase (DGAT1), a key enzyme in TGs formation, and four transcription factors [protein kinase A RIIβ (PKARIIβ), high-mobility group protein I-C (HMGIC), protein tyrosine phosphatase, nonreceptor type 1, group 1B phospholipase A2 (PLA2G1B)] involved in fat cell proliferation control. Four other genes [perilipin (PLIN), nuclear receptor coactivator 2 (NCOA2), lipase (LIPE), MCH receptor-1 (MCHR-1)] showed no differences in weight, but presented a greater FI, apparently compensated by a higher EE. Interestingly, the third melanocortin receptor (MC3R), while showing no change in weight in KO mice, has a lower FI compensated by a lower fat-free mass and a reduced activity. Generally, for this group of genes, lipolysis is enhanced and TG and free fatty acid (FFA) levels are lowered in KO mice [PLIN, NCOA2, LIPE, DGAT1, PKARIIβ, PLA2G1B, stearoyl-CoA desaturase (delta-9-desaturase)]. Conversely, in Tg mice for LIPE, TG and FFA levels are enhanced, together with atherosclerosis in Tg mice for resistin (RETN).

The third group of genes (Table 2 C) showed lower weight or no fat at all in KO or Tg models. The latter includes genes mostly related to human familial lipodystrophy, such as the lamin A (LMNA), the fatty liver dystrophy, fld (LPIN1), or the α-glycerol phosphate dehydrogenase genes. In this group of genes, a greater level of TGs in KO mice and a lower one in Tg mice are generally observed.

The fourth and last group of genes (Table 2 D) are those more related to CVD than to obesity for which few of them have been characterized. These include the APO gene family, the lecithin:cholesterol acyltransferase, the cholesteryl ester transfer protein (CETP), and the lipoprotein lipase (LPL) genes. Unexpectedly, the adrenergic receptors that, in the past years, were strong candidates for obesity showed very little effect on this phenotype in KO or Tg rodent models, probably because of compensatory effects of other genes. For instance, the triple KO mice for the adrenergic receptors beta, identified as Adrb3 KO-Adrb1, 2 KO in Table 2 D, have been shown to be cold intolerant with higher levels of FFAs and lipolysis. For most of the APO genes, and for some others, combined KO-KO, KO-Tg, or Tg-Tg mice have been produced. For example, Apoc1 Tg mice were also expressed in ApoE KO, or Ldlr KO, or Lep$^{ob/ob}$ KO mice to evaluate combined effects of these Tg manipulations on lipid profile (Table 2 D). In these cases the effects reported in the table referred to the overexpression of Apoc1 over the KO mice and not to a control wild-type mice. Hence, the lower weight observed in Apoc1 Tg-Lep$^{ob/ob}$ KO mice is in accordance with obese Lep$^{ob/ob}$ and showed that the Lep$^{ob/ob}$ KO mice are less obese when Apoc1 is overexpressed. However, the Apoc1 Tg-Lep$^{ob/ob}$ KO mice remain obese when contrasted to wild-type or normal weight mice.

## SHARED LOCI BETWEEN OBESITY AND CVD

Table 3 presents a summary of the convergence of the results from the three lines of evidence i.e., the genome scans for obesity or CVD, association studies of candidate genes, and KO and Tg rodent models. From Table 3, we can see that 10 chromosomes (1, 2, 3, 5, 6, 10, 11, 15, 17, and 18) out of the 23 human chromosome pairs showed convergent linkage results for obesity and CVD. Among these 10 chromosomes, chromosomes 5, 10, and 18 did not show any evidence with CVD from association studies in humans, or from Tg models in rodents. Chromosome 3 appeared to be the only chromosome showing the three lines of evidence on both its 3p and 3q arms.

The first chromosomal region showing convergent results from all three independent lines of evidence was 1p32-p22. In this region the LEPR

**Table 3** Summary of the Chromosomal Regions with Convergent Evidence from Linkage and Association Studies in Humans and from KO and Tg Rodent Models

| Region | Linkages | Association studies | Ko and Tg rodent models |
|---|---|---|---|
| 1p32-p22 | Leptin, TGs | LEPR obesity, fat, FFM | KO obesity, FI >, insulin >, glucose >; KO (fat) FI=, fat >, TGs >, IR, glucose > |
| 2p25.2-p21 | Leptin, fat, HDL-C | APOB BMI >, FHBL, LDL-C > Chol >, CHD >; POMC obesity (KO), leptin >; LPIN1 | Tg LDL >, TGs > |
| 3p26-p21.2 | BMI, FHPL | PPARG leptin >, weight >, WC >, ASF >, DBMI, FPLD2, TGs >, insulin <, LDL-C >, Chol >, ApoB >, IR < | KO weight >; KO no fat, TGs >, IR; KO (muscle) fat pads > CD, weight >, FI < HFD; TGs (fat) > HFD, IR, insulin >, glucose > |
| 3q26.32-q29 | BMI, LDL-3 | APM1 weight >, WC >, LDL >, Tot/HDL >, insulin >, IR > | Tg weight <, FI <, IS >, glucose >, TGs <, lipogenesis < |
| 5p15.2-p12 | APM1, HDL-C | SLC6A3 risk obesity > (in smokers) | KO activity > |
| 6q23.1-q27 | BMI, leptin, Lp(a) | ENPP1 leptin >, TGs > | |
| 10p15.1-p12.33 | Obesity, TGs | ESR1 obesity (android), C-peptide <; PRKCQ GAD2 weight >, FI >, RNA > | KO weight=, FI=, lipids= (resistant); Tg weight >, insulin >, glucose > |

| Locus | Markers | Gene findings | Model findings |
|---|---|---|---|
| 11q14.3-q24.3 | BMI, LDL-C | APOA1 BMI < (diabetics), HDL-C > (males)<br>APOA4 BMI >, fat >, WHR >, TGs ><br>BMI <, fat <, WC > (non-smokers)<br>APOC3 Chol >, TGs >, LDL-C > | Tg atherosclerosis: Lp(a) ><br>KO FI=, Chol <, TGs <, ApoCIII < |
| 15q21-q26 | TGs, LDL-C, HDL-C, FFM, FH | CYP19A1 obesity (abdominal), leanness<br>PLIN BMI=, lipolysis >, PLIN < | KO Chol <, TGs < weight >, FI=, fat > (abdominal), FFM < Chol >, HDL >, insulin ><br>KO weight= HFD, FI >, lean, lipolysis (constitutive), FFAs < |
| 17p12-q21.33 | Leptin, LPL-PPD | SREBF1 BMI=, Chol > | Tg no fat, lipids > (liver) |
| 18p11.23-q12.3 | FFM, Lp(a) | MC4R weight >, FI >, fat >, leptin >, insulin > | KO weight >, FI > |

*Abbreviations*: KO, knockout; Tg, transgenic; LEPR, leptin receptor; SREBF1, sterol regulatory element binding protein 1; PLIN, perilipin; APM1 (Acrp30, adiponectin), adipocyte complement related protein; PPARG, peroxisome proliferator receptor gamma; SLC6A3 (DAT), dopamine transporter; ESR1, estrogen receptor 1; PRKCQ, protein kinase C, theta; ENPP1 (PC-1), plasma cell membrane glycoprotein; GAD2, glutamic acid decarboxylase; CYP19A1, cytochrome P450 aromatase; TG, triglycerides; FFM, fat-free mass; HDL-C, high density lipoprotein-cholesterol; LDL-C, low density lipoprotein-cholesterol; CD, chow diet; HFD, high fat diet; FI, food intake; IR, insulin resistant; FPLD2, familial partial lypodystrophy 2; FHBL, familial hypobetalipoproteinemia; APOB, apolipoprotein B; BMI, body mass index; Chol, cholesterol; POMC, pro-opiomelanocortin; LPIN1, lipin; WC, waist circumference; Lp(a), lipoprotein(a); WHR, waist to hip ratio; LPL-PPD, lipoprotein lipase-luminogen PPD; MC4R, melanocortin receptor 4; FH, familial hypercholesteronemia.

gene is located. The LEPR is deeply involved in the regulation of body weight and EE and also in other functions such as in reproduction. Some studies in humans have related LEPR variations to body composition and obesity or to the lipids profile in humans. These results are also consistent with those from rodent models, where LEPR has been shown to be involved in weight and lipids regulations and also in insulin sensitivity.

Three important genes related either to obesity, CVD, or both traits are located on chromosome 2p25.2-p21. The apolipoprotein B (APOB) is involved in the transport of cholesterol between LDL, HDL, and VLDL lipids subfractions, whereas few studies have investigated its relation with obesity (Table 2 D). Variations in the APOB gene have been reported to be associated with some or the other lipids and TG fractions, with athero-sclerosis and ischemic heart disease risks, and with familial hypobetalipo-proteinemia. One study reported an association with BMI. No KO model is apparently available for APOB, but in the Tg model, higher levels of LDL and trigycerides have been observed. Moreover, Tg overexpression of APOB in mice overexpressing CETP also has shown a lipoprotein choles-terol distribution similar to that of normolipidemic humans. The second gene located within chromosomal region 2p25.2-p21 is the POMC gene (Table 2 A). POMC encodes, among other peptides, the α-MSH that is the natural agonist of the melanocortin receptors. The melanocortin system is located downstream of the leptin in the control of weight, and mutations in POMC induced strong obesity in humans and rodents. No study had reported on the possible role of POMC on the lipids profile. However, the adrenocorticotropic hormone, one of the other peptides encoded by POMC, has been shown to increase the expression of the scavenger receptor B or CD36 gene (268) known to be a key component in the reverse cholesterol transport pathway. Finally, the third gene located at 2p25.2-p21 is the lipin (LPIN1) gene. Mice carrying mutations in the fld gene encoding lipin have features of human lipodystrophy, a genetically heterogeneous group of dis-orders characterized by loss of body fat, fatty liver, hypertriglyceridemia, and insulin resistance. LPIN1 encodes a recently identified nuclear protein, which has not been investigated in humans either for obesity or CVD.

Chromosome 3 showed evidence of implications in both obesity and CVD on its two arms at 3p26-p21.2 and 3q26.32-q29, respectively. On chro-mosome 3p26-p21.2, the peroxisome proliferator alpha receptor gamma (PPARG) is a strong candidate gene for both obesity and CVD. Some recent reviews have been made on PPARG metabolism and genetics (2,269–272). The peroxisome proliferator alpha controls fat cell proliferation via princi-pally its receptor gamma 2 almost exclusively expressed in adipose tissue in contrast to the gamma 1 receptor ubiquitously expressed at relatively low levels. Antidiabetic agents such as thiazolidinediones acting as insulin sensi-tizers are high-affinity ligands of PPARG. Numerous studies have shown a strong relation between PPARG and obesity- or CVD-related phenotypes.

Two common variants (Pro115Gln, C161T) have been associated with BMI, leptin, or weight, and different lipid levels. The third most studied Pro12Ala substitution has been associated with phenotypes related to central fat depot such as waist circumference and abdominal subcutaneous fat, and to insulin levels. PPARG is also one of the genes at the origin of the familial partial lipodystrophy 2, as is the LMNA gene. KO mice for PPARG in muscle showed greater adiposity and weight, but lower FI on a regular CD. On a HFD, these mice showed a higher fat TG content and developed insulin resistance. On the q arm of chromosome 3 at 3q26.32-q29, the new gene APM1 encoding the adipose tissue–specific adiponectin has been shown to be involved in body-weight control in humans and rodents and also in lipids and insulin sensitivity.

Chromosomes 5 and 18 showed less evidence than previous chromosomes with CVD because no results from association studies or KO and Tg models can be found. Nevertheless, some interesting genes can be found in these chromosomal regions. The dopamine transporter SLC6A3 gene is located at chromosome 5p15.2-p12 that showed linkages with APM1 (adiponectin) and HDL-C levels. A variation in SLC6A3 has been associated in smokers with a greater risk of developing obesity, whereas KO mice invalidated for SLC6A3 showed greater activity than the wild type. Apparently, SLC6A3 has not been studied yet in relation to lipid metabolism. At 18p11.23-q12.3, an important gene for body-weight control is found: the MC4R. This chromosomal region is linked to the fat-free part of the body and with lipid (a). With POMC, MC4R is the second gene related to the melanocortin system highlighted by the present compilation. MC4R has been shown to be associated mainly with weight and FI. In humans, MC4R is the gene showing the greatest number of mutations and variations (well over 50) associated with obesity. More particularly, the two distinct mutations, four bases insertion (Tyr35X) or deletion (Lys211delCTCT), completely invalidated the receptor activity and induced, as in rodent KO, hyperphagia and obesity. Apparently, no study has ever investigated MC4R polymorphisms in relation to lipid metabolism.

On chromosome 6q23.1-q27 linked to BMI, leptin, and Lp(a), the plasma cell membrane glycoprotein, ENPP1, also called PC-1, and the estrogen receptor 1 (ESR1) are found. A variation in ENPP1 has been associated with higher leptin and TGs levels. No KO and Tg model is available for this gene. For its part, variation in ESR1 has been associated with android obesity and a lower C-peptide level. KO mice showed no change in weight and FI, but appeared to be resistant to inducing a greater lipid level. On chromosome 10, mice overexpressing the protein kinase C theta showed greater weight and greater insulin and glucose levels. No association study is available for either obesity or CVD for this gene. On the other hand, at 10p15.1-p12.33, the GAD2 gene encoding the glutamic acid decarboxylase is found. GAD2 is probably the first new obesity gene identified by position following a genome scan. GAD2 was shown to be associated with greater weight and FI in humans and with a lower fear level and greater anxiety in KO mice.

Chromosome 11 carries major players in the control of the lipids metabolism with the cluster of APO genes including APOA1, APOA4, and APOC3 genes. These genes, with APOB, are known to be responsible for cholesterol transport between the different lipid subfractions. APOA1 and APOA4 have been associated with a lower BMI in diabetics and nonsmokers, respectively, while APOA4 and APOC3 have both been associated with greater TGs levels. APOA1 has also been associated with a greater HDL-C level in males, and APOC3 with greater cholesterol and LDL-C levels. Tg APOA1 mice showed atherosclerosis and a higher level of Lp(a), whereas KO for APOA4 and APOC3 both showed lower cholesterol and TG levels. FI was unchanged in APOA4 KO mice.

Chromosome 15q21-q26 is particularly rich in linked CVD phenotypes (TGs, LDL-C, HDL-C, and familial hypercholesteronemia), but also shows linkage with the body composition–related variable fat-free mass. The most interesting gene located in this region is the PLIN. The PLIN is a small molecule that is linked to TGs and which preserves them to be used in lipolysis. When LPIN is inactivated, a constitutive lipolysis inducing leanness is observed. A variation in human PLIN has been associated with a greater lipolysis with no change in BMI. KO mice showed no weight change on a HFD, but a greater FI and a constitutive lipolysis. Consequently, these mice were leaner. A second interesting gene, CYP19A1, is also located in this region. CYP19A1 has been associated with abdominal obesity and leanness. KO mice showed more weight, fat, cholesterol, HDL, and insulin, with no change in FI and a lower fat-free mass. Finally, at 17p12-q21.33, linkages with leptin and the LPL-PPD are observed. In this region, the sterol regulatory element-binding protein 1 gene is found. It was shown to be associated with cholesterol but with no change in BMI, whereas Tg mice showed no fat at all, with a higher lipid content in liver.

The common metabolic picture for these 11 chromosomal regions and 18 genes related to obesity and CVD is complex. Numerous reviews covering either obesity or CVD mechanisms, or covering some of the most studied genes in some of the metabolic pathways involved have been published. In an exhaustive review of KO and Tg models producing obesity, leanness, or resistance to obesity, Fruhbeck and Gomez-Ambrosi (273) present a schematic representation of the main TG metabolism pathways in adipocytes. In this schema, the PLIN plays a final role in the production of TGs induced by the hormone-sensitive lipase. An important conclusion in Arch's (274) review of obesity in Tg animals is that obesity can develop without hyperphagia, and leanness without hypophagia. The CYP19A1 gene represents such a gene as shown in Table 2 A–D. Both PLIN and CYP19A1 are located on chromosome 15q21-q26 (Table 3), showing effects on body composition and CVD-related phenotypes. CYP19A1 catalyzes the conversion of androgens to estrogens via oxidative cleavage of the substrate's angular C-19 methyl group. Interestingly, on chromosome 6q23.1-q27, the ESR1 is also candidate for android obesity, as CYP19A1 at 15q21-q26 (Table 3).

The leptin pathway is obvious for its association with FI and EE controls. In his review, Inui (275) presented a simplified model of the interaction of leptin with neuropeptidergic effector molecules. In this model, the LEPR (LEPR; 1p32-p22) received a signal from leptin and interacted with MC4R (MC4R; 18p11.23-q12.3) that produced an anorexigenic signal to control appetite. Among other candidate molecules that control energy intake, expenditure, and/or partitioning, the α-MSH encoded by the POMC (POMC; 2p25.2-p21) is positively stimulated by leptin and acts as an anorexigenic molecule to reduce FI.

The peroxisome proliferator-activated receptor gamma (PPARG; 3p26-p21.2) and the adiponectin (APM1; 3q26.32-q29) are both involved in the regulation of insulin sensitivity and energy homeostasis as illustrated in the schematic of Gurnell (269) on the insulin action in muscle. APM1 has an insulin-sensitizing effect that counterbalances the factors (RETN and tumor necrosis factor alpha) that impair the insulin action in muscles. All three factors are modulated by PPARG and APM1, positively, and the two others, negatively.

Finally, some of the 18 genes are also involved in other apparently very different traits. For example, the dopamine transporter (SLC6A3) and the glutamic acid decarboxylase (GAD2) are candidates for some mental health diseases where SZ, BP, autism, and alcoholism are associated with SLC6A3, and memory learning, fear, and anxiety with GAD2. This does not seem to be uncommon. For example, the serotonin system is well known to be an important system in mental health but also in FI control. Recent reports have highlighted that the serotonin 5-$HT_{2C}$ receptor located on chromosome Xq24 is associated with obesity per se (276), with weight loss capacity (277), with antipsychotic-induced obesity (278,279), and with SZ (280–282).

## SUMMARY

Obesity and CVD are two complex traits with their specific genetic and environmental factors driving their expression, but also with common origins and modes of action, reflecting their belonging to the metabolic syndrome. In an attempt to identify some of the genetic factors involved in both obesity and CVD and eventually in the metabolic syndrome, linkage results from genome-wide scans on obesity- and CVD-related phenotypes have been pooled together: only the significant results have been retained. Eleven regions from 10 chromosomes showed linkages with both obesity and CVD. Association studies and KO and Tg rodent models of candidate genes within these linked chromosomal regions were then used to identify the genes more susceptible to be at the origin of the linkage. Some 18 genes have been identified. Among these genes, some have not been characterized either for their possible association with obesity or CVD in humans or for KO or Tg effects in rodent models. These 11 chromosomal regions and 18 candidate genes offer a good starting point to those who want to investigate the genetics of obesity, CVD, or the metabolic syndrome. The present results also highlight the usefulness of characterizing more extensively the effects of genetic variations in human or KO and Tg rodent models on a larger spectra of phenotypes (anthropometric and metabolic variables), particularly when studying metabolic syndrome–related traits.

## REFERENCES

1. Reaven GM. Banting lecture 1988. Role of insulin resistance in human disease. Diabetes 1988; 37(12):1595–1607.
2. Gurnell M, et al. The metabolic syndrome: peroxisome proliferator-activated receptor gamma and its therapeutic modulation. J Clin Endocrinol Metab 2003; 88(6):2412–2421.
3. Isomaa B, et al. Cardiovascular morbidity and mortality associated with the metabolic syndrome. Diabetes Care 2001; 24(4):683–689.
4. Qu D, et al. A role for melanin-concentrating hormone in the central regulation of feeding behaviour. Nature 1996; 380(6571):243–247.
5. Collins CA, Kym PR. Prospects for obesity treatment: MCH receptor antagonists. Curr Opin Investig Drugs 2003; 4(4):386–394.
6. Eurlings PM, et al. Identification of differentially expressed genes in subcutaneous adipose tissue from subjects with familial combined hyperlipidemia. J Lipid Res 2002; 43(6):930–935.
7. Beattie JH, et al. Obesity and hyperleptinemia in metallothionein (-I and -II) null mice. Proc Natl Acad Sci USA 1998; 95(1):358–363.
8. Do MS, et al. Metallothionein gene expression in human adipose tissue from lean and obese subjects. Horm Metab Res 2002; 34(6):348–351.
9. Chagnon YC, et al. The human obesity gene map: the 2002 update. Obes Res 2003; 11(3):313–367.
10. Chen HC, Farese RV Jr. Fatty acids, triglycerides, and glucose metabolism: recent insights from knockout mice. Curr Opin Clin Nutr Metab Care 2002; 5(4):359–363.
11. Fazio S, Linton MF. Mouse models of hyperlipidemia and atherosclerosis. Front Biosci 2001; 6:D515–D525.
12. Coleman DL. Obese and diabetes: two mutant genes causing diabetes-obesity syndromes in mice. Diabetologia 1978; 14(3):141–148.
13. Rice T, et al. Segregation analysis of abdominal visceral fat: the HERITAGE Family Study. Obes Res 1997; 5(5):417–424.
14. Ober C, Abney M, McPeek MS. The genetic dissection of complex traits in a founder population. Am J Hum Genet 2001; 69(5):1068–1079.

15. Cheng LS, et al. Segregation analysis reveals a major gene effect controlling systolic blood pressure and BMI in an Israeli population. Hum Biol 1998; 70(1):59–75.
16. Borecki IB, et al. Evidence for multiple determinants of the body mass index: the National Heart, Lung, and Blood Institute Family Heart Study. Obes Res 1998; 6(2):107–114.
17. Faith MS, et al. Evidence for independent genetic influences on fat mass and body mass index in a pediatric twin sample. Pediatrics 1999; 104(1 Pt 1):61–67.
18. Selby JV, et al. Genetic and behavioral influences on body fat distribution. Int J Obes 1990; 14(7):593–602.
19. Sellers TA, et al. Familial aggregation and heritability of waist to-hip ratio in adult women: the Iowa Women's Health Study. Int J Obes Relat Metab Disord 1994; 18(9):607–613.
20. Mitchell BD, et al. Genetic and environmental contributions to cardiovascular risk factors in Mexican Americans. The San Antonio Family Heart Study. Circulation 1996; 94(9):2159 2170.
21. Edwards KL, et al. Pleiotropic genetic effects on LDL size, plasma triglyceride, and HDL cholesterol in families. Arterioscler Thromb Vasc Biol 1999; 19(10): 2456–2464.
22. Brenn T. Genetic and environmental effects on coronary heart disease risk factors in northern Norway. The Cardiovascular Disease Study in Finnmark. Ann Hum Genet 1994; 58(Pt 4):369–379.
23. Perusse L, et al. Familial resemblance of plasma lipids, lipoproteins and post-heparin lipoprotein and hepatic lipases in the HERITAGE Family Study. Arterioscler Thromb Vasc Biol 1997; 17(11):3263–3269.
24. Shearman AM, et al. Evidence for a gene influencing the TG/HDL-C ratio on chromosome 7q32.3-qter: a genome-wide scan in the Framingham Study. Hum Mol Genet 2000; 9(9):1315–1320.
25. Hong Y, et al. Potential environmental effects on adult lipoprotein(a) levels: results from Swedish twins. Atherosclerosis 1995; 117(2):295–304.
26. Rainwater DL, et al. Characterization of the genetic elements controlling lipoprotein(a) concentrations in Mexican Americans. Evidence for at least three controlling elements linked to LPA, the locus encoding apolipoprotein(a). Atherosclerosis 1997; 128(2):223–233.
27. Scholz M, et al. Genetic control of lipoprotein(a) concentrations is different in Africans and Caucasians. Eur J Hum Genet 1999; 7(2):169–178.
28. Ordovas JM. HDL genetics: candidate genes, genome wide scans and gene-environment interactions. Cardiovasc Drugs Ther 2002; 16(4):273–281.
29. Bosse Y, et al. Compendium of genome-wide scans of lipid-related phenotypes: adding a new genome-wide search of apolipoprotein levels. J Lipid Res 2004; 45(12); 2174–2184.
30. Al-Kateb H, et al. Mutation in the ARH gene and a chromosome 13q locus influence cholesterol levels in a new form of digenic-recessive familial hypercholesterolemia. Circ Res 2002; 90(9):951–958.
31. Eden ER, et al. Use of homozygosity mapping to identify a region on chromosome 1 bearing a defective gene that causes autosomal recessive homozygous

hypercholesterolemia in two unrelated families. Am J Hum Genet 2001; 68(3):653–660.

32. Hunt SC, et al. Linkage of body mass index to chromosome 20 in Utah pedigrees. Hum Genet 2001; 109(3):279–285.

33. Varret M, et al. A third major locus for autosomal dominant hypercholesterolemia maps to 1p34.1-p32. Am J Hum Genet 1999; 64(5):1378–1387.

34. van der Kallen CJ, et al. Genome scan for adiposity in Dutch dyslipidemic families reveals novel quantitative trait loci for leptin, body mass index and soluble tumor necrosis factor receptor superfamily 1A. Int J Obes Relat Metab Disord 2000; 24(11):1381–1391.

35. Reed DR, et al. A genome-wide scan suggests a locus on chromosome 1q21-q23 contributes to normal variation in plasma cholesterol concentration. J Mol Med 2001; 79(5–6):262–269.

36. Comuzzie AG, et al. A major quantitative trait locus determining serum leptin levels and fat mass is located on human chromosome 2. Nat Genet 1997; 15(3): 273–276.

37. Hixson JE, et al. Normal variation in leptin levels in associated with polymorphisms in the proopiomelanocortin gene, POMC. J Clin Endocrinol Metab 1999; 84(9):3187–3191.

38. Soro A, et al. Genome scans provide evidence for low-HDL-C loci on chromosomes 8q23, 16q24.1–24.2, and 20q13.11 in Finnish families. Am J Hum Genet 2002; 70(5):1333–1340.

39. Newman DL, et al. Major loci influencing serum triglyceride levels on 2q14 and 9p21 localized by homozygosity-by-descent mapping in a large Hutterite pedigree. Hum Mol Genet 2003; 12(2):137–144.

40. Watanabe RM, et al. The Finland-United States investigation of non-insulin-dependent diabetes mellitus genetics (FUSION) study. II. An autosomal genome scan for diabetes-related quantitative-trait loci. Am J Hum Genet 2000; 67(5):1186–1200.

41. Yuan B, et al. Linkage of a gene for familial hypobetalipoproteinemia to chromosome 3p21.1–22. Am J Hum Genet 2000; 66(5):1699–1704.

42. Wu X, et al. A combined analysis of genomewide linkage scans for body mass index from the National Heart, Lung, and Blood Institute Family Blood Pressure Program. Am J Hum Genet 2002; 70(5):1247–1256.

43. Kissebah AH, et al. Quantitative trait loci on chromosomes 3 and 17 influence phenotypes of the metabolic syndrome. Proc Natl Acad Sci USA 2000; 97(26): 14478–14483.

44. Stone S, et al. A major predisposition locus for severe obesity, at 4p15-p14. Am J Hum Genet 2002; 70(6):1459–1468.

45. Rainwater DL, et al. A genome search identifies major quantitative trait loci on human chromosomes 3 and 4 that influence cholesterol concentrations in small LDL particles. Arterioscler Thromb Vasc Biol 1999; 19(3):777–783.

46. Comuzzie AG, et al. The genetic basis of plasma variation in adiponectin, a global endophenotype for obesity and the metabolic syndrome. J Clin Endocrinol Metab 2001; 86(9):4321–4325.

47. Peacock JM, et al. Genome scan for quantitative trait loci linked to high-density lipoprotein cholesterol: The NHLBI Family Heart Study. Arterioscler Thromb Vasc Biol 2001; 21(11):1823–1828.

48. Arya R, et al. Factors of insulin resistance syndrome-related phenotypes are linked to genetic locations on chromosomes 6 and 7 in nondiabetic Mexican-Americans. Diabetes 2002; 51(3):841–847.

49. Broeckel U, et al. A comprehensive linkage analysis for myocardial infarction and its related risk factors. Nat Genet 2002; 30(2):210–214.

50. Feitosa MF, et al. Quantitative-trait loci influencing body-mass index reside on chromosomes 7 and 13: the National Heart, Lung, and Blood Institute Family Heart Study. Am J Hum Genet 2002; 70(1):72–82.

51. Duggirala R, et al. Quantitative variation in obesity-related traits and insulin precursors linked to the OB gene region on human chromosome 7. Am J Hum Genet 1996; 59(3):694–703.

52. Borecki IB, Province MA, Rao DC. Power of segregation analysis for detection of major gene effects on quantitative traits. Genet Epidemiol 1994; 11(5): 409–418.

53. Mitchell BD, et al. A quantitative trait locus influencing BMI maps to the region of the beta-3 adrenergic receptor. Diabetes 1999; 48(9):1863–1867.

54. Almasy L, et al. Human pedigree-based quantitative-trait-locus mapping: localization of two genes influencing HDL-cholesterol metabolism. Am J Hum Genet 1999; 64(6):1686–1693.

55. Arya R, et al. Linkage of high-density lipoprotein-cholesterol concentrations to a locus on chromosome 9p in Mexican Americans. Nat Genet 2002; 30(1): 102–105.

56. Hager J, et al. A genome-wide scan for human obesity genes reveals a major susceptibility locus on chromosome 10. Nat Genet 1998; 20(3):304–308.

57. Pajukanta P, et al. Combined analysis of genome scans of Dutch and Finnish families reveals a susceptibility locus for high-density lipoprotein cholesterol on chromosome 16q. Am J Hum Genet 2003; 72(4):903–917.

58. Pajukanta P, et al. Genomewide scan for familial combined hyperlipidemia genes in Finnish families, suggesting multiple susceptibility loci influencing triglyceride, cholesterol, and apolipoprotein B levels. Am J Hum Genet 1999; 64(5):1453–1463.

59. Coon H, et al. A genome-wide screen reveals evidence for a locus on chromosome 11 influencing variation in LDL cholesterol in the NHLBI Family Heart Study. Hum Genet 2002; 111(3):263–269.

60. Hanson RL, et al. An autosomal genomic scan for loci linked to type II diabetes mellitus and body-mass index in Pima Indians. Am J Hum Genet 1998; 63(4):1130–1138.

61. Bosse Y, et al. Genome-wide linkage scan reveals multiple susceptibility loci influencing lipid and lipoprotein levels in the Quebec Family Study. J Lipid Res 2004; 45(3):419–426.

62. Knoblauch H, et al. A cholesterol-lowering gene maps to chromosome 13q. Am J Hum Genet 2000; 66(1):157–166.

63. Duggirala R, et al. A major susceptibility locus influencing plasma triglyceride concentrations is located on chromosome 15q in Mexican Americans. Am J Hum Genet 2000; 66(4):1237–1245.

64. Chagnon YC, et al. Genome-wide search for genes related to the fat-free body mass in the Quebec Family Study. Metabolism 2000; 49(2):203–207.

65. Ciccarese M, et al. A new locus for autosomal recessive hypercholesterolemia maps to human chromosome 15q25-q26. Am J Hum Genet 2000; 66(2):453–460.

66. Mahaney MC, et al. A quantitative trait locus on chromosome 16q influences variation in plasma HDL-C levels in Mexican Americans. Arterioscler Thromb Vasc Biol 2003; 23(2):339–345.

67. Imperatore G, et al. A locus influencing total serum cholesterol on chromosome 19p: results from an autosomal genomic scan of serum lipid concentrations in Pima Indians. Arterioscler Thromb Vasc Biol 2000; 20(12):2651–2656.

68. Klos KL, et al. Genome-wide linkage analysis reveals evidence of multiple regions that influence variation in plasma lipid and apolipoprotein levels associated with risk of coronary heart disease. Arterioscler Thromb Vasc Biol 2001; 21(6):971–978.

69. Elbein SC, Hasstedt SJ. Quantitative trait linkage analysis of lipid-related traits in familial type 2 diabetes: evidence for linkage of triglyceride levels to chromosome 19q. Diabetes 2002; 51(2):528–535.

70. Norman RA, et al. Autosomal genomic scan for loci linked to obesity and energy metabolism in Pima Indians. Am J Hum Genet 1998; 62(3):659–668.

71. Lee JH, et al. Genome scan for human obesity and linkage to markers in 20q13. Am J Hum Genet 1999; 64(1):196–209.

72. Ohman M, et al. Genome-wide scan of obesity in Finnish sibpairs reveals linkage to chromosome Xq24. J Clin Endocrinol Metab 2000; 85(9):3183–3190.

73. Lander E, Kruglyak L. Genetic dissection of complex traits: guidelines for interpreting and reporting linkage results. Nat Genet 1995; 11(3):241–247.

74. Maziade M, et al. A search for specific and common susceptibility loci for schizophrenia and bipolar disorder: a linkage study in 13 target chromosomes. Mol Psychiat 2001; 6(6):684–693.

75. Maziade M, et al. Shared and specific susceptibility loci for schizophrenia and bipolar disorder: a genome scan in eastern Quebec families. Mol Psychiat 2004:1–14.

76. Sklar P. Linkage analysis in psychiatric disorders: the emerging picture. Annu Rev Genomics Hum Genet 2002; 3:371–413.

77. Kohn Y, Lerer B. Genetics of schizophrenia: a review of linkage findings. Isr J Psychiat Relat Sci 2002; 39(4):340–351.

78. McCarthy MI. Growing evidence for diabetes susceptibility genes from genome scan data. Curr Diab Rep 2003; 3(2):159–167.

79. Stern MP. The search for type 2 diabetes susceptibility genes using whole-genome scans: an epidemiologist's perspective. Diabetes Metab Res Rev 2002; 18(2):106–113.

80. Goldin LR, et al. Analysis of metabolic syndrome phenotypes in Framingham Heart Study families from Genetic Analysis Workshop 13. Genet Epidemiol 2003; 25(suppl 1):S78–S89.

81. Montague CT, et al. Congenital leptin deficiency is associated with severe early-onset obesity in humans. Nature 1997; 387(6636):903–908.
82. Strobel A, et al. A leptin missense mutation associated with hypogonadism and morbid obesity. Nat Genet 1998; 18(3):213–215.
83. Ozata M, Ozdemir IC, Licinio J. Human leptin deficiency caused by a missense mutation: multiple endocrine defects, decreased sympathetic tone, and immune system dysfunction indicate new targets for leptin action, greater central than peripheral resistance to the effects of leptin, and spontaneous correction of leptin-mediated defects. J Clin Endocrinol Metab 1999; 84(10):3686–3695.
84. Ke Y, et al. Overexpression of leptin in transgenic mice leads to decreased basal lipolysis, PKA activity, and perilipin levels. Biochem Biophys Res Commun 2003; 312(4):1165–1170.
85. Matsuoka N, et al. Decreased triglyceride-rich lipoproteins in transgenic skinny mice overexpressing leptin. Am J Physiol Endocrinol Metab 2001; 280(2):E334–E339.
86. Clement K, et al. A mutation in the human leptin receptor gene causes obesity and pituitary dysfunction. Nature 1998; 392(6674):398–401.
87. Ukkola O, et al. Leptin receptor Gln223Arg variant is associated with a cluster of metabolic abnormalities in response to long-term overfeeding. J Intern Med 2000; 248(5):435–439.
88. Chagnon YC, et al. Linkages and associations between the leptin receptor (LEPR) gene and human body composition in the Quebec Family Study. Int J Obes Relat Metab Disord 1999; 23(3):278–286.
89. Chagnon Y, et al. Associations between the leptin receptor gene and adiposity in middle-aged Caucasian males from the HERITAGE Family Study. J Clin Endocrinol Metab 2000; 85(1):29–34.
90. Huan JN, et al. Adipocyte-selective reduction of the leptin receptors induced by antisense RNA leads to increased adiposity, dyslipidemia, and insulin resistance. J Biol Chem 2003; 278(46):45638–45650.
91. Yeo GS, et al. A frameshift mutation in MC4R associated with dominantly inherited human obesity. Nat Genet 1998; 20(2):111–112.
92. Vaisse C, et al. A frameshift mutation in human MC4R is associated with a dominant form of obesity. Nat Genet 1998; 20(2):113–114.
93. Farooqi IS, et al. Dominant and recessive inheritance of morbid obesity associated with melanocortin 4 receptor deficiency. J Clin Invest 2000; 106(2): 271–279.
94. Chagnon YC, et al. Linkage and association studies between the melanocortin receptors 4 and 5 genes and obesity-related phenotypes in the Quebec Family Study. Mol Med 1997; 3(10):663–673.
95. Huszar D, et al. Targeted disruption of the melanocortin-4 receptor results in obesity in mice. Cell 1997; 88(1):131–141.
96. Funakoshi A, et al. Gene structure of human cholecystokinin (CCK) type-A receptor: body fat content is related to CCK type-A receptor gene promoter polymorphism. FEBS Lett 2000; 466(2–3):264–266.

97. Schwartz GJ, et al. Decreased responsiveness to dietary fat in Otsuka Long-Evans Tokushima fatty rats lacking CCK-A receptors. Am J Physiol 1999; 277(4 Pt 2):R1144–R1151.

98. Menzaghi C, et al. A haplotype at the adiponectin locus is associated with obesity and other features of the insulin resistance syndrome. Diabetes 2002; 51(7):2306–2312.

99. Zietz B, et al. Gly15Gly polymorphism within the human adipocyte-specific apM-1gene but not Tyr111His polymorphism is associated with higher levels of cholesterol and LDL-cholesterol in Caucasian patients with type 2 diabetes. Exp Clin Endocrinol Diabetes 2001; 109(6):320–325.

100. Shklyaev S, et al. Sustained peripheral expression of transgene adiponectin offsets the development of diet-induced obesity in rats. Proc Natl Acad Sci USA 2003; 100(24):14217–14222.

101. Boutin P, et al. GAD2 on Chromosome 10p12 is a candidate gene for human obesity. PLoS Biol 2003; 1(3):E68.

102. Stork O, et al. Altered conditioned fear behavior in glutamate decarboxylase 65 null mutant mice. Genes Brain Behav 2003; 2(2):65–70.

103. Stork O, et al. Postnatal development of a GABA deficit and disturbance of neural functions in mice lacking GAD65. Brain Res 2000; 865(1):45–58.

104. Gelernter-Yaniv L, et al. Associations between a polymorphism in the 11 beta hydroxysteroid dehydrogenase type I gene and body composition. Int J Obes Relat Metab Disord 2003; 27(8):983–986.

105. Morton NM, et al. Improved lipid and lipoprotein profile, hepatic insulin sensitivity, and glucose tolerance in 11beta-hydroxysteroid dehydrogenase type 1 null mice. J Biol Chem 2001; 276(44):41293–41300.

106. Masuzaki H, et al. A transgenic model of visceral obesity and the metabolic syndrome. Science 2001; 294(5549):2166–2170.

107. Krude H, et al. Severe early-onset obesity, adrenal insufficiency and red hair pigmentation caused by POMC mutations in humans. Nat Genet 1998; 19(2): 155–157.

108. Yaswen L, et al. Obesity in the mouse model of pro-opiomelanocortin deficiency responds to peripheral melanocortin. Nat Med 1999; 5(9):1066–1070.

109. Argyropoulos G, et al. A polymorphism in the human agouti-related protein is associated with late-onset obesity. J Clin Endocrinol Metab 2002; 87(9): 4198–4202.

110. Vink T, et al. Association between an agouti-related protein gene polymorphism and anorexia nervosa. Mol Psychiat 2001; 6(3):325–328.

111. Graham M, et al. Overexpression of Agrt leads to obesity in transgenic mice. Nat Genet 1997; 17(3):273–274.

112. Pihlajamaki J, et al. Codon 54 polymorphism of the human intestinal fatty acid binding protein 2 gene is associated with dyslipidemias but not with insulin resistance in patients with familial combined hyperlipidemia. Arterioscler Thromb Vasc Biol 1997; 17(6):1039–1044.

113. Baier LJ, et al. An amino acid substitution in the human intestinal fatty acid binding protein is associated with increased fatty acid binding, increased fat oxidation, and insulin resistance. J Clin Invest 1995; 95(3):1281–1287.

114. Vassileva G, et al. The intestinal fatty acid binding protein is not essential for dietary fat absorption in mice. FASEB J 2000; 14(13):2040–2046.

115. Boord JB, Fazio S, Linton MF. Cytoplasmic fatty acid-binding proteins: emerging roles in metabolism and atherosclerosis. Curr Opin Lipidol 2002; 13(2):141–147.

116. Shaughnessy S, et al. Adipocyte metabolism in adipocyte fatty acid binding protein knockout mice (aP2-/-) after short-term high-fat feeding: functional compensation by the keratinocyte [correction of keritinocyte] fatty acid binding protein. Diabetes 2000; 49(6):904–911.

117. Hotamisligil GS, et al. Uncoupling of obesity from insulin resistance through a targeted mutation in aP2, the adipocyte fatty acid binding protein. Science 1996; 274(5291):1377–1379.

118. Baghaei F, et al. The CYP19 gene and associations with androgens and abdominal obesity in premenopausal women. Obes Res 2003; 11(4):578–585.

119. Baghaei F, et al. The lean woman. Obes Res 2002; 10(2):115–121.

120. Jones ME, et al. Aromatase-deficient (ArKO) mice accumulate excess adipose tissue. J Steroid Biochem Mol Biol 2001; 79(1 5):3–9.

121. Hewitt KN, et al. The aromatase knockout mouse presents with a sexually dimorphic disruption to cholesterol homeostasis. Endocrinology 2003; 144(9):3895–3903.

122. Hegele RA, et al. PPARG F388L, a transactivation-deficient mutant, in familial partial lipodystrophy. Diabetes 2002; 51(12):3586–3590.

123. Ristow M, et al. Obesity associated with a mutation in a genetic regulator of adipocyte differentiation. N Engl J Med 1998; 339(14):953–959.

124. Meirhaeghe A, et al. A genetic polymorphism of the peroxisome proliferator-activated receptor gamma gene influences plasma leptin levels in obese humans. Hum Mol Genet 1998; 7(3):435–440.

125. Meirhaeghe A, et al. Impact of the peroxisome proliferator activated receptor gamma2 Pro12Ala polymorphism on adiposity, lipids and non-insulin-dependent diabetes mellitus. Int J Obes Relat Metab Disord 2000; 24(2):195–199.

126. Kao WH, et al. Pro12Ala of the peroxisome proliferator-activated receptor-gamma2 gene is associated with lower serum insulin levels in nonobese African Americans: the Atherosclerosis Risk in Communities Study. Diabetes 2003; 52(6):1568–1572.

127. Robitaille J, et al. The PPAR-gamma P12A polymorphism modulates the relationship between dietary fat intake and components of the metabolic syndrome: results from the Quebec Family Study. Clin Genet 2003; 63(2):109–116.

128. Ek J, et al. Homozygosity of the Pro12Ala variant of the peroxisome proliferation-activated receptor-gamma2 (PPAR-gamma2): divergent modulating effects on body mass index in obese and lean Caucasian men. Diabetologia 1999; 42(7):892–895.

129. Norris AW, et al. Muscle-specific PPARgamma-deficient mice develop increased adiposity and insulin resistance but respond to thiazolidinediones. J Clin Invest 2003; 112(4):608–618.

130. Mottagui-Tabar S, et al. Evidence for an important role of perilipin in the regulation of human adipocyte lipolysis. Diabetologia 2003; 46(6):789–797.

131. Tansey JT, et al. Perilipin ablation results in a lean mouse with aberrant adipocyte lipolysis, enhanced leptin production, and resistance to diet-induced obesity. Proc Natl Acad Sci USA 2001; 98(11):6494–6499.

132. Castro-Chavez F, et al. Coordinated upregulation of oxidative pathways and downregulation of lipid biosynthesis underlie obesity resistance in perilipin knockout mice: a microarray gene expression profile. Diabetes 2003; 52(11): 2666–2674.

133. Martinez-Botas J, et al. Absence of perilipin results in leanness and reverses obesity in Lepr(db/db) mice. Nat Genet 2000; 26(4):474–479.

134. Picard F, et al. SRC-1 and TIF2 control energy balance between white and brown adipose tissues. Cell 2002; 111(7):931–941.

135. Garenc C, et al. The hormone-sensitive lipase gene and body composition: the HERITAGE Family Study. Int J Obes Relat Metab Disord 2002; 26(2): 220–227.

136. Talmud PJ, et al. Association of the hormone sensitive lipase-60C > G variant with fasting insulin levels in healthy young men. Nutr Metab Cardiovasc Dis 2002; 12(4):173–177.

137. Harada K, et al. Resistance to high-fat diet-induced obesity and altered expression of adipose-specific genes in HSL-deficient mice. Am J Physiol Endocrinol Metab 2003; 285(6):E1182–E1195.

138. Choy HA, Wang XP, Schotz MC. Reduced atherosclerosis in hormone-sensitive lipase transgenic mice overexpressing cholesterol acceptors. Biochim Biophys Acta 2003; 1634(3):76–85.

139. Marsh DJ, et al. Melanin-concentrating hormone 1 receptor-deficient mice are lean, hyperactive, and hyperphagic and have altered metabolism. Proc Natl Acad Sci USA 2002; 99(5):3240–3245.

140. Chen HC, et al. Increased insulin and leptin sensitivity in mice lacking acyl CoA: diacylglycerol acyltransferase 1. J Clin Invest 2002; 109(8):1049–1055.

141. Smith SJ, et al. Obesity resistance and multiple mechanisms of triglyceride synthesis in mice lacking Dgat. Nat Genet 2000; 25(1):87–90.

142. Chen HC, et al. Dissociation of obesity and impaired glucose disposal in mice overexpressing acyl coenzyme a: diacylglycerol acyltransferase 1 in white adipose tissue. Diabetes 2002; 51(11):3189–3195.

143. Cummings DE, et al. Genetically lean mice result from targeted disruption of the RII beta subunit of protein kinase A. Nature 1996; 382(6592):622–626.

144. Planas JV, et al. Mutation of the RIIbeta subunit of protein kinase A differentially affects lipolysis but not gene induction in white adipose tissue. J Biol Chem 1999; 274(51):36281–36287.

145. Anand A, Chada K. In vivo modulation of Hmgic reduces obesity. Nat Genet 2000; 24(4):377–380.

146. Elchebly M, et al. Increased insulin sensitivity and obesity resistance in mice lacking the protein tyrosine phosphatase-1B gene. Science 1999; 283(5407): 1544–1548.

147. Huggins KW, Boileau AC, Hui DY. Protection against diet-induced obesity and obesity-related insulin resistance in Group 1B PLA2-deficient mice. Am J Physiol Endocrinol Metab 2002; 283(5):E994–E1001.

148. Ntambi JM, et al. Loss of stearoyl-CoA desaturase-1 function protects mice against adiposity. Proc Natl Acad Sci USA 2002; 99(17):11482–11486.

149. Miyazaki M, et al. The biosynthesis of hepatic cholesterol esters and triglycerides is impaired in mice with a disruption of the gene for stearoyl-CoA desaturase 1. J Biol Chem 2000; 275(39):30132–30138.
150. Cohen P, et al. Role for stearoyl-CoA desaturase-1 in leptin-mediated weight loss. Science 2002; 297(5579):240–243.
151. Gunn TM, et al. The mouse mahogany locus encodes a transmembrane form of human attractin. Nature 1999; 398(6723):152–156.
152. Nagle DL, et al. The mahogany protein is a receptor involved in suppression of obesity. Nature 1999; 398(6723):148–152.
153. Speer G, et al. Vitamin D and estrogen receptor gene polymorphisms in type 2 diabetes mellitus and in android type obesity. Eur J Endocrinol 2001; 144(4):385–389.
154. Geary N, et al. Deficits in E2-dependent control of feeding, weight gain, and cholecystokinin satiation in ER-alpha null mice. Endocrinology 2001; 142(11):4751–4757.
155. Engert JC, et al. 5′ flanking variants of resistin are associated with obesity. Diabetes 2002; 51(5):1629–1634.
156. Tan MS, et al. Association of resistin gene 3′-untranslated region +62G→A polymorphism with type 2 diabetes and hypertension in a Chinese population. J Clin Endocrinol Metab 2003; 88(3):1258–1263.
157. Pravenec M, et al. Transgenic and recombinant resistin impair skeletal muscle glucose metabolism in the spontaneously hypertensive rat. J Biol Chem 2003; 278(46):45209–45215.
158. Boucher N, et al. A +2138InsCAGACC polymorphism of the melanocortin receptor 3 gene is associated in human with fat level and partitioning in interaction with body corpulence. Mol Med 2002; 8(3):158–165.
159. Chen AS, et al. Inactivation of the mouse melanocortin-3 receptor results in increased fat mass and reduced lean body mass. Nat Genet 2000; 26(1):97–102.
160. Butler AA, et al. A unique metabolic syndrome causes obesity in the melanocortin-3 receptor-deficient mouse. Endocrinology 2000; 141(9):3518–3521.
161. Shimada M, et al. Mice lacking melanin-concentrating hormone are hypophagic and lean. Nature 1998; 396(6712):670–674.
162. Segal-Lieberman G, et al. Melanin-concentrating hormone is a critical mediator of the leptin-deficient phenotype. Proc Natl Acad Sci USA 2003; 100(17):10085–10090.
163. Ludwig DS, et al. Melanin-concentrating hormone overexpression in transgenic mice leads to obesity and insulin resistance. J Clin Invest 2001; 107(3):379–386.
164. Serra C, et al. Transgenic mice with dominant negative PKC-theta in skeletal muscle: a new model of insulin resistance and obesity. J Cell Physiol 2003; 196(1):89–97.
165. Tsukiyama-Kohara K, et al. Adipose tissue reduction in mice lacking the translational inhibitor 4E-BP1. Nat Med 2001; 7(10):1128–1132.
166. Hong SH, et al. Association between HaeIII polymorphism of scavenger receptor class B type I gene and plasma HDL-cholesterol concentration. Ann Clin Biochem 2002; 39(Pt 5):478–481.

167.  Hsu LA, et al. Association between a novel 11-base pair deletion mutation in the promoter region of the scavenger receptor class B type I gene and plasma HDL cholesterol levels in Taiwanese Chinese. Arterioscler Thromb Vasc Biol 2003; 23(10):1869–1874.

168.  Osgood D, et al. Genetic variation at the scavenger receptor class B type I gene locus determines plasma lipoprotein concentrations and particle size and interacts with type 2 diabetes: the Framingham Study. J Clin Endocrinol Metab 2003; 88(6):2869–2879.

169.  Goudriaan JR, et al. CD36 deficiency increases insulin sensitivity in muscle, but induces insulin resistance in the liver in mice. J Lipid Res 2003; 44(12): 2270–2277.

170.  Febbraio M, et al. A null mutation in murine CD36 reveals an important role in fatty acid and lipoprotein metabolism. J Biol Chem 1999; 274(27): 19055–19062.

171.  Ibrahimi A, et al. Muscle-specific overexpression of FAT/CD36 enhances fatty acid oxidation by contracting muscle, reduces plasma triglycerides and fatty acids, and increases plasma glucose and insulin. J Biol Chem 1999; 274(38):26761–26766.

172.  Peterfy M, et al. Lipodystrophy in the fld mouse results from mutation of a new gene encoding a nuclear protein, lipin. Nat Genet 2001; 27(1):121–124.

173.  Moitra J, et al. Life without white fat: a transgenic mouse. Genes Dev 1998; 12(20):3168–3181.

174.  Hegele RA, et al. Association between nuclear lamin A/C R482Q mutation and partial lipodystrophy with hyperinsulinemia, dyslipidemia, hypertension, and diabetes. Genome Res 2000; 10(5):652–658.

175.  Cao H, Hegele RA. Nuclear lamin A/C R482Q mutation in Canadian kindreds with Dunnigan-type familial partial lipodystrophy. Hum Mol Genet 2000; 9(1):109–112.

176.  Hegele RA, et al. Genetic variation in LMNA modulates plasma leptin and indices of obesity in aboriginal Canadians. Physiol Genomics 2000; 3(1):39–44.

177.  Hegele RA, Huff MW, Young TK. Common genomic variation in LMNA modulates indexes of obesity in Inuit. J Clin Endocrinol Metab 2001; 86(6):2747–2751.

178.  Smith AC, et al. Hypercholesterolemia in children with Smith-Magenis syndrome: del (17) (p11.2p11.2). Genet Med 2002; 4(3):118–125.

179.  Shimomura I, et al. Insulin resistance and diabetes mellitus in transgenic mice expressing nuclear SREBP-1c in adipose tissue: model for congenital generalized lipodystrophy. Genes Dev 1998; 12(20):3182–3194.

180.  Shimano H, et al. Overproduction of cholesterol and fatty acids causes massive liver enlargement in transgenic mice expressing truncated SREBP-1a. J Clin Invest 1996; 98(7):1575–1584.

181.  Gudayol M, et al. Detection of a new variant of the mitochondrial glycerol-3-phosphate dehydrogenase gene in Spanish type 2 DM patients. Biochem Biophys Res Commun 1999; 263(2):439–445.

182.  St-Pierre J, et al. A sequence variation in the mitochondrial glycerol-3-phosphate dehydrogenase gene is associated with increased plasma glycerol

and free fatty acid concentrations among French Canadians. Mol Genet Metab 2001; 72(3):209–217.

183. Kozak LP, Kozak UC, Clarke GT. Abnormal brown and white fat development in transgenic mice overexpressing glycerol 3-phosphate dehydrogenase. Genes Dev 1991; 5(12A):2256–2264.

184. Xu Y, et al. A common Hpa I RFLP of apolipoprotein C-I increases gene transcription and exhibits an ethnically distinct pattern of linkage disequilibrium with the alleles of apolipoprotein E. J Lipid Res 1999; 40(1):50–58.

185. Shachter NS, et al. Combined hyperlipidemia in transgenic mice overexpressing human apolipoprotein Cl. J Clin Invest 1996; 98(3):846–855.

186. Jong MC, et al. In the absence of the low density lipoprotein receptor, human apolipoprotein C1 overexpression in transgenic mice inhibits the hepatic uptake of very low density lipoproteins via a receptor-associated protein-sensitive pathway. J Clin Invest 1996; 98(10):2259–2267.

187. Conde-Knape K, et al. Overexpression of apoC-I in apoE-null mice: severe hypertriglyceridemia due to inhibition of hepatic lipase. J Lipid Res 2002; 43(12):2136–2145.

188. Jong MC, et al. Protection from obesity and insulin resistance in mice overexpressing human apolipoprotein C1. Diabetes 2001; 50(12):2779–2785.

189. Wilson CJ, et al. Apolipoprotein C-II deficiency presenting as a lipid encephalopathy in infancy. Ann Neurol 2003; 53(6):807–810.

190. Kuniyoshi A, et al. A thymidine to cytosine substitution for codon 26 of exon 3 of apolipoprotein C-II gene in a patient with apolipoprotein C-II deficiency. Intern Med 1999; 38(2):140–144.

191. Shachter NS, et al. Overexpression of apolipoprotein CII causes hypertriglyceridemia in transgenic mice. J Clin Invest 1994; 93(4):1683–1690.

192. Lopez-Miranda J, et al. Influence of the SstI polymorphism at the apolipoprotein C-III gene locus on the plasma low-density-lipoprotein-cholesterol response to dietary monounsaturated fat. Am J Clin Nutr 1997; 66(1):97–103.

193. Henderson HE, et al. Association of a DNA polymorphism in the apolipoprotein C-III gene with diverse hyperlipidaemic phenotypes. Hum Genet 1987; 75(1):62–65.

194. Brown S, Ordovas JM, Campos H. Interaction between the APOC3 gene promoter polymorphisms, saturated fat intake and plasma lipoproteins. Atherosclerosis 2003; 170(2):307–313.

195. Maeda N, et al. Targeted disruption of the apolipoprotein C-III gene in mice results in hypotriglyceridemia and protection from postprandial hypertriglyceridemia. J Biol Chem 1994; 269(38):23610–23616.

196. Jong MC, et al. Apolipoprotein C-III deficiency accelerates triglyceride hydrolysis by lipoprotein lipase in wild-type and apoE knockout mice. J Lipid Res 2001; 42(10):1578–1585.

197. Masucci-Magoulas L, et al. A mouse model with features of familial combined hyperlipidemia. Science 1997; 275(5298):391–394.

198. Kamboh MI, Aston CE, Hamman RF. DNA sequence variation in human apolipoprotein C4 gene and its effect on plasma lipid profile. Atherosclerosis 2000; 152(1):193–201.

199. Allan CM, Taylor JM. Expression of a novel human apolipoprotein (apoC-IV) causes hypertriglyceridemia in transgenic mice. J Lipid Res 1996; 37(7): 1510–1518.

200. Pasagian-Macaulay A, et al. A dietary and behavioral intervention designed to lower coronary heart disease. Risk factors are unaffected by variation at the APOE gene locus. Atherosclerosis 1997; 132(2):221–227.

201. Wang CH, Zhou X. Meta-analysis for relationship between apoE gene polymorphism and coronary heart disease. Zhonghua Yu Fang Yi Xue Za Zhi 2003; 37(5):368–370.

202. Hubacek JA, et al. Genetic determination of plasma lipids and insulin in the Czech population. Clin Biochem 2001; 34(2):113–118.

203. Zhao SP, et al. Plasma lipoproteins in familial dysbetalipoproteinemia associated with apolipoproteins E2(Arg158→Cys), E3-Leiden, and E2(Lys146→Gln), and effects of treatment with simvastatin. Arterioscler Thromb 1994; 14(11): 1705–1716.

204. Viitanen L, et al. Apolipoprotein E gene promoter (-219G/T) polymorphism is associated with premature coronary heart disease. J Mol Med 2001; 79(12): 732–737.

205. Lambert JC, et al. Independent association of an APOE gene promoter polymorphism with increased risk of myocardial infarction and decreased APOE plasma concentrations—the ECTIM Study. Hum Mol Genet 2000; 9(1):57–61.

206. Matsushima Y, Hayashi S, Tachibana M. Spontaneously hyperlipidemic (SHL) mice: Japanese wild mice with apolipoprotein E deficiency. Mamm Genome 1999; 10(4):352–357.

207. Zhang SH, et al. Spontaneous hypercholesterolemia and arterial lesions in mice lacking apolipoprotein E. Science 1992; 258(5081):468–471.

208. Plump AS, et al. Severe hypercholesterolemia and atherosclerosis in apolipoprotein E-deficient mice created by homologous recombination in ES cells. Cell 1992; 71(2):343–353.

209. Namiki M, et al. Intramuscular gene transfer of interleukin-10 cDNA reduces atherosclerosis in apolipoprotein E-knockout mice. Atherosclerosis 2004; 172(1):21–29.

210. Boord JB, et al. Adipocyte fatty acid-binding protein, aP2, alters late atherosclerotic lesion formation in severe hypercholesterolemia. Arterioscler Thromb Vasc Biol 2002; 22(10):1686–1691.

211. Frank PG, et al. Genetic ablation of caveolin-1 confers protection against atherosclerosis. Arterioscler Thromb Vasc Biol 2004; 24(1):98–105.

212. Ishibashi S, et al. The two-receptor model of lipoprotein clearance: tests of the hypothesis in "knockout" mice lacking the low density lipoprotein receptor, apolipoprotein E, or both proteins. Proc Natl Acad Sci USA 1994; 91(10): 4431–4435.

213. Whitfield AJ, et al. Four novel mutations in APOB causing heterozygous and homozygous familial hypobetalipoproteinemia. Hum Mutat 2003; 22(2):178.

214. Burnett JR, et al. A novel nontruncating APOB gene mutation, R463W, causes familial hypobetalipoproteinemia. J Biol Chem 2003; 278(15):13442–13452.

215. Boekholdt SM, et al. Molecular variation at the apolipoprotein B gene locus in relation to lipids and cardiovascular disease: a systematic meta-analysis. Hum Genet 2003; 113(5):417–425.
216. Rajput-Williams J, et al. Variation of apolipoprotein-B gene is associated with obesity, high blood cholesterol levels, and increased risk of coronary heart disease. Lancet 1988; 2(8626–8627):1442–1446.
217. Linton MF, et al. Transgenic mice expressing high plasma concentrations of human apolipoprotein B100 and lipoprotein(a). J Clin Invest 1993; 92(6): 3029–3037.
218. Purcell-Huynh DA, et al. Transgenic mice expressing high levels of human apolipoprotein B develop severe atherosclerotic lesions in response to a high-fat diet. J Clin Invest 1995; 95(5):2246–2257.
219. Callow MJ, et al. Atherogenesis in transgenic mice with human apolipoprotein B and lipoprotein (a). J Clin Invest 1995; 96(3):1639–1646.
220. Grass DS, et al. Transgenic mice expressing both human apolipoprotein B and human CETP have a lipoprotein cholesterol distribution similar to that of normolipidemic humans. J Lipid Res 1995; 36(5):1082–1091.
221. Ma YQ, et al. Association of two apolipoprotein A-I gene MspI polymorphisms with high density lipoprotein (HDL)-cholesterol levels and indices of obesity in selected healthy Chinese subjects and in patients with early-onset type 2 diabetes. Clin Endocrinol (Oxf) 2003; 59(4):442–449.
222. Lawn RM, et al. Feedback mechanism of focal vascular lesion formation in transgenic apolipoprotein(a) mice. J Biol Chem 1996; 271(49):31367–31371.
223. Fiegenbaum M, Hutz MH. Further evidence for the association between obesity-related traits and the apolipoprotein A-IV gene. Int J Obes Relat Metab Disord 2003; 27(4):484–490.
224. Lefevre M, et al. Common apolipoprotein A-IV variants are associated with differences in body mass index levels and percentage body fat. Int J Obes Relat Metab Disord 2000; 24(8):945–953.
225. Fisher RM, et al. Effect of variation in the apo A-IV gene on body mass index and fasting and postprandial lipids in the European Atherosclerosis Research Study II. EARS Group. J Lipid Res 1999; 40(2):287–294.
226. Weinstock PH, et al. Decreased HDL cholesterol levels but normal lipid absorption, growth, and feeding behavior in apolipoprotein A-IV knockout mice. J Lipid Res 1997; 38(9):1782–1794.
227. Talmud PJ, et al. Genetic and environmental determinants of plasma high density lipoprotein cholesterol and apolipoprotein AI concentrations in healthy middle-aged men. Ann Hum Genet 2002; 66(Pt 2):111–124.
228. Fumeron F, et al. Alcohol intake modulates the effect of a polymorphism of the cholesteryl ester transfer protein gene on plasma high density lipoprotein and the risk of myocardial infarction. J Clin Invest 1995; 96(3):1664–1671.
229. Yamashita S, et al. Molecular mechanisms, lipoprotein abnormalities and atherogenicity of hyperalphalipoproteinemia. Atherosclerosis 2000; 152(2): 271–285.
230. Marotti KR, et al. Severe atherosclerosis in transgenic mice expressing simian cholesteryl ester transfer protein. Nature 1993; 364(6432):73–75.

231. Hayek T, et al. An interaction between the human cholesteryl ester transfer protein (CETP) and apolipoprotein A-I genes in transgenic mice results in a profound CETP-mediated depression of high density lipoprotein cholesterol levels. J Clin Invest 1992; 90(2):505–510.

232. Hayek T, et al. Hypertriglyceridemia and cholesteryl ester transfer protein interact to dramatically alter high density lipoprotein levels, particle sizes, and metabolism. Studies in transgenic mice. J Clin Invest 1993; 92(3):1143–1152.

233. Blake WL, et al. The development of fatty liver is accelerated in transgenic mice expressing cynomolgus monkey cholesteryl ester transfer protein. Biochem Biophys Res Commun 1994; 205(2):1257–1263.

234. Gautier T, et al. Apolipoprotein CI deficiency markedly augments plasma lipoprotein changes mediated by human cholesteryl ester transfer protein (CETP) in CETP transgenic/ApoCI-knocked out mice. J Biol Chem 2002; 277(35):31354–31363.

235. Kawano K, et al. Cholesteryl ester transfer protein and phospholipid transfer protein have nonoverlapping functions in vivo. J Biol Chem 2000; 275(38): 29477–29481.

236. Plump AS, et al. Increased atherosclerosis in ApoE and LDL receptor gene knock-out mice as a result of human cholesteryl ester transfer protein transgene expression. Arterioscler Thromb Vasc Biol 1999; 19(4):1105–1110.

237. Rainwater DL, et al. A DNA polymorphism for LCAT is associated with altered LCAT activity and high density lipoprotein size distributions in baboons. Arterioscler Thromb 1992; 12(6):682–690.

238. Kammerer CM, Hixson JE, Mott GE. A DNA polymorphism for lecithin: cholesterol acyltransferase (LCAT) is associated with high density lipoprotein cholesterol concentrations in baboons. Atherosclerosis 1993; 98(2):153–163.

239. Berard AM, et al. High plasma HDL concentrations associated with enhanced atherosclerosis in transgenic mice overexpressing lecithin-cholesteryl acyltransferase. Nat Med 1997; 3(7):744–749.

240. Foger B, et al. Cholesteryl ester transfer protein corrects dysfunctional high density lipoproteins and reduces aortic atherosclerosis in lecithin cholesterol acyltransferase transgenic mice. J Biol Chem 1999; 274(52):36912–36920.

241. Wittekoek ME, et al. A frequent mutation in the lipoprotein lipase gene (D9N) deteriorates the biochemical and clinical phenotype of familial hypercholesterolemia. Arterioscler Thromb Vasc Biol 1999; 19(11):2708–2713.

242. Hokanson JE. Functional variants in the lipoprotein lipase gene and risk cardiovascular disease. Curr Opin Lipidol 1999; 10(5):393–399.

243. Gerdes C, et al. Lipoprotein lipase variants D9N and N291S are associated with increased plasma triglyceride and lower high-density lipoprotein cholesterol concentrations: studies in the fasting and postprandial states: the European Atherosclerosis Research Studies. Circulation 1997; 96(3):733–740.

244. van Bockxmeer FM, et al. Lipoprotein lipase D9N, N291S and S447X polymorphisms: their influence on premature coronary heart disease and plasma lipids. Atherosclerosis 2001; 157(1):123–129.

245. Garenc C, et al. Evidence of LPL gene-exercise interaction for body fat and LPL activity: the HERITAGE Family Study. J Appl Physiol 2001; 91(3):1334–1340.

246. Garenc C, et al. Linkage and association studies of the lipoprotein lipase gene with postheparin plasma lipase activities, body fat, and plasma lipid and lipoprotein concentrations: the HERITAGE Family Study. Metabolism 2000; 49(4):432–439.

247. Ukkola O, et al. Genetic variation at the lipoprotein lipase locus and plasma lipoprotein and insulin levels in the Quebec Family Study. Atherosclerosis 2001; 158(1):199–206.

248. Ishimura-Oka K, et al. A missense (Asp250–Asn) mutation in the lipoprotein lipase gene in two unrelated families with familial lipoprotein lipase deficiency. J Lipid Res 1992; 33(5):745–754.

249. Yagyu H, et al. Overexpressed lipoprotein lipase protects against atherosclerosis in apolipoprotein E knockout mice. J Lipid Res 1999; 40(9):1677–1685.

250. Shimada M, et al. Suppression of diet-induced atherosclerosis in low density lipoprotein receptor knockout mice overexpressing lipoprotein lipase. Proc Natl Acad Sci USA 1996; 93(14):7242–7246.

251. Gonzalez-Sanchez JL, et al. K121Q PC-1 gene polymorphism is not associated with insulin resistance in a Spanish population. Obes Res 2003; 11(5): 603–605.

252. Hessle L, et al. Tissue-nonspecific alkaline phosphatase and plasma cell membrane glycoprotein-1 are central antagonistic regulators of bone mineralization. Proc Natl Acad Sci USA 2002; 99(14):9445–9449.

253. Epstein LH, et al. Dopamine transporter genotype as a risk factor for obesity in African-American smokers. Obes Res 2002; 10(12):1232–1240.

254. Gainetdinov RR, et al. Glutamatergic modulation of hyperactivity in mice lacking the dopamine transporter. Proc Natl Acad Sci USA 2001; 98(20): 11047–11054.

255. Dionne IJ, et al. Association between obesity and a polymorphism in the beta(1)-adrenoceptor gene (Gly389Arg ADRB1) in Caucasian women. Int J Obes Relat Metab Disord 2002; 26(5):633–639.

256. Rohrer DK, et al. Targeted disruption of the mouse beta1-adrenergic receptor gene: developmental and cardiovascular effects. Proc Natl Acad Sci USA 1996; 93(14):7375–7380.

257. Ehrenborg E, et al. The Q/E27 polymorphism in the beta2-adrenoceptor gene is associated with increased body weight and dyslipoproteinaemia involving triglyceride-rich lipoproteins. J Intern Med 2000; 247(6):651–656.

258. Ishiyama-Shigemoto S, et al. Association of polymorphisms in the beta2-adrenergic receptor gene with obesity, hypertriglyceridaemia, and diabetes mellitus. Diabetologia 1999; 42(1):98–101.

259. Mori Y, et al. The Gln27Glu beta2-adrenergic receptor variant is associated with obesity due to subcutaneous fat accumulation in Japanese men. Biochem Biophys Res Commun 1999; 258(1):138–140.

260. Garenc C, et al. Effects of beta2-adrenergic receptor gene variants on adiposity: the HERITAGE Family Study. Obes Res 2003; 11(5):612–618.

261. Meirhaeghe A, et al. Impact of polymorphisms of the human beta2-adrenoceptor gene on obesity in a French population. Int J Obes Relat Metab Disord 2000; 24(3):382–387.

262. Chruscinski AJ, et al. Targeted disruption of the beta2 adrenergic receptor gene. J Biol Chem 1999; 274(24):16694–16700.
263. Rohrer DK, et al. Cardiovascular and metabolic alterations in mice lacking both beta1- and beta2-adrenergic receptors. J Biol Chem 1999; 274(24): 16701–16708.
264. Clement K, et al. Genetic variation in the beta 3-adrenergic receptor and an increased capacity to gain weight in patients with morbid obesity. N Engl J Med 1995; 333(6):352–354.
265. Kadowaki H, et al. A mutation in the beta 3-adrenergic receptor gene is associated with obesity and hyperinsulinemia in Japanese subjects. Biochem Biophys Res Commun 1995; 215(2):555–560.
266. Susulic VS, et al. Targeted disruption of the beta 3-adrenergic receptor gene. J Biol Chem 1995; 270(49):29483–29492.
267. Jimenez M, et al. Beta(1)/beta(2)/beta(3)-adrenoceptor knockout mice are obese and cold-sensitive but have normal lipolytic responses to fasting. FEBS Lett 2002; 530(1–3):37–40.
268. Sun Y, Wang N, Tall AR. Regulation of adrenal scavenger receptor-BI expression by ACTH and cellular cholesterol pools. J Lipid Res 1999; 40(10): 1799–1805.
269. Gurnell M. PPARgamma and metabolism: insights from the study of human genetic variants. Clin Endocrinol (Oxf) 2003; 59(3):267–277.
270. Lee CH, Olson, Evans RM. Minireview: lipid metabolism, metabolic diseases, and peroxisome proliferator-activated receptors. Endocrinology 2003; 144(6): 2201–2207.
271. Walczak R, Tontonoz P. PPARadigms and PPARadoxes: expanding roles for PPARgamma in the control of lipid metabolism. J Lipid Res 2002; 43(2): 177–186.
272. Francis GA, et al. Nuclear receptors and the control of metabolism. Annu Rev Physiol 2003; 65:261–311.
273. Fruhbeck G, Gomez-Ambrosi J. Control of body weight: a physiologic and transgenic perspective. Diabetologia 2003; 46(2):143–172.
274. Arch JR. Lessons in obesity from transgenic animals. J Endocrinol Invest 2002; 25(10):867–875.
275. Inui A. Transgenic approach to the study of body weight regulation. Pharmacol Rev 2000; 52(1):35–61.
276. Yuan X, et al. Identification of polymorphic loci in the promoter region of the serotonin 5-HT2C receptor gene and their association with obesity and type II diabetes. Diabetologia 2000; 43(3):373–376.
277. Westberg L, et al. Association between a polymorphism of the 5-HT2C receptor and weight loss in teenage girls. Neuropsychopharmacology 2002; 26(6):789–793.
278. Basile VS, et al. 759C/T genetic variation of 5HT(2C) receptor and clozapine-induced weight gain. Lancet 2002; 360(9347):1790–1791.
279. Reynolds GP, Zhang ZJ, Zhang XB. Association of antipsychotic drug-induced weight gain with a 5-HT2C receptor gene polymorphism. Lancet 2002; 359(9323):2086–2087.

280. Iwamoto K, Kato T. RNA editing of serotonin 2C receptor in human post-mortem brains of major mental disorders. Neurosci Lett 2003; 346(3):169–172.

281. Dracheva S, et al. RNA editing and alternative splicing of human serotonin 2C receptor in schizophrenia. J Neurochem 2003; 87(6):1402–1412.

282. Castensson A, et al. Decrease of serotonin receptor 2C in schizophrenia brains identified by high-resolution mRNA expression analysis. Biol Psychiat 2003; 54(11):1212–1221.

# 9

# Risk Assessment and Treatment Standards of Obesity and Overweight in Relation to Cardiovascular Disease

**Lalita Khaodhiar**

*Beth Israel Deaconess Medical Center and Harvard Medical School, Center for the Study of Nutrition Medicine, Boston, Massachusetts, U.S.A.*

**Karen C. McCowen**

*Beth Israel Deaconess Medical Center and Harvard Medical School, Boston, Massachusetts, U.S.A.*

**George L. Blackburn**

*Beth Israel Deaconess Medical Center and Harvard Medical School, Center for the Study of Nutrition Medicine, Boston, Massachusetts, U.S.A.*

## INTRODUCTION

Obesity has long been associated with an increased risk for cardiovascular disease (CVD). It is widely known that obesity promotes the development of hypertension, diabetes mellitus, sleep apnea, and dyslipidemia—all recognized contributors to CVD (1). Research over the past decade has shown that obesity promotes a state of inflammation evidenced by elevated levels of C-reactive protein, interleukin 6, and tumor necrosis factor-$\alpha$ (TNF$\alpha$) (2,3). Inflammatory processes in atheromatous plaques (4) are associated with coronary disease, as are such hemorheological abnormalities as elevated plasma concentration of fibrinogen, vonWillebrand factor, factor VII, plasminogen activator inhibitor-1 (5,6), and high blood viscosity (7). Obesity also causes insulin resistance with consequent hyperinsulinemia. Whether elevated insulin levels are linked to atherosclerosis is subject to debate. Intra-abdominal fat, estimated by waist circumference, is associated with insulin resistance syndrome, sleep apnea, and inflammation—three factors that appear to be of critical importance in the link between obesity and CVD.

In this chapter, we will discuss the assessment of obesity, epidemiological and pathophysiological links between obesity and CVD risk factors, and the impact of weight loss on these variables. Treatment strategies that can lead to improvements in cardiovascular risk factors and obesity-related comorbidities will also be discussed.

## OBESITY ASSESSMENT AND RISK OF CVD

Persons who are overweight or obese are assessed by degree and type of obesity as well as overall cardiac risk status (Table 1A and B). The goal in managing such patients should be to achieve a healthy weight. A 5% to 10% reduction of excess body weight is an achievable reduction that contributes to control of cardiovascular risk factors. Long-term maintenance of a lower body weight can significantly improve longevity (9,10).

## Table 1

*(A) Major Emerging Cardiovascular Risk Factors*

| Modifiable | Nonmodifiable | Life habit |
|---|---|---|
| Elevated LDL-C | Age | Obesity |
| Low HDL-C | Male sex | Physical inactivity |
| Hypertension | Family history | Atherogenic diet |
| Diabetes mellitus | | |
| Cigarette smoking | | |

*(B) Emerging Cardiovascular Risk Factors*

| Lipid | Nonlipid |
|---|---|
| Triglycerides | Homocysteine |
| Lipoprotein remnants | Thrombogenic/hemostatic factors |
| Small LDL particles | Inflammatory markers |
| Lipoprotein (a) | Impaired fasting glucose |
| Metabolic syndrome | Metabolic syndrome |

*Abbreviations*: HDL-C, high-density lipoprotein cholesterol; LDL-C, low-density lipoprotein cholesterol; LDL, low-density lipoprotein.
*Source*: From Ref. 8.

## Definition and Degree of Overweight and Obesity

Overweight and obesity refer to a clinical continuum. Overweight can be seen as step 1, where excess fat makes up an average of 10% of total body weight. Obesity is step 2, where excess fat accounts for greater than 25% of total body weight in men, or greater than 30% in women. Body fat is determined by several methods, e.g., underwater weighing, dual photon X ray absorptiometry, and imaging studies [computerized tomography (CT) and magnetic resonance imaging (MRI)] (11). These tests, however, are too complex and costly for use in most clinical settings.

Body mass index (BMI), a measure easily and quickly obtained in clinical settings, is typically used to estimate body fat in office practice and in large epidemiologic studies. BMI, calculated by dividing an individual's weight (in kilograms) by the square of the height (in meters) (12,13), can also be read off a chart or nomogram (Fig. 1). In general, BMI correlates well with body fat in both men and women, and is relatively unaffected by height. Because it correlates significantly with morbidity and mortality, recommendations for treatment of obesity are based on the level of BMI (13). Epidemiologic data show a modest increase in risk of mortality for a BMI $>25 \, kg/m^2$, and a markedly increased one for a BMI $> 30 \, kg/m^2$ (Fig. 2) (15). Table 2 provides a classification of overweight and obesity by BMI, waist circumference, and associated disease risk. This classification system, developed by the World Health Organization (WHO) Obesity Task Force (16), has been adopted by the Expert Panel on the Identification, Evaluation, and Treatment of Overweight and Obesity in Adults, the National Heart, Lung, and Blood Institute (NHLBI) of the National Institutes of Health (NIH) (13).

## Prevalence of Obesity

Data from the National Center for Health Statistics indicate a marked increase in the prevalence of obesity (defined as a BMI $\geq 30 \, kg/m^2$), a rise from 12.8% in 1976–1980 to 22.5% in 1988–1994 to 30% between 1999 and 2002. Approximately 31% of American adults, about 59 million people, are considered obese, and 5% are extremely obese. Sixty-six percent of adults meet the criterion for overweight (BMI $\geq 25 \, kg/m^2$). The prevalence of obesity varies by age, sex, and racial group, ranging from 23% in non-Hispanic white men aged 20 to 39 to 51% in non-Hispanic black women aged 40 to 59 years. Overall the prevalence of obesity in adults is higher among women than men with non-Hispanic black women having the highest prevalence across racial/ethnic group (49% obesity, 14% extreme obesity) (17,18).

## Regional Fat Distribution

Regional fat distribution has become recognized as an important factor in determining health risk in obese individuals. Data from epidemiologic and

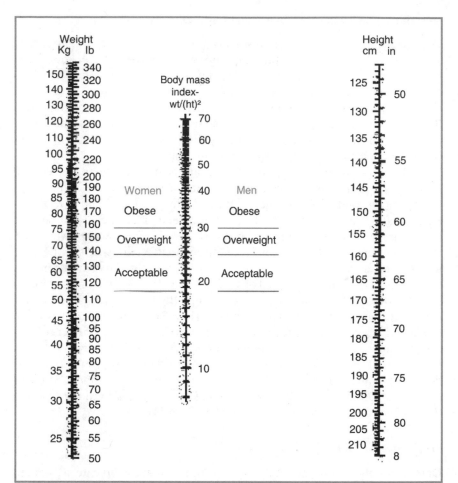

**Nomogram for determining body mass index** The nomogram is used by placing a ruler or other straight edge between the body weight in kilograms or pounds (the left-hand line) and the height in centimeters or inches (the right-hand line). The body mass index is read from the middle of the scale, in metric units.

**Figure 1**  BMI nomogram: For a quick determination of BMI (kg/m$^2$), use a straight edge to help locate the point on the chart where height (in. or cm) and weight (lbs or kg) intersect. The number on the dashed line closest to this point is read. For example, an individual who weighs 69 kg and is 173 cm tall has a BMI of approximately 23. *Abbreviation*: BMI, body mass index. *Source*: Health and Welfare Canada (1988). Canadian Guidelines for Healthy Weights. Report of an Expert Group Convened by Health Promotion Directorate, Health Services and Promotion Branch. Ottawa: Health and Welfare Canada.

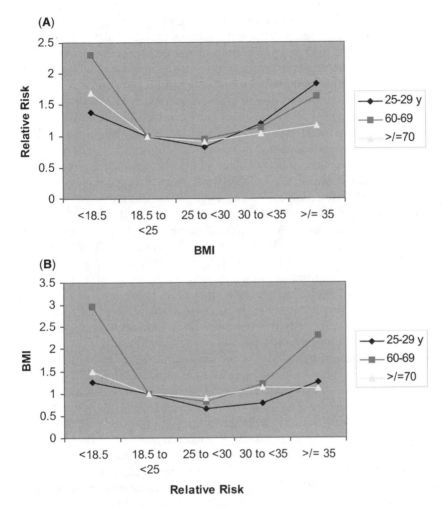

**Figure 2** Relationship between mortality and BMI: relative risks by age group and BMI level from the combined NHANES I, II, and III data set. (**A**) Overall. (**B**) Never smoker only. *Abbreviations*: BMI, body mass index; NHANES, National Health and Nutrition Examination Surveys. *Source*: From Ref. 14.

clinical studies have shown that excess abdominal fat is an independent predictor for cardiovascular risk and mortality (11,19,20). Risk factors include type 2 diabetes mellitus, impaired glucose tolerance (IGT), hypertension, dyslipidemia, and atherosclerosis of coronary, cerebral, and peripheral blood vessels.

The impact of regional fat distribution on health is related to both abdominal (upper body fat) and visceral fat located in the intra-abdominal cavity. Studies on the effects of fat distribution and the impact of visceral fat have been hampered by problems in measuring fat distribution. In general, anthropometric measurements [waist circumference, waist-to-hip ratio (WHR), or skinfold thickness] have been used to estimate central or upper body obesity. These measurements are simple and convenient for epidemiological studies, and provide useful estimates of the proportion of abdominal fat. They do not, however, distinguish between accumulations of deep abdominal (visceral) fat and subcutaneous abdominal fat. Imaging techniques such as CT or MRI provide more accurate data, but are costly and infeasible for use in large studies.

In clinical practice, abdominal fat is best determined by measuring the waist circumference or the ratio of waist circumference divided by hip circumference (WHR). Waist is defined as the smallest circumference of the torso midway between the inferior margin of the 12th rib and the iliac crest in a horizontal plane. Waist circumference should be taken with the subject standing, feet 25 to 30 cm apart, and weight evenly distributed. The clinician sits by the side of the subject and, with a nonstretchable tape measure, applies a snug fit that does not compress soft tissues. Hip circumference is measured horizontally around the pelvis at the level of the maximal protrusion of the buttocks (21). Measurements of skinfold thickness, considerably less accurate than measurements of circumferences, are not commonly used in clinical practice (19).

Bioelectrical impedance (BIA) is another noninvasive, simple, quick, and inexpensive method for measuring body composition. It is based on the principle that the resistance to an applied electric current is inversely related to the amount of fat-free mass within the body. It is currently used in diverse settings including private clinicians' office, health clubs, and hospitals. When done correctly on properly operating equipment, BIA accuracy is approximately ±3%. However it tends to overestimate fat-free mass in obese people (22).

In general, an individual is considered to be at high risk for cardiovascular morbidity at a BMI $\geq 35 \, \text{kg/m}^2$, with a waist circumference greater than 102 cm (40 in.) for men and 88 cm (35 in.) for women (23). These cutoff points, however, lose their predictive value in patients with a BMI $\geq 35 \, \text{kg/m}^2$. A WHR $\geq 1$ for men and $\geq 0.85$ for women is also used to identify patients with abdominal obesity, though the NHLBI and WHO consider waist circumference the preferred measurement (Table 2).

## Association of Obesity with Cardiovascular Morbidity and Mortality

Most epidemiological studies indicate that being overweight or obese is associated with higher overall mortality (9,24,25). The Nurses' Health Study showed that in women with a recently stable weight, who had never smoked, a BMI of 27 to 28.9 was associated with a relative risk (RR) of death of 1.6; a BMI of 29 to 31.9 with a RR of 2.1; and a BMI $\geq 32$ with an RR of 2.2

**Table 2**  Classification of Overweight and Obesity by BMI, Waist Circumference, and Associated Disease Risks

| | BMI (kg/m²) | Obesity class | Disease risk[a] relative to normal weight and waist circumference | |
| | | | Men ≤ 102 cm (≤40 in.) ≥102 cm (≥40 in.) | Women ≤ 88 cm (≤35 in.) ≥88 cm (≥35 in.) |
|---|---|---|---|---|
| Underweight | < 18.5 | | | |
| Normal | 18.5–24.9 | | | |
| Overweight | 25.0–29.9 | | Increased | High |
| Obesity | 30.0–34.9 | I | High | Very high |
| | 35.0–39.9 | II | Very high | Very high |
| Extreme obesity | ≥40 | III | Extremely high | Extremely high |

[a]Disease risk for type 2 diabetes, hypertension, and CVD.
Increased waist circumference can also be a marker for increased risk even in persons of normal weight.
*Source*: From Ref. 13.

compared with the leanest cohort (BMI <19) (26). Among women with a BMI ≥32, the RR of death from CVD was 4.1 compared with women with a BMI < 19. Similarly in never-smoking male alumni of Harvard University, BMI ≥ 26 was associated with an RR of death of 1.67 compared with those with a BMI < 22.5 (27). The leanest participants showed the lowest mortality without evidence for a J- or U-shaped curve when smokers and those with intercurrent illnesses were excluded. Some of the controversy related to the U-shaped curve died down after those with low BMI related to low lean body mass were removed from the analysis. Based on all-cause mortality, desirable BMI in Caucasians is probably between 18.5–25; ideal weight in other populations is not clear (28).

Although the relationship between obesity and coronary heart disease (CHD) is still uncertain, the Nutrition Committee of the American Heart Association has identified obesity as an independent risk factor (1,29). Several epidemiological data have shown that CVD risks are directly related to obesity. In the Nurses' Health Study, almost 1300 cases of CHD were ascertained over 14 years (30,31). After controlling for age, smoking habit, menopausal status, postmenopausal hormone use, and parental history of CHD, risk of CHD rose with increasing BMI ≥ 23. This was striking because it indicated elevated risk even within the "normal" range for BMI. For women with a BMI ≥ 29, the RR compared with those with BMI < 21 was 3.6. Similarly, a history of weight gain, even in women of normal weight, was strongly associated with the development of CHD. In addition, greater waist circumference and higher WHR were independently associated with a significantly increased age-adjusted risk of CHD. After adjusting for BMI and other cardiac risk factors (hypertension, diabetes, and high cholesterol level), women with a WHR $\geq 0.88$ had an RR of 3.25 for CHD compared with women with a WHR $< 0.72$. A waist circumference of 96.5 cm (38 in.) or more was associated with an RR of 3.06 (32). Although less research has been done on stroke, a variety of studies associate ischemic events with overweight (33–36).

National Health and Nutrition Examination Surveys (NHANES) reported a relative risk of 1.5 for CVD in later life for a woman with a BMI $\geq 29$ versus the referent population (BMI $< 21$) (37). Similar findings have been reported for men (38) as well as many other populations (with the notable exception of the Pima Indian tribe, in which rates of CHD are strangely low despite obesity and a plethora of other risk factors endemic in this group) (39).

In the Framingham cohort (40), obesity has been associated with myocardial hypertrophy independent of hypertension and with higher rates of heart failure. High metabolic activity of excessive fat induces an increase in total blood volume and cardiac output; this may lead to left ventricular dilation, increased left ventricular wall stress, compensatory left ventricular hypertrophy, and left ventricular diastolic dysfunction. Zarich et al. and Alpert have found moderate diastolic dysfunction, left ventricular hypertrophy, cardiomegaly, and impaired contractility in over 50% of patients with morbid obesity (41–43).

## EPIDEMIOLOGY OF CVD IN OBESITY

### Low Birth Weight

Fetal programming of thrifty phenotype may provide an explanation for subsequent obesity and obesity-related cardiovascular events. The Dutch Hunger Winter, which occurred at the end of World War II, from 1944 to 1945, represents a unique opportunity to study the effect of intrauterine malnutrition due to the availability of a relatively good food immediately prior to and following that period. In one study, oral glucose tolerance tests were performed on adult survivors. Postchallenge glycemia was higher in those exposed to famine in utero than in infancy. It was highest in those who were exposed in mid- and late-gestation, especially in those who subsequently became obese (44). Persons exposed to famine also had a more atherogenic lipid profile than controls, although this finding was independent of adult obesity (45). In contrast, high blood pressure has not been linked to prenatal malnutrition (46).

Roseboom et al. found a significantly higher prevalence of CHD in those adults exposed to famine in early utero (compared with controls), especially in those who manifested adulthood obesity (47). In some studies, low birth weight related to maternal undernutrition predicted increased visceral adiposity and insulin-resistant states in childhood and adulthood (48). Epidemiologic studies have shown an association between reduced fetal growth and insulin resistance, high blood pressure, high serum triglycerides (TG), and low concentrations of high-density lipoprotein (HDL) cholesterol. People who were small at birth and became obese (49–52) had the highest values of these coronary risk factors. These findings suggest fetal programming of a thrifty phenotype as an explanation for subsequent obesity and obesity-related cardiovascular risk factors.

## Hypertension

The association between obesity and hypertension is well documented. NHANES III data show that in men as well as women, the prevalence of hypertension rises progressively with increase in BMI (53). In adults with BMI $\geq 30\,kg/m^2$, the prevalence of high blood pressure is 38% in men and 32% in women; in those with BMI $< 25\,kg/m^2$, it is 18% in men and 16% in women (with respective RRs of 2.1 and 1.9). The Nurses' Health Study reported a similar relation between BMI and hypertension (54). Middle-aged women with a BMI $\geq 31\,kg/m^2$ had a 6.3 RR of hypertension compared with those with BMI $< 20\,kg/m^2$. Multivariate analysis showed that risk for hypertension rose 12% for every $1\,kg/m^2$ increase in BMI. Weight gain as low as 2.1 to 4.9 kg also increases risk. Each 10 lb (4.5 kg) weight gain increased the risk of hypertension by an estimated 20%. Women who gained more than 25 kg had a fivefold increase in risk. Conversely, those who lost more than 10 kg reduced their risk of hypertension by 26%. Similar findings from INTERSALT showed that an additional 10 kg of body weight was associated with increases in systolic and diastolic blood pressure of 3.0 and 2.3 mmHg, respectively (55). Data from the Framingham Heart Study suggest that approximately 65% to 75% of risk for hypertension can be directly attributed to excess weight (56).

Recent research has clarified the pathophysiologic mechanisms that underlie the association between obesity and hypertension (57). Obesity is associated with increases in regional blood flow, cardiac output, and arterial pressure. Although part of the increased cardiac output is due to additional blood flow required by excess fat, blood flow to other tissues (e.g., the heart, kidneys, and skeletal muscle) also increases. Vasodilation in these tissues appears to result from high metabolic rate and local accumulation of vasodilator metabolites (58). The maintenance of hypervolemia in the presence of hypertension implies a resetting of pressure natriuresis toward higher blood pressure (59). Obesity increases renal sodium reabsorption by activating renin-angiotensin and the sympathetic nervous system (60).

Hormones secreted from adipose tissue, such as leptin, may be partly responsible for sympathetic activation. Acute infusions of leptin increase renal sympathetic activity (61). Insulin may also play a role; it increases renal tubular resorption of sodium and boosts intracellular stores of free calcium in the vascular smooth muscle cells, thereby increasing vascular tone (62–64). Many cross-sectional studies demonstrate that insulin concentrations correlate with blood pressure. Other mediators of the effect of obesity on blood pressure include obstructive sleep apnea (OSA), which elevates catecholamines, and fetal malnutrition, which can promote the development of both obesity and hypertension. Prolonged obesity causes structural changes in the kidneys, which eventually lead to a loss of nephron function, further increases in blood pressure, and in some cases, severe renal disease.

### Diabetes Mellitus

Several epidemiologic studies have linked increased risk for type 2 diabetes with higher BMIs. In the Nurses' Health Study (65), a greater risk of diabetes was observed in women with BMI as low as 22. Women with a BMI in the average range ($24.0$–$24.9 \, kg/m^2$) had up to a fivefold elevated risk compared with women with a BMI $< 22 \, kg/m^2$. The risk of type 2 diabetes increased by more than 40-fold in those with a BMI over $31 \, kg/m^2$ (Fig. 3). This relation between BMI and diabetes was seen in black and white women, and in those up to 69 years of age. Changes in body weight during adulthood were also a strong predictor of risk for diabetes. Women who gained 20 kg or more had a 12-fold increased risk compared with

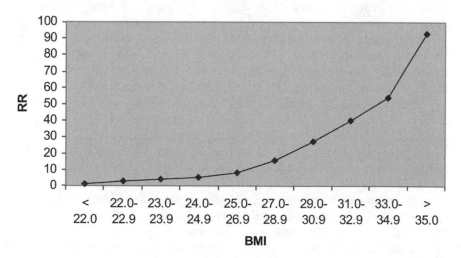

**Figure 3** Attained body mass index and relative risk for type 2 diabetes mellitus in U.S. women aged 30 to 55 years. *Source*: From Ref. 65.

women whose weight changes were less than 5 kg. Conversely, a weight loss of 20 kg or more reduced the risk of diabetes by 87%.

Similar results were reported in men. In the Professionals' Health Study, RR for diabetes was 4.2 in men with a BMI $> 35$ kg/m$^2$ compared with those with a BMI $< 23$ kg/m$^2$. Men who gained 15 kg or more after age 21 had a 3.4 times higher risk than those with stable weight.

The association of higher BMI with increased risk of type 2 diabetes has been shown in diverse populations, including those with high and low rates of diabetes. Studies of the Pima Indian tribe (66–68), with its very high prevalence of diabetes, show that the incidence of diabetes is strongly related to preceding obesity with approximately 0.8 cases per 1000 person-years for a BMI $< 20$ kg/m$^2$ compared with 72 cases per 1000 person-years for a BMI $\geq 40$. Interestingly, diabetes was extremely rare in this tribe in the 1940s, when the diet consisted of complex carbohydrates with very low amounts of fat. Exposure of the Pima Indians to a more typical Western high-calorie, high-fat diet and a more sedentary lifestyle has led to obesity and a prevalence of adult diabetes that exceeds 50%.

Obesity is a major risk factor for the development of type 2 diabetes, particularly in the presence of low birth weight (69,70). It decreases insulin sensitivity, compounding underlying (possibly inherited) insulin resistance. Ultimately, beta cell failure results in hyperglycemia and frank diabetes mellitus. Obesity may account for 50% or more of the variance in insulin sensitivity in the general population; abdominal fat bears a particularly strong relation to insulin resistance.

Excessive visceral adiposity and increased intramyocellular fat have been specifically linked to insulin resistance. Rates of lipolysis from omental fat is significantly increased compared with subcutaneous fat; thus high levels of free fatty acid (FFA) and TNFα are released by excess adipocytes. The elevation of FFA levels causes hyperinsulinemia by inhibiting muscle glucose utilization, increasing hepatic glucose output, and stimulating insulin secretion from pancreatic β cells (71–73). The presence of fat deposits in muscle cells has been similarly associated with reductions in insulin-mediated glucose uptake (74,75). A potential additional link between obesity and diabetes is through OSA. As with hypertension, sleep apnea–related excess catecholamine can lead to insulin resistance (76).

## Dyslipidemia

Obesity and insulin resistance strongly affect lipoprotein metabolism and lead to higher fasting plasma TG and lower plasma HDL cholesterol levels (77). Low-density lipoprotein (LDL) cholesterol is slightly elevated or normal, but small, dense atherogenic LDL particles are usually increased (78,79). Weight loss reduces TG and LDL, and increases HDL; while HDL increases are more pronounced in women, LDL changes are of greater magnitude in men (1). Rates of cholesterol production correlate with excess body mass, increasing approximately 20 mg/day/kg rise in body fat (80,81). In the Framingham Offspring Study, increased BMI is associated with lower HDL and higher LDL. A $10 \text{ kg/m}^2$ increment in BMI lowered LDL cholesterol levels by 3.2 mg/dL (in women) and 10 mg/dL (in men) (82). Cross-sectional data indicate that this magnitude of weight difference may cause a 10 mg/dL rise in LDL cholesterol with more small and dense atherogenic LDL particles (83). As with other coronary risk factors, visceral adiposity has an impact on many of these relations. One study found negative correlations between deep abdominal fat mass and HDL, or the HDL/LDL ratio, in obese, premenopausal women (84).

Visceral obesity and hyperinsulinemia cause excess production of very low density lipoprotein (VLDL), which is TG rich in the liver. Enhanced lipolytic activity of visceral adipocytes increases FFA flux to the liver and stimulates VLDL secretion (85). The activity of lipoprotein lipase, the enzyme that transforms TG-rich chylomicrons to HDL, and VLDL to LDL, also declines with insulin resistance (86). These alterations in VLDL metabolism can lead to slower VLDL clearance, reduced HDL production, and an increase in smaller, denser LDL particles (77,87). In addition, obesity-related insulin resistance decreases affinity for the LDL receptor and may impair clearance of LDL particles (88).

## Obstructive Sleep Apnea

Obesity is known to be a major risk factor for sleep-disordered breathing (apnea and hypopnea). One large study showed a 4.2 odds ratio for the presence of OSA with each 1 standard deviation increase in BMI. For WHR and body weight, the respective odds ratios were 3.4 and 2.0 (89). Up to 60% to 70% of sleep apnea sufferers are obese, and among the morbidly obese, OSA occurs at a 12- to 20-fold rate of frequency (90). Interestingly, OSA patients have a greater proportion of visceral fat than obese controls without sleep apnea (91). Vgontzas et al. found that indices of sleep-disordered breathing were correlated with visceral fat, not BMI or total fat. In a Swedish cohort of middle-aged men, risk of CVD was increased in OSA, independent of age, BMI, blood pressure, and smoking habit (92). OSA has been linked to chronically elevated blood pressure (93) and insulin resistance (94).

Studies have consistently shown that patients with OSA have high levels of sympathetic nerve traffic. Mechanisms that contribute to the maintenance of higher sympathetic activity and blood pressure include chemoreflex and baroreflex dysfunction (95), altered cardiovascular variability (96–98), vasoconstrictor effects of nocturnal endothelin release, and endothelial dysfunction (99). When blood pressure was measured using 24-hour ambulatory monitors, nocturnal desaturation was associated with a rise in daytime blood pressure independent of BMI (100). Pankow et al. found that higher ratios of night-to-day blood pressure (nondipping phenomenon) in patients with severe OSA compared with participants with mild disease.

In the Wisconsin Sleep Cohort Study, a longitudinal study of more than 700 patients, a significant dose response was found between measures of sleep-disordered breathing at baseline and the presence of hypertension at four-year follow-up (101). In a cross-sectional study of 2677 adults who underwent sleep studies, OSA was a significant predictor of both systolic and diastolic blood pressure independent of age, BMI, and sex. Each additional apnea per hour of sleep increased the odds of hypertension by 1%, and each 10% decrease in oxygen saturation increased the odds by 13% (102). Perhaps the strongest evidence that sleep apnea may mediate some of the effects of obesity on hypertension comes from a canine model of OSA. Experimental OSA resembling the human condition resulted in sustained daytime hypertension after three months. In contrast, repeated arousals from sleep without airway occlusion did not result in daytime hypertension (103).

## TREATMENT OF OBESITY TO LOWER CARDIOVASCULAR RISK

### Effect of Weight Control on Risk Reduction

Weight loss studies in obese persons generally focus on surrogate end points of CVD. Many nutrition intervention trials have been performed in patients selected for high coronary risk, or with a need for secondary prevention of myocardial infarction rather than elevated BMI. One interesting trial randomized Indian patients after acute myocardial infarction to either a "usual care" group or one that received frequent weight loss advice and a diet low in saturated fat and rich in fruits, vegetables, nuts, and grains. Over one year, the diet group lost more weight, and had a larger reduction in cardiac events and lower mortality than controls (104). In France, randomization to a Mediterranean diet (replacing animal fat with polyunsaturated vegetable oil rich in $\omega$-3 fats, and increasing intake of legumes, fruits, vegetables, and bread) reduced all-cause mortality, coronary death, and recurrent myocardial infarction in survivors of a first heart attack (105). In a Norwegian trial, where patients at high risk for CHD were advised to change their diet by increasing polyunsaturated fat at the expense of saturated fat, and to stop smoking, incidence of myocardial infarction and cardiac death was also reduced (106). Such outcomes indicate that implementation of these dietary strategies might be particularly beneficial in obese patients at increased coronary risk, even if they fail to lose weight (107).

Many studies have focused on the effects of weight loss through dietary restriction (with or without exercise) as a means to control obesity-related comorbidities. The vast majority of these have shown that weight loss in obese persons results in improvements in blood pressure, dyslipidemia, and diabetes. Almost all of these diet studies are short term, however, with high rates of recidivism. Although most dieters regain lost weight over time, those who exercise concurrently appear better able to achieve sustained success.

Many obese people have had recurrent cycles of weight loss followed by regain (weight cycling). Although some studies suggest that a history of weight cycling in itself may be a risk factor for cardiac events, this premise is still controversial (108,109). In a prospective cohort study of over 33,000 women in Iowa, increasing CVD and cardiovascular death were seen across the quartiles of increasing weight cycling (110). Although this finding was confounded to some extent by unhealthy behaviors in frequent weight cyclers, statistical significance remained when these behaviors were factored out. Evidence shows that methods of weight control, which prolong successful weight loss, such as bariatric surgery, are immensely valuable for permanent reduction of coronary risk factors in the obese population.

## Methods of Weight Loss

The three major components of weight loss therapy are diet, physical activity, and behavior modification. The lifestyle changes should be attempted for at least six months before considering weight loss medications. Pharmacotherapy should be considered as an adjunct to lifestyle changes for patients with a BMI $\geq 27$ with obesity-related comorbidities or BMI $\geq 30$ without comorbidities. Patients with morbid obesity may be candidates for bariatric surgery (Table 3).

### Behavior Modification

Hypocaloric dieting invariably produces weight loss and a decrease in abdominal adiposity, at least over the short term. Most people, however, regain the lost weight after a certain period of time. Surveys of dieters suggest that maintenance of 10% weight loss is possible for five years or more in many Americans (111). Both low-calorie diets (LCDs: 800–1500 kcal/day) and the very low calorie diet (VLCD: 250–800 kcal/day) produce similar amount of weight loss over a year (112). An exercise program without a hypocaloric diet has produced weight loss in some trials. The combination of low-calorie diet and aerobic exercise has been shown to produce better long-term weight loss maintenance than either strategy alone. One study showed that diet combined with various types of exercise (or no exercise) produced weight losses ranging from 13.5 to 17.4 kg over 48 weeks, but participants regained 35% to 55% of their weight in the year after treatment. Those who reported regular exercise in the four months preceding the follow-up assessment regained significantly less weight than the nonexercisers (113). Similarly, a meta-analysis of studies published in the past 25 years showed

**Table 3** A Guide to Selecting Treatment

| | BMI category | | | | | |
|---|---|---|---|---|---|---|
| Treatment | <.24.9 | 25–26.9 | 27 29.9 | 30–35 | 35–39.9 | >40 |
| Diet, exercise, and behavior therapy | | With comor-bidity | With comor-bidity | + | + | + |
| Pharmaco-therapy | | | With comor-bidity | + | + | + |
| Surgery | | | | | With comor-bidity | + |

Prevention of weight gain with lifestyle therapy is indicated in any patients with a BMI $\geq 25\,kg/m^2$, even without comorbidities, while weight loss is not necessarily recommended for those with a BMI of 25–29.9 kg/m² or a high waist circumference, unless they have two or more comorbidities.
Combined therapy with an LCD, increased physical activity, and behavior therapy provides the most successful intervention for weight loss and weight maintenance.
Consider pharmacotherapy only if a patient has not lost 1 lb/week after six months of combined lifestyle therapy.
*Abbreviations*: LCD, low-calorie diet; BMI, body mass index.
*Source*: Adapted from Ref. 13.

that 15-week diet or diet-plus-exercise programs produced weight loss of about 11 kg. After one year, those in the diet-only group maintained about a 6.6 kg of their weight loss compared with 8.6 kg in the diet-plus-exercise group (114).

### Pharmacotherapy

Medications to reduce appetite may be effective in the short term, but lost weight is usually regained when they are discontinued, implying a need for long-term use. Possible association of fenfluramine/phentermine with pulmonary hypertension and valvular heart disease has led to caution in the medical treatment of obesity (115,116).

Sibutramine, a serotonin and norepinephrine reuptake blocker, has been approved by the Food and Drug Administration (FDA) for weight control in those with marked adult weight gain or a BMI $\geq 27$ mg/k². A dose-related effect on weight loss has been found, but not all studies have shown efficacy (117–119). Sibutramine increases satiety and thermogenesis of brown adipose tissue in animal models. Although it may cause an increase in mean blood pressure, data indicate no compromise of blood pressure in obese patients with well-controlled hypertension (119–121). Nevertheless, the medication is not recommended for use in patients with a history of coronary artery disease (CAD), congestive heart failure, cardiac arrhythmia, or stroke.

Orlistat, an FDA-approved inhibitor of intestinal and pancreatic lipases, works by inhibiting fat absorption from the gastrointestinal tract. Several trials, of one to two years duration, demonstrate efficacy at a dose of 120 mg three times daily, and favorable effects on cardiovascular risk factors (compared with placebo) when combined with a reduced calorie diet (122–132). Avoiding a high-fat diet can minimize side effects.

Bariatric Surgery

Bariatric surgery is the only treatment that offers successful long-term weight loss; often, over 50% of excess weight can be lost in the first two years (133). There are two types of major procedures—intestinal malabsorption and gastric restriction (134). A National Institutes of Health consensus conference in 1991 recommended surgery as the treatment of choice for patients with a BMI $\geq 40\,kg/m^2$, or $\geq 35\,kg/m^2$ with obesity-related comorbidities (135).

Data from randomized trials show that gastroplasty results in more successful long-term weight maintenance than dieting (136,137). Surgical patients who reduced excess weight by 75% over a mean of 10 months saw dramatic changes in their metabolic profiles—a 24% increase in HDL, a 35% decrease in TG, and a 62% decrease in fasting insulin (138). Gastric restriction also improves hypertension and cardiomyopathy associated with obesity. One year after surgery, a group of 12 obese individuals with a mean weight loss of 55 kg had significant improvement in cardiac ventricular compliance and function (139). Similarly, a gastric stapling procedure produced improvements in cardiac chamber size and left ventricular function in a study of 34 patients (140). While there have been no long-term randomized trials of reduced morbidity and mortality with this approach, observational studies demonstrate that the incidence of diabetes, hypertension, and dyslipidemia can be significantly reduced (141–148).

Gastric bypass is also an effective treatment for OSA in patients with clinically significant obesity. Weight loss from surgery results in clinical symptoms of daytime sleepiness, and respiratory disturbance as seen on overnight sleep study (149,150).

## Effect of Weight Loss on Obesity-Related Cardiovascular Risk Factors

Effect of Weight Loss on Blood Pressure

Lifestyle modification—which includes diet intervention, physical activity, behavior therapy, or combination therapy—can significantly reduce blood pressure in hypertensive and nonhypertensive people with obesity. At six months, the Trial of Antihypertensive Interventions and Management (TAIM) (151,152) reported a 12 mmHg decrease in diastolic blood pressure in patients who lost 4.5 kg or more compared with 7 mmHg in those who lost less than 2.5 kg. The effect was comparable to that produced by

25 mg of chlorthalidone or 50 mg of atenolol. Moreover, weight loss potentiated the effect of antihypertensive drugs.

In Phase II of the TAIM, 587 patients with mild hypertension were followed for a mean of 4.5 years. Of those receiving placebo, low-dose diuretic, or beta-blockers, a 2 to 3 kg weight loss reduced the need for additional antihypertensive medications by 23% (153). A meta-analysis by MacMahon et al. (154), which included five randomized controlled trials, indicated that weight loss of 10 kg in hypertensive patients resulted in a reduction of 6.8 mmHg in systolic, and 3.4 mmHg in diastolic blood pressure. In the Dietary Intervention Study in Hypertension (155) and the Hypertension Control Program (156), overweight patients with uncomplicated, well-controlled hypertension were withdrawn from drug treatment. Subsequent modest weight loss from diet therapy resulted in a significant reduction in the redevelopment of hypertension over one to four years.

Weight loss is also effective in preventing hypertension in nonhypertensive, overweight individuals. Cutler reviewed four randomized controlled trials in which 872 nonhypertensive adults and adolescents engaged in weight loss programs using dietary intervention and/or exercise (157). Weight loss of 1 kg in adults reduced both systolic and diastolic blood pressure by approximately 0.45 mmHg; weight loss of 1 kg in adolescents resulted in a 5 mmHg reduction in blood pressure. Modest weight reduction (a mean of 2.7 kg), in conjunction with low salt and alcohol intake and increased physical activity, reduced the five-year incidence of hypertension by 52% (158). Data from the Trial of Hypertension Prevention Phase I (TOHP I) and Phase II (TOHP II), two large randomized controlled trials, produced similar results. Modest weight loss by behavioral means in subjects with borderline hypertension (systolic blood pressure < 140 mmHg and diastolic 83–89 mmHg) reduced the incidence of hypertension by 20% to 50% at 18 months, and by 19% at three years (159,160).

Improvement in blood pressure after bariatric surgery has been consistently reported. Foley et al. reported preoperative hypertension resolved in 66% of 67 patients at the time of their last follow-up (145). In another study, 45 morbidly obese patients with diastolic hypertension underwent gastric surgery; 12 months later, hypertension had resolved in 22 of them (54%), and had improved in six patients (15%) (144). The resolution of hypertension depended on the severity of preoperative hypertension and the amount of postoperative weight loss. Patients who required no antihypertensive medications preoperatively, and those who lost more weight, tended to do better regardless of preoperative weight.

### Effects of Weight Loss on Type 2 Diabetes Mellitus

Weight loss produced by diet and/or exercise improves insulin sensitivity and reduces blood glucose levels in both obese diabetic and nondiabetic individuals. Initiation of a hypocaloric diet frequently improves hyperglycemia, an outcome that suggests a beneficial effect from restricted caloric intake independent of weight loss. In a study of a VLCD in obese patients with type 2 diabetes, 87% of the reduction in plasma glucose levels was observed within the first 10 days of caloric restriction, while 60% of weight loss occurred between days 10 and 40 (161).

In another study, 93 obese type 2 diabetic patients were assigned to either 400 or 1000 kcal (162). At a comparable degree of weight loss (11%), subjects on lower calorie diets had lower fasting glucose levels and greater insulin sensitivity. When subjects switched from 400 to 1000 kcal, glycemic control and insulin sensitivity worsened despite continued weight loss. Subjects on 1000 kcal from the beginning of the study, however, showed further improvement in glycemic control and additional weight loss.

Moderate weight loss in obese patients with type 2 diabetes can significantly improve glycemic control, as shown by a reduction in $HbA_1C$ levels; some patients are able to discontinue insulin or oral therapy. Depending on the level of weight maintenance, such improvements can last many years. In one randomized, controlled study of diet and exercise in overweight African-Americans with type 2 diabetes, weight loss of 3% in the intervention group at six months was accompanied by a reduction of $HbA_1C$ by 2.4% (163). In another study of newly diagnosed diabetes, those who attended regular group education sessions run by nurse-specialists in diabetes and a dietitian lost 5 kg more weight at six months than did those who had no structured education. Their $HbA_1C$ was also 2% lower than that of subjects in the unstructured education group (164). Long-term study of weight loss in diabetes demonstrated long-lasting improvement of glycemic control in patients who maintained reduction of at least 5% of initial body weight at three years, whereas those who maintained less than 5% had worsening glycemia (165).

Although diet and exercise are mainstays of treatment for type 2 diabetes, there are wide variations in patient response. A 48-month retrospective study on 135 patients on diet therapy indicated that only 41% of those who lost at least 9 kg had plasma glucose concentration below 10 mmol/L (166). Some of these individuals, however, decreased their plasma glucose levels after losing only 2.3 kg. Improvements in glycemic control occurred early in the course of weight loss; patients who remained hyperglycemic after reductions of 2.3 to 9.1 kg were unlikely to improve with additional weight loss.

These results might be due to relatively higher insulin resistance in patients who responded to diet therapy, and severe insulin deficiency in patients who did not. Other studies have shown that initial fasting plasma glucose is a strong predictor of response to diet therapy. The U.K. Prospective Diabetic Study reported that patients with initial fasting blood glucose of 6 to 8 mmol/L (108–144 mg/dL) needed to lose 10 kg (16% of initial body weight) to achieve a normal fasting plasma glucose of less than 6 mmol/L, whereas 26 kg weight loss (41% of initial body weight) was required in those with initial blood glucose greater than 14 mmol/L (252 mg/dL) (167).

In addition to benefits of weight loss in diabetes treatment, recent studies have shown that modest weight reduction is effective in preventing type 2 diabetes. The Finnish Diabetes Prevention Study, a diet and exercise program, produced a 58% reduction in diabetes compared with control (168,169). The U.S. Diabetes Prevention Program, a randomized clinical trial of more than 3200 overweight subjects at high risk for diabetes, (i.e., with IGT) also showed a 58% reduction in diabetes from 11% per year in the control group to 4.8% per year in the lifestyle modification group, which lost 5% to 7% of initial body weight (170,171).

In a majority of patients, gastric bypass surgery can substantially control type 2 diabetes. In one large study, 608 morbidly obese patients underwent Roux-en-Y gastric bypass; prior to surgery, 165 patients had type 2 diabetes and 165 had IGT (147,148). Of those with diabetes, 121 of 146 patients (83%) maintained normal fasting blood glucose and HbA$_1$C levels at the end of follow-up (up to 14 years), while 25 remained diabetic. Among patients with IGT, only two progressed to overt disease. Postoperative normalization of blood glucose was observed within a few days, before the occurrence of weight loss. By the end of the first week, the majority of the patients were able to stop insulin or oral hypoglycemic drugs.

### Effect of Weight Loss on Plasma Lipids

Modest weight loss, induced by either diet or exercise, is associated with increases in HDL-C, and decreases in serum TG, serum total cholesterol, and LDL-cholesterol (172). A meta-analysis by Dattilo and Kris-Etherton associated weight reduction with significant decreases in total cholesterol, LDL-cholesterol, VLDL, and TG; during active weight loss, HDL increased by 0.007 mmol/L for every kilogram weight lost (173). The NHLBI reviewed 14 randomized controlled trials on the effect of weight loss induced by diet and/or physical activity on plasma lipid levels (13). A 5% to 13% weight loss in the intervention group was accompanied by changes of 0% to 18% in total cholesterol; –2% to –44% in TG; –3% to –22% in LDL; and –7% to +27% in HDL.

Most of these trials lasted about 4 to 12 months, excluding the period of acute caloric deprivation. Waki et al. (174) reported that the beneficial effects of weight loss continued for longer duration; healthy obese women who lost a mean 16.7 kg had decreased serum total cholesterol, LDL-C, and TG, and increased HDL-C to total cholesterol ratio after 17 months of follow-up.

Bariatric surgery normalized plasma TG, increased plasma HDL-C levels, and reduced total cholesterol to HDL-C ratio in morbidly obese patients within six months of Roux-en-Y gastric bypass (146,175). Despite some weight regain, the improved lipid profiles were sustained for five to seven years. Brolin et al. (141,142), Wolf (138,146,175), and Cowan and Buffington (143) reported significant reduction in total TG and total cholesterol, and increase in HDL-C levels within 6 to 12 months of gastric surgery, with improvements sustained through five years.

Effect of Weight Loss on CVD

The beneficial effects of weight loss on cardiovascular risk factors are well established, but the effects of weight loss on the progression of CAD have not been widely studied. Available data indicate that weight loss can help reduce cardiovascular events and cardiovascular mortality (176). In the Lifestyle Heart Trial, patients with CAD were prescribed a lifestyle program that included a low-fat vegetarian diet, exercise, stress management training, smoking cessation, and group support (177,178). The treatment group lost more weight and had a significant reduction in total cholesterol and LDL-C. Its members also showed significant regression in coronary lesions assessed by CT and quantitative angiography at one and five years. In contrast, the control group showed no change in weight or lipid profiles and had progression of stenotic lesions. At five years, the control group had suffered more than twice the number of cardiac events. Although one cannot conclude that weight loss per se causes regression in coronary artery lesions, the study proves that lifestyle modifications can have an impact on CHD.

## CONCLUSION

Obesity is a widespread problem with serious health consequences. It is linked to chronic diseases that include CVD, hypertension, diabetes, and dyslipidemia. Central fat distribution, in particular, is an important independent predictor of cardiovascular morbidity and mortality. Weight loss, by whatever means, is clearly associated with improvements in obesity-related comorbidity.

The challenge remains of how to reduce the increasing prevalence of obesity and its sequelae in both children and adults. Unfortunately, rates of relapse are high after initial periods of success, particularly if initial weight loss occurs rapidly. If there is to be any chance of permanency, emphasis must be placed on lifestyle alterations that are personally and culturally acceptable. Perhaps the greatest challenge for weight loss practitioners is to target obese children and adolescents. They will grow up to become the obese hypertensive, diabetic, hypercholesterolemic patients in the offices of tomorrow's physicians. Finally, both a population approach and an individual approach are needed. The population-based effort should focus on the community including schools and the media, while the individual strategy should focus on a multidisciplinary approach consisting of physicians, exercise specialists, dietitians, nurses, and other health care personnel.

## REFERENCES

1. Krauss RM, Winston M, Fletcher BJ, Grundy SM. Obesity: impact on cardiovascular disease. Circulation 1998; 98:1472–1476.
2. Das UN. Is obesity an inflammatory condition? Nutrition 2001; 17:953–966.
3. Ziccardi P, Nappo F, Giugliano G, et al. Reduction of inflammatory cytokine concentrations and improvement of endothelial functions in obese women after weight loss over one year. Circulation 2002; 105:804–809.
4. Folsom AR, Aleksic N, Catellier D, Juneja HS, Wu KK. C-reactive protein and incident coronary heart disease in the Atherosclerosis Risk In Communities (ARIC) study. Am Heart J 2002; 144:233–238.
5. Juhan-Vague I, Alessi MC. PAI-1, obesity, insulin resistance and risk of cardiovascular events. Thromb Haemost 1997; 78:656–660.
6. De Pergola G, Pannacciulli N. Coagulation and fibrinolysis abnormalities in obesity. J Endocrinol Invest 2002; 25:899–904.
7. Hall JE, Crook ED, Jones DW, Wofford MR, Dubbert PM. Mechanisms of obesity-associated cardiovascular and renal disease. Am J Med Sci 2002; 324: 127–137.
8. Linton MF, Fazio S. A practical approach to risk assessment to prevent coronary artery disease and its complications. Am J Cardiol 2003; 92:19i–26i.
9. Fontaine KR, Redden DT, Wang C, Westfall AO, Allison DB. Years of life lost due to obesity. JAMA 2003; 289:187–193.
10. Peeters A, Bonneux L, Barendregt J, Nusselder W. Methods of estimating years of life lost due to obesity. JAMA 2003; 289:2941; author reply 2941–2942.
11. Bray GA, Ryan DH. Clinical evaluation of the overweight patient. Endocrine 2000; 13:167–186.
12. Willett WC, Dietz WH, Colditz GA. Guidelines for healthy weight. N Engl J Med 1999; 341:427–434.
13. Clinical guidelines on the identification, evaluation, and treatment of overweight and obesity in adults: executive summary. Expert Panel on the Identification, Evaluation, and Treatment of Overweight in Adults. Am J Clin Nutr 1998; 68:899–917.
14. Flegal KM, Graubard BI, Williamson DF, Gail MH. Excess deaths associated with underweight, overweight, and obesity. JAMA 2005; 293:1861–1867.
15. Lew EA. Mortality and weight: insured lives and the American Cancer Society studies. Ann Intern Med 1985; 103:1024–1029.
16. World Health Organization. Obesity: Preventing and managing the global epidemic, Report of WHO Consultation on Obesity. Geneva, 1998.
17. National Center for Health Statistics. Prevalence of overweight and obesity among adults, 1999, 2000.
18. Hedley AA, Ogden CL, Johnson CL, Carroll MD, Curtin LR, Flegal KM. Prevalence of overweight and obesity among US children, adolescents, and adults, 1999–2002. JAMA 2004; 291:2847–2850.
19. Bray GA. Clinical evaluation of the obese patient. Baillieres Best Pract Res Clin Endocrinol Metab 1999; 13:71–92.
20. Pi-Sunyer FX. Weight loss and mortality in type 2 diabetes. Diabetes Care 2000; 23:1451–1452.

21. Yanovski SZ. A practical approach to treatment of the obese patient. Arch Fam Med 1993; 2:309–316.
22. Baumgartner RN, Ross R, Heymsfield SB. Does adipose tissue influence bioelectric impedance in obese men and women? J Appl Physiol 1998; 84: 257–262.
23. Janssen I, Katzmarzyk PT, Ross R. Body mass index, waist circumference, and health risk: evidence in support of current National Institutes of Health guidelines. Arch Intern Med 2002; 162:2074–2079.
24. Bender R, Trautner C, Spraul M, Berger M. Assessment of excess mortality in obesity. Am J Epidemiol 1998; 147:42–48.
25. Allison DB, Fontaine KR, Manson JE, Stevens J, VanItallie TB. Annual deaths attributable to obesity in the United States. JAMA 1999; 282: 1530–1538.
26. Manson JE, Willett WC, Stampfer MJ, et al. Body weight and mortality among women. N Engl J Med 1995; 333:677–685.
27. Lee IM, Manson JE, Hennekens CH, Paffenbarger Jr RS. Body weight and mortality. A 27-year follow-up of middle-aged men. JAMA 1993; 270:2823–2828.
28. Seidell JC, Visscher TL, Hoogeveen RT. Overweight and obesity in the mortality rate data: current evidence and research issues. Med Sci Sports Exerc 1999; 31:S597–S601.
29. Eckel RH, Krauss RM. American Heart Association call to action: obesity as a major risk factor for coronary heart disease. AHA Nutrition Committee. Circulation 1998; 97:2099–2100.
30. Manson JE, Colditz GA, Stampfer MJ, et al. A prospective study of obesity and risk of coronary heart disease in women. N Engl J Med 1990; 322: 882–889.
31. Willett WC, Manson JE, Stampfer MJ, et al. Weight, weight change, and coronary heart disease in women. Risk within the 'normal' weight range. JAMA 1995; 273:461–465.
32. Rexrode KM, Carey VJ, Hennekens CH, et al. Abdominal adiposity and coronary heart disease in women. JAMA 1998; 280:1843–1848.
33. Field AE, Coakley EH, Must A, et al. Impact of overweight on the risk of developing common chronic diseases during a 10-year period. Arch Intern Med 2001; 161:1581–1586.
34. Folsom AR, Prineas RJ, Kaye SA, Munger RG. Incidence of hypertension and stroke in relation to body fat distribution and other risk factors in older women. Stroke 1990; 21:701–706.
35. Wilson PW, D'Agostino RB, Sullivan L, Parise H, Kannel WB. Overweight and obesity as determinants of cardiovascular risk: the Framingham experience. Arch Intern Med 2002; 162:1867–1872.
36. Rexrode KM, Hennekens CH, Willett WC, et al. A prospective study of body mass index, weight change, and risk of stroke in women. JAMA 1997; 277:1539–1545.
37. Harris TB, Ballard-Barbasch R, Madans J, Makuc DM, Feldman JJ. Overweight, weight loss, and risk of coronary heart disease in older women. The NHANES I Epidemiologic Follow-up Study. Am J Epidemiol 1993; 137: 1318–1327.

38. Harris TB, Launer LJ, Madans J, Feldman JJ. Cohort study of effect of being overweight and change in weight on risk of coronary heart disease in old age. BMJ 1997; 314:1791–1794.

39. Nelson RG, Sievers ML, Knowler WC, et al. Low incidence of fatal coronary heart disease in Pima Indians despite high prevalence of non-insulin-dependent diabetes Circulation 1990; 81:987–995.

40. Hubert HB, Feinleib M, McNamara PM, Castelli WP. Obesity as an independent risk factor for cardiovascular disease: a 26-year follow-up of participants in the Framingham Heart Study. Circulation 1983; 67:968–977.

41. Zarich SW, Kowalchuk GJ, McGuire MP, Benotti PN, Mascioli EA, Nesto RW. Left ventricular filling abnormalities in asymptomatic morbid obesity. Am J Cardiol 1991; 68:377–381.

42. Alpert MA. Obesity cardiomyopathy: pathophysiology and evolution of the clinical syndrome. Am J Med Sci 2001; 321:225–236.

43. Alpert MA. Management of obesity cardiomyopathy. Am J Med Sci 2001; 321:237–241.

44. Ravelli AC, van der Meulen JH, Michels RP, et al. Glucose tolerance in adults after prenatal exposure to famine. Lancet 1998; 351:173–177.

45. Roseboom TJ, van der Meulen JH, Osmond C, Barker DJ, Ravelli AC, Bleker OP. Plasma lipid profiles in adults after prenatal exposure to the Dutch famine. Am J Clin Nutr 2000; 72:1101–1106.

46. Roseboom TJ, van der Meulen JH, Ravelli AC, et al. Blood pressure in adults after prenatal exposure to famine. J Hypertens 1999; 17:325–330.

47. Roseboom TJ, van der Meulen JH, Osmond C, et al. Coronary heart disease after prenatal exposure to the Dutch famine, 1944–45. Heart 2000; 84: 595–598.

48. Yajnik C. Interactions of perturbations in intrauterine growth and growth during childhood on the risk of adult-onset disease. Proc Nutr Soc 2000; 59:257–265.

49. Fall CH, Osmond C, Barker DJ, et al. Fetal and infant growth and cardiovascular risk factors in women. BMJ 1995; 310:428–432.

50. Barker M, Robinson S, Osmond C, Barker DJ. Birth weight and body fat distribution in adolescent girls. Arch Dis Child 1997; 77.381–383.

51. Forsen T, Eriksson JG, Tuomilehto J, Osmond C, Barker DJ. Growth in utero and during childhood among women who develop coronary heart disease: longitudinal study. BMJ 1999; 319:1403–1407.

52. Osmond C, Barker DJ. Fetal, infant, and childhood growth are predictors of coronary heart disease, diabetes, and hypertension in adult men and women. Environ Health Perspect 2000; 108(suppl 3):545–553.

53. Field AE, Byers T, Hunter DJ, et al. Weight cycling, weight gain, and risk of hypertension in women. Am J Epidemiol 1999; 150:573–579.

54. Huang Z, Willett WC, Manson JE, et al. Body weight, weight change, and risk for hypertension in women. Ann Intern Med 1998; 128:81–88.

55. Dyer AR, Elliott P. The INTERSALT study: relations of body mass index to blood pressure. INTERSALT Co-operative Research Group. J Hum Hypertens 1989; 3:299–308.

56. Garrison RJ, Kannel WB, Stokes J 3rd, Castelli WP. Incidence and precursors of hypertension in young adults: the Framingham Offspring Study. Prev Med 1987; 16:235–251.

57. Hall JE, Kuo JJ, Da Silva AA, De Paula RB, Liu J, Tallam L. Obesity-associated hypertension and kidney disease. Curr Opin Nephrol Hypertens 2003; 12: 195–200.

58. Hall JE. The kidney, hypertension, and obesity. Hypertension 2003; 41: 625–633.

59. Hall JE. Mechanisms of abnormal renal sodium handling in obesity hypertension. Am J Hypertens 1997; 10:49S–55S.

60. Reisin E. Sodium and obesity in the pathogenesis of hypertension. Am J Hypertens 1990; 3:164–167.

61. Hall JE, Hildebrandt DA, Kuo J. Obesity hypertension: role of leptin and sympathetic nervous system. Am J Hypertens 2001; 14:103S–115S.

62. Skott P, Hother-Nielsen O, Bruun NE, et al. Effects of insulin on kidney function and sodium excretion in healthy subjects. Diabetologia 1989; 32:694–699.

63. DeFronzo RA, Cooke CR, Andres R, Faloona GR, Davis PJ. The effect of insulin on renal handling of sodium, potassium, calcium, and phosphate in man. J Clin Invest 1975; 55:845–855.

64. Andersen UB, Skott P, Bruun NE, Dige-Petersen H, Ibsen H. Renal effects of hyperinsulinaemia in subjects with two hypertensive parents. Clin Sci (Lond) 1999; 97:681–687.

65. Colditz GA, Willett WC, Rotnitzky A, Manson JE. Weight gain as a risk factor for clinical diabetes mellitus in women. Ann Intern Med 1995; 122: 481–486.

66. Knowler WC, Pettitt DJ, Saad MF, et al. Obesity in the Pima Indians: its magnitude and relationship with diabetes. Am J Clin Nutr 1991; 53:1543S–1551S.

67. Knowler WC, Saad MF, Pettitt DJ, Nelson RG, Bennett PH. Determinants of diabetes mellitus in the Pima Indians. Diabetes Care 1993; 16:216–227.

68. Knowler WC, Pettitt DJ, Saad MF, Bennett PH. Diabetes mellitus in the Pima Indians: incidence, risk factors and pathogenesis. Diabetes Metab Rev 1990; 6:1–27.

69. Martyn CN, Hales CN, Barker DJ, Jespersen S. Fetal growth and hyperinsulinaemia in adult life. Diabet Med 1998; 15:688–694.

70. Hales CN, Barker DJ, Clark PM, et al. Fetal and infant growth and impaired glucose tolerance at age 64. BMJ 1991; 303:1019–1022.

71. Boden G, Shulman GI. Free fatty acids in obesity and type 2 diabetes: defining their role in the development of insulin resistance and beta-cell dysfunction. Eur J Clin Invest 2002; 32(suppl 3):14–23.

72. Yu C, Chen Y, Cline GW, et al. Mechanism by which fatty acids inhibit insulin activation of insulin receptor substrate-1 (IRS-1)-associated phosphatidylinositol 3-kinase activity in muscle. J Biol Chem 2002; 277:50230–50236.

73. Shulman GI. Cellular mechanisms of insulin resistance in humans. Am J Cardiol 1999; 84:3J–10J.

74. Forouhi NG, Jenkinson G, Thomas EL, et al. Relation of triglyceride stores in skeletal muscle cells to central obesity and insulin sensitivity in European and South Asian men. Diabetologia 1999; 42:932–935.

75. Perseghin G, Scifo P, De Cobelli, et al. Intramyocellular triglyceride content is a determinant of in vivo insulin resistance in humans: a 1H-13C nuclear magnetic resonance spectroscopy assessment in offspring of type 2 diabetic parents. Diabetes 1999; 48:1600–1606.

76. Ip MS, Lam B, Ng MM, Lam WK, Tsang KW, Lam KS. Obstructive sleep apnea is independently associated with insulin resistance. Am J Respir Crit Care Med 2002; 165:670–676.

77. Despres JP. Dyslipidaemia and obesity. Baillieres Clin Endocrinol Metab 1994; 8:629–660.

78. Ruotolo G, Howard BV. Dyslipidemia of the metabolic syndrome. Curr Cardiol Rep 2002; 4:494–500.

79. Ravussin E, Klimes I, Sebokova E, Howard BV. Lipids and insulin resistance: what we've learned at the Fourth International Smolenice Symposium. Ann N Y Acad Sci 2002; 967:576–580.

80. Nestel PJ, Whyte HM, Goodman DS. Distribution and turnover of cholesterol in humans. J Clin Invest 1969; 48:982–991.

81. Schreibman PH, Dell RB. Human adipocyte cholesterol. Concentration, localization, synthesis, and turnover. J Clin Invest 1975; 55:986–993.

82. Anderson KM, Wilson PW, Garrison RJ, Castelli WP. Longitudinal and - secular trends in lipoprotein cholesterol measurements in a general population sample. The Framingham Offspring Study. Atherosclerosis 1987; 68:59–66.

83. Reaven GM, Chen YD, Jeppesen J, Maheux P, Krauss RM. Insulin resistance and hyperinsulinemia in individuals with small, dense low density lipoprotein particles. J Clin Invest 1993; 92:141–146.

84. Despres JP, Nadeau A, Tremblay A, et al. Role of deep abdominal fat in the association between regional adipose tissue distribution and glucose tolerance in obese women. Diabetes 1989; 38:304–309.

85. Frayn KN. Visceral fat and insulin resistance—causative or correlative? Br J Nutr 2000; 83(suppl 1):S71–S77.

86. Coppack SW, Evans RD, Fisher RM, et al. Adipose tissue metabolism in obesity: lipase action in vivo before and after a mixed meal. Metabolism 1992; 41:264–272.

87. Howard BV. Insulin resistance and lipid metabolism. Am J Cardiol 1999; 84:28J–32J.

88. Garg A. Insulin resistance in the pathogenesis of dyslipidemia. Diabetes Care 1996; 19:387–389.

89. Young T, Palta M, Dempsey J, Skatrud J, Weber S, Badr S. The occurrence of sleep-disordered breathing among middle-aged adults. N Engl J Med 1993; 328:1230–1235.

90. Sugerman HJ, Fairman RP, Baron PL, Kwentus JA. Gastric surgery for respiratory insufficiency of obesity. Chest 1986; 90:81–86.

91. Vgontzas AN, Papanicolaou DA, Bixler EO, et al. Sleep apnea and daytime sleepiness and fatigue: relation to visceral obesity, insulin resistance, and hypercytokinemia. J Clin Endocrinol Metab 2000; 85:1151–1158.

92. Peker Y, Hedner J, Norum J, Kraiczi H, Carlson J. Increased incidence of cardiovascular disease in middle-aged men with obstructive sleep apnea: a 7-year follow-up. Am J Respir Crit Care Med 2002; 166:159–165.

93.  Pankow W, Lies A, Lohmann FW. Sleep-disordered breathing and hypertension. N Engl J Med 2000; 343:966; author reply 967.
94.  Punjabi NM, Sorkin JD, Katzel LI, Goldberg AP, Schwartz AR, Smith PL. Sleep-disordered breathing and insulin resistance in middle-aged and overweight men. Am J Respir Crit Care Med 2002; 165:677–682.
95.  Narkiewicz K, Pesek CA, Kato M, Phillips BG, Davison DE, Somers VK. Baroreflex control of sympathetic nerve activity and heart rate in obstructive sleep apnea. Hypertension 1998; 32:1039–1043.
96.  Narkiewicz K, Montano N, Cogliati C, van de Borne PJ, Dyken ME, Somers VK. Altered cardiovascular variability in obstructive sleep apnea. Circulation 1998; 98:1071–1077.
97.  Narkiewicz K, van de Borne PJ, Pesek CA, Dyken ME, Montano N, Somers VK. Selective potentiation of peripheral chemoreflex sensitivity in obstructive sleep apnea. Circulation 1999; 99:1183–1189.
98.  Narkiewicz K, Somers VK. Sympathetic nerve activity in obstructive sleep apnoea. Acta Physiol Scand 2003; 177:385–390.
99.  Kato M, Roberts-Thomson P, Phillips BG, et al. Impairment of endothelium-dependent vasodilation of resistance vessels in patients with obstructive sleep apnea. Circulation 2000; 102:2607–2610.
100.  Pankow W, Nabe B, Lies A, et al. Influence of sleep apnea on 24-hour blood pressure. Chest 1997; 112:1253–1258.
101.  Peppard PE, Young T, Palta M, Skatrud J. Prospective study of the association between sleep-disordered breathing and hypertension. N Engl J Med 2000; 342:1378 1384.
102.  Lavie P, Herer P, Hoffstein V. Obstructive sleep apnoea syndrome as a risk factor for hypertension: population study. BMJ 2000; 320:479–482.
103.  Brooks D, Horner RL, Kozar LF, Render-Teixeira CL, Phillipson EA. Obstructive sleep apnea as a cause of systemic hypertension. Evidence from a canine model. J Clin Invest 1997; 99:106–109.
104.  Singh RB, Rastogi SS, Verma R, et al. Randomised controlled trial of cardioprotective diet in patients with recent acute myocardial infarction: results of one year follow up. BMJ 1992; 304:1015–1019.
105.  de Lorgeril M, Salen P, Martin JL, Monjaud I, Delaye J, Mamelle N. Mediterranean diet, traditional risk factors, and the rate of cardiovascular complications after myocardial infarction: final report of the Lyon Diet Heart Study. Circulation 1999; 99:779–785.
106.  Hjermann I, Velve Byre K, Holme I, Leren P. Effect of diet and smoking intervention on the incidence of coronary heart disease. Report from the Oslo Study Group of a randomised trial in healthy men. Lancet 1981; 2:1303–1310.
107.  Blackburn GL. Making good decisions about diet: weight loss is not weight maintenance. Cleve Clin J Med 2002; 69:864–865, 869.
108.  Phinney SD. Weight cycling and cardiovascular risk in obese men and women. Am J Clin Nutr 1992; 56:781–782.
109.  Prentice AM, Jebb SA, Goldberg GR, et al. Effects of weight cycling on body composition. Am J Clin Nutr 1992; 56:209S–216S.

110. Folsom AR, French SA, Zheng W, Baxter JE, Jeffery RW. Weight variability and mortality: the Iowa Women's Health Study. Int J Obes Relat Metab Disord 1996; 20:704–709.

111. McGuire MT, Wing RR, Hill JO. The prevalence of weight loss mainte nance among American adults. Int J Obes Relat Metab Disord 1999; 23: 1314–1319.

112. Wadden TA, Foster GD, Letizia KA. One-year behavioral treatment of obesity: comparison of moderate and severe caloric restriction and the effects of weight maintenance therapy. J Consult Clin Psychol 1994; 62:165–171.

113. Wadden TA, Vogt RA, Foster GD, Anderson DA. Exercise and the maintenance of weight loss: 1-year follow-up of a controlled clinical trial. J Consult Clin Psychol 1998; 66:429–433.

114. Miller WC, Koceja DM, Hamilton EJ. A meta-analysis of the past 25 years of weight loss research using diet, exercise or diet plus exercise intervention. Int J Obes Relat Metab Disord 1997; 21:941–947.

115. Connolly HM, Crary JL, McGoon MD, et al. Valvular heart disease associated with fenfluramine-phentermine. N Engl J Med 1997; 337:581–588.

116. Connolly HM, McGoon MD. Obesity drugs and the heart. Curr Probl Cardiol 1999; 24:745–792.

117. Bray GA, Ryan DH, Gordon D, Heidingsfelder S, Cerise F, Wilson K. A double-blind randomized placebo-controlled trial of sibutramine. Obes Res 1996; 4:263–270.

118. Bray GA, Blackburn GL, Ferguson JM, et al. Sibutramine produces dose-related weight loss. Obes Res 1999; 7:189–198.

119. McNulty SJ, Ur E, Williams G. A randomized trial of sibutramine in the management of obese type 2 diabetic patients treated with metformin. Diabetes Care 2003; 26:125–131.

120. McMahon FG, Weinstein SP, Rowe E, Ernst KR, Johnson F, Fujioka K. Sibutramine is safe and effective for weight loss in obese patients whose hypertension is well controlled with angiotensin-converting enzyme inhibitors. J Hum Hypertens 2002; 16:5–11.

121. McMahon FG, Fujioka K, Singh BN, et al. Efficacy and safety of sibutramine in obese white and African American patients with hypertension: a 1-year, double-blind, placebo-controlled, multicenter trial. Arch Intern Med 2000; 160:2185–2191.

122. Harp JB. Orlistat for the long-term treatment of obesity. Drugs Today (Barc) 1999; 35:139–145.

123. Krempf M, Louvet JP, Allanic H, Miloradovich T, Joubert JM, Attali JR. Weight reduction and long-term maintenance after 18 months treatment with orlistat for obesity. Int J Obes Relat Metab Disord 2003; 27:591–597.

124. Tong PC, Lee ZS, Sea MM, et al. The effect of orlistat-induced weight loss, without concomitant hypocaloric diet, on cardiovascular risk factors and insulin sensitivity in young obese Chinese subjects with or without type 2 diabetes. Arch Intern Med 2002; 162:2428–2435.

125. Hanefeld M, Sachse G. The effects of orlistat on body weight and glycaemic control in overweight patients with type 2 diabetes: a randomized, placebo-controlled trial. Diabetes Obes Metab 2002; 4:415–423.

126. Broom I, Wilding J, Stott P, Myers N. Randomised trial of the effect of orlistat on body weight and cardiovascular disease risk profile in obese patients: UK Multimorbidity Study. Int J Clin Pract 2002; 56:494–499.
127. Miles JM, Leiter L, Hollander P, et al. Effect of orlistat in overweight and obese patients with type 2 diabetes treated with metformin. Diabetes Care 2002; 25:1123–1128.
128. Kelley DE, Bray GA, Pi-Sunyer FX, et al. Clinical efficacy of orlistat therapy in overweight and obese patients with insulin-treated type 2 diabetes: a 1-year randomized controlled trial. Diabetes Care 2002; 25:1033–1041.
129. Reaven G, Segal K, Hauptman J, Boldrin M, Lucas C. Effect of orlistat-assisted weight loss in decreasing coronary heart disease risk in patients with syndrome X. Am J Cardiol 2001; 87:827–831.
130. Lindgarde F. The effect of orlistat on body weight and coronary heart disease risk profile in obese patients: the Swedish Multimorbidity Study. J Intern Med 2000; 248:245–254.
131. Heck AM, Yanovski JA, Calis KA. Orlistat, a new lipase inhibitor for the management of obesity. Pharmacotherapy 2000; 20:270–279.
132. Sjostrom L, Rissanen A, Andersen T, et al. Randomised placebo-controlled trial of orlistat for weight loss and prevention of weight regain in obese patients. European Multicentre Orlistat Study Group. Lancet 1998; 352: 167–172.
133. Macgregor AM, Rand CS. Gastric surgery in morbid obesity. Outcome in patients aged 55 years and older. Arch Surg 1993; 128:1153–1157.
134. Mun EC, Blackburn GL, Matthews JB. Current status of medical and surgical therapy for obesity. Gastroenterology 2001; 120:669–681.
135. NIH conference. Gastrointestinal surgery for severe obesity. Consensus Development Conference Panel. Ann Intern Med 1991; 115:956–961.
136. Andersen T, Backer OG, Stokholm KH, Quaade F. Randomized trial of diet and gastroplasty compared with diet alone in morbid obesity. N Engl J Med 1984; 310:352–356.
137. Andersen T, Stokholm KH, Backer OG, Quaade F. Long-term (5-year) results after either horizontal gastroplasty or very-low-calorie diet for morbid obesity. Int J Obes 1988; 12:277–284.
138. Wolf AM, Beisiegel U, Kortner B, Kuhlmann HW. Does gastric restriction surgery reduce the risks of metabolic diseases? Obes Surg 1998; 8:9–13.
139. Alaud-din A, Meterissian S, Lisbona R, MacLean LD, Forse RA. Assessment of cardiac function in patients who were morbidly obese. Surgery 1990; 108:809–818; discussion 818–820.
140. Alpert MA, Terry BE, Kelly DL. Effect of weight loss on cardiac chamber size, wall thickness and left ventricular function in morbid obesity. Am J Cardiol 1985; 55:783–786.
141. Brolin RE, Kenler HA, Wilson AC, Kuo PT, Cody RP. Serum lipids after gastric bypass surgery for morbid obesity. Int J Obes 1990; 14:939–950.
142. Brolin RE, Bradley LJ, Wilson AC, Cody RP. Lipid risk profile and weight stability after gastric restrictive operations for morbid obesity. J Gastrointest Surg 2000; 4:464–469.

143. Cowan GS Jr, Buffington CK. Significant changes in blood pressure, glucose, and lipids with gastric bypass surgery. World J Surg 1998; 22:987–992.

144. Carson JL, Ruddy ME, Duff AE, Holmes NJ, Cody RP, Brolin RE. The effect of gastric bypass surgery on hypertension in morbidly obese patients Arch Intern Med 1994; 154:193–200.

145. Foley EF, Benotti PN, Borlase BC, Hollingshead J, Blackburn GL. Impact of gastric restrictive surgery on hypertension in the morbidly obese. Am J Surg 1992; 163:294–297.

146. Gleysteen JJ. Results of surgery: long-term effects on hyperlipidemia. Am J Clin Nutr 1992; 55:591S–593S.

147. Pories WJ, MacDonald KG Jr, Morgan EJ, et al. Surgical treatment of obesity and its effect on diabetes: 10-y follow-up. Am J Clin Nutr 1992; 55:582S–585S.

148. Pories WJ, Swanson MS, MacDonald KG, et al. Who would have thought it? An operation proves to be the most effective therapy for adult-onset diabetes mellitus. Ann Surg 1995; 222:339–350; discussion 350–332.

149. Rasheid S, Banasiak M, Gallagher SF, et al. Gastric bypass is an effective treatment for obstructive sleep apnea in patients with clinically significant obesity. Obes Surg 2003; 13:58–61.

150. Dixon JB, Schachter LM, O'Brien PE. Sleep disturbance and obesity: changes following surgically induced weight loss. Arch Intern Med 2001; 161:102–106.

151. Wassertheil-Smoller S, Oberman A, Blaufox MD, Davis B, Langford H. The Trial of Antihypertensive Interventions and Management (TAIM) Study. Final results with regard to blood pressure, cardiovascular risk, and quality of life. Am J Hypertens 1992; 5:37–44.

152. Wassertheil-Smoller S, Blaufox MD, Oberman AS, Langford HG, Davis BR, Wylie-Rosett J. The Trial of Antihypertensive Interventions and Management (TAIM) study. Adequate weight loss, alone and combined with drug therapy in the treatment of mild hypertension. Arch Intern Med 1992; 152:131–136.

153. Davis BR, Blaufox MD, Oberman A, et al. Reduction in long-term antihypertensive medication requirements. Effects of weight reduction by dietary intervention in overweight persons with mild hypertension. Arch Intern Med 1993; 153:1773–1782.

154. MacMahon S, Cutler J, Brittain E, Higgins M. Obesity and hypertension: epidemiological and clinical issues. Eur Heart J 1987; 8(suppl B):57–70.

155. Langford HG, Blaufox MD, Oberman A, et al. Dietary therapy slows the return of hypertension after stopping prolonged medication. JAMA 1985; 253:657–664.

156. Stamler R, Stamler J, Grimm R, et al. Nutritional therapy for high blood pressure. Final report of a four-year randomized controlled trial—the Hypertension Control Program. JAMA 1987; 257:1484–1491.

157. Cutler JA. Randomized clinical trials of weight reduction in nonhypertensive persons. Ann Epidemiol 1991; 1:363–370.

158. Stamler R, Stamler J, Gosch FC, et al. Primary prevention of hypertension by nutritional-hygienic means. Final report of a randomized, controlled trial. JAMA 1989; 262:1801–1807.

159. Stevens VJ, Corrigan SA, Obarzanek E, et al. Weight loss intervention in phase 1 of the Trials of Hypertension Prevention. The TOHP Collaborative Research Group. Arch Intern Med 1993; 153:849–858.

160. Effects of weight loss and sodium reduction intervention on blood pressure and hypertension incidence in overweight people with high-normal blood pressure. The Trials of Hypertension Prevention, phase II. The Trials of Hypertension Prevention Collaborative Research Group. Arch Intern Med 1997; 157:657–667.

161. Henry RR, Wiest-Kent TA, Scheaffer L, Kolterman OG, Olefsky JM. Metabolic consequences of very-low-calorie diet therapy in obese non-insulin-dependent diabetic and nondiabetic subjects. Diabetes 1986; 35:155–164.

162. Wing RR, Blair EH, Bononi P, Marcus MD, Watanabe R, Bergman RN. Caloric restriction per se is a significant factor in improvements in glycemic control and insulin sensitivity during weight loss in obese NIDDM patients. Diabetes Care 1994; 17:30–36.

163. Agurs-Collins TD, Kumanyika SK, Ten Have TR, Adams-Campbell LL. A randomized controlled trial of weight reduction and exercise for diabetes management in older African-American subjects. Diabetes Care 1997; 20: 1503–1511.

164. Heller SR, Clarke P, Daly H, et al. Group education for obese patients with type 2 diabetes: greater success at less cost. Diabet Med 1988; 5:552–556.

165. Mancini M, Di Biase G, Contaldo F, Fischetti A, Grasso L, Mattioli PL. Medical complications of severe obesity: importance of treatment by very-low-calorie diets: intermediate and long-term effects. Int J Obes 1981; 5: 341–352.

166. Watts NB, Spanheimer RG, DiGirolamo M, et al. Prediction of glucose response to weight loss in patients with non-insulin-dependent diabetes mellitus. Arch Intern Med 1990; 150:803–806.

167. UK Prospective Diabetes Study 7: response of fasting plasma glucose to diet therapy in newly presenting type II diabetic patients, UKPDS Group. Metabolism 1990; 39:905–912.

168. Tuomilehto J, Lindstrom J, Eriksson JG, et al. Prevention of type 2 diabetes mellitus by changes in lifestyle among subjects with impaired glucose tolerance. N Engl J Med 2001; 344:1343–1350.

169. Uusitupa M, Louheranta A, Lindstrom J, et al. The Finnish Diabetes Prevention Study. Br J Nutr 2000; 83(suppl 1):S137–S142.

170. Molitch ME, Fujimoto W, Hamman RF, Knowler WC. The diabetes prevention program and its global implications. J Am Soc Nephrol 2003; 14:S103–S107.

171. Knowler WC, Barrett-Connor E, Fowler SE, et al. Reduction in the incidence of type 2 diabetes with lifestyle intervention or metformin. N Engl J Med 2002; 346:393–403.

172. Pi-Sunyer FX. Short-term medical benefits and adverse effects of weight loss. Ann Intern Med 1993; 119:722–726.

173. Dattilo AM, Kris-Etherton PM. Effects of weight reduction on blood lipids and lipoproteins: a meta-analysis. Am J Clin Nutr 1992; 56:320–328.

174. Waki M, Heshka S, Heymsfield SB. Long-term serum lipid lowering, behavior modification, and weight loss in obese women. Nutrition 1993; 9:23–28.

175. Gleysteen JJ, Barboriak JJ, Sasse EA. Sustained coronary-risk-factor reduction after gastric bypass for morbid obesity. Am J Clin Nutr 1990; 51:774–778.
176. Van Gaal LF, Wauters MA, De Leeuw IH. The beneficial effects of modest weight loss on cardiovascular risk factors. Int J Obes Relat Metab Disord 1997; 21(suppl 1):S5–S9.
177. Ornish D, Brown SE, Scherwitz LW, et al. Can lifestyle changes reverse coronary heart disease? The Lifestyle Heart Trial. Lancet 1990; 336:129–133.
178. Ornish D, Scherwitz LW, Billings JH, et al. Intensive lifestyle changes for reversal of coronary heart disease. JAMA 1998; 280:2001–2007.

# 10

# The Roles of Dietary Fats in Reducing Weight and Cardiovascular Risk Factors in Overweight and Obese Individuals

**Kathy McManus**

*Department of Nutrition, Brigham and Women's Hospital,
Boston, Massachusetts, U.S.A.*

**Kris M. Mogensen**

*Metabolic Support Service, Brigham and Women's Hospital,
Boston, Massachusetts, U.S.A.*

## INTRODUCTION

Dietary fat has been thought to be an important factor in weight loss and cardiovascular heart disease (CHD). The type of fat clearly has an effect on the risk of heart disease. The effects of the amount and type of fat on weight loss are less substantiated. This chapter will discuss quantity and quality of dietary fatty acids in the nutrition interventions for obese patients.

## TYPES OF DIETARY FATS

### Saturated Fats

Saturated fats include three major cholesterol-raising fatty acids that have carbon chain lengths of 12 (lauric acid), 14 (myristic acid), and 16 (palmitic acid). Animal fats provide about two-thirds of the saturated fat in the American diet (1). These fats include butterfat (contained in butter, whole

**Table 1** Food Sources of Dietary Fat

| Type of fat | Food sources |
| --- | --- |
| Saturated fat | Butterfat, butter, cream, whole milk, cheese, ice cream, beef, chicken, pork, lamb, palm kernel oil, palm oil, coconut oil |
| *trans* Fat | Stick margarine, vegetable shortening, foods containing "partially hydrogenated vegetable oil," deep fried foods, most commercial baked goods, many "fast" foods |
| Omega-6 polyunsaturated fat | Safflower oil, sunflower oil, corn oil, soybean oil |
| Omega-3 polyunsaturated fat | Fish oil, canola oil, flaxseeds and flaxseed oil, commercial supplements |
| Conjugated linoleic acid | Meats, dairy products, commercial supplements |
| Monounsaturated fat | Olive oil, canola oil, peanut oil, most nuts, peanut butter, avocado |

milk, cream, ice cream, and cheese) and the fat of beef, pork, lamb, and poultry (Table 1). The remaining saturated fat comes from various plant products. Three plant oils—palm oil, palm kernel oil, and coconut oil— are high in saturated fatty acids. One of the pioneering epidemiologic studies demonstrating a correlation between the intake of saturated fat as a percentage of calories and coronary death rates ($r = 0.84$) was published by Ancel Keys (2). In Keys' sample populations, many of the countries with lower saturated fat intakes (i.e., $\leq 8\%$ of total calories) were those around the Mediterranean Sea. In the same study, the percentage of energy from total fat had little relationship with cardiovascular mortality. Table 2 summarizes the physiologic effects of saturated fat.

**Table 2** Physiologic Effects of Dietary Fats

| Type of fat | Physiologic effects |
| --- | --- |
| Saturated fat | Raise TC and LDL-C |
| *trans* Fat | Raise TC and LDL-C, lowers HDL |
| Omega-6 polyunsaturated fatty acids | Lower TC, LDL-C, and HDL-C |
| Omega-3 polyunsaturated fatty acids | Lower TG; promote decreased platelet aggregation, decreased inflammatory response, decreased blood pressure |
| Monounsaturated fat | Lower LD-C; in Type 2 diabetes mellitus improved TG levels when substituted for carbohydrate |

*Abbreviations*: TC, total cholesterol; LDL-C, low-density lipoprotein cholesterol; HDL-C, high-density lipoprotein cholesterol; TG, triglyceride.

## *trans* Fats

Research indicates that *trans* fatty acids increase low-density lipoprotein cholesterol (LDL-C) levels as much as saturated fatty acids, and in some cases, substantially lower high-density lipoprotein cholesterol (HDL-C) (3–6). The Nurse's Health Study showed that women who ate 3% of daily calories as *trans* fat were 53% more likely to develop cardiovascular disease over a 14-year period than those who ate ≤1% of daily energy as *trans* fats (7). Table 2 summarizes the physiologic effects of *trans* fats.

    *trans* Fats are formed through the process of hydrogenation, the addition of hydrogen atoms, which converts a vegetable oil to a more solid fat. Hydrogenation converts some of the polyunsaturated fat to monounsaturated fat. The latter occurs in two forms—oleic acid (a *cis* fatty acid) and *trans* fatty acids, one of which is elaidic acid. Main sources of *trans* fats in the diet are listed in Table 1.

## Polyunsaturated Fats

Polyunsaturated fats are defined as fatty acids that have two or more double bonds between carbons. These fats are typically plant derived and are generally liquid at room temperature. There are two subclassifications of polyunsaturated fats, omega-6 and omega-3, which refer to the location of the first double bond from the methyl end of the fatty acid (8). Table 2 summarizes the physiologic effects of omega-6 and omega-3 polyunsaturated fats. Both types of polyunsaturated fats offer cardiovascular benefits.

    Linoleic acid is the main source of $n$-6 polyunsaturated fat in the diet. Omega-6 fatty acids decrease cholesterol levels through effects on both LDL-C and HDL-C (8,9). Studies have shown that replacing saturated fat and *trans* fat with polyunsaturated fats significantly decreases the risk of coronary heart disease (10). Sources of omega-6 polyunsaturated fats are listed in Table 1.

    Dietary omega-3 fatty acids are found in fish oils and certain plant oils such as canola oil and borage oil. Fish oils contain eicosapentaenoic acid (EPA) and docosahexaenoic acid (DHA) naturally; the omega-3 fatty acids derived from plant sources (primarily α-linolenic acid) are metabolized to form EPA and DHA. Fish oil in particular has been found to be effective at reducing triglyceride (TG) levels. EPA and DHA offer other cardioprotective effects such as decreased platelet aggregation, inflammatory responses, and blood pressure (8–10). For reduction of cardiac and all-cause mortality, optimum intake of EPA and DHA combined is between 0.5 and 1.8 g/day (either from fatty fish or commercial supplements) and for α-linolenic acid, 1.5 and 3 g/day (11).

    There has been increasing interest in dietary conjugated linoleic acid (CLA), another polyunsaturated fatty acid. This fatty acid is discussed in detail at the end of this chapter.

## Monounsaturated Fats

Monounsaturated fats are plant-derived fats that contain only one double bond. These fats have been shown to reduce LDL-C while having no effect on HDL-C, although this effect is not as significant as with polyunsaturated fatty acids (8). In non–insulin dependent diabetic patients with hypertrigly-ceridemia, replacing carbohydrates (CHO) with monounsaturated fatty acids has been shown to improve TG levels (12). Food sources of monoun-saturated fats are listed in Tables 1 and 2 summarizes the physiologic effects of monounsaturated fats.

## LOW-FAT VS. MODERATE-FAT DIETS AND WEIGHT LOSS

Obesity is a multifactorial, complex metabolic disorder. It is apparent that the major cause is an overconsumption of energy and/or deficit of energy expenditure.

In general, the scientific community had favored the belief that fat in the American diet was the major cause/reason for overconsumption of calories.

During the 1980s and 1990s, dietary guidelines recommended that no more than 30% of energy intake come from fat (13,14). However, there are limited data from controlled studies on the appropriate amount of fat in the diet to promote long-term weight reduction and their effects on cardiovas-cular risk. Despite numerous weight loss programs and guides, and the pro-liferation and successful marketing of low-fat prepared foods, the epidemic of obesity has increased.

The low-fat hypothesis is that by reducing fat, energy intake will decrease and subsequently weight loss will be achieved. An alternative theory is that by reducing intake of all macronutrients and leaving the proportions unchanged, weight loss will be more effective. In clinical studies with con-trolled diets, the nutrient composition did not affect weight loss (15–18). Over different time periods, altering the percentage of calories from the macronu-trients (fat, protein, and CHO) within a 1200 cal/day diet did not change the rate of weight loss. Thus, calories determine weight loss.

In one 12-week study of 35 obese women comparing the effect of vary-ing amounts of dietary fat (10%, 20%, 30%, and 40% of energy) on body weight, with calories for energy reduction constant (1200 cal/day), Powell et al. (19) showed that all four dietary interventions resulted in the loss of significant amounts of weight. There were no significant differences among any of the four dietary treatment groups in the amount or rate of weight loss.

A meta-analysis (20) of trials of low-fat diets, administered for a pri-mary reason other than weight loss, showed mean dietary fat reduction from 38% to 27%, and a mean 3.2 kg weight loss. These studies, mostly with short duration, support the long-standing hypothesis that low-fat diets reduce passive overconsumption of calories that could occur in higher fat diets

(21,22). However, this interpretation of results from low-fat studies has been challenged (23,24). Methodological concerns for certain studies used in the meta-analysis include the often greater intensity of the intervention in the low-fat compared to "no intervention" control groups, and lack of randomized control groups. Clinical studies of diets for weight loss show that weight loss is maximal at three to six months (25–27). After such relatively short treatment periods, several studies found that participants lost similar amounts of weight on a low-fat diet without instruction for energy reduction or an energy-reduced, higher-fat diet (19,25,28).

One long-term trial that did receive similar intensity of dietary education was published by Jeffrey et al. (25) This study randomized 75 obese women. The two dietary treatments included low-fat counseling, limiting fat to no more than 20 g/day with no restriction of energy versus traditional calorie-restriction counseling and limiting energy to no more than 1000 to 1200 cal/day, depending upon baseline weight. At the end of the study, participants in the fat-counseling group reported reducing their fat intake from 37% of energy to 23% at six months, with a moderate increase thereafter. Among the 74 women completing the study, mean weight losses of 4.6 kg for the low-fat group and 3.7 kg for the low-caloric group were observed between baseline and six months. After six months, however, both groups regained weight, and by 18 months the average weight for both groups was above baseline. There were no significant group differences in weight loss or regain.

In contrast, Toubro and Astrup (29) compared an ad libitum low-fat (20–25% energy) diet with a higher fat (unspecified fat content), energy-restricted diet to prevent regain of weight loss. Initial weight loss of 14 kg was induced over two to four months by high-protein intake with 60 mg ephedrine and 600 mg caffeine daily. After a one-year weight-maintenance program with one to three group-counseling sessions per month, the low-fat group regained 0.3 kg compared to 4.1 kg in the higher fat, energy-reduced group ($P = 0.08$). After an additional year of follow-up, which was unsupervised, overall weight regain was 5.4 kg and 11.4 kg in the low-fat and higher fat groups, respectively ($P = 0.03$). This study suggests that a low-fat diet can support long-term weight reduction better than the calorie-controlled diet.

In another study, in which both treatment groups received similar intensity of interventions, McManus et al. (30) randomized 101 overweight men and women to a diet with 35% of energy from fat (mostly unsaturated fat) or a diet with 20% of energy from fat. At the conclusion of the 18-month trial, 31 participants in the moderate-fat group and 30 in the low-fat group were available for measurements. Analysis showed that the weight loss was significantly greater in the moderate-fat group, with a loss of 4.1 kg versus a gain of 2.9 kg in the low-fat group. In addition, there was a significantly greater participation rate in the moderate-fat group (54%) versus the low-fat group (20%).

There have been a number of meta-analyses examining various trials on fat reduction diets. In 1998, Bray and Popkin (31) published data from 28 clinical trials including both normal-weight and overweight individuals with varying periods of duration. The study concluded that a 10% reduction in the proportion of energy from fat was associated with 16 g/day reduction in body weight. Over a period of one year, this would predict a weight loss of 6 kg if fat intake was reduced by 10% of energy. In a review that included an assessment of weight-loss trials that lasted more than one year, Willett and Leibel (24) reported that the weighted mean difference between low-fat and control groups for randomized trials is –0.25 kg. None of the reviewed studies that included fat reduction as the intervention for weight loss achieved clinically significant weight loss (approximately 5% of baseline weight).

A meta-analysis by Yu-Poth et al. (32) published in 1999 showed a correlation between a decrease in percent of energy from fat and decrease in body weight. This meta-analysis had similar limitations because, of the 37 selected studies, only four were of greater than one-year duration. In addition, many of the studies did not have comparable control interventions and some of the studies had multiple interventions.

In 2002, Pirozzo et al. (33) assessed the effects of advice on low-fat diets as a means of achieving sustained weight loss, using all available randomized clinical trials. This review focused primarily on participants who were overweight or clinically obese and were dieting for the purpose of weight reduction. Because the researchers were particularly interested in the ability of participants to sustain weight loss over a longer period of time, they focused on studies of free-living men and women who were given dietary advice rather than the provision of food or money to purchase food. Two researchers independently applied the inclusion criteria to the studies identified. Data were extracted by three independent reviewers and meta-analysis performed using a random-effects model. Weighted mean differences of weight loss were calculated for treatment and control groups at 6, 12, and 18 months. For studies of 18 months or more, the weighted mean difference was +3.7 kg (95% CI—1.8–9.2). The review suggests that low-fat diets are no better than low-calorie diets in achieving long-term weight loss in overweight or obese people.

## CARDIOVASCULAR EFFECTS OF LOW-FAT AND HIGHER-FAT DIETS

There have been a number of dietary interventions for cardiovascular disease focused on reducing total fat. The Medical Research Council study (34) involved 123 male post–myocardial infarct patients instructed to limit fat to 22% of energy. The Diet and Reinfarction Trial (35) devoted one arm of intervention to fat reduction. Post–myocardial infarct males ($n = 1015$) reduced fat to 32% of energy. After three and two years, respectively, the approach of total fat reduction did not find a significant reduction in serum cholesterol or CHD events in these trials.

Low-fat, high-CHO diets generate higher fasting TGs and lower serum cholesterol levels than high-fat diets (36). The decrease in total cholesterol (TC) is mostly due to a decrease in LDL-C, but part is due to a decrease in HDL-C. Mensink and Katan (36) reviewed 27 well-controlled trials involving 682 subjects and showed that HDL-C decreased by 0.012 mmol/L (0.5 mg/dL) for every 1% of energy from saturated fatty acids that was replaced by CHO. Other meta-analyses by Hegsted et al. (37) and Yu et al. (38) support this conclusion.

## LOW-CARBOHYDRATE, HIGH-FAT DIETS

Low-CHO, high-fat diets have been gaining in popularity. Many weight-loss books in the popular press, for example the Atkins diet (39), focus on this type of diet with claims of promoting changes in metabolism so that adipose tissue is used for energy, facilitating rapid weight loss (40). However, there are little data supporting these claims and few studies assessing long-term outcomes.

### Low-Carbohydrate, High-Fat Diets and Weight Loss

In a study of 10,014 people participating in the United States Department of Agriculture's Continuing Survey of Food Intake by Individuals (41), 4% were following diets that contained less than 30% of energy intake from CHO. This group had significantly higher body mass indexes (BMIs) compared to those following moderate CHO (30–55% of energy from CHO) or high CHO diets (>55% energy from CHO). This adds to the concern that these types of diets may not be as effective as promoted in the popular press.

Recent studies have assessed the efficacy of low-CHO, high-fat diets. Table 3 gives a brief summary of the characteristics of the diets used in these studies and key results. Westman et al. (42) studied 51 healthy overweight or obese subjects following a low-CHO diet for six months. The subjects were not asked to limit their energy intake and they received counseling on CHO restriction and exercise. The mean energy intake was $1447\pm350$ kcal; the authors estimated that maintenance energy requirements were $1905\pm239$ kcal. The mean change in body weight from baseline was a loss of $10.3\%\pm5.9\%$ ($P < 0.001$). Adherence to the diet plan correlated significantly with weight loss.

In another six-month study, Samaha et al. (43) studied a group of 132 severely obese (mean BMI of 43) subjects randomized to follow a low-CHO or a low-fat diet for six months. The low-CHO diet contained 30 g of CHO or less per day; the low-fat diet limited fat intake to 30% or less of total energy intake. At the end of the study, those following a low-CHO diet

**Table 3** Summary of Recent Low-Carbohydrate, High-Fat Dietary Intervention Studies

| Study | Group | Energy intake (cal, mean ± SD) | Macronutrient distribution (% CHO/% fat/% protein) | Key results |
|---|---|---|---|---|
| Westman et al. (42) | Control diet | No control diet | N/A | |
| | Study diet | 1447 ± 350 | 6/61/32 | After 6mo: 10.3% weight loss; ↓ TC, LDL-C, TG; ↑ HDL-C |
| Samaha et al. (43) | Control diet | 1576 ± 760 | 51/33/16 | After 6mo: greater weight loss and improved TG in study vs. control diet; no differences in other lipid levels; ↓ FBS in diabetic subjects on study diet |
| | Study diet | 1630 ± 894 | 37/41/22 | |
| Stern et al. (44) | Control diet | 1822 ± 1008 | 50/34/16 | After 12mo: no significant difference in weight loss between study groups; improved TG in study diet vs. control; ↓ HDL-C in control vs. study diet; no differences in other lipid levels; ↓ Hgb A$_{1c}$ in diabetic subjects on study diet |
| | Study diet | 1462 ± 776 | 33/57/20 | |
| Yancy et al. (45) | Control diet | 1502 ± 162.1 | 52/29/19 | After 24wk: greater weight loss with the study vs. control diet; greater improvement in TG and HDL-C in study vs. control diet |
| | Study diet | 1461 ± 325.7 | 8/68/26 | |
| Foster et al. (46) | Control diet | Women: 1200–1500, Men: 1500–1800 | 60/25/16 | After 12mo: no significant difference in weight loss between study groups; no significant differences between groups in lipid levels; improved TG and HDL-C in study diet vs. control; no significant differences in other lipid levels |
| | Study diet | Atkins diet; calorie information not available | Unknown | |

*Abbreviations*: SD, standard deviation; TC, total cholesterol; LDL-C, low-density lipoprotein cholesterol; TG, triglyceride; HDL-C, high-density lipoprotein cholesterol; FBS, fasting blood glucose; Hgb A$_{1c}$, hemoglobin A$_{1c}$.

lost more weight than those on the low-fat diet (mean, $5.8 \pm 8.6$ kg vs. $1.9 \pm 4.2$ kg; 95% CI 1.6–6.3 kg, $P = 0.002$). These results remained significant when repeat analysis was done including the baseline weights of those patients who dropped out (mean, $5.7 \pm 8.6$ kg vs. $1.8 \pm 3.9$ kg; 95% CI 1.6–6.2 kg, $P = 0.002$) (44).

Another short-term study was conducted by Yancy et al. (45) that consisted of 120 overweight, hyperlipidemic subjects randomized to follow either a low-CHO, ketogenic diet or a low-fat, low-cholesterol, reduced-calorie diet for 24 weeks. The low-CHO, ketogenic diet subjects were instructed to eat 20 g of CHO or less daily and were allowed unlimited amounts of meat, poultry, or fish, and limited amounts of dairy products and vegetables. Those subjects on the low-fat, low-cholesterol, reduced-calorie diet were instructed to follow a diet consisting of less than 30% fat, less than 10% saturated fat, and less than 300 mg cholesterol/day. Energy intake was calculated as 500 to 1000 cal less than estimated maintenance requirements. At the end of six months, 76% of the subjects following the low-CHO, ketogenic diet completed the study, compared to only 57% of the low-fat, low-cholesterol, reduced-calorie group ($P = 0.02$). Both groups lost more fat mass than fat-free mass, but the low-CHO group lost significantly more total weight compared to the low-fat, low-cholesterol, reduced-calorie group (12.9% vs. 6.7%; $P < 0.001$).

In a study of one-year duration, Foster et al. (46) assessed the efficacy of following the Atkins diet (39) versus a conventional weight-loss diet. Results at three and six months were similar to the results of Samaha et al. (43), with those subjects following the low-CHO, high-fat diet losing significantly more weight than those on the conventional diet. However, there were no significant differences in weight change between groups at 12 months. In the one-year follow-up study to Samaha et al. (43), Stern et al. (44) also found that there was no significant difference in total weight lost between the low-CHO, high-fat diet and a conventional weight-loss diet. Interestingly, those following the low-fat diet lost weight throughout the entire year, whereas the subjects following the low-CHO diet simply maintained the weight they lost during the first six months of the study. Energy restriction may be the most important factor for long-term weight loss rather than adjustments in macronutrient distribution.

## Low-Carbohydrate, High-Fat Diets and Lipid Levels

With changes in weight, it is expected that there will be changes in lipid levels. There are concerns with low-CHO, high-fat diets that there will be a negative impact on lipid levels (47). Westman et al. (42) found that this was not the case with subjects experiencing significant improvements in TC, LDL-C, HDL-C, and TG by the end of the study. In the short term, subjects following low-CHO diets have significantly greater improvements in TG levels compared to low-fat diets (43,45). In one short-term study (45), those following the low-CHO diet also experienced a significant increase in HDL-C from baseline and compared to the low-fat diet group.

Long-term results are important to assess efficacy of low-CHO, high-fat diets in improving lipid levels. At the one-year mark, subjects following low-CHO, high-fat diets continue to have significantly improved TG levels compared to those following low-fat diets (44,46). Foster et al. (46) found that those on the low-CHO, high-fat diet experienced significant increases in HDL-C at 3, 6, and 12 months, but subjects in the study by Stern et al. (44) experienced a significant decrease with HDL-C compared to the control diet.

These studies suggest that the low-CHO, high-fat diets may not be as detrimental to lipid profiles at 6 and 12 months as expected. However, more long-term studies are required to confirm these findings.

## Low-Carbohydrate, High-Fat Diets and Insulin Sensitivity

Samaha et al. (43), Foster et al. (46), and Stern et al. (44) assessed changes in insulin sensitivity, but in different ways. In all subjects and in diabetic subjects, Samaha et al. (43) found that those following a low-CHO, high-fat diet had a significant improvement in fasting blood glucose. Insulin levels were significantly lower for subjects who were following the low-CHO, high-fat diet and were not receiving medication for diabetes; in those requiring medication, there were no significant differences. Neither diet had a significant impact on glycosylated hemoglobin levels in diabetic subjects. Stern et al. (44) assessed the same parameters as Samaha et al. (43); the only significant difference was seen in the glycosylated hemoglobin levels in diabetic subjects following the low-CHO, high-fat diet. These results were significant only after controlling for baseline differences between the groups. Foster et al. (46) used oral glucose-tolerance tests to assess changes in insulin sensitivity. There were no significant differences between diet treatment groups. Both groups had improved insulin sensitivity from baseline at six months, but these changes were not significant at 12 months.

## Low-Carbohydrate, High-Fat Diets and Hypertension

Low-CHO, high-fat diets have not consistently improved blood pressure. Westman et al. (42) found a significant improvement from baseline blood pressure after six months of a low-CHO, high-fat diet, but Samaha et al. (43) did not confirm these results. Foster et al. (46) found no significant difference between treatment groups, but did show significant differences from baseline diastolic blood pressure at 6 and 12 months in the low-CHO, high-fat group and at three months in the conventional diet group. In Stern et al. (44), there were no significant differences in blood pressure. Of note, subjects lost what is considered a clinically significant amount of weight in the Westman et al. (42) study (about 10% of baseline weight), where low-CHO, high-fat diet subjects in Samaha et al. (43), Foster et al. (46), and Stern et al. (44) lost only approximately 4% of their baseline weight. This could be the reason for the lack of change in blood pressure in those studies (48).

## Overall Efficacy of Low-Carbohydrate, High-Fat Diets

With the gaining popularity of low-CHO, high-fat diets, more research is required to determine clinical efficacy, particularly for those electing to follow these diets for more than 6 to 12 months. Although there are significant improvements in weight at six months, the differences between low-CHO, high-fat diets and conventional weight-loss diets disappear at the one-year mark. Long-term follow-up of people following low-CHO, high-fat diets would be helpful to determine if changes in lipid levels and glucose levels can be sustained, as well as including other important outcomes such as incidence of cardiac events. There are other concerns about the risks associated with the high protein load associated with low-CHO, high-fat diets, particularly in diabetic subjects with impaired renal function (49). Until more information regarding safety and efficacy is available, these types of diets should not be routinely recommended to the general public.

## DIETARY PATTERNS

### The Mediterranean Diet and Cardiovascular Effects

Diets consumed by Mediterranean populations have been a subject of interest since antiquity, with many recent investigations focused on their health benefits. The term "traditional Mediterranean diet" reflects food patterns typical of Crete, much of the rest of Greece, and southern Italy in the 1960s. The Mediterranean diet of the early 1960s is described by the following broad characteristics: an abundance of plant foods which are minimally processed, seasonally fresh, and grown locally. Red meat is consumed in small amounts. Olive oil is the principal source of fat. Cheese and yogurt are consumed daily in low to moderate amounts, zero to four eggs consumed weekly. Fresh fruit is the typical daily dessert, with sweets containing concentrated sugars or honey eaten a few times per week; wine is consumed in low to moderate amounts, usually with meals. This diet is low in saturated fat (7–8% of energy), with total fat ranging from less than 28% to more than 40% of energy.

There appear to be a number of factors in the traditional Mediterranean diet of the 1960s that promote cardiovascular risk reduction, including a low intake of red meat, daily use of olive oil, regular consumption of fish, and abundant intake of plant foods, including fruits, vegetables, nuts, and grains.

A major hallmark of the Mediterranean diet pyramid is its recommendation of a much lower intake of red meat compared with the typical U.S. dietary recommendations. The most compelling evidence that regular meat consumption increases the risk of coronary heart disease mortality comes from studies that compared Seventh Day Adventists. Multivariate analyses showed significant associations between beef consumption and fatal ischemic heart disease in men (relative risk = 2.31 for subjects who ate beef greater than three times per week compared with vegetarians) (50). The Mediterranean diet incorporates fish as a main protein source and numerous clinical trials have demonstrated the effects of omega-3 fatty acids found in fish as a secondary prevention of coronary heart disease (51,52).

Although a reduction in total fat intake is commonly suggested as an important means to reduce heart disease, there is little evidence to suggest that fat per se is the cause. The lack of a clear association between total fat intake and heart disease rates in international studies was noted in the Seven Countries Study by Keys (2), who observed that regions with the highest fat intake, Finland and Crete, demonstrated the highest and lowest rates of heart disease, respectively. Keys (2) compared the percentage of energy from fat to the 10-year risk of coronary death in 15 populations in seven countries. Many of the countries around the Mediterranean Sea, consuming the Mediterranean diet, had low incidence of heart disease compared to the countries that consumed typical Western diets.

One study that specifically evaluated the effect of a Mediterranean-type diet on heart disease was the Lyon Heart Study (53). The treatment group was advised to follow a Mediterranean diet with increased amounts of fruits, vegetables, beans, and breads. The men were also advised to eat less meat, butter, and cream. The study used a specially prepared margarine that contained alpha linolenic acid. Alpha linolenic acid is a short-chain omega-3 fatty acid, which is metabolized in the body to long-chain omega-3 fatty acids (including EPA and DHA). Alpha linolenic acid has both antithrombotic and antiarrhythmic properties, which may explain its effects in reducing heart disease in populations throughout the world.

The protective effect of the Mediterranean diet pattern was maintained up to four years after the first heart attack. Those eating the Mediterranean diet were 50% to 70% less likely to develop a second heart attack compared to the control group. The control diet included prudent heart-healthy recommendations to reduce both total and saturated fat—similar to an American Heart Association diet.

Another healthful food used in the daily diets in the Mediterranean regions are nuts. A number of large epidemiologic studies support the reduction of risk for heart disease in nut eaters. Fraser et al. (54) examined 30,000 members of the Seventh Day Adventist Church and reported that people who ate nuts one to four times per week had 25% less risk of dying from heart disease compared to those who ate nuts less than once per week.

Similarly, Hu et al. (55) reported in the Nurse's Health Study that women who ate 150 g or more of nuts each week had 35% less risk of developing heart disease than those who never ate nuts. In the Iowa Women's Health Study, Ellsworth et al. (56) reported that women who ate nuts twice per week (about 60 g) reduced their risk of heart disease by 60% compared to women who did not eat nuts.

In Mediterranean traditions, wine is enjoyed in moderation and usually with meals. Many adverse influences of heavy alcohol consumption are well recognized, but moderate consumption has both beneficial and harmful effects. Overwhelming epidemiologic data indicate that moderate alcohol consumption reduces the risk of coronary heart disease. In a summary by Moore and Pearson (57), a protective effect was seen in both case–control and cohort studies. The reduction in CHD risk was approximately 30% to 70%.

Although conclusive evidence for the weight-loss diet that will reduce risk of cardiovascular disease has not been trailed in a randomized intervention study, it appears that a diet model incorporating an energy-controlled diet based on the Mediterranean pattern is a prudent approach.

## CURRENT RESEARCH

### CLA

CLA is a derivative of linoleic acid, a polyunsaturated fatty acid, that has double bonds either in the *cis* or *trans* configuration typically in positions 8 and 10, 9 and 11, 10 and 12, or 11 and 13 (58–60). Food sources of CLA are listed in Table 1. Interest in CLA is growing because of its potential in decreasing body fat and weight; improving lipid profiles, hypertension, and hyperinsulinemia; and preventing cancer in animal and human studies (59,60). This section will focus on the weight and cardiovascular effects of CLA.

#### CLA and Weight Loss

In animal studies, CLA supplementation has had the most impact on body fat deposition as opposed to body weight. Rahman et al. (61) conducted a short-term study of CLA supplementation in Otsuka Long-Evans Tokushima Fatty (OLETF) rats, which are obese and develop non–insulin dependent diabetes. After just 48 hours, those rats supplemented with 7.5% CLA had no significant difference in body weight, but experienced a 27% reduction in perirenal white adipose tissue (PWAT) and epididymal white adipose tissue (EWAT) weights compared to the control. Ohnuki et al. (62) fed mice diets containing 0%, 0.25%, 0.5% or 1% CLA for four or eight weeks. At four and eight weeks, mice receiving CLA supplemented diets had significantly lower body weights and PWAT and EWAT weights compared to the mice receiving the 0% CLA diet. Yamasaki et al. (63) conducted a similar study using rats, but modified the total fat intake to 4%, 7%, or 10% of food weight while keeping CLA constant at 1.5% of food weight; control rats received the same percentage of total fat, but no CLA. Overall, rats on the CLA-supplemented diets had less PWAT and EWAT compared to rats on the control diets, but there were no significant differences in body weight. The rats on the 4% fat diet with CLA had the least amount of PWAT and EWAT compared to control. Supplementing a high-fat diet with CLA may offer some benefit in decreasing fat deposition. Terpstra et al. (64) reported that mice fed a high-fat diet (20% food weight) supplemented with CLA (1.5% food weight) had lower overall body weight and body fat compared to mice fed a high-fat diet without supplemental CLA.

There may be an isomeric response to CLA supplementation. The *trans* 10 *cis* 12 (t10 c12) isomer of CLA is thought to be more metabolically potent than the c9, t11 isomer (65–67). Clement et al. (66) fed mice a diet supplemented with 2.4% sunflower oil (control diet), 2% sunflower oil plus 0.4% linoleic acid, 2% sunflower oil plus 0.4% c9, t11 CLA, or 2% sunflower oil plus 0.4% t10, c12 CLA for four weeks. Although there were no significant differences in body weight, those mice receiving the t10, c12 CLA supplemented diet had significantly decreased periuteral white adipose tissue compared to all other study groups. Henrikson et al. (65) studied the effect of an ad lib chow diet supplemented with gavage feeding of 76% c9, t11 CLA/24% t10, c12 CLA, 90% t10, c12 CLA/10% c9, t11 CLA, a 50:50 mix of the isomers, or plain corn oil on obese Zucker rats. The rats received 1.5 g CLA (or corn oil) for three weeks. The rats receiving the 90% t10, c12 CLA- or 10% c9, t11 CLA-supplemented diet had significantly less weight gain compared to all groups, including control. Those rats receiving the 50:50 mix gained significantly less weight compared to the control group only. The 90% t10, c12 CLA/10% c9, t11 CLA group also had significantly less abdominal fat compared to all groups.

There may also be a genetic-specific response to CLA supplementation. For example, Sisk et al. (68) found that lean and obese Zucker rats respond differently to CLA-supplemented diets. The obese rats fed a diet supplemented with 0.5% CLA gained significantly more weight and had greater inguinal and retroperitoneal fat pad weights compared to lean rats fed the same diet. In other species, response to CLA has been variable, with inconsistent results (58).

Human studies have shown an effect on body composition as in the animal studies, but not a significant impact on body weight. Blankson et al. (69) assessed the effect of CLA supplementation at different levels in overweight and obese humans. Sixty subjects were randomized to receive placebo or 1.7, 3.4, 5.1, or 6.8 g CLA/day in three divided doses. After 12 weeks, there were no significant differences in weight or BMI, but those receiving 1.7, 3.4, and 6.8 g CLA/day had a significant decrease in body fat mass compared to baseline as well as the placebo-treated group. When all CLA-supplemented subjects were pooled and compared to placebo-treated group, body fat mass was significantly reduced. Despite these changes in body composition, the subjects did not experience a significant change in weight or BMI.

Riserus et al. (70) assessed the effect of supplementing obese men with symptoms of the metabolic syndrome with 4.2 g CLA/day. After four weeks, those receiving supplementation with CLA had a significant decrease in sagittal abdominal diameter compared to the placebo-treated group. The CLA-supplemented group also experienced a significant decrease in waist circumference and waist-to-hip ratio from baseline measurements, but the differences were not significant compared to measurements in the placebo-treated group. As in the study by Blankson et al. (69), there were no significant differences in weight or BMI at the end of the study.

Kamphuis et al. (71) took a different approach to CLA, and started supplementation in overweight subjects after they had lost weight following a very low calorie diet. Although the CLA-supplemented group had greater feelings of satiety and fullness compared to placebo-treated group, there were no significant differences in maintenance of weight loss, with both groups experiencing weight regain.

Both animal and human studies have shown a varied response in body composition and weight change as a result of CLA supplementation. The potential for CLA supplementation to have an effect on upper-body obesity is encouraging, given the increased risk of coronary artery disease associated with this type of obesity. Further research is required to fully assess the effect of CLA as well as the effect of isomeric-specific functions on body weight and composition in humans.

### CLA and Lipid Levels

In the short-term study in OLETF rats (61), two days of CLA supplementation significantly reduced TC and HDL-C, but not TG, compared to control rats. Nagao et al. (67) found that supplementing OLETF rats with CLA for four weeks resulted in significantly lower serum TG compared to control; no other serum lipids were measured. However, in the study by Sisk et al. (68), there were no significant differences in both lean and obese Zucker rats fed diets supplemented with CLA compared to control diet.

As with CLA and body composition, there seems to be an isomer-specific response with CLA supplementation. Nagao et al. (67) reported on a 10-day study in OLETF rats comparing a diet supplemented with one of two isomers of CLA. Those rats receiving the 10t, 12c-CLA isomer had significantly lower serum TG compared to those receiving the 9c, 11t-CLA-supplemented diet, supporting the theory that the isomer of CLA is important, not just general CLA supplementation.

In humans, effect on serum lipids has been variable. In a study of four weeks duration (70), there were no significant differences in TC, LDL-C, or TG between subjects who received CLA or placebo. The only significant difference was an increase in HDL-C in the placebo group. Duration of CLA supplementation may be important, and perhaps four weeks was inadequate to see an effect. Subjects supplemented with either 1.7 or 3.4 g CLA daily for 12 weeks experienced significantly lowered TC, LDL-C, and HDL-C, but no change in TG levels (69). However, other studies do not support these results. For example, in a study by Riserus et al. (72), 60 men with abdominal obesity were randomized to receive 3.4 g mixed-isomer CLA, purified t10, c12 CLA, or placebo for 12 weeks. At the end of the study, the subjects receiving the mixed-isomer CLA and the t10, c12 CLA had significantly lower HDL-C levels compared to the placebo group; there was a trend ($P = 0.06$) toward higher VLDL TG in both treated groups.

As with body weight and body composition, the effect of CLA supplementation on blood lipid levels in both animal and human studies has been inconsistent. Thus, definitive recommendations for supplementation to treat hyperlipidemia cannot be made at this time.

## CLA and Insulin Sensitivity

Houseknecht et al. (73) fed Zucker diabetic fatty rats a 1.5% CLA diet versus a control diet or control diet plus 0.2% troglitazone for 14 days. At the end of the study, those rats fed on the CLA-supplemented and troglitazone-supplemented diets had significantly lower insulin levels compared to the control rats, but were still hyperinsulinemic compared to lean Zucker rats that were also fed the control diet. These rats also had improved glucose tolerance compared to the fatty rats fed the control diet. The authors proposed that CLA has similar insulin sensitizing properties as troglitazone. Nagao et al. (74) studied Zucker diabetic fatty rats receiving a 1% CLA diet versus 1% linoleic acid diet (control) for eight weeks. At the end of the study, the control rats had severe hyperinsulinemia. The study rats, although still hyperinsulinemic compared to lean Zucker rats, had plasma insulin levels significantly lower than the control rats. These rats also had significantly lower plasma glucose levels than the control rats. Xu et al. (75) fed mice a diet supplemented with 0.5% CLA versus a control diet (no CLA) for four days for one group and seven weeks for another. At the end of both time periods, there were no significant differences in fasting insulin levels. The seven-week arm of the study was repeated using rats, which also revealed no significant differences in insulin levels (75).

As in other parameters, isomer-specific actions were studied in animals. Obese Zucker rats fed the t10 c12 isomer of CLA had significantly improved plasma glucose levels compared to rats fed diets supplemented with other isomers of CLA. Plasma insulin levels were significantly reduced in the rats receiving the 50:50 mix of both CLA isomers and the t10 c12 isomer of

CLA alone (65). In mice, however, t10, c12 CLA supplementation led to severe hyperinsulinemia compared to control, c9, t11 CLA-supplemented, and linoleic acid–supplemented mice. There were no significant differences in plasma glucose levels in all groups (66).

Supplementing humans with CLA has not been as effective as in animal studies in improving blood glucose levels or insulin sensitivity. Belury et al. (76) conducted a small-scale study of 21 adults with diet-controlled type 2 diabetes. Subjects were randomized to receive 6 g of mixed-isomer CLA ($n = 11$) or safflower oil ($n = 10$) daily for eight weeks. After eight weeks, 81% of the CLA-supplemented group had decreases in fasting plasma glucose, compared to 20% in the safflower oil group. A larger study by Riserus et al. (72) did not support these results. The t10, c12 CLA–treated group had decreased insulin sensitivity compared to the control group; there were no differences between the mixed-isomer CLA group and the t10, c12 CLA group or the mixed-isomer CLA group and placebo group. The t10, c12 CLA group also had significantly higher insulin, glucose, and hemoglobin A1c levels compared to baseline. Upon further analysis of those subjects, it was found that both CLA treated-groups had significantly higher levels of measures of oxidative stress [8-iso-prostaglandin F (PGF) 2α and 15-K-dihydro-PGF 2α] compared to placebo (77). The t10, c12 CLA group had higher levels than the mixed-isomer CLA-supplemented group. The authors concluded that the oxidative stress induced by CLA supplementation (particularly the t10 c12 isomer) contributed to the insulin resistance.

### CLA and Hypertension

Nagao et al. conducted two studies (74,78) that assessed the effect of CLA supplementation on hypertension. One study was conducted in OLETF rats (78) and one in Zucker diabetic fatty rats (74). In OLETF rats, t10, c12, CLA supplementation was correlated with a significant lower rise in blood pressure with the onset of obesity when compared to rats receiving the control diet or c9, t11 CLA supplementation. In Zucker diabetic fatty rats, supplementation with mixed-isomer CLA resulted in a significantly lower rise in blood pressure with the onset of obesity compared to control rats. It remains to be seen if similar results will be found in human studies.

### Complications Associated with CLA Supplementation

The main complication reported in animal studies has been fatty liver. For example, in the study by Ohnuki et al. (62), mice fed a 1% CLA, but not 0.25% or 0.5% CLA diets, had significantly higher hepatic TG levels after four weeks and eight weeks on the diet compared to control feeding. Clement et al. (66) found that mice fed the t10 c12 isomer developed severe liver enlargement compared to control feeding and supplementation with t9, c11 CLA supplementation. Other studies have found no hepatic injury (63,67). In humans, adverse effects have been related to insulin resistance

**Table 4**  Potential Benefits and Risks of Supplementation with CLA

| Human studies | Animal studies |
|---|---|
| *Potential benefits of CLA supplementation* | |
| Decreased upper-body obesity | Decreased visceral fat deposition |
| Improved waist-to-hip ratio | Decreased triglyceride levels, particularly with t10 c12 CLA isomer |
| Decreased TC, LDL-C | Improved glucose levels |
| | Decreased insulin levels |
| | Decreased blood pressure |
| *Potential risks of CLA supplementation* | |
| Decreased HDL-C | Fatty liver |
| Insulin resistance, particularly with t10 c12 CLA isomer | |
| Increased oxidative stress, particularly with t10 c12 CLA isomer | |

*Abbreviations*: CLA, conjugated linoleic acid; TC, total cholesterol; LDL-C, low-density lipoprotein cholesterol; HDL-C, high-density lipoprotein cholesterol; t10 c12 CLA, *trans* 10 *cis* 12 conjugated linoleic acid.

and increased oxidative stress; lowered HDL-C levels could also be considered an adverse effect (70,72).

## Overall Efficacy of CLA

Overall efficacy of CLA supplementation on obesity and cardiovascular risk factors has yet to be determined. Table 4 summarizes potential risks and benefits of CLA supplementation. In animal studies, there seems to be genetic or species-specific responses to CLA supplementation as well as isomer-specific effects. In humans, there are similar issues in terms of both positive and negative studies and the question of isomer-specific effects that favor one isomer of CLA over another. Further study of adverse effects in humans is also required. Thus, recommendations for CLA supplementation cannot be made at this time.

## CONCLUSIONS

Modification of the type of fat in the diet can have a significant impact on cardiac risk factors. Based on the current literature and expert guidelines, Table 5 summarizes recommendations that can be followed for dietary fat intake. The low-CHO, high-fat diets offer the potential of immediate results for weight loss, but the implications of following this type of diet over a long-term period have yet to be studied. The use of supplemental fatty acids such as CLA also requires further research before clinicians can recommend routine supplementation. Following a healthy eating pattern such as the

**Table 5** Recommended Intake for Dietary Fat—Summary Based on Current Literature and Expert Guidelines

| Type of fat | Amount |
| --- | --- |
| Total fat intake | 20–35% of total energy intake |
| Saturated fat | ≤8% of total energy intake |
| *trans* Fat | < 1% of total energy intake |
| Total polyunsaturated fat | ≤10% of total energy intake |
| Omega-3 fatty acids | 0.5–1.8 g EPA + DHA (combined)/day, 1.5–3 g α-linoleic acid/day |
| Monounsaturated fats | 12–22% of total energy intake |

*Abbreviations*: EPA, cicosapentaenoic acid; DHA, docosahexaenoic acid.

Mediterranean diet may be a more prudent approach because not only does this diet promote consumption of healthy fats, but also promotes a more balanced diet compared to the low-CHO, high-fat diets.

## REFERENCES

1. Block G, Dresser CM, Hartman AM, Carroll MD. Nutrient sources in the American diet: quantitative data from the NHANES II survey. II. Macronutrients and fats. Am J Epidemiol 1985; 122:27–40.
2. Keys A. Seven Countries: A Multivariate Analysis of Death and Coronary Heart Disease. Cambridge, MA: Harvard University Press, 1980.
3. Mensink RP, Katan MB. Effect of dietary *trans* fatty acids on high-density and low-density lipoprotein cholesterol levels in healthy subjects. N Engl J Med 1990; 323:439–445.
4. Mensink RP, Zock PL, Katan MB, Hornstra G. Effects of dietary *cis* and *trans* fatty acids on serum lipoprotein [a] levels in humans. J Lipid Res 1992; 33: 1493–1501.
5. Zock PL, Katan MB. Hydrogenation alternatives: effects of *trans* fatty acids and stearic acid versus linoleic acid on serum lipids and lipoproteins in humans. J Lipid Res 1992; 33:399–410.
6. Lichtenstein AH, Ausman LM, Carrasco W, Jenner JL, Ordovas JM, Schaefer EJ. Hydrogenation impairs the hypolipidemic effect of corn oil in humans: hydrogenation, *trans* fatty acids, and plasma lipids. Arterioscler Thromb 1993; 13:154–161.
7. Hu F, Stampfer M, Manson J, et al. Dietary fat intake and the risk of coronary heart disease in women. N Engl J Med 1997; 337:1491–1499.
8. Schaefer EJ. Lipoproteins, nutrition, and heart disease. Am J Clin Nutr 2002; 75:191–212.
9. Kris-Etherton P, Daniels SR, Eckel RH, et al. Summary of the scientific conference on dietary fatty acids and cardiovascular health. Conference summary from the nutrition committee of the American Heart Association. Circulation 2001; 103:1034–1039.

10.  Hu FB, Manson JE, Willett WC. Types of dietary fat and risk of coronary heart disease: a critical review. J Am Coll Nutr 2001; 20:5–19.
11.  Kris-Etherton PM, Harris WS, Appel LJ. Fish consumption, fish oil, omega-3 fatty acids, and cardiovascular disease. Circulation 2002; 106:2747–2757.
12.  Kris-Etherton PM. Monounsaturated fatty acids and the risk of cardiovascular disease. Circulation 1999; 100:1253–1258.
13.  Krauss RM, Eckel RH, Howard B, et al. AHA Dietary Guidelines: revision 2000: a statement for healthcare professionals from the Nutrition Committee of the American Heart Association. Circulation 2000; 102:2284–2299.
14.  National Cholesterol Education Program. Report of the Expert Panel on Detection, Evaluation, and Treatment of High Blood Cholesterol in Adults (ATP II). Washington, D.C.: US Department of Health and Human Services, 1993.
15.  Shah M, Garg A. High fat and high carbohydrate diets and energy balance. Diabetes Care 1996; 199:1142–1152.
16.  Kinsell LW, Schlierf G. Alimentary and nonalimentary hyperglyceridemia. Ann NY Acad Sci 1965; 13:603–613.
17.  Leibel RL, Hirsch J, Appel BE, Checani GC. Energy intake required to maintain body weight is not affected by wide variation in diet composition. Am J Clin Nutr 1992; 55:350–355.
18.  Yang MU, Barbosa-Saldivar JL, Pi-Sunyer FX, Van Itallie TB. Metabolic effects of substituting carbohydrate for protein in a low-calorie diet: a prolonged study in obese patients. Int J Obes 1981; 5:231–236.
19.  Powell JJ, Tucker L, Fisher AG, Wilcox K. The effects of different percentages of dietary fat intake, exercise, and calorie restriction on body composition and body weight in obese females. Am J Health Promot 1994; 8:442–448.
20.  Astrup A, Ryan L, Grunwald GK. The role of dietary fat in body fatness; evidence from a preliminary meta-analysis of ad libitum low-fat dietary intervention studies. Br J Nutr 2000; 83(suppl 1):S25–S32.
21.  Jequier E, Bray GA. Low fat diets are preferred. Am J Med 2002; 113:41S–46S.
22.  Bray GA, Lovejoy JC, Most-Windhauser M, et al. A 9-month randomized clinical trial comparing fat-substituted and fat-reduced diets in healthy obese men: the Ole Study. Am J Clin Nutr 2002; 76:928–934.
23.  Willet WC. Is dietary fat a major determinant of body fat? Am J Clin Nutr 1998; 67:556S–562S.
24.  Willett WC, Leibel RL. Dietary fat is not a major determinant of body fat. Am J Med 2002; 113:47S–59S.
25.  Jeffrey RW, Hellerstedt WL, French SA, Baxter JE. A randomized trial of counseling for fat restriction versus calories restriction in the treatment of obesity. Int J Obes 1995; 19:132–137.
26.  Kasim SE, Martino S, Kim PN, et al. Dietary and anthropometric determinants of plasma lipoproteins during a long-term low-fat diet in healthy women. Am J Clin Nutr 1993; 57:146–153.
27.  Shepard L, Kristal AR, Kushi LH. Weight loss in women participating in a randomized trial of low fat diets. Am J Clin Nutr 1991; 54:821–828.
28.  Shah M, McGovern P, French S, Baxter J. Comparison of a low-fat, complex carbohydrate diet with a low-energy diet in moderately obese women. Am J Clin Nutr 1994; 59:980–984.

29. Toubro S, Astrup A. Randomized comparison of diets for maintaining obese subjects weight after major weight loss: ad lib, low fat, high carbohydrate diet vs. fixed energy intake. Br Med J 1997; 314:29–34.
30. McManus K, Antinoro L, Sacks F. A randomized trial of a moderate fat, low energy diet compared with a low fat, low energy diet for weight loss in overweight adults. Int J Obes Rel Met Disord 2001; 25:1503–1511.
31. Bray GA, Popkin BM. Dietary fat intake does affect obesity. Am J Clin Nutr 1998; 68:1157–1173.
32. Yu-Poth S, Zhao G, Etherton T, Naglak M, Jonnalagadda S, Kris-Etherton PM. Effects of the National Cholesterol Education Program's Step I and Step II dietary intervention programs on cardiovascular disease risk factors: a meta-analysis. Am J Clin Nutr 1999; 69:632–646.
33. Pirozzo S, Summerbell C, Cameron C, Glasziou P. Advice on low fat diets for obesity. Cochrane Database Syst Rev 2002; [2]:CDC03640.
34. Ball KP, Honington E, McAllen PM, et al. Low fat diet in myocardial infarction: a controlled trial. Lancet 1965; 2:501–504.
35. Burr ML, Fehily AM, Gilbert SF, et al. Effects of changes in fat, fish, and fiber intakes on death and myocardial infarction. Diet and Reinfarction Trial (DART). Lancet 1989; 2:757–761.
36. Mensink RP, Katan MB. Effect of dietary fatty acids on serum lipids and lipoproteins—a meta-analysis of 27 trials. Arterioscler Thromb 1992; 12:911–919.
37. Hegsted DM, Ausman LM, Johnson JA, Dellal GE. Dietary fat and serum lipids: an evaluation of the experimental data. Am J Clin Nutr 1993; 57:875–883.
38. Yu S, Derr J, Etherton TD, Kris-Etherton PM. Plasma cholesterol-predictive equations demonstrate that stearic acid is neutral and monounsaturated fatty acids are hypocholesterolemic. Am J Clin Nutr 1995; 61:1129–1135.
39. Atkins RC. Dr. Atkins' New Diet Revolution. New York: Avon Books, 2002.
40. Bravata DeM, Sanders L, Huang J, et al. Efficacy and safety of low-carbohydrate diets. A systematic review. JAMA 2003; 289:1837–1850.
41. Kennedy ET, Bowman SA, Spence JT, Freedman M, King J. Popular diets: correlation to health, nutrition, and obesity. J Am Diet Assoc 2001; 101:411–420.
42. Westman EC, Yancy WS, Edman JS, Tomlin KF, Perkins CE. Effect of a 6-month adherence to a very low carbohydrate diet program. Am J Med 2002; 113:30–36.
43. Samaha FF, Iqbal N, Seshadri P, et al. A low-carbohydrate as compared with a low-fat diet in severe obesity. N Engl J Med 2003; 348:2074–2081.
44. Stern L, Iqbal N, Seshadri P, et al. The effects of low-carbohydrate versus conventional weight loss diets in severely obese adults: one-year follow-up of a randomized trial. Ann Intern Med 2004; 140:778–785.
45. Yancy WS, Olsen MK, Guyton JR, Bakst RP, Westman EC. A low-carbohydrate, ketogenic diet versus a low-fat diet to treat obesity and hyperlipidemia. Ann Intern Med 2004; 140:769–779.
46. Foster GD, Wyatt H, Hill JO, et al. A randomized trial of a low-carbohydrate diet for obesity. N Engl J Med 2003; 348:2082–2090.
47. St. Jeor ST, Howard BV, Prewitt TE, Bovee V, Bazzarre T, Eckel RH for the AHA Nutrition Committee. Dietary protein and weight reduction. A statement for healthcare professionals from the Nutrition Committee of the Council on

Nutrition, Physical Activity, and Metabolism of the American Heart Association. Circulation 2001; 104:1869–1874.

48. Clinical guidelines on the identification, evaluation, and treatment of overweight and obesity in adults—the evidence report: executive summary. Obes Res 1998; 6(suppl 2):51S–63S [Erratum, Obes Res 1998;6:464].

49. Duggirala MK, Mundell WC, Mikkilineni P. Low-carbohydrate diets as compared with low-fat diets (correspondence). N Engl J Med 2003; 349:1000–1002.

50. Fraser GE. Associations between diet and cancer, ischemic heart disease, and all cause mortality in non-Hispanic white California Seventh-Day Adventists. Am J Clin Nutr 1999; 70(suppl 3):5325–5385.

51. GISSI-Prevenzione Investigators. Dietary supplementation with n-3 polyunsaturated fatty acids and vitamin E after myocardial infarction: results from the GISSI-Prevenzione trial. Lancet 1999; 354:447–455.

52. Singh RB, Niaz MA, Sharma JP, Kumar R, Rastogi V, Moshiri M. Randomized, double-blind, placebo controlled trial of fish oil and mustard oil in patients with suspected acute myocardial infarction: the Indian Experiment of Infarct Survival 4. Cardiovasc Drugs Ther 1997; 11:485–491.

53. de Lorgeril M, Salen P, Martin JL, Monjaud I, Delaye J, Mamelle N. Mediterranean diet, traditional risk factors, and the rate of cardiovascular complications after myocardial infarction: final report of the Lyon Diet Heart Study. Circulation 1999; 99:779–785.

54. Fraser G, Sabate J, Beeson LW, Strahan MT. A possible effect of nut consumption on risk of coronary heart disease. Arch Intern Med 1992; 152:1416–1424.

55. Hu FB, Stampfer MJ, Manson JE, et al. Frequent nut consumption and risk of coronary heart disease in women: prospective cohort study. BMJ 1998; 317:1341–1345.

56. Ellsworth JL, et al. Frequent nut intake and risk of death from coronary heart disease and all causes in postmenopausal women: the Iowa Women's Health Study. Nutr Metabol Cardiovasc Dis 2001; 11:362–372.

57. Moore RD, Pearson TA. Moderate alcohol consumption and coronary artery disease: a review. Medicine 1986; 65:242–267.

58. Larsen TM, Toubro S, Astrup A. Efficacy and safety of dietary supplements containing CLA for the treatment of obesity: evidence from animal and human studies. J Lipid Res 2003; 44:2234–2241.

59. Whigham LD, Cook ME, Atkinson RL. Conjugated linoleic acid: implications for human health. Pharmacol Res 2000; 42:503–510.

60. Belury MA. Dietary conjugated linoleic acid in health: physiological effects and mechanisms of action. Ann Rev Nutr 2002; 22:505–531.

61. Rahman SM, Wang Y-M, Han S-Y, et al. Effects of short-term administration of conjugated linoleic acid on lipid metabolism in white and brown adipose tissues of starved/refed Otsuka Long-Evans Tokushima Fatty rats. Food Res Int 2001; 34:515–520.

62. Ohnuki K, Haramizu S, Ishihara K, Fushiki T. Increased energy metabolism and suppressed body fat accumulation in mice by a low concentration of conjugated linoleic acid. Biosci Biotechnol Biochem 2001; 65:2200–2204.

63. Yamasaki M, Ikeda A, Oji M, et al. Modulation of body fat and serum leptin levels by dietary conjugated linoleic acid in Sprague-Dawley rats fed various fat-level diets. Nutrition 2003; 19:30–35.

64. Terpstra AHM, Beynen AC, Everts H, Kocsis S, Katan MB, Zock PL. The decrease in body fat in mice fed conjugated linoleic acid is due to increases in energy expenditure and energy losses in the excreta. J Nutr 2002; 132:940–945.

65. Henrikson EJ, Teachey MK, Taylor ZC, et al. Isomer-specific actions of conjugated linoleic acid on muscle glucose transport in the obese Zucker rat. Am J Physiol Endocrinol Metab 2003; 285:E98–E105.

66. Clement L, Poirier H, Niot I, et al. Dietary *trans*-10, *cis*-12 conjugated linoleic acid induces hyperinsulinemia and fatty liver in the mouse. J Lipid Res 2002; 43:1400–1409.

67. Nagao K, Wang Y-M, Inoue N, et al. The 10*trans*, 12*cis* isomer of conjugated linoleic acid promotes energy metabolism in OLETF rats. Nutrition 2003; 19:652–656.

68. Sisk MB, Hausman DB, Martin RJ, Azain MJ. Dietary conjugated linoleic acid reduces adiposity in lean but not obese Zucker rats. J Nutr 2001; 131: 1668–1674.

69. Blankson H, Stakkestad JA, Fagertun H, Thom E, Wadstein J, Gudmundsen O. Conjugated linoleic acid reduces body fat mass in overweight and obese humans. J Nutr 2000; 130:2943–2948.

70. Riserus U, Berglund L, Vessby B. Conjugated linoleic acid (CLA) reduced abdominal adipose tissue in obese middle-aged men with signs of the metabolic syndrome: a randomized controlled trial. Int J Obes 2001; 25:1129–1135.

71. Kamphuis MMJW, Lejeune MPGM, Saris WHM, Westerterp-Plantenga MS. Effect of conjugated linoleic acid supplementation after weight loss on appetite and food intake in overweight subjects. Eur J Clin Nutr 2003; 57:1268–1274.

72. Riserus U, Arner P, Brismar K, Vessby B. Treatment with dietary trans10cis12 conjugated linoleic acid causes isomer-specific insulin resistance in obese men with the metabolic syndrome. Diabetes Care 2002; 25:1516–1521.

73. Houseknecht KL, Vanden Heuvel JP, Moya-Camarena SY, et al. Dietary conjugated linoleic acid normalizes impaired glucose tolerance in the Zucker diabetic fatty fa/fa rat. Biochem Biophys Res Commun 1998; 244:678–682.

74. Nagao K, Inous N, Wang Y-M, Yanagita T. Conjugated linoleic acid enhances plasma adiponectin level and alleviates hyperinsulinemia and hypertension in Zucker diabetic fatty (fa/fa) rats. Biochem Biophys Res Commun 2003; 310: 562–566.

75. Xu X, Storkson J, Kim S, Sugimoto K, Park Y, Pariza MW. Short-term intake of conjugated linoleic acid inhibits lipoprotein lipase and glucose metabolism but does not enhance lipolysis in mouse adipose tissue. J Nutr 2003; 133: 663–667.

76. Belury MA, Mahon A, Banni S. The conjugated linoleic acid (CLA) isomer, t10c12-CLA, is inversely associated with changes in body weight and serum leptin in subjects with type 2 diabetes mellitus. J Nutr 2003; 133:257S–260S.

77. Riserus U, Basu S, Jovings S, Nordin Fredrikson G, Ärnlov J, Vessby B. Supplementation with conjugated linoleic acid causes isomer-dependent oxidative stress and elevated C-reactive protein. Circulation 2002; 106:1925–1929.

78. Nagao K, Inoue N, Wang Y-M, et al. The 10trans, 12cis isomer of conjugated linoleic acid suppresses the development of hypertension in Otsuka Long-Evans Tokushima fatty rats. Biochem Biophys Res Commun 2003; 306:134–138.

# 11

# Dietary Intervention and Monitoring of Obese Patients with Cardiovascular Disease

**Kris M. Mogensen**

*Metabolic Support Service, Brigham and Women's Hospital, Boston, Massachusetts, U.S.A.*

**Barbara B. Hodges**

*Baystate Medical Center, Springfield, Massachusetts, U.S.A.*

**Natalie M. Egan and Jenny Hegmann**

*Program for Weight Management, Brigham and Women's Hospital, Boston, Massachusetts, U.S.A.*

## INTRODUCTION

Dietary intervention for obese patients with cardiovascular disease (CVD) presents a challenge because of the many different diets available to promote weight loss and to improve blood lipid levels. Weight-loss diets can be classified as low-calorie diet (LCD), defined as providing 800 to 1500 cal/day, or very low calorie diet (VLCD), defined as providing 800 cal or less per day. It is beyond the scope of this chapter to cover every weight-loss and/or lipid-lowering diet. This chapter will review the following LCDs: the National Cholesterol Education Project (NCEP) diet, the Dietary Approaches to Stop Hypertension (DASH) diet, glycemic index (GI), plant-based diets, and the post–gastric bypass diet; VLCDs will also be reviewed.

## NATIONAL CHOLESTEROL EDUCATION PROJECT (NCEP)

The National Heart, Lung, and Blood Institute started the NCEP in 1985. This program is designed to educate both practitioners and the public about the risks associated with high cholesterol and appropriate interventions for hypercholesterolemia with the ultimate goal to decrease morbidity and mortality associated with coronary heart disease (CHD) (1).

The first guidelines for managing high cholesterol were published in 1988 (2) and have subsequently undergone two revisions (3,4). The third report of the NCEP expert panel on detection, evaluation, and treatment of high blood cholesterol in adults [Adult Treatment Panel III (ATP III)] was published in 2002 (4). As with the prior two reports, the ATP III guidelines include comprehensive guidelines for medical and nutritional therapy for the management of high cholesterol in order to prevent the development of CHD, as well as guidelines for those with existing CHD. The ATP III report also includes new guidelines for the management of those people with multiple risk factors for the development of CHD.

Nutritional guidelines have been modified since the ATP II report. In the ATP II report (3), two levels of dietary modification were recommended: the "step 1" diet was designed for the initial dietary intervention for hypercholesterolemia, and the "step 2" diet was a more restrictive diet for either those who did not respond to the step 1 diet or those with pre-existing CHD. Table 1 describes the characteristics of the step 1 and step 2 diets. With the ATP III report, the dietary recommendations have been modified. The step 1 diet is still recommended for the general population as a preventative measure against the development of CHD. For those who are determined to be at risk for CHD or those with existing CHD, the recommended clinical management is referred to as therapeutic lifestyle changes (TLC). This approach not only incorporates dietary guidelines (still following the basic tenets of the step 2 diet), but also physical activity and other important lifestyle interventions to decrease the risk of CHD. Table 2 summarizes the TLC diet recommendations. The full ATP III report (4) also provides detailed recommendations for lifestyle changes and drug therapy.

**Table 1** National Cholesterol Education Project "Step" Diets

|                    | Step 1 diet                | Step 2 diet                |
| ------------------ | -------------------------- | -------------------------- |
| Carbohydrate       | ≥55% total energy intake   | ≥55% total energy intake   |
| Fat                | ≤30% total energy intake   | ≤30% total energy intake   |
| Protein            | 15% total energy intake    | 15% total energy intake    |
| Saturated fat      | 8–10% total energy intake  | <7% total energy intake    |
| Polyunsaturated fat| ≤10% total energy intake   | ≤10% total energy intake   |
| Monounsaturated fat| ≤15% total energy intake   | ≤15% total energy intake   |
| Cholesterol        | <300 mg/day                | <200 mg/day                |

**Table 2**   National Cholesterol Education Project TLC Diet

| | |
|---|---|
| Saturated fat | <7% total energy intake |
| Polyunsaturated fat | Up to 10% of total energy intake |
| Monounsaturated fat | Up to 10% of total energy intake |
| *Total fat* | 25–35% of total energy intake |
| Carbohydrate | 50–60% of total energy intake |
| Fiber | 20–30 g/day |
| Protein | 15% of total energy intake |
| Cholesterol | <200 mg/day |
| *Total energy* | Balance energy intake and activity level to maintain healthy weight or prevent weight gain |

*Abbreviation:* TLC, therapeutic lifestyle changes.

## Outcomes with the TLC Diet

The TLC dietary guidelines have been developed based on epidemiological studies, animal studies, and clinical trials. Lichtenstein et al. (5) evaluated the effectiveness of the TLC/step 2 diet compared to a conventional western diet in subjects with mild hypercholesterolemia. Those subjects following the TLC diet had significantly decreased low-density lipoprotein cholesterol (LDL-C) and high-density lipoprotein cholesterol (HDL-C) compared to those on the control diet. There was a trend toward higher triglyceride (TG) levels in the intervention diet group compared to the conventional diet group. There were no significant changes in body weight because the diets were designed to promote weight maintenance.

A criticism of the NCEP dietary guidelines is the promotion of high-carbohydrate intake as a result of decreased fat intake, which could promote hypertriglyceridemia. Aude et al. (6) compared the NCEP step 2 diet to a modified low-carbohydrate diet to promote weight loss in overweight subjects. After 12 weeks, the subjects on the modified low-carbohydrate diet lost significantly more weight than the NCEP diet subjects. Total cholesterol (TC) was significantly decreased from baseline in both groups, but there were no between-group differences. The NCEP diet group also had significantly decreased HDL-C and LDL-C. The modified low-carbohydrate group had significantly decreased TG. Chapter 10 gives an extensive review of the role of dietary fat in weight loss and in managing lipid levels.

## Overall Efficacy of the TLC Diet

With appropriate dietary instruction, the TLC diet can be effective in achieving the goals of the NCEP. Because these guidelines are still relatively new, it will take some time to see more research comparing the full TLC guidelines to other dietary interventions for improving cardiovascular risk as well as for promoting weight loss in obese patients.

## DIETARY APPROACHES TO STOP HYPERTENSION (DASH) DIET

The DASH study has received much attention because of the significant impact the diet modification had on hypertension and the uniqueness of the study population (7). A concerted effort was made to recruit African-Americans because of the high incidence of hypertension in this group and women because of their underrepresentation in many studies. As a result of these efforts, 60% of the study participants were African-American and 49% were women. Table 3 summarizes the basic eating pattern for the DASH diet (8).

The study design included a three-week run-in period for participants to follow the control diet, which was a diet low in fruits, vegetables, and dairy products with approximately 37% of energy from fat. After three weeks of following the control diet, participants were randomized to one of three dietary interventions: control diet, fruits-and-vegetables diet, or combination diet, which was high in fruits, vegetables, and low-fat dairy products, and low in total fat, saturated fat, and cholesterol. Participants followed the diets for eight weeks. Adequate energy was provided to promote weight maintenance.

### DASH Diet and Weight Loss

In the original DASH diet study (7), study participants did not lose weight. Weights were monitored carefully and energy intake increased accordingly if subjects were losing weight. In the Diet, Exercise, and Weight Loss Intervention Trial (9), a low-calorie DASH diet was used in conjunction with

**Table 3** Description of the DASH Diet

Seven to eight servings of whole grains/day
Four to five servings of fruits/day
Four to five servings of vegetables/day
Two to three servings of nonfat or low-fat dairy products/day
Two or less servings of meats, poultry, and fish/day
Four to five servings/week of nuts, seeds, and legumes
Two to three servings/day of fats and oils
Five servings/week of sweets
Eating plan is based on 2000 cal/day diet; total servings will increase or decrease based on a specific patient's estimated energy requirements.

*Abbreviation*: DASH, dietary approaches to stop hypertension.

aerobic exercise to promote weight loss in overweight, hypertensive subjects taking one antihypertensive medication versus a control group receiving no intervention. After nine weeks, the study group lost an average of 5.5 kg, compared to only 0.6 kg in the control group. The study subjects had significant help with adhering to the intervention; all food was provided and exercise sessions were scheduled and supervised. The study subjects were considered to be highly motivated; 97% of the participants reported no deviation from the study diet and attended 86% of the scheduled exercise sessions.

The PREMIER Clinical Trial (10) used counseling to implement dietary and activity changes in three study groups: a control group receiving one counseling session at the beginning of the six-month study and no further intervention, a behavioral intervention group that received counseling on well-established lifestyle modifications to improve blood pressure (the "established" group), and a third group that received lifestyle counseling with specific dietary instruction on the DASH diet and additional weight-loss strategies ("established + DASH" group). Both the intervention groups attended 14 group and four individual counseling sessions. All groups lost weight at the end of six months, but the established group and the established + DASH group lost significantly more weight than the control group: $1.1 \pm 3.2$ kg for the control group, $4.9 \pm 5.5$ and $5.8 \pm 5.8$ kg for the established and established + DASH groups, respectively. However, there were no significant differences between the two intervention groups. This suggests that either diet can be effective to promote weight loss in conjunction with exercise and intensive counseling.

## Effect of DASH Diet on Lipid Levels

Based on the nutrient composition of the DASH diet, Obarzanek et al. (11) analyzed the effect on serum lipid levels in the original DASH diet study group. Nincty-five percent of the study group provided fasting blood samples at the beginning and end of the study. Those following the DASH diet had significant reductions in TC, LDL-C, and HDL-C. In subgroup analysis by race, the results remained significant; in subgroup analysis by gender, women did not have significant decreases in LDL-C.

## DASH Diet and Hypertension

The DASH diet has been shown to improve blood pressure both alone (7,12,13) and in conjunction with a low-sodium diet (14), and also as part of a total lifestyle change that included aerobic exercise and weight loss (9,10). The proposed mechanism for these improvements is the high intake of potassium and calcium promoting natriuresis and offsetting the blood pressure effects of sodium, respectively (15).

## Overall Efficacy of DASH Diet

The DASH diet is low in fat, saturated fat, and cholesterol, and is high in fruits, vegetables, and low-fat dairy products. It has been shown to significantly reduce blood pressure both alone and with dietary sodium restriction in overweight and obese individuals. When used in conjunction with other types of lifestyle modification to improve blood pressure, the DASH diet can be effective in promoting weight loss.

## GLYCEMIC INDEX (GI)

The traditional dietary approach to treating the obese patient with CVD is reducing both fat and total energy intake. Because fat is more energy dense than carbohydrate, this approach can be considered beneficial for both CVD and obesity by eliminating unhealthy fats and by decreasing total energy intake, respectively. Pawlak and Ludwig (16) describe the lower rates of obesity in countries with similar per capita dietary fat intake as the United States. While fat intake in the United States has been decreasing over the last 30 years, the incidence of obesity continues to rise. Limitation or attempted elimination of fat intake has led to an increase in carbohydrate intake, particularly refined carbohydrates, starchy foods, and simple sugars (16). This has led to research into the various types of carbohydrates consumed and the effect on obesity, weight loss, and lipid profile.

## Description

The GI was proposed in 1981 by Jenkins et al. (17) as an alternative method to classify carbohydrate-containing foods. This method of classifying carbohydrates grew from the "dietary fiber hypothesis" that was proposed in the late 1970s. This hypothesis suggests that high-fiber foods are absorbed slowly in the intestinal tract, thus offering metabolic benefits including improved postprandial blood glucose and insulin levels. There are also potential cardiovascular benefits associated with the consumption of high-fiber foods. The GI gives a more specific classification of carbohydrates by assigning a numerical value reflecting the postprandial glucose and insulin concentration expected after eating that particular food item (17). The formula to calculate GI is the following: GI = (incremental area under glucose response curve to 50 g carbohydrate from test food/incremental area under glucose response curve to 50 g carbohydrate standard) × 100. A higher GI food will, therefore, produce a greater rise in postprandial glucose and insulin levels compared to a lower GI food (16). The limitation of using the GI of individual foods is that these foods are typically consumed as part of a meal, rather than individually. The glycemic load (GL) can be used to calculate the effect of a mixed meal on blood glucose and insulin levels.

The formula to calculate GL is the following: GL = GI (food, meal, diet) × carbohydrate content (food, meal, diet). The GL can also be used to determine the effect of individual foods that may have a particular macronutrient composition and a different effect on blood glucose and insulin levels than expected based on GI alone (18).

The proposed mechanism of a high-GI intake promoting obesity is based on the metabolic effects of a high-GI meal. Consumption of high-GI foods leads to a significant rise in blood glucose with a subsequent increase in insulin release and inhibition of glucagon production. This imbalance leads to a high insulin-to-glucagon ratio, with the end result of hypoglycemia occurring approximately two to four hours after the high-GI meal. The resulting hypoglycemia leads to hunger and potentially excessive food intake, eventually leading to obesity. A low-GI meal does not lead to these metabolic consequences. This process has been reviewed in detail in a recent article by Ludwig (18).

### Efficacy of the Low-GI Diet

Studies in the adult population do not show dramatic differences in weight loss, lipid levels, or insulin sensitivity when compared to conventional weight-loss diets, but there are improvements in these factors when the study subjects are compared to baseline levels (19–21). The possibility of a high-GI/GL diet contributing to the inflammatory process that is a risk factor for heart disease is an area that certainly warrants more attention and interventional studies. For example, it was proposed that the GI of the diet may contribute to elevated high-sensitivity C-reactive protein (hs-CRP). Lui et al. (22) studied the relationship between diet and hs-CRP. The authors measured hs-CRP concentrations and calculated the dietary GL and overall dietary GI of 244 healthy females. There was a strong association between a high GL and hs-CRP; this response was greater in women with a body mass index (BMI) $\geq 25\,\mathrm{kg/m^2}$.

There are limitations of using the GI in a clinical setting. The GI/GL concept is complex and requires patients to learn a great deal about the GI of specific foods as well as how to calculate the GL. Certain concepts require sophisticated nutritional knowledge, for example, learning that some high-GI foods can fit into an overall low-GI diet as long as these foods are sufficiently low in calories, high in vitamins and minerals, and must be consumed in very large quantities to reach the amount required to induce the high-GI effect (17).

The GI should be considered an educational tool for patients. It can be used to instruct patients on the benefits of selecting less refined carbohydrates to promote glucose control and thus, promote satiety. Given the complexity of learning to implement the low-GI diet, appropriate patient selection will be important to promote success. Future research is important to further assess the benefits associated with following this diet, but practitioners also need to develop educational materials that will make implementation of the low-GI diet achievable for patients of all educational levels.

## PLANT-BASED DIETS: VEGETARIAN AND DR. DEAN ORNISH

There are many components of a vegetarian and plant-based diet that may be beneficial in the treatment of obesity and CVD. When plant foods are substituted for animal foods, there is a reduction in the intake of cholesterol and saturated fat and an increase in the intake of fiber, soluble fiber, antioxidants, and phytochemicals. Of the many plant-based diets, this section will focus on two: the vegetarian diet and Dr. Dean Ornish's Reversal Diet.

### Vegetarian Diets

The term vegetarian refers to a variety of diets that limit or omit some or all animal products. Vegan diets omit all animal and animal-derived foods. Lactovegetarian diets omit all animal and animal-derived foods except for milk and milk products. Lactoovovegetarian diets omit all animal and animal derived foods except for milk, milk products, and eggs (23). Because of these differences among vegetarian diets, they can vary greatly in energy, fat, and cholesterol content. These diets require careful planning as dietary fat, saturated fat, cholesterol (except in vegan diet), and energy content can easily exceed recommended intake levels if nuts, coconut, cooking oils, eggs, butter, cheese, full-fat milk products are frequently and abundantly consumed as part of the vegetarian diet.

Vegetarian diets can be inadequate in protein, so those following this diet should choose beans, lentils, split peas, nuts, and milk or egg products to meet their daily requirements. Eating legumes (e.g., beans and lentils) daily as part of a vegetarian diet may help patients increase their intake of soluble fiber and improve cardiovascular risk and glycemic control (23).

The following nutrients are a possible concern for vegetarians: calcium, zinc, iron, vitamins D and B12, and omega-3 fatty acids. To assure adequate intake of these and other nutrients as well as assure caloric deficit to produce weight loss in the obese patient, all vegetarian diets used to promote weight loss should be designed by a registered dietitian (23).

#### Outcomes with Vegetarian Diets

Vegetarians have a decreased risk of obesity compared to omnivores (i.e., those who eat all foods). In a study (24) of over 55,000 women, women following an omnivorous diet had a significantly higher BMI as well as prevalence of overweight or obesity compared to those following a semivegetarian (defined as lactoovovegetarians who occasionally eat fish), lactovegetarian, or vegan diets. Those following vegetarian eating patterns had significantly lower energy, fat, and protein intake and higher fruit, vegetable, and fiber consumption compared to the omnivorous group. Diets rich in fiber promote satiety, which is a proposed mechanism for the decreased energy intake, leading to the decreased prevalence of overweight and obesity in all of the vegetarian groups.

Vegetarian diets can also have a significant impact on cardiac risk factors. In the Oxford Vegetarian Study, a prospective study of 6000 vegetarians and 5000 nonvegetarian controls in the United Kingdom, subjects following vegan diets had significantly lower TC and LDL-C compared to meat eaters. Subjects following lactovegetarian or lactovegetarian plus fish diets also had lower TC and LDL-C compared to meat eaters, but these levels were not as low as those of the vegans. There were no differences in HDL-C levels (25). The properly designed vegetarian diet is low in saturated fat, promoting desirable lipid levels. In addition, a regular intake of legumes contributes to lowering of blood cholesterol levels through the presence of soluble fiber and isoflavones that may lower blood cholesterol by inhibiting either cholesterol absorption or bile acid reabsorption (23,26). Soy protein ($\geq 25\,g/day$) can also lower cholesterol levels (23). Vegetarians have lower rates of diabetes and hypertension compared to nonvegetarians, further decreasing risk of CVD (23).

## Dr. Dean Ornish's Reversal Diet

Dr. Dean Ornish's Reversal Diet is a modified lactoovovegetarian diet that derives only 10% of its calories from fat. It encourages foods in their natural form, or "whole" foods. Because of the diet's stringent fat restriction, foods that contain even moderate amounts of fat, saturated fat, and/or cholesterol are excluded. Meat, poultry, egg yolks, fish, shellfish, and low-fat or full-fat milk products, nuts, and avocados are omitted. Protein is derived from mostly nonfat sources such as legumes, with the exception of full-fat soybean products (to provide essential fatty acids), egg whites, and nonfat milk products, the latter two being the only animal products allowed. The consumption of processed foods, concentrated sugars, caloric sweeteners, alcohol, caffeine, and refined grain products is discouraged. All oils are excluded with the exception of 3 g/day of flaxseed oil or fish oil to provide omega-3 essential fatty acid. Fruits and vegetables are eaten without restrictions, with an emphasis on dark green leafy vegetables, dark yellow and orange fruits and vegetables, and cruciferous vegetables. Besides dietary changes, Ornish's reversal program includes moderate exercise, daily stress management, such as meditation and stretching exercises, and twice weekly group support sessions (27).

The diet's foundation of soluble-fiber rich foods, such as whole grains, oats, beans, fruits, and vegetables, can be an effective strategy to improve cholesterol and blood glucose levels. The diet is low energy-dense, allowing patients to eat ad libitum and to satisfaction while consuming fewer calories.

## Outcomes with Dr. Dean Ornish's Reversal Diet

Subjects who followed Ornish's reversal program demonstrated significant regression of coronary atherosclerosis, weight loss, and fewer cardiac events than controls following a less restrictive, low-fat diet (28,29). In these studies, HDL-C decreased, but there was clear improvement in coronary atherosclerosis, cardiac perfusion, and cardiac events. In contrast, the control group coronary atherosclerosis progressed and more than twice as many cardiac events occurred.

In a comparison of four popular diets (Atkins, Zone, Weight Watchers, and Ornish), the Ornish diet resulted in a statistically significant weight loss, reduced waist circumference, TC, LDL-C, CRP, and insulin at one year (30).

A comprehensive review of popular diets found that overweight subjects who eat very low fat (10%), high-carbohydrate, high-fiber diets eat fewer calories and lose weight (31). Blood pressure, insulin, and glucose also decrease in most subjects, which may be attributed to dietary changes, exercise, or weight loss.

Very low fat diets that limit meats and other animal proteins may be low in vitamin $B_{12}$, vitamin E, zinc, and other micronutrients found in these foods and may need to be supplemented (23). The Ornish diet is nutritionally adequate for all nutrients except vitamin $B_{12}$ (31).

Although the research is encouraging, questions remain with regard to long-term efficacy and risk reduction. Compliance to such strict dietary and lifestyle regimen may not be easily adopted and maintained, even among motivated individuals. It is also difficult to assess how much effect the stress reduction exercises, group support, and physical activity influenced Ornish's results. For optimal efficacy, patients must adopt not just the diet, but also the lifestyle changes.

## POST–GASTRIC BYPASS DIET

The post–gastric bypass diet is a very specialized LCD that takes into account the anatomic changes as a result of this surgery that may cause significant food intolerance and nutrient deficiencies, as well as the need to limit total energy intake. Food and liquid intake is minimized due to the small size of the stomach following gastric bypass. For this reason it is essential to consume the recommended foods in the correct amounts to prevent vitamin and mineral deficiency.

### Dietary Progression

The recommended progression of the diet after gastric bypass takes place in stages. Rate of advancement is dependent on the discretion of the physician and registered dietitian overseeing the patient as well as patient tolerance. The basic stages of dietary progression are outlined in Table 4 (32). Certain

**Table 4**   Dietary Progression After Gastric Bypass

---

Clear liquids: Water, noncaloric, noncaffeinated, noncarbonated beverages
Full liquids: Liquids containing high biological value protein
Pureed/ground/diced foods: Red meat, poultry, fish, tofu, fruits, and vegetables
Small meals/small snacks: All foods—caution with raw vegetables
Low-fat solids: All foods as tolerated

---

foods are poorly tolerated and close monitoring by a registered dietitian is essential to facilitate appropriate diet progression and minimize food intolerances (33,34).

The proper macronutrient composition of the post–bariatric surgery diet is essential to balanced nutrition. Adequate protein intake is essential after weight-loss surgery and especially after gastric bypass surgery to assist in wound healing, maintain visceral proteins, and help prevent hair loss. Oral protein goals can be estimated by using 1 to 1.5 g/kg ideal body weight (IBW) (35). Sixty grams per day can also be used as an ideal goal and then individualized based on patient needs and diagnostic values (36). Protein sources should be of high biologic value and preferably include foods such as eggs, milk, or meat. Protein–energy malnutrition can be seen after bariatric surgery in patients with dysfunctional eating habits or those with protracted vomiting (37).

Carbohydrates provide energy to the cells in the body, particularly the brain, which is the only carbohydrate-dependent organ in the body. An estimated average requirement for carbohydrate has been established based on the average amount of glucose utilized by the brain. The current recommended dietary allowance for carbohydrate is 130 g/day for adults and children (38). Complex carbohydrates should be recommended over simple carbohydrates after weight-loss surgery because they tend to have greater nutritional value and will not cause dumping syndrome as seen with simple sugars. Dumping syndrome is precipitated by ingestion of high-sugar foods and is caused by rapid emptying of food into the jejunum where the hyperosmolarity of intestinal contents results in an influx of fluid and subsequent distention (34).

The percent of energy that is consumed as fat can vary greatly while still meeting daily energy needs, therefore specific recommendations are not set for adults (35). It is recommended that patients adhere to the American Heart Association guidelines and take in approximately 30% of total calories as fat (39). Small amounts should be included at each meal because larger quantities can trigger dumping syndrome in gastric bypass patients. If the patient demonstrates signs of essential fatty acid deficiency (dry flaky skin and/or hair loss), additional supplementation of essential fatty acids may be necessary.

Adequate hydration can be a challenge after bariatric surgery. On the basis of body weight, obese patients need greater amounts of fluid than their lean counterparts to maintain normal fluid balance (40). The general formula for hydration for these patients is 1 mL/kcal estimated energy expenditure or 30 to 40 mL/kg (41). Typical postoperative bariatric surgery recommendations include drinking no more than eight ounces of fluid per hour, thus, an average of six to nine 8-ounce glasses of fluid per day is an acceptable goal.

Micronutrient deficiencies are most typically observed in patients after bariatric surgeries that involve malabsorption. Vitamin and mineral deficiencies are rarely seen after purely restrictive operations such as the laparoscopic adjustable gastric band. Gastric bypass operations cause weight loss by restricting food intake and by the malabsorption of ingested nutrients. For these reasons, vitamin and mineral deficiencies are relatively common after bariatric surgery. Most often, the duodenum and jejunum are affected by bariatric surgery, explaining the most common vitamin and mineral deficiencies that occur after weight-loss surgery. Iron, folate and vitamin $B_{12}$ deficiencies are most common, although intake of calcium and fat-soluble vitamins are also of concern (42). Consistent multivitamin ingestion is recommended for all gastric bypass patients and frequent laboratory testing is essential in diagnosing and treating vitamin and mineral deficiencies.

## Outcomes Associated with Bariatric Surgery

Chapter 14 reviews the weight and cardiovascular outcomes associated with bariatric surgery.

## VERY LOW-CALORIE DIETS (VLCDs)

A VLCD can be defined as a hypocaloric diet containing less than 800 cal/day or less than 12 kcal/kg of IBW/day (43). This differs from the definition of an LCD that typically contains 800 to 1500 cal/day. VLCDs cannot be defined by caloric content alone; The National Task Force on the prevention and treatment of obesity outlined four other characteristic criteria of VLCDs (43). These additional characteristics are listed in Table 5.

The birth of VLCDs took place in the early 1970s with the introduction of the protein sparing modified fast (PSMF) (43). This diet consisted of 650 to 800 cal/day provided by protein foods of high biologic value with additional supplementation of multivitamins, potassium and calcium (44). Generally protein was administered at a level of 1.5 g/kg of IBW and was typically obtained from lean meat, fish and fowl while carbohydrate ingestion was prohibited (43,44). Proponents of the PSMF argue that the diet teaches patients to successfully handle conventional foods and facilitates a smooth transition from the reducing diet to a maintenance diet consisting of conventional foods (44).

**Table 5**  National Task Force on the Prevention and Treatment of Obesity Characteristics of VLCDs

---

VLCDs are hypocaloric but are relatively enriched in protein (0.8–1.5 g/kg IBW/ day). Generally a minimum protein content of 50 g/day

VLCDs are designed to include the full complement of the recommended daily allowance for vitamins, minerals, electrolytes and fatty acids, but not for calories

VLCDs are given in a form that completely replaces usual food intake. The most common forms are liquid formulations. Food based on PSMFs are also used and considered VLCDs

VLCDs are usually given for a prolonged period, usually 12–16 weeks

---

*Abbreviations*: IBW, ideal body weight; PSMF, protein sparing modified fast; VLCD, very low calorie diets.
*Source*: From Ref. 2.

The mechanism of action of the PSMF requires review of carbohydrate metabolism and fatty acid utilization in the body. During starvation or periods of very low carbohydrate intake, ketone bodies serve as an alternative oxidative fuel for peripheral tissues to spare carbohydrate and protein. Adherence to a very low carbohydrate diet mimics starvation such that fatty acid catabolism is increased and fatty acid synthesis is depressed. The increase in fatty acid catabolism causes nonesterified fatty acids (NEFA) to be released into the blood in large quantities. When the NEFA levels increase, the malonyl CoA levels drop, allowing NEFA to more readily enter the mitochondria and be metabolized. As a result, the liver is provided with more acetyl CoA than it can use for its own energy needs. The liver converts this excess acetyl CoA into ketone bodies. The brain is unable to use NEFA for its energy needs due to the blood brain barrier, but the brain can readily use ketone bodies. In prolonged starvation, the brain may obtain as much as 30% to 40% of its energy needs from ketone bodies (45).

Today the PSMF has re-evolved using higher fat protein sources such as those recommended in the Atkins diet. A review of the Atkins diet and other low-carbohydrate diets can be found in Chapter 10.

The late 1970s brought the liquid VLCD to the forefront. These preparations were initially made largely from collagen and thus contained proteins of low biologic value. This diet led to reports of ventricular dysrhythmias and sudden death and prompted a formal investigation by the Public Health Service (43). Today, liquid VLCD regimens typically consist of an egg-based or a milk-based protein. The typical product provides 45 to 100 g/day of high biologic value protein and up to 100 g/day of carbohydrate (43). VLCDs use vitamin and mineral supplements to meet recommended daily intakes. Extensive evaluation of patients utilizing the "modern" VLCDs for 16 weeks or less has not shown an increased incidence for cardiac ventricular dysrhythmias or prolongation of the QT interval (46). Patients who are eligible for VLCD diet programs should exceed desirable body weights by 30 pounds or have a BMI of $\geq 30 \, \text{kg/m}^2$ (47).

The mechanism of action for VLCDs is initially based on fluid loss and then energy deficit. Several mechanisms of action promote fluid loss early in a VLCD. Insulin, which causes sodium retention by the kidney, decreases and the natriuretic hormone glucagon increases. Also, the increased excretion of ketones will lead to extra sodium and potassium loss together with water. Once a new mineral balance is achieved, weight loss is dependent on the energy deficit compensated by the release of fatty acids as energy substrate from the fat stores. Under these conditions the lean body mass loss is at a fixed level of about 25% (46).

## Weight Loss with VLCDs

The primary benefit of VLCDs is that they can produce large weight losses within a 12 to 24 week period (43). They are often chosen by patients for their ease in preparation and the limiting of daily food choices. The National Task Force on the Prevention and Treatment of Obesity provided an overview of the published scientific information on the efficacy and safety of VLCDs (43). It was found that a VLCD resulted in an average loss of 1.5 to 2.0 kg/wk in women and 2.0 to 2.5 kg/wk in men with average losses of 20 kg over 12 weeks. This was accompanied by an attrition rate of approximately 15%.

When compared to LCDs, it was found that VLCDs produce larger initial weight losses than LCDs, especially when combined with behavioral therapy. However, long-term maintenance of weight loss with both forms of dietary therapy is relatively poor. While long-term weight loss is slightly improved with behavioral therapy and exercise, it is not clear whether VLCDs provide a better long-term response than LCDs with the same behavioral and exercise training (43).

## Effect of VLCDs on Serum Lipids

The effect of VLCDs on lipid levels is of significant clinical interest. TC, LDL-C, and TG all decrease with VLCD treatment. Serum cholesterol has been shown to decrease to its lowest point at four to six weeks after beginning the VLCD. For morbidly obese subjects, TC decreased at a rate of 0.07 mmol/kg/m$^2$ decrease in BMI ($P < 0.001$) (47). This has also been identified as a 5% to 25% decrease over the first four to six weeks of the VLCD (43).

Serum TG levels have been shown to decrease approximately 15% to as much as 50% during VLCD treatment, depending on initial levels. Serum TG values decrease to their lowest point by two weeks and remain low for the duration of the weight-loss phase. Decreases in TG are significantly correlated ($P < 0.001$) with baseline values and changes in BMI, after adjustment for baseline values (47).

The response of HDL-C to the VLCD is uncertain. Some studies have shown decreases similar to that of TC over the short term while other studies have shown long-term increases (43). Anderson et al. (47) noted a biphasic serum HDL-C response in obese women with HDL-C decreasing initially, but returning to prediet levels by the 12th week of VLCD treatment.

### Effect of VLCDs on Blood Pressure

Hypertension can be controlled by maintaining a healthy weight, being physically active, and following an eating plan that is lower in sodium. During typical VLCDs, blood pressure in hypertensive patients will decrease by 8% to 13% (43). Systolic blood pressure decreases approximately 8% to 12% and diastolic blood pressure decreases 9% to 13% (47).

### Effect of VLCDs on Glucose Control

VLCDs show promising results in glycemic control for both normoglycemic and hyperglycemic individuals. Type II diabetics have shown a decrease of 38% to 58% in serum glucose as well as decreases in hemoglobin $A_{1C}$ and urinary C-peptide levels following VLCD treatment (47). The long-term effects on glycemic control are largely unknown. Wing et al. (48) found that one year after diabetic women underwent eight weeks of a VLCD, fasting blood glucose and hemoglobin $A_{1C}$ levels were significantly improved compared with women who underwent eight weeks of a balanced LCD, despite the fact that both groups regained similar amounts of weight. There is speculation that the VLCD improves insulin secretion, possibly due to beta cell restoration while following the diet (43).

Insulin resistance is an evolving cardiovascular risk factor in the United States, today. This situation has evolved with the marked increase in the number of individuals diagnosed with type 2 diabetes mellitus and a dramatic increase in obesity (49). The ATP III of the NCEP has defined criteria for the identification of the metabolic syndrome as a clustering of cardiovascular risk factors that are closely associated with insulin resistance, and it is estimated that 57 million adults in the United States meet these criteria (4). The metabolic syndrome is reviewed in detail in Chapter 3. Case et al. (49) found in patients using a VLCD that a weight loss of 6.5% of initial body weight in individuals with the metabolic syndrome resulted in substantial reductions in systolic (11 mmHg) and diastolic (6 mmHg) blood pressure, glucose (17 mg/dL), TG (94 mg/dL), and TC (37 mg/dL) after four weeks. Further strategies to identify these individuals should be undertaken, because those with the metabolic syndrome would benefit most from a medically supervised weight-loss program (49).

## Special Considerations for Monitoring

Any patient considering a VLCD should undergo a complete medical evaluation prior to beginning the VLCD. The evaluation should include a comprehensive medical history and physical examination, as well as an obesity-specific component determining weight history, dietary intake, and degree of medical risk posed by obesity (43). Initial laboratory measurements should include a complete blood count, comprehensive metabolic panel, urinalysis, and thyroid function test (47). An electrocardiogram should also be obtained to seek evidence of abnormal cardiac function, dysrhythmias, or prolonged QT interval (43,47). For women of childbearing age, a pregnancy test should also be performed because VLCDs are not recommended for women who are pregnant. Certain medical conditions (Table 6) are considered contraindications for VLCD use (43). Limited information is available regarding the medical monitoring during a VLCD. At a minimum, all patients should have weight, pulse, and blood pressure assessed every one to two weeks during the course of the modified fast and during refeeding. It is also prudent to check serum electrolyte levels during the first two weeks of the VLCD when initial diuresis would be most likely to produce abnormalities (43).

Patients utilizing a VLCD may experience some common short-term symptoms. Some of these include fatigue, weakness, dizziness, constipation, diarrhea, nausea, headache, and cold intolerance (47). Most of these can be treated by dietary adjustments such as increasing fluid intake, increasing caloric consumption, and/or increasing fiber intake. Side effects such as hair loss, dry skin, brittle nails, menstrual irregularities, and peroneal neuropathy may subside with refeeding to maintenance calories (47). The development of gallstones during VLCD is of concern because 10% to 25% of

**Table 6**  Contraindications for VLCDs

| |
|---|
| Systemic infections or diseases leading to protein wasting |
| Certain types of cardiac disease |
|    Unstable angina |
|    Recent myocardial infarction |
|    Malignant dysrhythmias |
| Recent or recurrent cerebrovascular accident |
| Transient ischemic attacks |
| Renal disease |
| Hepatic disease |
| Certain psychiatric disorders |
|    Bulimia nervosa |
|    Anorexia nervosa |
|    Recent alcohol and/or drug abuse |

*Abbreviation*: VLCDs, very low caloric diets.

persons following a VLCD can develop this complication. Ursodeoxycholic acid is highly effective in preventing gallstone formation in patients having dietary-induced weight reduction (50).

## CONCLUSION

As the rate of obesity continues to increase worldwide, the number of approaches to control obesity and its adverse effects will also continue to rise. The American Dietetic Association reports that People in the United States spend $30 billion annually on weight-loss foods, products, and services (51). For this reason, it is essential that health care providers understand basic dietary approaches, such as those described above, to achieve weight loss. This understanding will help patients achieve the best possible outcome for their health and overall lifestyle. When considering any weight-loss regimen for a patient, always start by encouraging healthy lifestyle behaviors coupled with smaller food portion size and regular physical activity. Encourage all patients to make healthy eating a part of their daily routine. Restricting specific foods or entire food groups in the name of weight loss may actually lead to long-term health problems rather than producing a long-term solution to obesity. Consultation with a registered dietitian will ensure that patients receive safe, effective, evidence-based approaches to weight management.

## REFERENCES

1. About the National Heart, Lung, and Blood Institute: National Cholesterol Education Program. http://www.nhlbi.nih.gov/about/ncep/ (accessed 6/9/2005).
2. National Cholesterol Education Program. High blood cholesterol in adults: report of the expert panel on detection, evaluation, and treatment. NIH Pub. No. 88–2925. Bethesda, MD: National Heart, Lung, and Blood Institute, 1988.
3. National Cholesterol Education Program. Second report of the expert panel on detection, evaluation, and treatment of high blood cholesterol in adults. NIH Pub. No. 93–3095. Bethesda, MD: National Heart, Lung, and Blood Institute, 1993.
4. National Cholesterol Education Program. Third report of the expert panel on detection, evaluation, and treatment of high blood cholesterol in adults. NIH Pub. No. 02–5215. Bethesda, MD: National Heart, Lung, and Blood Institute, 2002.
5. Lichtenstein AH, Ausman LM, Jalbert SM et al. Efficacy of a Therapeutic Lifestyle Change/Step 2 diet in moderately hypercholesterolemic middle-aged and elderly female and male subjects. J Lipid Res 2002; 43:264–273.
6. Aude YW, Agatston AS, Lopez-Jimenez, et al. The national cholesterol education program diet vs. a diet lower in carbohydrates and higher in protein and monounsaturated fat: a randomized trial. Arch Intern Med 2004; 164: 2141–2146.

7.  Appel LJ, Moore TJ, Obarzanek E, et al. A clinical trial of the effects of dietary patterns on blood pressure. DASH Collaborative Research Group. N Engl J Med 1997; 336:1117–1124.
8.  National Heart, Lung, and Blood Institute. Facts about the DASH eating plan. NIH Pub. No. 03–4082. Bethesda, MD: National Heart, Lung, and Blood Institute, 2003.
9.  Miller 3rd ER, Erlinger TP, Young DR, et al. Results of the Diet, Exercise, and Weight Loss Intervention Trial (DEW-IT). Hypertension 2002; 40:612–618.
10. Writing Group of the PREMIER Collaborative Research Group. Effects of comprehensive lifestyle modification on blood pressure control: main results of the PREMIER clinical trial. JAMA 2003; 289:2083–2093.
11. Obarzanek E, Sacks FM, Vollmer WM, et al. Effects on blood lipids of a blood pressure-lowering diet: the Dietary Approaches to Stop Hypertension (DASH) Trial. Am J Clin Nutr 2001; 74:80–89.
12. Moore TJ, Vollmer WM, Appel LJ, et al. Effect of dietary patterns on ambulatory blood pressure: results from the Dietary Approaches to Stop Hypertension (DASH) Trial. DASH Collaborative Research Group. Hypertension 1999; 34:472–477.
13. Lopes HF, Martin KL, Nashar K, Morrow JD, Goodfriend TL, Egan BM. DASH diet lowers blood pressure and lipid-induced oxidative stress in obesity. Hypertension 2003; 41:422–430.
14. Sacks FM, Svetkey LP, Vollmer WM, et al. Effects on blood pressure of reduced dietary sodium and the Dietary Approaches to Stop Hypertension (DASH) diet. N Engl J Med 2001; 344:3–10.
15. Akita S, Sacks FM, Svetkey LP, Conlin, Kimura G. DASH-Sodium Trial Collaborative Research Group. Effects of the Dietary Approaches to Stop Hypertension (DASH) diet on the pressure-natriuresis relationship. Hypertension 2003; 42:8–13.
16. Pawlak DB, Ebbeling CB, Ludwig DS. Should obese patients be counselled to follow a low-glycaemic index diet? Yes. Obesity Rev 2002; 3:235–243.
17. Jenkins DJA, Kendall CWC, Augustin LSA, et al. Glycemic index: overview of implications in health and disease. Am J Clin Nutr 2002; 76:266S–273S.
18. Ludwig DS. The glycemic index: physiological mechanisms relating to obesity, diabetes, and cardiovascular disease. JAMA 2002; 287:2414–2423.
19. Bouché C, Rizkalla SW, Luo J, et al. Five-week, low-glycemic index diet decreases total fat mass and improves plasma lipid profile in moderately overweight nondiabetic men. Diabetes Care 2002; 25:822–828.
20. Sloth B, Krog-Mikkelsen I, Flint A, et al. No difference in body weight decrease between a low-glycemic-index and a high-glycemic-index diet but reduced LDL cholesterol after 10-wk ad libitum intake of the low-glycemic-index diet. Am J Clin Nutr 2004; 80:331–347.
21. Ebbeling CB, Leidig MM, Sinclair KB, Seger-Shippee LG, Feldman HA, Ludwig DS. Effects of an ad libitum low-glycemic load diet on cardiovascular disease risk factors in obese young adults. Am J Clin Nutr 2005; 81:976–982.
22. Liu S, Manson JE, Buring JE, Stampfer MJ, Willett WC, Ridker PM. Relation between a diet with a high glycemic load and plasma concentrations of

high-sensitivity C-reactive protein in middle-aged women. Am J Clin Nutr 2002; 75:492–498.

23. Position of the American Dietetic Association and Dietitians of Canada: Vegetarian diets. J Am Diet Assoc 2003; 103:748–765.

24. Newby PK, Tucker LK, Wolk A. Risk of overweight and obesity among semivegetarian, lactovegetarian, and vegan women. Am J Clin Nutr 2005; 81: 1267–1274.

25. Appleby PN, Thorogood M, Mann JI, Key TJA. The Oxford Vegetarian Study: an overview. Am J Clin Nutr 1999; 70(suppl 1):525S–531S.

26. Leterme P. Recommendations by health organizations for pulse consumption. Br J Nutr 2002; 88(suppl 3):S239–S242.

27. Ornish D. Dr Dean Ornish's Program for Reversing Heart Disease. New York: Ballantine Books 1990.

28. Ornish D, Brown SE, Scherwitz LW, et al. Can lifestyle changes reverse coronary heart disease? The Lifestyle Heart Trial. Lancet 1990; 336:129–133.

29. Ornish D. Scherwitz LW, Billings JH, et al. Intensive lifestyle changes for reversal of coronary heart disease. JAMA 1998; 280:2001–2007.

30. Dansinger ML, Gleason JA, Griffith JL, Selker HP, Schaefer EJ. Comparison of the Atkins, Ornish, Weight Watchers, and Zone diets for weight loss and heart disease risk reduction: a randomized trial. JAMA 2005; 293:43–53.

31. Freedman MR, King J, Kennedy E. Popular diets: a scientific review. Obesity Res 2001; 9(suppl 1):1S–40S.

32. Saltzman E, Anderson W, Apovian CM, et al. Criteria for patient selection and multidisciplinary evaluation and treatment of the weight loss surgery patient. Obes Res 2005; 13:234–243 (includes online appendix).

33. Elliot K. Nutritional considerations after bariatric surgery. Crit Care Nursing Quart 2003; 26:133–138.

34. Collene AL, Hertzler SH. Metabolic outcomes of gastric bypass. Nutr Clin Pract 2003; 18:136–140.

35. Moize V, Gelicbter A, Gluck ME, et al. Obese patients have inadequate protein intake related to protein intolerance up to 1 year following Roux-en-Y gastric bypass. Obes Surg 2003; 13:23–28.

36. Marcason W. What are the dietary guidelines following bariatric surgery? J Am Diet Assoc 2004; 104:487–488.

37. Kim JJ, Tarnoff ME, Shikora SA. Surgical treatment for extreme obesity: evolution of a rapidly growing field. Nutr Clin Pract 2003; 18:109–123.

38. Institute of Medicine. Dietary Reference Intakes for Macronutrients. Washington DC: National Academies Press 2002.

39. Lichtenstein AH, Van Horn L. Very low fat diets. Circulation 1998; 98: 935–939.

40. Marotta RB, Floch MH. Diet and nutrition in ulcer disease. Med Clin North Am 1991; 75:967–979.

41. Whitmire SJ. Fluid and Electrolytes. In: Gottschlich MM, Fuhrman MP, Hammond KA, Holcombe BJ, Seidner DL, eds. The Science and Practice of Nutrition Support: A Case-Based Core Curriculum. Dubquqe, Iowa: Kendall/Hunt Publishing Company, 2001:56.

42. Stocker DJ. Management of the bariatric surgery patient. Endocrinol Metab Clin North Am 2003; 32:437–457.
43. National Task Force on the Prevention and Treatment of Obesity, National Institutes of Health. Very low-calorie diets. JAMA 1993; 270:967–974.
44. Wadden TA, Stunkard AJ, Brownell KD, Day SC. A comparison of two very-low-calorie diets: protein-sparing-modified fast versus protein-formula-liquid diet. Am J Clin Nutr 1985; 41:533–539.
45. Zeman FJ, Hansen RJ. Diabetes Mellitus, Hypoglycemia, and Other Endocrine Disorders. In: Zeman FJ, ed. Clinical Nutrition and Dietetics. 2nd ed. New York: Macmillan Publishing Company, 1991:408–409.
46. Saris WHM. Very-low-calorie diets and sustained weight loss. Obes Res 2001; 9(suppl 4):295S–301S.
47. Anderson JW, Hamilton CC, Brinkman-Kaplan V. Benefits and risks of an intensive very-low-calorie diet program for severe obesity. Am J Gastroenterol 1992; 87:6–15.
48. Wing RR, Marcus MD, Salata R, Epstein LH, Miaskiewicz S, Blair EH. Effects of a very-low-calorie diet on long-term glycemic control in obese type 2 diabetic subjects. Arch Intern Med 1991; 151:1334–1340.
49. Case CC, Jones PH, Nelson K, O'Brian Smith E, Ballantyne CM. Impact of weight loss on the metabolic syndrome. Diabetes Obesity Metab 2002; 4:407–414.
50. Shiffman ML, Kaplan GD, Brinkman-Kaplan V, Vickers FF. Prophylaxis against gallstone formation with ursodeoxycholic acid in patients participating in a very-low-calorie diet program. Ann Intern Med 1995; 122:899–905.
51. Position of the American Dietetic Association: Weight management. J Am Diet Assoc 2002; 102:1145–1155.

# 12

# Lifestyle Modification in the Obese Patient with Cardiovascular Disease

**Rena R. Wing**

*The Miriam Hospital/Brown Medical School, Providence, Rhode Island, U.S.A.*

**Douglas A. Raynor**

*The State University of New York, Geneseo, New York, U.S.A.*

## INTRODUCTION

Lifestyle intervention has the potential to be extremely effective in the prevention and treatment of cardiovascular disease (CVD) in overweight and obese patients. However, unfortunately, physicians often miss the opportunity or may be unaware of effective strategies to help their patients with weight control (1). The purpose of this chapter is to try to improve this situation by identifying key lifestyle approaches that may be beneficial for overweight patients with CVD.

## EVIDENCE THAT LIFESTYLE MODIFICATION CAN PRODUCE IMPORTANT HEALTH BENEFITS

Fewer than half of obese patients report that their physician has advised them to lose weight (1). This reluctance on the part of the physician may originate from concerns about the futility of weight loss—that few patients are successful at long-term weight reduction or that modest weight losses may not be effective in improving health. In fact, there is now evidence to dispel both of these beliefs.

There are many good examples of the benefits of lifestyle intervention in the treatment and prevention of disease (2–5). Of particular note is the Diabetes Prevention Program (DPP) (3), a multicenter study testing whether lifestyle intervention or metformin could prevent or delay the development of type 2 diabetes in those at a high risk for this disease. The study randomly assigned 3234 individuals [mean age = 51; mean body mass index (BMI) = 34; 68% were women; 45% were members of minority groups] to placebo, metformin, or lifestyle intervention. The lifestyle intervention was designed to achieve a 7% or greater weight loss and at least 150 minutes/wk of physical activity, using activities similar in intensity to brisk walking. To accomplish these goals, participants were assigned a "case manager" who met with them individually, with weekly contacts for the first 16–24 weeks and then in-person meetings at least once every two months (on average monthly). Participants and their case managers completed a 16-session core curriculum that provided education regarding diet, exercise, and behavior modification. Participants were given a fat gram goal, designed to reduce their fat intake to 25% of calories; if weight loss was not achieved by lowering fat alone, a calorie goal was also introduced. The emphasis of the physical activity intervention was on brisk walking, but other activities of similar intensity could also be applied to achieving the goal.

Weight loss in the lifestyle intervention averaged 7 kg at six months; these weight losses were maintained from 6 to 12 months, but then participants gradually regained to a weight loss of approximately 4 kg at three years (Fig. 1). Fifty percent of participants achieved the 7% weight-loss goal at week 24 and 38% achieved the goal at their final visit (at study end). Based on self-report logs, 74% met the 150-minute activity goal at week 24 and 58 % at the final visit. On average, participants reported 225 minutes of activity at both time points.

The weight losses and activity levels achieved in DPP are in fact modest, but they produced dramatic effects on the risk of developing diabetes. DPP was stopped early (after an average of 2.8 years of follow-up) because the results were clear. The incidence of diabetes in the trial was 11.0, 7.8, and 4.8 cases per 100 person-years in the placebo, metformin,

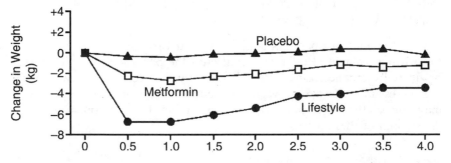

**Figure 1**  Weight losses of participants in the DPP. *Abbreviation*: DPP, Diabetes Prevention Program. *Source*: From Ref. 3.

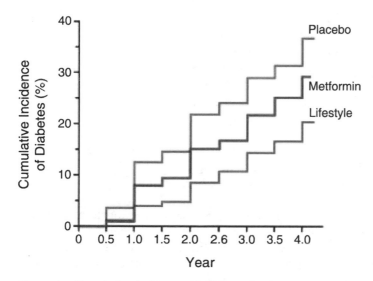

**Figure 2** Cumulative incidence of diabetes in the DPP according to study group. *Abbreviation*: DPP, Diabetes Prevention Program. *Source*: From Ref. 3.

and lifestyle groups, respectively. The lifestyle intervention reduced the risk of diabetes by 58% compared to placebo; metformin reduced the risk by 31%. Thus the lifestyle intervention was twice as effective as metformin (Fig. 2).

DPP focused on preventing diabetes, which in the long term should also help to delay the onset of CVD. However, there are also good examples of the benefits of lifestyle intervention in those who already have CVD. For example, Ornish et al. (6) randomly assigned 28 patients with angiographically documented coronary heart disease to a very intensive lifestyle program (including a low fat vegetarian diet, smoking cessation, stress management, and exercise) or to usual-care control. Over the year-long program, those in the lifestyle group had a 10 kg weight loss versus a 1.4 kg gain in controls ($P < 0.0001$); their exercise increased from 11 to 38 minutes/day, while it remained at about 20 minutes in controls, and their fat intake decreased from 31.5% to 6.8% of calories, while fat intake remained at approximately 30% in controls. These major lifestyle changes produced decreases in all of the CVD risk factors studied, and more importantly regression of coronary atherosclerosis as measured by quantitative coronary arteriography. Clearly, not all patients would be willing or motivated to make such drastic lifestyle changes, but when they do occur, the health benefits can be dramatic.

## EVIDENCE THAT LIFESTYLE CHANGES CAN PRODUCE LONG-TERM MAINTENANCE OF WEIGHT LOSS: THE NWCR

Another concern often raised is that "no one ever succeeds at weight loss." To counter this belief and learn about the strategies associated with successful long-term weight-loss maintenance, Wing and Hill established the National Weight Control Registry (NWCR) (7,8). For entry into the registry, the criteria is that one should have lost at least 30 lb and should have maintained it for at least one year. There are now over 4000 individuals in the registry (80% women and 97% Caucasian), and they far exceed the minimum criteria. On average, registry members have lost 60 lb (reducing from a BMI of 35 to 25) and have kept it off almost six years. Thus they are clearly successful by any criterion one would suggest. Members of the registry have been identified by newspaper and magazine articles describing findings from the registry and encouraging others to join. Thus findings from the registry may not generalize to the broader population of successful weight losers.

Registry members note that they have tried to lose weight many times in the past unsuccessfully (7). This finding should be encouraging to overweight persons who have tried to lose weight, because it suggests that they too may be successful on their next attempt. Registry members indicate that what distinguished this effort from prior efforts was greater commitment to behavior change and weight loss, stricter dieting, and a greater emphasis on physical activity.

Registry members report using many different approaches to achieve this successful weight loss. Almost all participants (89%) indicated that their successful weight loss experience involved the combination of diet plus physical activity. About half used some type of formal weight-loss program or received some professional assistance with their weight loss; the other half did it entirely on their own. Common diet strategies included restricting intake of certain types of foods (88%), limiting quantity of food (44%), and counting calories (44%).

Whereas there is marked variability in the approaches used for weight loss, there is more similarity in the approaches used to maintain the weight loss. Maintenance strategies include eating a low-calorie, low-fat diet; having high levels of physical activity; and regularly monitoring body weight.

At entry into the registry participants complete the Block Food Frequency Questionnaire (9) to describe what they are currently eating to maintain their weight loss. Participants report consuming 1381 kcal/day, with 24% of calories from fat, 19% from protein, and 56% from carbohydrates (7). Because food-frequency questionnaires typically underestimate calorie intake by approximately 30% (10), we estimate that registry members are probably consuming approximately 1800 kcal/day. Very few registry members report maintaining their weight loss with a low carbohydrate intake (11). Defining low carbohydrate as less than 24% carbohydrate (this would be equivalent to consuming 90 g or less of carbohydrate on a 1500 kcal diet), we found that less than 1% of registry members are maintaining their weight with a low-carbohydrate approach.

Recently we reported that 78% of registry participants consume breakfast everyday of the week, whereas only 4% report never consuming breakfast (12). The most common breakfast appears to be cereal and fruit; 60% say they have cereal for breakfast usually/often and 55% say they usually/often have fruit.

Another common strategy for weight-loss maintenance is frequent monitoring of body weight. Over 44% of registry members report weighing themselves at least daily and an additional 31% report weighing themselves at least once a week. We believe that frequent weighing may allow successful weight losers to make quick adjustments if increases in body weight are observed.

Finally, the third distinctive characteristic of registry members is their high level of physical activity. Participants in the registry completed the Paffenberger Physical Activity Questionnaire (13); women reported an average of 2545 kcal/wk of physical activity and men reported 3293 kcal/wk (8). This would be equivalent to walking about 25 to 30 miles/wk and would equal about an hour of physical activity per day. Thus this level far exceeds the public health recommendation to accumulate at least 30 minutes of activity on 5 days/wk (14).

Over 90% of registry members report doing physical activity as part of their weight-maintenance regimen; most (49%) report a combination of walking plus other activities; 28% report just walking; and 14% report only other types of activities. Common activities include cycling, weight lifting, and aerobics.

An important finding of particular relevance to health professionals working with CVDs is that medical triggers are a common and effective source of motivation for successful weight-loss maintainers. When asked about the events that triggered their successful weight-loss effort, 22.9% of NWCR members report a medical trigger (e.g., "doctor told me to lose weight, family member had a heart attack"). These individuals had significantly larger weight losses than those with nonmedical triggers or those reporting no trigger (mean weight loss of 36.4 and 31.9 kg, respectively). Moreover, when followed prospectively over two years, those with medical triggers regained less weight than those with nonmedical or no triggers (15).

## DESCRIPTION OF BEHAVIORAL TREATMENT PROGRAM FOR OBESITY

Given the benefits of lifestyle intervention for the treatment and prevention of disease, it is important that clinicians have an understanding of these approaches. The following section provides an overview of basic behavioral approaches and their results. For more detailed information, one is referred to the Handbook of Obesity Treatment (16) and the Handbook of Obesity: Clinical Applications (17). The LEARN Manual (18) provides a self-help behavioral weight-loss program for use by overweight patients.

## Overview of the Program

Lifestyle interventions are designed to help individuals change their diet and physical activity behaviors, and maintain these new behaviors long term. Growing out of learning theory (19,20), these programs assume (a) that changing diet and exercise behaviors will change energy balance and thereby produce weight loss and (b) that to change eating and exercise behaviors, it is important to change the environmental antecedents (cues) and consequences (reinforcers) that influence these behaviors.

Typically, behavioral programs are offered in a group format, with weekly lessons for six months and then biweekly or monthly meetings throughout the next year. Group sizes vary from 10 to 20. A group of participants begin the program together and stay together over time (closed group format), in contrast to the approach used by many commercial weight-loss programs. Therapists are usually trained in nutrition, exercise physiology, or clinical psychology, and in some programs a team of therapists with these different backgrounds may be used. Each lesson begins with a private weigh-in and a brief review of the self-monitoring records; the group meeting then includes a review of the prior lesson and presentation of a new topic for the day. Discussion about the topic is encouraged and participants share their own personal experiences relevant to the topic. Homework may be assigned to allow participants to practice the skills they have learned.

Key strategies incorporated in behavioral programs include the following:

**Self-monitoring:**   Patients in behavioral weight-loss programs are asked to record (self-monitor) all of the foods they eat or drink, the calories and fat grams in those foods, and their level of physical activity. Such self-monitoring is designed to make patients aware of their current behaviors and allows them to see small changes as they occur. For example, patients may see that they are consuming most of their calories in the evening after dinner and thus target this area for change. Others might be made aware of their frequent restaurant visits and the calories consumed in those eating episodes. Patients are typically asked to record their dietary intake every week for the first six months of the program and then at least one week/mo after that. Physical activity can be recorded in minutes, in calories, or by counting steps with a pedometer. Recording of physical activity is often continued on monthly calendars throughout the entire program. Several studies (21,22) have suggested that self-monitoring is the single most important strategy for initial and long-term behavior change.

**Goal setting:**   As soon as patients start to self-monitor, they want to know what goals they are trying to achieve. Short-term goals that can be attained by the participant are stressed (23). Behavioral weight-loss programs typically use a weight-loss goal of 1 to 2 lb/week. To accomplish this, patients are instructed to reduce calories by approximately 1000 kcal/day. In most behavioral programs, patients weighing less than 200 lb are encouraged to eat 1200 to 1500 kcal/day and those over 200 lb to eat 1500 to 1800 kcal/day. Many programs also assign a fat gram goal, designed to produce a 20% to 30% fat diet. Physical activity goals are increased gradually as patients become more fit, with an eventual goal of 150 to 200 minutes/wk of activity or 1000 to 2000 kcal/wk.

**Stimulus control:** A key premise of behavioral approaches is that antecedents or cues in the environment are important determinants of behavior. Thus to change behavior, it is important to change these cues. The goal is to increase cues for the behaviors being encouraged and decrease the cues for inappropriate behavior. For example, high-calorie, ready-to-eat foods that are out in the kitchen or stored in the refrigerator may cause patients to overeat; thus patients are taught to remove these cues from their homes and to increase cues for healthy eating (keeping fresh vegetables readily accessible). The same is true for physical activity; again, patients are encouraged to increase the cues for healthy behaviors (keep sneakers by the door) and to minimize cues for sedentary behaviors (reduce the number of television sets in the home).

**Cognitive restructuring:** The cues for inappropriate eating and sedentary behaviors extend beyond physical cues to social and cognitive cues. Patients often talk to themselves with statements such as "I've had a hard day; I deserve a treat." Such statements, including excuses, rationalizations, and negative comparisons with others, may then lead to overeating. Behavioral programs teach participants to recognize that they are having these negative thoughts, to try to understand the function they are serving, and to counter these thoughts with more positive ones (24).

**Social support:** Several studies have suggested that group programs produce better weight losses than individual programs (25). They are also clearly more cost effective. Consequently most lifestyle intervention programs are conducted in group settings, and patients are taught to use the other members of the group for support in changing their behaviors (26). Also, as part of the program, participants learn strategies to deal with family members and coworkers who may try to sabotage their efforts or nag them when inappropriate behaviors occur.

**Problem solving:** Patients in behavioral weight-loss programs are helped to identify the barriers that get in their way of adopting new healthier behaviors. They then use problem-solving techniques (27) to brainstorm solutions to these barriers and select an approach to try to see if they can overcome or reduce the barrier. Because patients present with different problems, these techniques allow individualization of the program within the context of a group meeting.

**Relapse prevention:**   Based on Marlatt and Gordon's theory of relapse prevention (28,29), patients are taught that lapses are inevitable. Given this, the important skills are to anticipate such lapses, recognize the situations in which they are likely to occur, and plan strategies that will allow the patient to deal effectively with the lapse. The goal is to keep lapses from leading to relapses.

### Results Obtained in Behavioral Weight-Loss Programs

Wing et al. (30) recently reviewed 12 behavioral weight-loss studies published from 1990 to 2000. Because many of these studies compared a variety of different approaches to weight loss, one treatment condition was selected from each study. In studies comparing a low-calorie diet (LCD) versus a very low calorie diet (VLCD), the low calorie group was selected because this more accurately reflects the usual behavioral program. Similarly, treatment groups that included diet plus aerobic exercise were selected because this is the recommended approach. In other studies, the most successful condition was selected; thus this review is highly selective and would overestimate the average effects of behavioral programs. Keeping these limitations in mind, the results (Table 1 and Fig. 3) are interesting to consider. At six months, weight losses averaged 10.4 kg (or 11% of initial body weight). As seen from the figure, most studies cluster around this 10 kg level (the two exceptions have 3–4 month treatments rather than the typical six months). Results are well maintained from 6 to 12 months and then patients begin to regain weight. The seven studies with 18-month data reported a mean weight loss of 8.2 kg at this time. Only two studies had 24-month data; average weight loss was 7.1 kg at 24 months; and none of the studies extended beyond two years. Thus, in the strongest behavioral programs, participants achieve a weight loss of approximately 10% and maintain a

**Table 1**   Summary of Results of Selected Behavioral Weight-Loss Trials, 1990–2000

| | |
|---|---|
| Number of treatment trials | 12 |
| Initial treatment | |
|     Duration (mo) | 5.6 mo |
|     Weight loss (kg) | 10.4 kg |
| Final follow-up | |
|     Duration (mo) | 17.6 mo |
|     Weight loss (kg) | 8.1 kg |
| % of initial weight loss retained | 82% |

*Source*: From Ref. 30.

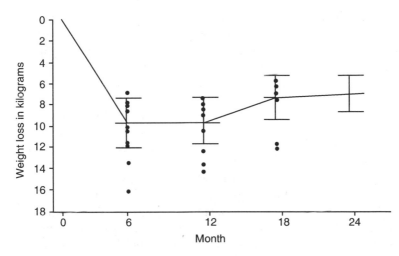

**Figure 3**   Results of selected behavioral weight-loss programs, 1990–2000. *Source*: From Ref. 30.

weight loss of 7% at two years. Although modest, DPP (3) and other studies (2,5) show that such weight losses can have dramatic health benefits.

## Predictors of Outcome

One of the striking findings in behavioral weight-loss programs is the variability in weight-loss outcomes, especially at 12 or 18 months. The standard deviation for weight loss at 18 months is typically 5 to 8 kg (31–33). Thus, some patients do very well in behavioral weight-loss programs, whereas others are unsuccessful. Ideally, it would be nice to be able to tell prior to starting the program who was going to be successful and who was not (and therefore should be dissuaded from joining). Unfortunately, baseline characteristics are not consistently associated with outcomes (34). Heavier patients tend to lose more weight than thinner ones (35), and in some studies, men have lost more weight than women [this difference is usually removed by adjusting for baseline weight (36)]. In DPP, older participants were more successful at meeting both the physical activity and the weight-loss goals. African-Americans have been found to lose less weight than Caucasians in studies with balanced LCDs and with VLCD regimens (37,38). It is unclear whether this difference reflects metabolic difference between ethnic groups or the cultural relevance of the treatment program. Higher depression and binge eating scores at baseline have been associated with increased risk of dropping out of treatment, but not consistently with weight-loss outcomes (34,39).

Of particular relevance is the question of whether medical status at baseline affects the outcome of behavioral weight-loss programs. In the NWCR, participants who identified medical triggers for their weight loss achieved larger weight losses and better maintenance of weight loss (15). In other studies, however, poorer health has been associated with poorer outcomes. Karlsson et al. (40) found that poorer health status at baseline using the Sickness Impact Profile was related to weight regain. Diabetics have been found to have poorer weight losses than the nondiabetics in behavioral weight-loss studies (41) as well as pharmacologic intervention studies (42). Further, Clark et al. (43) found that patients with untreated hypertension or higher baseline systolic blood pressure had poorer attendance at behavioral weight-loss programs, whereas hyperlipidemia and total number of medical diagnoses were unrelated to outcome. The relationship between baseline health status and outcome in a weight-loss program may be complicated by the medications used to treat the disease and by the extent to which the measure of health status reflects general adherence to self-care behaviors.

Whereas baseline variables have not been consistently related to outcome, the participants' initial weight losses are often predictive of subsequent outcome. Wadden et al. (44) found that weight losses at week 8 of a program correlated significantly ($r = 0.45$) with weight loss at one-year follow-up. Similarly, weight losses at six months predict overall weight loss at month 30 (45). Thus, it is important to get patients off to a good start in weight-loss interventions. There is also extensive evidence that patients who make the greatest changes in diet and exercise, and maintain these changes long term are the ones who maintain the greatest reductions in body weight (34). The issue thus becomes how best to help patients make these long-term behavior changes.

## STRATEGIES TO HELP PARTICIPANTS CHANGE THEIR EATING BEHAVIORS

To produce weight loss, it is necessary to help patients change their diet and exercise behaviors. The approaches used by behaviorists to effect these changes are discussed in the following sections.

### The Dietary Prescription

As noted previously, the typical dietary recommendation in behavioral programs is a caloric intake of 1200 to 1500 kcal/day with 20% to 30% of calories from fat. There have been several studies investigating the effects of greater caloric reduction, with VLCD regimens. VLCDs are diets of less than 800 kcal/day, typically consumed as liquid formula or lean meat, fish, and fowl. These regimens, used with carefully selected patients and medical monitoring, have been shown to produce weight losses of approximately

9 kg in 12 weeks (46,47). Moreover, when an 8- to 12-week period of VLCD was used in the context of a 24-week behavioral weight-loss program, weight losses of 18 to 19 kg were obtained (48,49). Although these initial weight losses are outstanding, the problem has been in the maintenance of weight loss. Even programs that have combined VLCDs with behavioral strategies, reasoning that the behavioral training would help in the maintenance of weight loss, have been ineffective at reducing weight regain. For example, Wing et al. (50) randomly assigned 93 patients with type 2 diabetes to a behavioral treatment program that either prescribed a balanced LCD (LCD; 1000–1200 kcal/day) throughout the 52-week program or included two 12-week periods of VLCDs (weeks 1–12 and 24–36). After six months, the VLCD group had lost significantly more weight than the LCD group (16.4 kg vs. 12.3 kg). However, by week 52 the differences were no longer significant (14.2 kg vs. 10.5 kg for VLCD vs. LCD, respectively; $P = 0.057$). Treatment stopped after a year, but patients were reexamined one year later; the weight losses of the VLCD group were now 7.2 kg versus 5.7 kg in the LCD group. Because this and other studies (51) have failed to find significant long-term benefits of using the VLCDs and these diets are costly to administer, most programs have returned to using LCDs with calorie goals of 1200 to 1500 kcal/day.

Reducing dietary fat intake has been shown to be an important strategy of long-term successful weight losers (7), and in correlational studies, dietary fat reduction is a stronger predictor of long-term weight loss than reduction in total calories (52). However, only one randomized trial has examined whether reducing calories alone (without specifically trying to restrict fat intake) is more or less successful than a program that focuses on lowering both calories and fat. Pascale et al. (53) randomly assigned 90 subjects (half had diabetes and half had a family history of diabetes) to either a low-calorie program or a program targeting both calories and dietary fat. The low-calorie group was given a 1000 to 1500 kcal/wk goal and the participants monitored their caloric intake only; the calorie plus fat group had the same 1000 to 1500 kcal goal and in addition were given a fat gram goal designed to produce a less than 20% fat diet; these participants monitored calories and fat grams. Among patients with diabetes, those given the calorie plus fat goal had better weight losses than those given only calorie goals (−7.7 kg vs. −4.6 kg at 16 weeks; −5.2 kg vs. −1.0 kg at 52 weeks), but no differences were seen in patients with a family history of diabetes.

Schlundt et al. (54) also found evidence supporting the use of low-calorie/low-fat regimen. In this study, 60 overweight subjects were randomly assigned to a low-calorie/low-fat regimen (1200–1500 kcal with 20 g fat) or to a low-fat regimen (20 g of fat) with no calorie restriction and ad libitum carbohydrate intake. After 20 weeks, weight losses were significantly better in the calorie plus fat restriction condition (−8.8 kg vs. −4.6 kg); weight losses at 9 to 12 month follow-up were also significantly better in patients given calorie and fat restriction (−5.5 kg vs. −2.6 kg) but only included 58% of the cohort.

Recently there has been increased interest in the benefits and risks of low-carbohydrate diets (where patients are allowed to eat as much protein and fat as they want as long as carbohydrates are restricted) (55,56). Most studies on this topic have been short term and have not examined low-carbohydrate diet regimens within the context of behavioral weight-loss programs. Moreover, in studies comparing low-carbohydrate and low-calorie/low-fat approaches, many nonspecific aspects of the diet regimen (e.g., the degree of structure provided) have not been equated. Foster et al. (56) reported results of a one-year clinical trial comparing a low-carbohydrate, high-protein, high-fat diet (Atkins diet) (57) with a low-calorie, high-carbohydrate, low-fat approach. Both groups received a book describing the specific approach and met once with a nutritionist. The style of the books, however, was quite different with the Atkins book providing a more structured approach and a more enthusiastic sales pitch. Sixty female overweight participants entered the trial; 42 completed six months, and 37 completed 12 months. Analyses, using intent-to-treat and assuming that dropouts had returned to their baseline weight, indicated that the low-carbohydrate group lost more weight at six months (–7.0% vs. –3.2% of body weight), but the differences at 12 months were not significant (–4.4% vs. –2.5% of body weight). Thus, in the only year-long study to date, overall adherence to both regimens was poor and at the end of the study, no differences in weight loss were observed.

## Structure of the Diet Regimen

Although many studies have focused on the number of calories or the macronutrient composition of the diet used for weight loss, these aspects of the diet may be less important than the structure of the regimen. Foster et al. (58) found equivalent weight losses on VLCDs of 400, 600, or 800 kcal/day, suggesting that the structure of these diets, rather than their actual calorie prescription, may be critical. Jeffery et al. (59) examined this empirically by randomly assigning patients to standard behavioral programs (SBT), which differed in the degree of structure provided regarding the diet. Participants in this study ($N = 202$) were randomly assigned to one of five conditions. Group 1 was given no treatment and was simply followed over time. Group 2 was given a SBT, with a 1000 or 1500 kcal diet (depending on initial body weight) and encouraged to limit dietary fat. Group 3 received the identical behavioral program and had the same diet goals as group 2, but to provide greater structure to the diet, participants in group 3 were given a box of food each week that contained exactly what they should eat for five breakfasts and five dinners. Group 4 was identical to group 2, but included a financial incentive for weight loss. Group 5 received the same behavioral program as group 2, but included both food provision and financial incentives.

The results clearly showed the benefits of the food provision. Whereas incentives had no effect on weight loss, the groups given food provision had significantly better weight losses at 6, 12, and 18 months (–10.1, –9.1, and –6.4 kg) than the groups given standard behavioral treatment (SBT) without food provision (–7.7, –4.5, and –4.1 kg).

To determine whether the benefits of food provision were due to the provision of the food itself, the fact that it was given free, or the structure provided by the meal plans given with the food, these investigators conducted another study (60). Women in this study ($N = 163$) were randomly assigned to a SBT, SBT plus meal plans and grocery lists, SBT plus food provided on cost-sharing basis, or SBT plus food provided free. This study confirmed the benefits of food provision, but indicated that the most important component of food provision was not the actual food, but rather the meal plans indicating what to eat for each meal. Participants in group 1 of this study lost 8.0 kg at six months, whereas groups 2 to 4 lost 12.0, 11.7, and 11.4 kg, respectively. Groups 2 to 4 were all statistically superior to group 1, but did not differ from each other.

Several studies using Slimfast (61) and other meal replacement products (32) have also shown benefits to more structured dietary approaches. Having patients use meal replacement products such as Slimfast for breakfast and lunch and frozen entrees for dinner may simplify the diet prescription and consequently improve adherence and weight loss. Wing et al. (60) found that these more structured approaches led to more regular eating patterns, storage of healthier foods in the home, and reduction of many of the barriers to weight reduction, such as finding time to plan meals, controlling eating when not hungry, and estimating portion sizes.

Table 2 summarizes the goal and key strategies for modifying dietary intake in lifestyle interventions.

## STRATEGIES TO HELP PARTICIPANTS CHANGE THEIR PHYSICAL ACTIVITY

Exercise alone has been shown to produce only modest weight loss (62,63), but the combination of exercise plus diet is most effective for long-term weight control. This next section describes the approach to exercise that is typically used in behavioral weight-loss programs.

### The Exercise Prescription

Behavioral weight-loss programs have traditionally encouraged participants to increase their activity to a level of 1000 kcal/wk. In the DPP (3), the exercise goal was 150 minutes of activity per week, but given that 1 mile

**Table 2** Modifying Dietary Intake and Physical Activity

| Goal | Strategies to achieve goal |
| --- | --- |
| Reduce calorie intake to 1200–1500 kcal/day | Use structured meal plans<br>Incorporate meal replacement products<br>Self-monitor calorie and dietary fat intake<br>Rearrange home environment to increase cues for healthy choices and decrease cues for unhealthy choices |
| Increase physical activity to 1000–2000 kcal/wk | Self-monitor physical activity in calories, minutes, or steps<br>Stress home-based activity<br>Accumulate exercise through multiple short bouts<br>Make activity convenient by providing home exercise equipment<br>Decrease sedentary activity<br>Increase cues for activity and decrease cues for inactivity |

equals about 100 cal, and takes about 15 minutes to complete, these prescriptions are actually quite similar. Recently, several studies have suggested that higher expenditure goals may be needed for long-term maintenance of weight loss. In the NWCR, participants report approximately 2800 kcal/wk of physical activity; Jakicic et al. (64) found that participants who reported more than 200 minutes/wk (mean = 2500 kcal/wk) had better maintenance of weight loss at the end of an 18-month program than participants reporting 150 minutes or less of activity per week. To test this empirically, Jeffery et al. (31) randomly assigned 202 participants to standard behavioral weight-loss programs, with an exercise goal of either 1000 or 2500 kcal/wk. The first question examined in this study was whether it was possible to achieve these higher calorie levels in a group of overweight participants. The authors found that they were able to come very close to this goal; on average, participants in the higher exercise group reported exercise expenditures of 2399 kcal/wk at six months, 2249 kcal/wk at 12 months, and 2317 kcal/wk at 18 months. These levels were significantly greater than the levels achieved in the 1000 kcal group (1500–1800 kcal/wk). Although weight losses in the two conditions were similar at six months (–9.0 for 2500 kcal group vs. –8.1 for 1000 kcal group), the higher exercise prescription led to significantly greater weight losses at 12 months (–8.5 kg vs. –6.1 kg) and 18 months (–6.7 kg vs. –4.1 kg) (33).

Another recent study (33) failed to find significant differences between participants assigned to 1000 kcal or 2000 kcal/wk exercise prescriptions or to moderate or higher intensity prescriptions. However, the groups with the 2000 cal/wk goal had an average weight loss of –8.5 kg whereas those with the 1000 kcal goal averaged –6.6 kg. A post hoc analyses showed that participants who exercised more than 200 minutes per week had significantly greater weight losses than those averaging 150 minutes or less per week.

Fewer studies have examined the type of physical activity to recommend. Most programs focus on aerobic activities, but resistance training might increase lean body mass and thus help blunt the decrease in metabolic rate that accompanies weight loss. Although this makes sense theoretically, most studies have found no difference in weight loss for participants assigned to aerobic or resistance activities. For example, Wadden et al. (32) randomly assigned 128 participants to SBT with no exercise, aerobic exercise, resistance exercise, or the combination of aerobic plus resistance. Weight losses in the four conditions were comparable at week 24, 48, and at follow-up at week 100.

## Strategies to Improve Adherence to Physical Activity

Behaviorists have also studied strategies that might promote long-term adherence to physical activity. Because lack of time is the most frequently reported barrier to physical activity, one approach is to recommend multiple short bouts of physical activity, rather than one long bout. Patients who say that it would be impossible to find a 30 to 60 minute period in the day for exercise, may be more receptive to the idea of just taking a 10-minute walk in the morning, at lunch, and after dinner, and "accumulating" 30 minutes of activity.

Jakicic et al. (64,65) studied the benefits of short versus long bouts of physical activity. Participants in a behavioral weight-loss program were given the same overall exercise goals but were randomly assigned to complete their activity in one long bout (40 minutes) each day, 5 days/wk or in multiple short bouts (four 10-minute bouts). In the first study (65), short bouts led to better exercise adherence and better weight losses at six months. In the second study (64), short bouts were helpful initially, but at 18 months the weight losses were not significantly different (–5.8 kg for long bout vs. –3.7 kg for short bout). Importantly, both the short- and the long-bout group had comparable improvement in fitness as well. Thus, prescribing exercise in multiple short bouts may be helpful initially as overweight individuals begin to exercise, and may be a useful option for long-term exercise.

Another question studied by behavioral researchers has been whether adherence is better in structured, supervised exercise programs or when the participant is encouraged to exercise on their own at home. Researchers have shown that both approaches can improve physical fitness (66), but home-based exercise seems preferable for long-term weight-loss maintenance (67,68), Perri et al. randomly assigned 49 participants to complete a moderate intensity walking program (30 minutes/day on 5 days/wk) either on their own at home or by attending supervised exercise sessions. Weight losses were similar at six months (−10.4 kg for home-based and −9.3 kg for supervised) but at 15 months, the home-based group maintained a weight loss of –11.6 kg whereas the supervised group had regained some weight and now averaged –7.0 kg.

Finally, home-based exercise may be made even more convenient by providing participants with their own exercise equipment (64). Participants who were given treadmills and instructed to exercise in multiple short bouts had better weight-loss outcomes over an 18-month program than participants given the same exercise prescription, but without the treadmills (–7.4 kg for treadmill group vs. –3.7 kg for those without the treadmill). Other studies have also found a correlation between the number of pieces of exercise equipment in the home and the physical activity level (69).

All of these strategies suggest that making exercise more convenient (by allowing participants to exercise at home, in multiple short bouts, and providing easy access to exercise equipment) improves adherence to exercise and consequently long-term weight-loss maintenance.

### Decreasing Sedentary Behavior

Although there has been tremendous attention directed toward understanding the role of physical activity in the behavioral treatment of obesity, there is an increasing recognition that sedentary behavior may also be important in the energy balance equation. Both cross-sectional and prospective epidemiological studies indicate that the amount of time spent in specific sedentary behaviors (e.g., television viewing), independent of time spent engaging in physical activities, may increase the risk of developing obesity and other health-related problems (70,71). Although to our knowledge there have been no published experimental studies with adults, several randomized, controlled trials have demonstrated that interventions aimed at reducing television viewing and other sedentary behaviors may help prevent weight gain (72) or reduce obesity (73) in children.

Epstein et al. (73) compared the effects of behavioral weight-loss programs targeting decreased sedentary activity, increased physical activity, or the combination of decreasing sedentary behaviors and increasing physical activity in the treatment of overweight children aged 8 to 12. All three approaches improved physical fitness, but at one-year follow-up, the group that had been taught to decrease their sedentary behaviors had greater decreases in percent overweight. In replicating this research, Epstein et al. (74) found that both decreasing sedentary behavior and increasing physical activity produced similar weight losses. Research examining similar approaches in adults is clearly needed.

### COMPLICATING FACTORS IN THE TREATMENT OF OBESITY IN PATIENTS WITH CVD

Many patients with established CVD present with co-occurring psychological or behavioral risk factors that may complicate treatment of obesity. In this section, we will discuss a few selected topics germane to treating obesity in patients with CVD, including depression, smoking, and medication regimens.

Although research on the relation between depression and obesity is inconsistent (75), depression is associated with CVD and may occur more commonly among those individuals with severe obesity (76) and in those seeking weight-control treatment (77). The presence of depression among obese patients is particularly concerning given that depression may be related to early attrition in behavioral weight-loss programs (43,78), and to weight regain among individuals already successful at long-term weight loss (79). However, there are many studies that suggest that participation in a behavioral weight-loss program can help reduce depressive symptomatology. Those who lose the most weight show the greatest improvement in mood, but even those who lose little or regain, show positive changes in mood (39,80). Although the specific mechanisms for this effect are unknown, it is possible that participation in a weight-loss program contributes to decreases in negative mood via increases in social support, self-efficacy, and outcome expectancies, or physical activity. Indeed, a growing body of research suggests that exercise may be an effective therapy for depression (81), in addition to promoting weight control and cardiovascular functioning.

It is also important to consider the possible co-occurrence of smoking and obesity when promoting lifestyle changes in CVD patients. Patients presenting with both problems should be encouraged to stop smoking first, because the health benefits of quitting smoking outweigh the benefits of weight loss, or the costs associated with gaining a moderate amount of weight (mean of 8–10 lb) (82). However, because the fear of postcessation weight gain is a major impediment to quitting smoking, particularly among women (83), some smoking cessation interventions have been tailored to address this issue. Perkins et al. (84) randomly assigned 219 weight-concerned women to one of three different smoking cessation interventions: a standard smoking program, a smoking program with a cognitive–behavioral intervention to reduce weight concerns, or a smoking program with a behavioral weight control intervention. Results showed that the smoking program, which focused on reducing weight concerns, improved smoking cessation and decreased postcessation weight gain relative to the other conditions over 12 months. Similarly, increasing physical activity in those attempting smoking cessation may be helpful. In a study with 281 sedentary female smokers, Marcus et al. (85) found that women who were randomly assigned to a smoking cessation program coupled with a physical activity intervention had improved smoking cessation and decreased weight gain over 12 months.

Medication management is another important factor to consider when treating obese patients with CVD who are making healthy lifestyle changes. Obese patients with CVD are often taking medications for hyperlipidemia, hypertension, and/or diabetes; weight reduction may allow these patients to reduce or eliminate these medications. Although this is clearly a benefit of weight reduction, it complicates treatment by necessitating frequent monitoring of these parameters and adjustments in medication as needed. In patients with diabetes, for example, glucose levels decrease dramatically within three to seven days of caloric restriction (86). Thus, reducing insulin and oral hypoglycemic agents prior to or in the first few weeks of a behavioral weight-loss program is often necessary to prevent abrupt onset of hypoglycemia.

## CONCLUSIONS

Lifestyle interventions are effective in producing initial weight losses of 7% to 10% of body weight. Although these weight losses are modest, and patients may regain weight over time, even modest weight losses have a dramatic impact on CVD risk. The most effective lifestyle change programs involve the combination of dietary modification and increases in physical activity. Behavioral techniques, including self-monitoring, stimulus control, and goal setting may help patients initiate and sustain these new diet and exercise behaviors.

## REFERENCES

1. Sciamanna CN, Tate DF, Lang W, Wing RR. Arch Intern Med 2000; 160: 2334–2339.
2. Whelton PK, Appel LJ, Espeland MA, et al., for the TONE Collaborative Research Group. JAMA 1998; 279(11):839–846.
3. The Diabetes Prevention Program Research Group. N Engl J Med 2002; 346: 393–403.
4. Tuomilehto J, Lindstrom J, Eriksson J, et al., for the Finnish Diabetes Prevention Study Group. N Engl J Med 2001; 344:1343–1350.
5. Stevens VJ, Corrigan SA, Obarzanek E, et al. Arch Intern Med 1993; 153: 849–858.
6. Ornish D, Brown SE, Scherwitz LW, et al. Lancet 1990; 336:129–133.
7. Klem ML, Wing RR, McGuire MT, Seagle HM, Hill JO. Am J Clin Nutr 1997; 66:239–246.
8. Wing RR, Hill JO. Successful weight loss maintenance. Annu Rev Nutr 2001; 21:323–341.
9. Block G, Hartman AM, Dresser CM, Carroll MD, Gannon J, Gardner L. Am J Epidemiol 1986; 124:453–469.
10. Subar AF, Kipnis V, Troiano RP, et al. Am J Epidemiol 2003; 158:1–13.
11. Wyatt HR, Seagle HM, Grunwald GK, et al. Obes Res 2000; 8(S1):87S.
12. Wyatt HR, Grunwald GK, Mosca CL, Klem M, Wing RR, Hill JO. Obes Res 2002; 10(2):78–82.
13. Paffenbarger RS Jr, Hyde RT, Wing AL, Hsieh CC. N Engl J Med 1986; 314: 605–613.

14. Pate RR, Pratt M, Blair SN, et al. JAMA 1995; 273:402–407.
15. Gorin AA, Phelan S, Hill JO, Wing RR. Prev Med 2004; 39:612–616.
16. Wadden T, Stunkard A, eds. Handbook of Obesity Treatment. New York: The Guilford Press, 2002.
17. Bray G, Bouchard C, eds. Handbook of Obesity: Clinical Applications. New York: Marcel Dekker, Inc., 2004.
18. Brownell KD. The LEARN Program for Weight Control. Dallas, TX: American Health Publishing Company, 1991.
19. Skinner BF. The Behavior of Organisms: An Experimental Analysis. New York: Appleton-Century-Crofts, 1938.
20. Bandura A. Social learning theory. Englewood Cliffs, NJ: Prentice-Hall, 1977.
21. Wadden TA, Letizia KA. Wadden TA, VanItallie TB, eds. Treatment of the Seriously Obese Patient. New York: The Guilford Press, 1992:383–410.
22. Guare JC, Wing RR, Marcus MD, Epstein LH, Burton LR, Gooding WE. Diabetes Care 1989; 12:500–503.
23. Bandura A, Simon KM. Cognit Ther Res 1977; 1:177–193.
24. Beck AT. Cognitive therapy and the emotional disorders. New York: International Universities Press, 1976.
25. Renjilian DA, Perri MG, Nezu AM, McKelvey WF, Shermer RL, Anton SD. J Consult Clin Psychol 2001; 69(4):717–721.
26. Wing R, Jeffery R. J Consult Clin Psychol 1999; 67(1):132–138.
27. D'Zurilla TJ, Goldfried MR. J Abnorm Psychol 1971; 78:107–126.
28. Marlatt GA, Gordon JR. Davidson PO, Davidson SM, eds. Behavioral Medicine: Changing Health Lifestyles. New York: Brunner/Mazel, 1979:410–452.
29. Marlatt GA, Gordon JR. Relapse Prevention: Maintenance Strategies in Addictive Behavior Change. New York: Guilford, 1985.
30. Wing RR. Behavioral approaches to the treatment of obesity. In: Bray G, Bouchard C, eds. Handbook of Obesity: Clinical Applications. New York: Marcel Dekker, Inc., 2004.
31. Jeffery RW, Wing RR, Sherwood NE, Tate DF. Am J Clin Nutr 2003; 89: 684–689.
32. Wadden TA, Vogt RA, Andersen RE, et al. Consult Clin Psychol 1997; 65: 269–277.
33. Jakicic J, Marcus BH, Gallagher KI, Napolitano M, Lang W. JAMA 2003; 290(10):1323–1330.
34. Wing RR, Phelan S. Eckel RH, ed. Obesity Mechanisms and Clinical Management. Philadelphia: Lippincott Williams & Wilkins, 2003.
35. Wadden TA, Foster GD, Wang J, et al. Am J Clin Nutr 1992; 56:274S–277S.
36. French SA, Jeffery RW, Wing RR. Addict Behav 1994; 19(2):147–158.
37. Kumanyika SK, Obarzanek E, Stevens VJ, Hebert PR, Whelton PK. Am J Clin Nutr 1991; 53:1631–1638.
38. Anglin K, Wing RR. Diabetes Care 1996; 19(5):409–413.
39. National Task Force on the Prevention and Treatment of Obesity. Arch Intern Med 2000; 160:2581–2589.
40. Karlsson J, Hallgren P, Kral JG, Lindross AK, Sjostrom L, Sullivan M. Appetite 1994; 23:15–26.
41. Guare JC, Wing RR, Grant A. Obes Res 1995; 3:329–335.

42. Khan M, St. Peter J, Breen G, Hartley G, Vessey J. Diabetes 1999; 48(suppl 1): A308.
43. Clark MN, Niaura RS, King TK, Pera V Addict Behav 1996; 21(4):509–513.
44. Wadden TA, Vogt RA, Foster GD, Anderson DA. J Consult Clin Psychol 1998; 66(2):429–433.
45. Jeffery RW, Wing RR, Mayer RR. J Consult Clin Psychol 1998; 66:641–645.
46. National Task Force on the Prevention and Treatment of Obesity. JAMA 1993; 270(8):967–974.
47. Wadden TA, Stunkard AJ, Brownell KD. Ann Intern Med 1983; 99:675–684.
48. Wadden TA, Stunkard AJ. J Consult Clin Psychol 1986; 54:482–488.
49. Wing RR, Marcus MD, Salata R, Epstein LH, Miaskiewicz S, Blair EH. Arch Intern Med 1991; 151:1334–1340.
50. Wing RR, Blair E, Marcus M, Epstein LH, Harvey J. Am J Med 1994; 97: 354–362.
51. Wadden TA, Foster GD, Letizia KA. J Consult Clin Psychol 1994; 62:165–171.
52. Harris JK, French SA, Jeffery RW, McGovern PG, Wing RR. Obes Res 1994; 2(4):307–313.
53. Pascale RW, Wing RR, Butler BA, Mullen M, Bononi P. Diabetes Care 1995; 18(9):1241–1248.
54. Schlundt DG, Hill JO, Pope-Cordle J, Arnold D, Virts KL, Katahn M. Int J Obes 1993; 17:623–629.
55. Samaha FF, Iqbal N, Seshadri P, et al. N Engl J Med 2003; 348(21):2074–2081.
56. Foster G, Wyatt HR, Hill JO, et al. N Engl J Med 2003; 348(21):2082–2090.
57. Atkins RC. Dr. Atkins' New Diet Revolution. New York: Avon Books, 1998.
58. Foster GD, Wadden TA, Peterson FJ, Letizia KA, Bartlett SJ, Conill AM. Am J Clin Nutr 1992; 55:811–817.
59. Jeffery RW, Wing RR, Thorson C, et al. Consult Clin Psychol 1993; 61: 1038–1045.
60. Wing RR, Jeffery RW, Burton LR, Thorson C, Sperber Nissinoff K, Baxter JE. Int J Obes 1996; 20:56–62.
61. Flechtner-Mors M, Ditschuneit HH, Johnson TD, Suchard MA, Adler G. Obes Res 2000; 8(5):399–402.
62. Wing RR. Med Sci Sports Exerc 1999; 31:S547–S552.
63. National Heart Lung & Blood Institute. Obes Res 1998; 6(S2):51S–210S.
64. Jakicic J, Wing R, Winters C. JAMA 1999; 282(16):1554–1560.
65. Jakicic JM, Wing RR, Butler BA, Robertson RJ. Int J Obes 1995; 19:893–901.
66. Dunn AL, Marcus BH, Kampert JB, Garcia ME, Kohl HW, Blair SN. JAMA 1999; 281:327–334.
67. Andersen R, Frankowiak S, Snyder J, Bartlett S, Fontaine K. JAMA 1998; 281(4):335–340.
68. Perri MG, Martin AD, Leermakers EA, Sears SF, Notelovitz M. J Consult Clin Psychol 1997; 65:278–285.
69. Jakicic JM, Wing RR, Butler BA, Jeffery RW. Am J Health Promotion 1997; 11:363–365.
70. Hu FB, Li TY, Colditz GA, Willett WC, Manson JE. JAMA 2003; 290(14):1785–1791.
71. Jakes RW, Day NE, Khaw KT, et al. Eur J Clin Nutr 2003; 57(9):1089–1096.

72. Robinson TN. Pediatr Clin North Am 2001; 48(4):1017–1025.
73. Epstein LH, Valoski AM, Vara LS, et al. Health Psychol 1995; 14:109–115.
74. Epstein LH, Paluch RA, Gordy CC, Dorn J. Arch Pediatr Adolesc Med 2000; 154:220–226.
75. Friedman MA, Brownell KD. Psychol Bull 1995; 117(1):3–20.
76. Stunkard AJ, Faith MA, Allison KC. Biol Psychol 2003; 54(3):330–337.
77. Fitzgibbon ML, Stolley MR, Kirschenbaum DS. Health Psychol 1993; 12(5):342–345.
78. Marcus MD, Wing RR, Guare JC, Blair EH, Jawad A. Diabetes Care 1992; 15(2):253–255.
79. Maguire MT, Wing RR, Klem ML, Lang W, Hill JO. J Consult Clin Psychol 1999; 67(2):177–185.
80. Wadden TA, Womble LG, Stunkard AJ, Anderson DA. Wadden TA, Stunkard AJ, eds. Handbook of Obesity Treatment. New York: Guilford Press, 2002: 144–169.
81. Blumenthal JAB, Moore K, Craighead WE, et al. Arch Intern Med 1999; 159(19):2349–2356.
82. Perkins KA. J Consult Clin Psychol 1993; 61(5):768–777.
83. Perkins KA, Levine MD, Marcus MD, Shiffman S. J Subst Abuse Treat 1997; 14(2):173–182.
84. Perkins KA, Marcus MD, Levine MD, et al. J Consult Clin Psychol 2001; 69(4):604–613.
85. Marcus BH, Albrecht AE, King TK, et al. Arch Intern Med 1999; 159(11): 1229–1234.
86. Kelley DE, Wing R, Buonocore C, Sturis J, Polonsky K, Fitzsimmons M. J Clin Endocrinol Metab 1993; 77:1287–1293.

## 13

# Use of Antiobesity Medications in Overweight Patients with Cardiovascular Disease: Implications of Drug Selection and Patient Monitoring

**Supawan Buranapin**

*Boston University School of Medicine, Boston, Massachusetts, U.S.A.*

**Caroline Apovian**

*Boston University School of Medicine and Center of Nutrition and Weight Management, Boston Medical Center, Boston, Massachusetts, U.S.A.*

## INTRODUCTION AND GUIDELINES

Weight loss and long-term weight maintenance of 5% to 10% of initial weight are considered adequate to improve cardiovascular risk factors and other obesity-related conditions. Lifestyle modification remains the most important tool in obesity management through the combination of dietary modification, an increase in physical activity, formal exercise regimens, and behavioral and cognitive therapy. As adjunctive treatment, antiobesity medications have been approved and recommended for

1. Patients who have a BMI $\geq 27 \, \text{kg/m}^2$ in the presence of two or more than two obesity-related medical conditions including established coronary heart disease, type 2 diabetes mellitus, hypertension, dyslipidemia, cerebrovascular disease, severe osteoarthritis, and sleep apnea and
2. Patients with a BMI $\geq 30 \, \text{kg/m}^2$.

The initial goal of the obesity treatment should be a 10% weight reduction in six months through lifestyle modification. If lifestyle change techniques are not enough to meet therapeutic goals, drug therapy may be considered (1,2). If the patient is not able to lose at least 2 kg in the first four weeks after initial therapy, the medication dose may be adjusted, discontinued, or substituted with a different medication. If significant weight loss is maintained, the medication may be continued as long as it remains effective, and the side effects are tolerable (3) (except for those drugs only approved for short-term use: see Section on Phentermine).

## CLASSIFICATIONS

Medications that have been approved by Food and Drug Administration (FDA) and in use in the United States can be classified into two groups: anorectic drugs, which suppress appetite or increase satiety, and malabsorptive drugs, which decrease fat absorbtion.

### Anorectic Drugs

Anorectic medications work by increasing serotonin, norepinephrine, dopamine, or a combination of these neurotransmitters in nerve terminals of the hypothalamic-feeding center. These are sympathomimetic drugs, which include

1.  Noradrenergic drugs such as phentermine, diethylpropion, phendimetrazine, mazindol, and benzphentamine. Phentermine has been the most prescribed weight-loss medication in this group and
2.  Serotonin and norepinephrine reuptake inhibitors: sibutramine (Meridia®).

#### Phentermine

Phentermine has been available since the 1960s and is the most popular of the noradrenergic drugs. It was approved by the FDA in 1972 for short-term treatment of obesity (≤12 weeks). It is available in a time-release resin under the brand name "Ionamin®" (15 or 30 mg) or a more quickly released hydrochloride form with 15, 30, or 37.5 mg doses in various brands and a generic form (4).

**Mechanism of action:** The mechanism of action of Phentermine involves suppression of appetite by increasing norepinephrine levels in the hypothalamus resulting in decreased food consumption.

**Efficacy and study support:** Since the 1960s, clinical trials have demonstrated that the combination of phentermine and a hypocaloric diet produces significantly more weight loss than a hypocaloric diet alone.

Munro et al. (5) studied 108 overweight and obese women between the ages of 21 and 60 years without cardiovascular or endocrine diseases by randomly treating with placebo, continuous phentermine [30 mg/day of the phentermine resin (Duromine)], or alternating four-week periods with the active and placebo capsule for 36 weeks. All three groups received instruction to adhere to a carbohydrate restricted 1000 cal/day diet. No dietary advice was given thereafter, but patients were followed every four weeks. The study reported significantly more weight loss in the phentermine-treated group than in the placebo group (4.8 kg), $P < 0.001$. There was no difference in weight loss between the intermittent (13 kg) or the continuous phentermine-treatment groups (12.2 kg). The most significant weight loss occurred in the first six months, although the phentermine-treated patients continued to lose weight at a slower rate between six and nine months of treatment. The adverse effects were minor, with only 8% of the drug-treated patients and 3% of the placebo-treated group dropping out because of perceived stimulant adverse effects such as insomnia, irritability, tension, anxiety, and agitation.

Truant et al. (6) conducted a controlled 20-week randomized double-blind prospective study of phentermine resin (Ionamin). The group was composed of 110-obese subjects between the ages of 21 and 65 years, without endocrine or metabolic disorders. The researchers found that both the continuous phentermine resin use groups and the intermittent use groups had substantially greater mean weight loss than did the placebo group during all treatment periods (losing 20.3 and 18.4 pounds vs. 11.5 pounds, respectively). Subjects who received continuous therapy with phentermine resin sustained a greater weight loss than those who received interrupted therapy; however, the difference was not statistically significant. There were neither serious adverse events nor evidence of tolerance or dependence detected.

Weintraub et al. (7) conducted a double-blind, controlled clinical trial comparing phentermine resin (30 mg in the morning), fenfluramine hydrochloride (20 mg three times a day), and a combination of phentermine resin (15 mg in the morning) and fenfluramine hydrochloride (30 mg before evening meal), with placebo in 81 obese patients. Subjects were 18 to 55 years old and at 130% to 180% of ideal body weight, and had no history of diabetes mellitus, hypertension, or hyperlipidemia. The study included a three-week run-in period of diet only, 16 weeks of drug plus diet (20 kcal/kg of ideal body weight: 900–1800 kcal/day), and a four-week taper of the medication. Patients were followed up every one to four weeks. The researchers demonstrated that weight loss in those receiving the combination (10.1%) was significantly greater than in those receiving placebo (4.9%) and equivalent to those receiving either drug alone (11% for phentermine and 8.4% for fenfluramine). Participants receiving placebo had increased hunger ratings compared to baseline, whereas the active-treatment group participants had marked decreases in hunger. Concerning adverse events, the phentermine and fenfluramine groups reported significantly more complaints than the placebo group. The combination group reported significantly fewer cardiovascular and central nervous system (CNS) complaints than the phentermine treatment group, but this was not significantly different from the fenfluramine group.

One hundred and seventy-five obese women ($>20\%$ ideal body weight) aged 20 to 60 years without endocrine or cardiovascular disease were included in a double-blind 36-week trial to assess the weight-loss properties of fenfluramine, 20 mg three times a day, and phentermine, 30 mg once daily, combined with a carbohydrate restricted, 1000-calorie diet. Subjects were randomly allocated into five groups allowing for comparison of treatment with intermittent phentermine, continuous and intermittent fenfluramine, alternate fenfluramine/phentermine, and intermittent fenfluramine/phentermine. There was a 6.8% withdrawal rate from the study because of side effects. Continuous fenfluramine produced the same mean weight loss as intermittent phentermine therapy (26.1 and 26.3 lbs, respectively). No significant advantage was gained by giving the two drugs alternately. Intermittent fenfluramine was less effective than phentermine and more likely to produce side effects. Clinically appreciable CNS stimulation to phentermine was not encountered (8).

Of note, fenfluramine was later withdrawn from the market along with dexfenfluramine because of evidence associating the drugs with cardiac valvulopathies. No such associations were found with the use of phentermine alone, and phentermine remains FDA approved for short-term treatment of obesity.

Only one study has addressed the cardiovascular risk reduction potential of phentermine (9). A partial crossover design was used to evaluate the impact of a nine-month weight reduction program on plasma lipid, dietary intake, and abdominal obesity using phentermine hydrochloride (Fastin) plus a low energy diet (5040 kJ/day) in 417 obese postmenopausal Caucasian women with BMI 30 to 38 kg/m$^2$. Both groups received drug and diet treatment over six months. However, group 1 received the intervention treatment from months 4 to 9, while group 2 received the intervention treatment from months 1 to 6, so that the weight-stable group 1 subjects could serve as a control for the weight-losing group 2 subjects in a comparison of body composition. Patients were followed for a total of nine months. Both groups had comparable weight loss, low-density lipoprotein cholesterol (LDL-C) and triacylglycerol reduction, and rise in plasma high-density lipoprotein cholesterol (HDL-C). There was also a comparable decrease in the total/HDL-C ratio in both groups. All subjects showed a decrease in abdominal fat, as measured by anthropometry and dual energy X-ray absorptiometry (DEXA), as well as decreased food consumption. Group 1 demonstrated changes in all parameters after month 4 (the first month of intervention treatment), whereas group 2 demonstrated changes in all parameters in the first month. These changes were maintained over nine months of follow up. This study suggests that phentermine not only produces weight loss but also reduces cardiovascular risk factors (abdominal obesity and dyslipidemia) in six months of treatment and nine months of total follow up.

**Dosage and administration:** The usual dose of phentermine is 8 mg three times a day 30 minutes before each meal with the last dose being taken at least four to six hours before bedtime to prevent insomnia, or 15 to 37.5 mg once daily before breakfast, or one to two hours after breakfast for $\leq 12$ weeks (1).

**Contraindications:** The use of phentermine is contraindicated in patients with uncontrolled hypertension and those with cardiovascular diseases as well as those with hyperthyroidism and glaucoma. Phentermine should be used with caution in patients with anxiety disorders or other agitated conditions due to the stimulant effects. Because the pharmacology and chemical structure of phentermine are closely related to that of amphetamines, it may be physically and psychologically addictive. Therefore the use of phentermine in patients with a history of drug abuse should be discouraged. Phentermine should not be taken with or within two weeks of discontinuing monoamine oxidase inhibitors (MAOIs) such as eldepryl, noradryl, or parnate as well as tricyclic antidepressants because of the risk of marked sympathomimetic effects, especially hypertensive crisis. The use of phentermine is discouraged in patients taking selective serotonin reuptake inhibitors because of the association of primary pulmonary hypertension and cardiac valve abnormalities with combinations of phentermine and other serotonergic drugs (fenfluramine and dexfenfluramine).

**Potential drug interactions:** Phentermine may interact with MAOIs, guanethidine, CNS stimulants, alcohol, sibutramine, tricyclic antidepressants (10). Phentermine may decrease the hypotensive effect of clonidine, guanethidine, and methyldopa and augment the metabolic effect of thyroid hormone (1).

**Adverse effects and monitoring:** The common side effects of phentermine are dry mouth, constipation, palpitations, increased heart rate and blood pressure, headache, nervousness, and insomnia. Serious but uncommon side effects are chest pain, shortness of breath, skin rash, blurred vision, confusion or hallucinations, and uncontrolled body movements or seizures. Patients taking phentermine should be monitored for pulse rate and blood pressure before initiating treatment and every two weeks for the first three months and every one to three months thereafter (9).

Sibutramine

Sibutramine is in another class of anorectic drugs that suppress appetite or increase satiety resulting in reduced food consumption. It has been approved for the treatment of obesity in the United States since 1997.

**Mechanism of action:**   It is through inhibition of both norepinephrine and serotonin reuptake as well as through a weak inhibition of dopamine reuptake. The increase in norepinephrine and serotonin in CNS leads to increased satiety and decreased food intake. One study demonstrated that sibutramine limits the decline in metabolic rate and consequent fall in energy expenditure that occurs with weight loss (11). Because of these dual actions, the authors predicted that sibutramine would lead to both weight loss and weight maintenance. Sibutramine does not act as a classic anorectic drug because it does not inhibit the initiation of eating but does enhance and prolong the feeling of fullness that usually develops after eating (12). Sibutramine has been shown to result in earlier termination of a meal and the avoidance of intermeal snacks (13).

### Efficacy and study support
*Simple obesity without endocrine and cardiovascular diseases.*   A meta-analysis has shown that three times as many sibutramine-treated patients achieved a 5% and 10% weight loss as did placebo-treated control patients (14).

Jones et al. (15) published a one-year clinical trial comparing sibutramine 10 to 15 mg/day to placebo in 485 patients. They demonstrated significantly greater weight loss in the sibutramine-treated groups (4.8 kg in the 10 mg dose and 6.1 kg in the 15 mg dose group) than in the placebo-treated groups (1.8 kg).

Smith and Goulder in 2001 (16) performed a randomized placebo-controlled trial of sibutramine 10 to 15 mg once daily for one year given with dietary advice in 485 mild to moderately obese subjects. Those treated with sibutramine 10 and 15 mg had a greater mean weight loss compared with placebo at each monthly assessment. Weight loss was dose related, and maximal weight loss occurred by month 6 in all treatment groups. Changes in body weight from baseline to end point were −1.6 kg for those taking placebo, −4.4 kg for those taking sibutramine 10 mg, and −6.4 kg for those taking sibutramine 15 mg. During the four weeks after treatment cessation, there were small weight increases in all treatment groups. There were statistically significant changes in triglycerides compared with placebo at month 6 for the sibutramine-treated group. Uric acid levels were also significantly reduced at month 6 for both the sibutramine-treated groups compared with placebo.

Bray et al. in 1999 (17) conducted a multicenter study randomizing 1047 obese patients to 24 weeks of treatment with one to six doses of sibutramine (1, 5, 10, 15, 20, and 30 mg) or placebo once daily. Weight loss was dose related and statistically significant compared with placebo across all time points for 5- to 30-mg/day dosage of sibutramine. Weight loss achieved at week 4 was predictive of weight loss achieved at week 24. Patients losing weight demonstrated an increase in HDL-C and reduction in serum triglycerides, total cholesterol, LDL-C, fasting plasma glucose, and uric acid.

In a weight maintenance trial called Sibutramine Trial of Obesity Reduction and Maintenance (STORM) (18), sibutramine was shown to reduce waist circumference in the first six months, and this effect was maintained over the two-year study period. Analysis of the type of fat lost in the first six months of the STORM trial (19) showed that the greatest loss occurred in the visceral compartment with a 24% reduction in abdominal fat and a 17% reduction in subcutaneous fat.

*Continuous and intermittent therapy.* A study in Germany (20) compared sibutramine 15 mg/day continuously for 48 weeks with 15 mg/day of sibutramine intermittently during week 1 to 12, 19 to 30, and 37 to 48, and with sibutramine 15 mg/day for the first four weeks of a run-in period followed by a placebo period for week 5 to 48. Mean weight loss was 3.8 kg in patients receiving continuous sibutramine therapy and 3.3 kg in patients receiving sibutramine intermittent therapy ($P = 0.28$) with a mean weight gain of 0.2 kg in placebo group. HDL-C increased in all treatment groups (15.3% in the continuous group, 10.0% in the intermittent group, and 7.1% in the placebo group). Triglyceride levels were substantially decreased in both the active-treatment groups compared with placebo group. LDL-C decreased in continuous and placebo groups but not in the intermittent group. There was no change in total cholesterol in all the three groups. Subgroup analyses revealed that there was a slight reduction in blood pressure in the 5% and 10% weight reduction groups. In contrast, patients with less than 5% weight loss exhibited a slight increase in blood pressure.

*For Weight Maintenance.* The STORM trial (18) was a double-blind, randomized, placebo-controlled study in eight European centers over 18 months, with 467 subjects to evaluate the effects of sibutramine on weight maintenance after an initial weight loss (>5%). Subjects who continued on in the study had first lost weight in a six-month open-label weight-loss phase in which all subjects were given sibutramine 10 mg/day, specific diet, and exercise and behavioral therapy. Subjects who were then placed in the placebo group regained weight two months after randomization, although they continued a lifestyle change program. By 24 months, they had regained almost 80% of the weight loss achieved during the initial weight-loss phase. In the sibutramine group, weight loss was maintained for 12 months with a slight increase in weight thereafter. At 24 months, the sibutramine group had maintained over 85% of the weight loss achieved at the end of the weight-loss phase. This data suggests that sibutramine is effective for both weight loss and weight maintenance.

*Predictor of long-term success.* Initial weight loss in response to sibutramine treatment is an important predictor of long-term success. Subjects losing less than 2 to 3 kg in three months were less likely to achieve any significant weight loss at two to three years (21), whereas those who lost more than 3 kg in the first month achieved on average a 10.5 kg weight loss in one year. Two-thirds of subjects achieved a weight loss of ≥5%, and one-third achieved a weight loss of ≥10% after losing 2 kg or more at week 4 of treatment. Weight loss was enhanced if intensive lifestyle therapy was provided (13).

*Diabetes Mellitus.*  Sibutramine is effective in achieving weight loss in patients with type 2 diabetes, but weight loss usually occurs more slowly for these patients than for nondiabetic patients (22). In type 2 diabetic obese patients (23), sibutramine 15 mg daily combined with a customized diet of 500 kcal/day, less than the individual's energy needs for 12 weeks, resulted in significantly more weight loss than in placebo plus diet. There was a decrease in all measurements including body weight, BMI, and waist circumference at the end of 12 weeks. Nineteen percent of subjects in the sibutramine-treated group lost 5% or more of their initial weight versus 0% in the placebo group, $P < 0.001$. Sibutramine-treated patients lost more fat mass as measured by DEXA than those in the placebo group (1% vs. 0.1%, $P < 0.05$). Mean peak blood glucose concentrations after a standard test meal decreased by 1.1 mmol/L in the sibutramine group and increased by 0.5 mmol/L in the placebo group. Mean fasting plasma glucose decreased by 0.3 mmol/L in the sibutramine group and increased by 1.4 mmol/L in the placebo group. HbA1c decreased by 0.3% in the sibutramine group and remained unchanged in the placebo group. More sibutramine-treated patients (33%) than placebo-treated patients (5%) achieved decreases in HbA1c of 1% or more. No significant differences in blood pressure were found between treatment groups.

Gokcel et al. (24) conducted a trial in female subjects with poorly controlled type 2 diabetes (HbA1c > 8%) on oral hypoglycemic therapy in which subjects received either placebo twice daily or sibutramine 10 mg bid for six months. Subjects in the sibutramine group showed a significantly greater reduction in body weight, fasting plasma glucose, two-hour postprandial blood glucose, insulin resistance, waist circumference, BMI, HbA1c, diastolic blood pressure, pulse rate, uric acid level, and most parameters of the lipid profile [total cholesterol, LDL-C, triglycerides, lipoprotein (a), and apolipoprotein B]. There were no changes in HDL-C, systolic blood pressure, or apolipoprotein A1.

In obese type 2 diabetic patients treated with metformin (25), sibutramine (15–20 mg/day) treatment for 12 weeks induced significantly more weight loss than placebo. Glycemic control improved in parallel with weight loss, and subjects who lost ≥10% of initial body weight showed significant decreases in both HbA1c and fasting plasma glucose. HDL-C increased slightly with the higher dose of sibutramine, whereas triglycerides fell with both doses, especially, in patients who lost ≥10% body weight. Sibutramine treatment raised sitting diastolic blood pressure (DBP) by ≥5 mmHg in a higher percentage of subjects than placebo did, but this effect was less evident in subjects who lost ≥10% of their initial weight.

In type 2 diabetic obese patients treated with sulfonylureas (26), treatment with sibutramine 15 mg/day plus a hypocaloric diet for six months produced twice as much weight loss than treatment with placebo plus diet. BMI and waist circumference also decreased to a greater extent with sibutramine than with the placebo. Mean reduction in HbA1c paralleled weight loss in both groups ($-0.78 \pm 0.17$ % in the sibutramine group and $-0.73 \pm 0.23$% in the placebo group, $P = 0.84$).

*Hypertension.* In the Netherlands, a 12 week randomized, double-blind placebo-controlled multicenter trial was conducted, which involved giving sibutramine 10 mg daily for 12 weeks to obesity-stabilized hypertensive patients with or without antihypertensive medication (27). The results demonstrated significantly greater weight reduction in the sibutramine group than in the placebo group from week 2 onwards with a mean 4.4 kg weight loss in the sibutramine group and a 2.2 kg weight loss in the placebo group. Reduction in excessive body weight was associated with a reduction in blood pressure in both groups (5.7 mmHg in the placebo and 4.0 mmHg in the sibutramine group, $P = 0.21$).

A 52-week multicenter trial compared sibutramine and placebo in the treatment of obese patients with a history of hypertension controlled with a calcium channel blocker with or without combined diuretics (28). This trial demonstrated that weight loss occurred during the first six months of the trial and was maintained over 12 months in the sibutramine-treated group. The number of sibutramine-treated patients who lost 5% or 10% of initial weight was significantly higher than the number in the placebo-treated group. Sibutramine-induced weight loss was associated with improvement in serum triglycerides, HDL-C, glucose, and uric acid. There was a small but significant increase in diastolic blood pressure (2.0 mmHg) and pulse rate (4.9 beats/min), but not systolic blood pressure.

In patients with hypertension well controlled on beta-blockers (DBP < 95 mmHg) (29), sibutramine 20 mg once daily for 12 weeks produced a greater weight reduction than placebo. This was accompanied by a greater reduction in serum triglycerides and VLDL-C. Mean supine and upright DBP and systolic blood pressure (SBP) were not statistically different between the two groups. However, there was a significant increase in pulse rate in the sibutramine group (5.6 beats/min) as compared to the placebo group (2.2 beats/min).

For hypertensive patients well treated with angiotensin-converting enzyme inhibitors (30), treatment with sibutramine 20 mg once daily for 52 weeks produced significantly more weight loss than placebo. Blood pressure remained well controlled in both groups. However, the difference in SBP and DBP between the placebo- and sibutramine-treated groups was significant by approximately 3 mmHg. Sibutramine also increased pulse rate (5.7 beats/min). Greater favorable changes in lipid profile, serum glucose, and uric acid in the sibutramine group could be accounted for by greater weight losses. The authors concluded that sibutramine is safe and effective and helps in achieving weight loss without compromising blood pressure control.

*Dyslipidemia.* In patients with dyslipidemia (triglycerides $\geq$250 mg/dL and $\leq$1000 mg/dL and serum HDL-C $\leq$ 45 mg/dL in women or $\leq$40 mg/dL in men), sibutramine 20 mg once daily plus the step 1 American Heart Association diet for 24 weeks resulted in significantly greater mean weight loss than placebo. Forty two percent and 12% of the sibutramine group lost 5% and 10% of baseline weight, respectively, compared with 8% and 3%, respectively, in the placebo group. There were also significant changes in serum triglycerides and HDL-C in the sibutramine group compared with the placebo group (31). Mean decreases in triglycerides among the 5% and 10% responders in the sibutramine group were 33.4 and 72.3 mg/dL, respectively, compared with a mean increase of 31.7 mg/dL among all patients receiving placebo. Mean increases in serum HDL-C for the 5% and 10% weight-loss responders in the sibutramine group were 4.9 and 6.7 mg/dL, respectively, compared with an increase of 1.7 mg/dL among all patients in the placebo group.

*Insulin resistance.* In studies by McLaughlin et al. (32,33), normotensive, nondiabetic insulin-resistant (IR) obese patients, as defined by higher steady-state plasma glucose (SSPG) concentration ($219 \pm 7$ mg/dL) than that in insulin-sensitive (IS) patients ($69 \pm 6$ mg/dL), had significantly higher plasma glucose, insulin, and free fatty acid (FFA), and higher plasma triglycerides as well as higher ratios of total to HDL-C than IS patients at baseline. After the introduction of sibutramine 15 mg/day with an energy-restricted diet for four months, weight loss was comparable in both groups. However, SSPG concentration decreased significantly after weight loss only in the IR group, and it was associated with a significant decline in daylong plasma glucose, insulin, and fasting triglyceride concentrations. The decline was not accompanied by a decrease in daylong plasma FFA responses. None of these variables changed in the IS group. These results indicate that weight loss is effective in reducing CHD risk in insulin-resistant, obese women.

**Dosage and administration:** The initial starting dose of sibutramine is 10 mg once daily in the morning. This can be increased to 15 mg/day after a four-week interval with less than a 4 lb weight loss or decreased to 5 mg/day, if patients do not tolerate the 10 mg dose.

**Indications:** Sibutramine has been approved by the FDA for weight loss and weight maintenance for up to two years in combination with diet control and behavioral modification. Sibutramine reaches a maximum effect after six months of therapy and can help maintain weight loss for up to two years.

**Contraindications:** Sibutramine should not be used in combination with MAOIs or within two weeks of discontinuing MAOIs due to the risk of increased norepinephrine activity leading to hypertensive crisis or excess serotonin activity resulting in serotonin syndrome. Patients who have poorly controlled hypertension ($\geq 145/90$ mmHg), coronary artery disease, congestive heart failure, arrhythmias, or cerebrovascular disease are not candidates for therapy with sibutramine. It should not be used in patients with anorexia nervosa and bulimia, those on selective serotonin reuptake or certain migraine drugs (the triptans), or patients with narrow angle glaucoma (10). Safety in pregnant or lactating women and people with renal or hepatic disease has not been established; therefore it is not recommended for those groups (34).

**Potential drug interactions:** Sibutramine negatively interacts with SSRIs, MAOIs, centrally active anorexiants, sumatriptan, dihydroergotamine, dextromethorphan, meperidine, pentazocine, fentanyl, lithium, and tryptophan. It is metabolized by the cytochrome P-450 isoenzyme 3A4. Its metabolism may be inhibited by ketoconazole and erythromycin; however, the clinical significance of these interactions is small (1).

**Adverse effects and monitoring:** The most medically significant side effects of sibutramine are an increase in blood pressure and heart rate, although these are usually mild. These side effects resulted in discontinuing drug therapy in about 5% of patients (35). Other common side effects are dry mouth, insomnia, headache, abdominal pain, constipation, and metallic taste. Pulse and blood pressure should be monitored before treatment and every two weeks for the first three months and every one to three months thereafter (18). Treatment should be stopped in patients who experience an increase in heart rate of 10 beats/min or an increase in either SBP or DBP of more than 10 mmHg on two consecutive visits (36,37).

Zannad et al. compared sibutramine 10 mg with sibutramine 20 mg or placebo for six months of treatment (38) on ventricular dimensions and heart valves in obese patients during weight reduction. The researchers found that left ventricular mass was reduced in all groups. The reductions in both the sibutramine groups were statistically significant compared with baseline, but a pairwise comparison with placebo was not statistically significant. There was no difference in overall status of the cardiac valves. No differences were observed with respect to blood pressure and electrocardiographic intervals among groups, but a significant increase in pulse rate (7 beats/min) was noted for patients on sibutramine treatment.

## Malabsorptive Drugs: Orlistat

### Mechanism of Action of Orlistat

Orlistat acts locally in the gastrointestinal (GI) tract by binding to gastric, carboxylester, lipoprotein, and pancreatic lipases, the enzymes that are essential for digestion of long-chain triglycerides, causing these enzymes to become inactive. This results in failure to hydrolyze dietary fat (triglyerides)

into absorbable FFA and monoacylglycerols. Orlistat received FDA approval for obesity treatment in April 23, 1999. Orlistat's mechanism of action
is complete in the GI tract and very little of the drug is absorbed systemically. Orlistat inhibits dietary fat absorption of up to 30% of fat calories
ingested, thus reducing calorie and fat intake (150–180 kcal/day). Patients
are strongly encouraged to eat a low-fat diet, because the consumption of
more than 20 g of fat/meal or 70 g of fat/day can induce adverse GI events
that include oily stools, flatus with discharge, and fecal urgency (39).

### Efficacy and Study Support

**For simple obesity:**  In double-blind, placebo-controlled trials, orlistat
was found to have had moderate efficacy for weight loss in adults. Orlistat-
treated subjects who completed trials lasting for one year lost approximately
9% of their pretreatment weight as compared with 5.8% among those treated
with placebo (40). Orlistat has been found to slow the rate of weight regain
during a second year of use. Orlistat-treated subjects regained less weight
than placebo did (35.2% vs. 62.4% of weight regained, a difference of about
2.5 kg) (41–43).

A randomized double-blind placebo-controlled multicenter study in
796 obese patients compared placebo three times a day with 60 mg of orlistat
tid or 120 mg of orlistat tid in conjunction with a reduced-energy diet for the
first year and a weight maintenance diet during the second year (44).
Patients treated with orlistat lost significantly more weight ($7.08 \pm 0.54$ kg
for 60 mg and $7.94 \pm 0.57$ kg for 120 mg orlistat group) than those treated
with placebo ($4.14 \pm 0.56$ kg) in year 1 and sustained more of this weight loss
during the second year. More patients treated with orlistat lost 5% or more
of their initial weight in year 1 compared with placebo. Reductions in all
lipid parameters were observed in all treatment groups during the placebo
lead-in period. After one year, total cholesterol and LDL-C levels were significantly lower in patients treated with 60 and 120 mg of orlistat compared
with placebo. These effects were maintained during the second year of treatment. Diastolic blood pressure increased slightly in the placebo group during the first year of treatment, but decreased in both orlistat groups. During
the second year of treatment, SBP was significantly reduced in the 120-mg
orlistat group compared with placebo, whereas changes in DBP did not differ significantly among groups. There were no significant differences among
treatment groups in serum triglycerides or glucose levels at any time. Fasting
insulin was lower in the 120-mg orlistat group than in placebo group after 52
weeks of treatment.

Davidson et al. conducted a randomized, double-blind, placebo-
controlled multicenter study in obese adults comparing orlistat and placebo
plus diet for two years. During the first year, orlistat-treated subjects lost
more weight than placebo-treated subjects, and this was associated with
improvements in fasting LDL-C and insulin levels. The results suggest that

orlistat effectively improves the constellation of metabolic risk factors that comprise the insulin resistance (metabolic) syndrome. For the second year, subjects treated with orlistat 120 mg three times a day regained less weight than those treated with orlistat 60 mg three times a day (41). There was also a small but significantly greater lowering of SBP and DBP between randomization and week 52 of treatment in the orlistat 120 mg group compared to placebo. After two years of treatment with orlistat 120 mg, LDL-C levels were reduced significantly below initial values compared with placebo. The greater improvements in total and LDL cholesterol were independent of the greater weight loss in the orlistat group. This independent cholesterol-lowering effect of orlistat is thought to be related to the partial inhibition of fat absorption from the GI tract (45).

Another 54 week randomized, double-blind placebo-controlled trial in 531 obese patients showed a mean weight loss in the orlistat group that was significantly greater than in the placebo group. Orlistat was associated with greater improvements than placebo in SBP and DBP, oral glucose tolerance test, fasting glucose, total cholesterol, LDL-C, and waist circumference (46).

In a multicenter, 18-month, double-blind study conducted in 81 hospital centers in France (47), orlistat 120 mg three times a day in conjunction with a mildly reduced energy diet compared with placebo plus diet had resulted in greater weight loss and a greater decrease in fasting blood glucose and LDL-C, whereas improvements in HDL-C, triglycerides, and blood pressure were not significantly different between the two treatment groups.

**Predictor of long-term success:** A retrospective analysis of pooled data from two multicenter, randomized, placebo-controlled clinical trials in 29 centers throughout Europe (48) was performed. The data showed that weight loss >5% of initial body weight after 12 weeks of orlistat 120 mg tid plus a hypocaloric diet was a good predictor of two-year weight loss. Weight loss of ≥2.5 kg during the first four weeks of lead-in and ≥10% after six months did not add significantly to the prediction of two-year outcomes. Patients who lost ≥5% of their weight at 12 weeks of treatment lost significantly more weight after two years than other patients. For those who achieved ≥5% weight loss at 12 weeks, the overall health benefits were not significantly greater in patients who lost ≥10% body weight at six months compared with those who did not achieve a 10% weight loss by month 6.

**Diabetes mellitus:** In terms of weight reduction and improvement in glycemic control (49), orlistat plus diet for one year was more effective in the treatment of obese patients with type 2 diabetes than placebo plus diet. Improvement in glycemic control was reflected as a decrease in HbA1c and fasting plasma glucose and the reduction of the dose of any oral sulfonylurea medication. Orlistat therapy also resulted in significantly greater improvements than placebo in several lipid parameters including reductions in total cholesterol, LDL-C, triglycerides, apolipoprotein B, and the LDL-C/HDL-C ratio.

Concerning glucose tolerance and type 2 diabetes, Heymsfield et al. pooled data from similar orlistat multicenter randomized, double-blind placebo-controlled trials to determine whether small amounts of weight loss improved glucose tolerance and decreased the rate of onset of type 2 diabetes in obese patients. This meta-analysis included only those patients who were assigned to treatment with orlistat 120 mg three times a day or placebo for two years. After two years of treatment, patients taking orlistat lost more weight than patients taking placebo. Among subjects with impaired glucose tolerance at baseline, glucose levels normalized in more subjects after orlistat treatment (71.6%) than after placebo treatment (49.1%). A smaller percentage of subjects with impaired glucose tolerance at baseline progressed to diabetes in the orlistat group (3.0%) as compared to the placebo (7.6%) group. Therefore the addition of orlistat to a conventional weight-loss regimen significantly improved oral glucose tolerance and diminished the rate of progression to the development of impaired glucose tolerance and type 2 diabetes (50).

Kelly et al. (51) conducted a one-year multicenter randomized, double-blind placebo-controlled trial of orlistat 120 mg three times a day or placebo combined with a reduced-calorie diet in overweight or obese patients with type 2 diabetes. Subjects were type 2 diabetic patients treated with insulin alone or combined with oral hypoglycemic agents but with suboptimal metabolic control (HbA1c 7.5–12%). After one year, the orlistat-treated group lost more weight than the placebo-treated group. Orlistat also produced greater decreases in HbA1c, fasting plasma glucose, and the required doses of insulin and other diabetic medications as well as greater improvement than placebo in serum total cholesterol, LDL-C, and LDL/HDL-C ratio.

**Hypertension:** A moderate weight loss of 5 kg is associated with a significant reduction in blood pressure in obese patients with or without hypertension (52,53). In a study by Sjostrom dealing with the effects of diet plus orlistat versus placebo for two years (43), SBP and DBP were significantly decreased in the orlistat group compared with the placebo-treated group. The greater reductions in blood pressure were consistent with the greater degree of weight loss in orlistat-treated group. A meta-analysis of five randomized, double-blind placebo-controlled trials demonstrated that patients who had diastolic hypertension (≥90 mmHg) showed a 7.9 mmHg reduction in DBP when treated with orlistat compared with a 5.5 mmHg reduction in the placebo-treated group for one year of treatment (54).

**Dyslipidemia:** In hypercholesterolemic patients (55), orlistat 120 mg three times a day plus a hypocaloric diet treatment for 24 weeks resulted in significantly more weight loss than placebo plus diet. The intervention was also associated with significantly greater changes in total cholesterol and LDL-C than placebo. For any category of weight loss, the change in LDL-C was greater in the orlistat-treated patients than in the placebo-treated patients, indicating that orlistat had a direct cholesterol-lowering effect that was independent of weight reduction.

Lucas et al. found that hypercholesterolemic patients treated with orlistat lost more weight and had a greater decrease in plasma total and LDL cholesterol, triglycerides, glucose, and insulin concentrations compared with the diet-only treated patients. Following orlistat-assisted weight loss, type IIB lipid disorder patients experienced a greater triglyceride and insulin decrease and HDL-C increase than type IIA lipid disorder patients. They also experienced a significantly greater decrease in the ratio of LDL-C/HDL-C (56).

**Metabolic syndrome:** In metabolic syndrome as defined by plasma triglycerides more than 195 mg/dL and HDL cholesterol less than 39 mg/dL, orlistat plus diet for one year produced significantly more weight loss than placebo plus diet. There was also a significant reduction in plasma insulin and triglycerides, an increase in HDL-C and a decrease in LDL-C/HDL-C ratio. It can therefore be concluded that orlistat attenuates coronary heart disease risk factors in obese patients with metabolic syndrome (57).

## Dosage and Administration

The recommended dose of orlistat is 120 mg three times a day with meals or up to one hour before or after meals. Patients considering orlistat should be instructed on a well-balanced, hypocaloric diet with fat content limited to approximately 30% of total calories to prevent aggravating the GI side effects of the drug.

## Contraindications

Contraindications for the use of orlistat are chronic malabsorption syndrome, cholestasis, and known hypersensitivity to orlistat or its components. There are no adequate and well-controlled studies of orlistat in pregnancy. It is not known if orlistat is secreted in breast milk; therefore, orlistat should not be used in pregnant and breast-feeding women (45).

## Potential Drug Interactions

Orlistat markedly decreased peak and trough blood cyclosporine concentrations in transplant patients (10). In a short-term study, orlistat did not result in any change in warfarin pharmacokinetics or pharmacodynamics. However, because of a potential decrease in vitamin K absorption, patients stabilized on warfarin should be closely monitored for changes in coagulation parameters (45). The warfarin-anticoagulant effect may increase over time (58). One small study showed that orlistat used concomitantly with pravastatin increased the lipid-lowering effect of pravastatin (59).

## Adverse Effects and Monitoring

The adverse events of orlistat include oily spotting, abdominal pain, flatus with discharge, fecal urgency/incontinence, steatorrhea (oily stool), and increased frequency of defecation, which are related to its pharmacological action. These effects are usually of mild to moderate intensity, transient, and can spontaneously resolve within a few weeks to one month. Nevertheless, such side effects lead to discontinuation in nearly 9% of patients as compared to 5% among placebo-treated group (39). One study found that the concomitant use of natural fiber (psyllium mucilliod), 6 g dissolved in a glass of water, in obese patients receiving orlistat 120 mg three times a day is helpful in reducing the incidence of these GI side effects (60).

Treatment with orlistat is not related to an increased risk of gallstone formation based on current studies. Some patients may excrete excessive urinary oxalate upon using orlistat; therefore it should be used cautiously in patients with a history of hyperoxaluria or calcium oxalate stones. Absorption of the fat-soluble vitamins (A, D, E, and K) and beta-carotene may decrease during orlistat therapy.

In the Sjostrom et al. (43) study, 11.9% of patients in the orlistat group and 5.3% in the placebo group had two or more consecutive low fat-soluble vitamin concentrations recorded in the first year of treatment. Treatment with orlistat was associated with a slightly higher incidence of reduced fat-soluble vitamin concentration in the Davidson study as well (41). Patients should be encouraged to take a multivitamin daily while taking orlistat, two hours before or after taking the orlistat dose (61).

## COMBINATION THERAPY WITH SIBUTRAMINE AND ORLISTAT

Because the mechanisms of action are different, it is reasonable to combine orlistat with sibutramine to increase efficacy. A study of 34-obese women treated with sibutramine for one year showed achievement of a mean weight loss of 11.6%. The subjects were then randomly assigned by a double-blind method to either a sibutramine plus placebo group or sibutramine plus orlistat group. The sibutramine plus orlistat group demonstrated no additional weight loss during 16 weeks of combined therapy (62). This finding suggests that the combination of sibutramine and orlistat is unlikely to have additional effects that will yield mean losses ≥15% of initial weight as desired by many obese patients. However, the sample size in the study was small. More data is needed to support or refute the use of combination therapy with sibutramine and orlistat.

## A COMPARISON STUDY OF ORLISTAT AND SIBUTRAMINE

One study compared sibutramine 10 mg bid with orlistat 120 mg tid and metformin 850 mg bid in 150 females for six months of therapy (63). All three groups showed significant reductions in BMI, fasting and postprandial blood glucose, and insulin resistance as assessed by the homeostasis model for assessment of insulin resistance, total cholesterol, VLDL-C, and LDL-C, triglyceride, lipoprotein (a), and apolipoprotein B, uric acid levels, pulse, and SBP and DBP. None of the groups showed significant changes in HDL-C or apolipoprotein A1. There was a significantly greater fall in BMI in the sibutramine group (13.57%) as compared to the two other groups (9.06% in the orlistat group and 9.90% in the metformin group) with $P < 0.0001$. According to this study, it can be concluded that 10 mg bid of sibutramine is more effective than orlistat or metformin therapy in terms of weight reduction.

## COMPARISONS AMONG THE THREE FDA-APPROVED ANTIOBESITY AGENTS—SIBUTRAMINE, ORLISTAT, AND PHENTERMINE

A meta-analysis of randomized clinical trials of medications for obesity (64) presented the effect size and 95% confidence intervals (CI) for drug–placebo comparisons. The outcomes suggested that sibutramine produced the largest mean effect size suggesting that sibutramine overall produced the most weight loss. Nevertheless, the 95% CI of the effect size of sibutramine and orlistat overlapped with the 95% CI of phentermine. Therefore it was concluded that no drug or class of drugs demonstrated clear superiority over other classes. Increasing lengths of drug treatment periods did not lead to more weight losses. Thus longer treatments appear to promote weight maintenance but further weight loss beyond the typical plateau at six months is unlikely.

## COMMENTS AND CONCLUSIONS

Weight maintenance is an important step after weight loss to ensure reduction in cardiovascular risk and requires ongoing contact with a physician, other weight-loss counselors (dietitians, exercise therapists, etc.), exercise, social support, and extended treatment. In the long term, the most effective approach to controlling obesity may be to view it as a chronic disease (65). As such, it requires long-term treatment, and obese patients must be willing to make major changes in eating habits, lifestyle, and physical activity to achieve long lasting results (66).

The greatest benefit of pharmacotherapy may reside in facilitating maintenance rather than the induction of weight loss. Therefore weight-loss medications should be used long term in the same manner as agents used for hypertension and diabetes. However, there are several barriers to the long-term use of antiobesity agents, including costs and side effects (67).

Because obesity is a chronic condition, pharmacotherapy should be initiated with the expectation that long-term use will most likely be needed (68). Numerous studies indicate that just as blood pressure may increase when antihypertensive drugs are discontinued, patients may regain weight

**Table 1**  Summary of Pharmacological Therapy for Obesity

| Medication | Mechanism of action | Dosage | Contraindications | Common adverse effects |
|---|---|---|---|---|
| Phentermine (Adipex®, Ionamin®): Approved by the FDA in 1973 for short-term use (≤3 mo) | Norepinephrine reuptake inhibitor | 15–37.5 mg once daily before breakfast or 1–2 hrs after breakfast | Uncontrolled HTN severe cardiovascular disease; hyperthyroidism glaucoma; combinations with MAOI, TCA | Dry mouth; constipation; palpitations; increased blood pressure; headache; nervousness; insomnia |
| Sibutramine (Meridia®): Approved by the FDA in 1997 for long-term use (up to two years) | Serotonin and norepinephrine reuptake inhibitor; weak dopamine reuptake inhibitor | Starting dose 10 mg once daily in the AM Maximum dose 10 mg twice per day. Also comes in 5 and 15 mg doses | Combinations with MAOI; uncontrolled HTN coronary artery disease; congestive heart failure; arrhythmias; cerebrovascular disease; narrow angle glaucoma | Increased blood pressure; increased heart rate; dry mouth; insomnia; headache; abdominal pain; constipation; metallic taste |
| Orlistat (Xenical®): Approved by the FDA in 1999 for long-term use (up to two years) | Lipase inhibitor: binds to gastric, carboxyl ester, lipoprotein, and pancreatic lipase in GI tract resulting in inhibition of 30% dietary fat absorption | 120 mg three times a day with meals or up to 1 hr before or after meals | Chronic malabsorption syndrome; cholestasis; hypersensitivity to orlistat | Oily spotting; abdominal pain; flatus with discharge; fecal urgency; fecal incontinent; steatorrhea |

after discontinuing weight-loss medications. Therefore, careful consideration of the known and possible risks of long-term medical therapy must
be weighed against potential improvements in the patient's risk of obesity-
related diseases.

Approved prescription medications for weight loss appear to have
similar efficacy in controlled studies. Therefore an empirical choice of a specific medication should be based on consideration of underlying medical
conditions or contraindications to particular drugs, concurrent medications,
need for monitoring, approval for long-term use, cost, and the preference of
the patient (10). Table 1 gives a summary of the pharmacologic agents
reviewed in this chapter.

Identification of patients with a response would enable the risk and
costs of drug treatment to be concentrated among those who are most likely
to be benefit. In addition to preintervention body weight, success during the
first month of therapy usually predicts ultimate weight loss (69). In patients
without a weight loss of at least 2 kg in the first four weeks of treatment,
compliance with medication, diet, and exercise recommendations should
be reassessed, and the possible need for an adjustment in the dosage should
be considered. If there continues to be minimal response to the medication,
the clinician should consider discontinuing the drug or substituting another
medication (68).

Currently, several studies are ongoing to identify the new targets for
pharmacological regulation of body weight gain. It is possible that in the
future, patients will be treated with multiple antiobesity agents, affecting different mechanisms responsible for appetite, thermogenesis, as well as fuel
utilization to develop safe and effective ways to lose weight, or with gene
therapy to regulate body weight and prevent obesity in high-risk patients.

Based on the data presented in this chapter, antiobesity agents can be
safe and effective adjunctive treatment for overweight and obese subjects
with mild to moderate cardiovascular disease as long as they are used with
caution and frequent monitoring for adverse events.

## REFERENCES

1. Campbell ML, Mathys ML. Pharmacologic options for the treatment of obesity. Am J Health Syst Pharm 2001; 58:1301–1308.
2. The practical guide: identification, evaluation, and treatment of overweight and
   obesity in adults. Bethesda MD: National Heart, Lung, and Blood Institute,
   North American Association for the study of obesity. NIH Publication no.
   00–4084.
3. Weigle DS. Pharmacological therapy of obesity: past, present, and future.
   J Clin Endocrinol Metab 2003; 88:2462–2469.
4. Glazer, Gary. Long term pharmacotherapy of obesity 2000: a review of efficacy
   and safety. Arch Intern Med 2001; 161:1814–1824.

5. Munro JF, Maccuish AC, Wilson EM, Duncan LJP. Comparison of continuous and intermittent anorectic therapy in obesity. BMJ 1968; 1:352–354.
6. Truant AP, Olon LP, Cobb S. Phentermine resin as an adjunct in medical weight reduction: a controlled, randomized, double-blind prospective study. Current Therapeutic Research 1972; 14:726–737.
7. Weintraub M, Hasday JD, Mushlin AI, Lockwood DH. A double-blind clinical trial in weight control: use of fenfluramine and phentermine alone and in combination. Arch Intern Med 1984; 144:1143–1148.
8. Steel JM, Munro JF, Duncan LJ. A comparison trial of different regimens of fenfluramine and phentermine in obesity. Practitioner 1973; 211:232–236.
9. Cordero-MacIntyre ZR, Lohman TG, Rosen J, et al. Weight loss is correlated with an improved lipoprotein profile in obese postmenopausal women. J Am Col Nutr 2000; 19:275–284.
10. Yanovski, S, Yanovski JA. Drug therapy: obesity. N Engl J Med 2002; 346: 591–602.
11. Hensen DL, Toubro S, Stock MJ, Macdonald IA, Astrup AV. Thermogenic effect of sibutramine in humans. Am J Clin Nutr 1998; 68:1180–1186.
12. Hensen DL, Toubro S, Stock MJ, Macdonald IA, Astrup A. The effect of sibutramine on energy expenditure and appetite during chronic treatment without dietary restriction. Int J Obes Relat Metab Disord 1999; 23:1016–1024.
13. Finer N. Sibutramine: its mode of action and efficacy. Int J Obes Relat Metab Disord 2002; 26(suppl 4):S29–S33.
14. Van Gaal LF, Peiffer FW. The importance of obesity in diabetes and its treatment with sibutramine. J Obes Relat Metab Disord 2001; 25(suppl 4): S24–S28.
15. Jones SP, Smith IG, Kelly F, Gray JA. Long term weight loss with sibutramine. Int J Obes Relat Metab Disord 1995; 19(suppl 2):S41.
16. Smith IG, Goulder MA. Randomized placebo-controlled trial of long term treatment with sibutramine in mild to moderate obesity. J Fam Pract 2001; 50: 505–512.
17. Bray GA, Blackburn GL, Ferguson JM, et al. Sibutramine produces dose-related weight loss. Obes Res 1999; 7:189–198.
18. James WP, Astrup A, Finer N, Hilsted J, Kopelman P, Rossner S, Saris WH, Van Gaal LF. Effect of sibutramine on weight maintenance after weight loss: a randomized trial. STORM Study Group. Sibutramine trial of obesity reduction and maintenance. Lancet 2000; 356:2119–2125.
19. Van Gaal LF, Wauters MA, Peiffer FW, De leeuw IH. Sibutramine and fat distribution: is there a role for pharmacotherapy in abdominal/visceral fat reduction? J Obes Relat Metab Disord 1998; 22(suppl 1):S38–S40.
20. Wirth A, Krause J. Long-term weight loss with sibutramine: a randomized controlled trial. JAMA 2001; 286:1331–1339.
21. Finer N. Sibutramine in clinical practice. Int J Obes Relat Metab Disord 2001; 25(suppl 4):S12–S15.
22. Krejs GJ. Metabolic benefits associated with sibutramine therapy. J Obes Relat Metab Disord 2002; 26(suppl 4):S34–S37.
23. Finer N, Bloom SR, Forst GS, Banks LM, Griffiths J. Sibutramine is effective for weight loss and diabetic control in obesity with type 2 diabetes: a

randomized, double-blind, placebo-controlled study. Diabestes Obes Metab 2000; 2:105–112.

24. Gokcel A, Karakose H, Ertorer EM, Tanaci N, Tutunca NB, Guvener N. Effects of sibutramine in obese female subjects with type 2 diabetes and poor blood glucose control. Diabetes Care 2001; 24:1957–1960.

25. McNulty SJ, Ur E, Williams G. A randomized trial of sibutramine in the management of obese type 2 diabetic patients treated with metformin. Diabetes Care 2003; 26:125–131.

26. Serrano-Rios M, Melchionda N, Moreno-Carretero E, Spanish Investigators. Role of sibutramine in the treatment of obese type 2 diabetic patients receiving sulfonylurea therapy. Diabet Med 2002; 19:119–124.

27. Hazenberg BP. Randomized, double-blind, placebo-controlled, multicenter study of sibutramine in obese hypertensive patients. Cardiology 2000; 94: 152–158.

28. McMahon FG, Fujioka K, Singh BN, et al. Efficacy and safety of sibutramine in obese white and African American patients with hypertension: a 1-year, double-blind, placebo-controlled, multicenter trial. Arch Intern Med 2000; 160: 2185–2191.

29. Sramek JJ, Leibowitz MT, Weinstein SP, et al. Efficacy and safety of sibutramine for weight loss in obese patients with hypertension well controlled by beta adrenergic-blocking agents: a placebo-controlled, double-blind, randomized trial. J Hum Hypertens 2002; 16:13–19.

30. McMahon FG, Weinstein SP, Rowe E, Ernst KR, Johnson F, Fujioka K, Sibutramine in hypertensives clinical study group. Sibutramine is safe and effective for weight loss in obese patients whose hypertension is well controlled with angiotensin-converting enzyme inhibitors. J Hum Hypertens 2002; 16:5–11.

31. Dujovne CA, Zavoral JH, Rowe E, Mendel CM. Effects of sibutramine on body weight and serum lipids: a double-blind, randomized, placebo-controlled study in 322 overweight and obese patients with dyslipidemia. Am Heart J 2001; 142:489–497.

32. McLaughlin T, Abbasi F, Lamendola C, Kim HS, Reaven GM. Metabolic changes following sibutramine-assisted weight loss in obese individuals: role of plasma free fatty acids in the insulin resistance of obesity. Metab: Clin Exp 2001; 50:819–824.

33. McLaughlin T, Abbasi F, Kim HS, Lamendola C, Schaaf P, Reaven GM. Relationship between insulin resistance, weight loss and coronary heart disease risk in healthy, obese women. Metab: Clin Exp 2001; 50:795–800.

34. Abbott Laboratories: Meridia (sibutramine hydrochloride monohydrate). Product information. In: Physician's desk reference. Montvale, NJ: Thompson PDR, 2003:475–480.

35. Fujioka K, Seaton TB, Rowe E, Jelinek CA, Raskin P, Lebovitz HE. Weight loss with sibutramine improves glycemic control and other metabolic parameters in obese patients with type 2 diabetes mellitus. Diabetes Obes Metab 2000; 2:175–187.

36. Wooltorton Eric. Obesity drug sibutramine (meridia): hypertension and cardiac arrythmias. Can Med Assoc J 2002; 166:1307–1308.

37. Narkiewicz K. Sibutramine and its cardiovascular profile. Int J Obes Relat Metab Disord 2002; 26(suppl 4):S38–S41.
38. Zannad F, Gille B, Grentzinger A, et al. Effects of sibutramine on ventricular dimensions and heart valves in obese patients during weight reduction. Am Heart J 2002; 144:508–515.
39. Fabricatore AN, Wadden TA. Treatment of obesity: an overview. Clin Diabetes 2003; 21:67–72.
40. Heck AM, Yanovski JA, Calis KA. Orlistat, a new lipase inhibitor for the management of obesity. Pharmacotherapy 2000; 20:270–279.
41. Davidson MH, Hauptman J, DiGirolamo M, et al. Weight control and risk factor reduction in obese subjects treated for 2 years with orlistat: a randomized controlled trial. JAMA 1999; 281:235–242.
42. Hill JO, Hauptman J, Anderson JW, et al. Orlistat, a lipase inhibitor, for weight maintenance after conventional dieting: a 1-y study. Am J Clin Nutr 1999; 69: 1108–1116.
43. Sjostrom L, Rissanen A, Andersen T, et al. Randomized placebo-controlled trial of orlistat for weight loss and prevention of weight regain in obese patients. Lancet 1998; 352:167–172.
44. Hauptman J, Lucas C, Boldrin MN, Collins H, Segal K. Orlistat in the long-term treatment of obesity in primary care settings. Arch Fam Med 2000; 9:160–167.
45. Ballinger A, Peikin SR. Orlistat: its current status as an anti-obesity drug. Eur J Pharmacol 2002; 440:109–117.
46. Broom I, Wilding J, Stott P, Myers N, UK Multimorbidity study group. Randomized trial of the effect of orlistat on body weight and cardiovascular disease risk profile in obese patients: UK multimorbidity study. Int J Clin Prac 2002; 56:494–499.
47. Krempf M, Louvet JP, Allanic H, Miloradovich T, Joubert JM, Attali JR. Weight reduction and long term maintenance after 18 months treatment with orlistat for obesity. Int J Obes Relat Metab Disord 2003; 27:591–597.
48. Rissanen A, Lean M, Rossner S, Segal KR, Sjostrom L. Predictive value of early weight loss in obesity management with orlistat: an evidence-based assessment of prescribing guidelines. Int J Obes Relat Metab Disord 2003; 27: 103–109.
49. Hollander PA, Elbein SC, Hirsch IB, et al. Role of orlistat in the treatment of obese patients with type 2 diabetes: a 1-year randomized double-blind study. Diabetes Care 1998; 21:1288–1294.
50. Heymsfield, SB, Segal KR, Hauptman J, et al. Effects of weight loss with orlistat on glucose tolerance and progression to type 2 diabetes in obese adults. Arch Intern med 2000; 160:1321–1326.
51. Kelly DE, George A, Pi-Sunger FX, et al. Clinical efficacy of orlistat therapy in overweight and obese patients with insulin-treated type 2 diabetes: a 1-year randomized controlled trial. Diabetes Care 2002; 25:1033–1041.
52. Langford HG, Davis BR, Blaufox D, et al. Effect of drug and diet treatment of mild hypertension on diastolic blood pressure. The TAIM Research Group. Hypertension 1991; 17:210–217.

53. Whelton PK, Appel LJ, Espeland MA, et al. Sodium reduction and weight loss in the treatment of hypertension in older persons: a randomized controlled trial of nonpharmacologic interventions in the elderly (TONE). TONE Collaborative Research Group. JAMA 1998; 279:839–846.
54. Zavoral JH. Treatment with orlistat reduces cardiovascular risk in obese patients. J Hypertens 1998; 16:2013–2017.
55. Muls E, Kolanowski J, Scheen A, Gaal LV for the ObelHyx study group. The effects of orlistat on weight and on serum lipids in obese patients with hypercholesterolemia: randomized, double-blind, placebo-controlled, multicenter study. Int J Obes Relat Metab Disord 2001; 25:1713–1721.
56. Lucas CP, Boldrin MN, Reaven GM. Effect of orlistat added to diet (30% of calories from fat) on plasma lipids, glucose, and insulin in obese patients with hypercholesterolemia. Am J Cardiol 2003; 91:961–964.
57. Reaven G, Segal K, Hauptman J, Boldrin M, Lucas C. Effect of orlistat-assisted weight loss in decreasing coronary heart disease risk in patients with syndrome X. Am J Cardiol 2001; 87:827–831.
58. Cada DJ, Baker DE, Levien T. Orlistat. Hosp Pharm 1999; 34:1195–1213.
59. Schrefer J ed. Mosby GenRx: a comprehensive reference for generic and brand prescription drugs. 11th ed. St. Louis: Mosby, 2001.
60. Cavaliere H, Floriano I, Medeiros-Neto G. Gastrointestinal side effects of orlistat may be prevented by concomitant prescription of natural fibers (psyllium mucilloid). Int J Obes Relat Metab Disord 2001; 25:1095–1099.
61. Physicians' desk reference. 55th ed. Montvale, NJ: Medical economics, 2001.
62. Wadden TA, Berkowitz RI, Womble LG, Sarwer DB, Arnold ME, Steinberg CM. Effects of sibutramine plus orlistat in obese women following 1 year of treatment by sibutramine alone: a placebo-controlled trial. Obes Res 2000; 8:431–437.
63. Gokcel A, Gumurdulu Y, Karakose H, et al. Evaluation of safety and efficacy of sibutramine, orlistat and metformin in the treatment of obesity. Diabestes Obes Metab 2002; 4:49–55.
64. Haddock CK, Poston WSC, Dill PL, Foreyt JP, Ericsson M. Pharmacotherapy for obesity: a quantitative analysis of four decades of published randomized clinical trials. Int J Obes Relat Metab Disord 2002; 26:262–273.
65. Krauss RM, Winston M. Obesity: impact on cardiovascular disease. Circulation 1998; 98:1472–1476.
66. Aronne LJ. Obesity. Med Clin N Am 1998; 82:161–181.
67. Bray GA. Use and abuse of appetite-suppressant drugs in the treatment of obesity. Ann Intern Med 1993; 119:707–713.
68. National task force on the prevention and treatment of obesity. Long-term pharmacotherapy in the management of obesity. JAMA 1996; 276:1907–1915.
69. National Institutes of Health/National heart Lung and Blood Institute: clinical guidelines on the identification, evaluation, and treatment of overweight and obesity in adults: the evidence report. Obes Res 1998; 6(suppl 2):S51–S210.

# 14

# Bariatric Surgery and Reduction of Cardiovascular Risk Factors

**Malcolm K. Robinson and J. Efren Gonzalez**

*Metabolic Support Service and the Department of Surgery, Brigham and Women's Hospital, Harvard Medical School, Boston, Massachusetts, U.S.A.*

**Danny O. Jacobs**

*Department of Surgery, Duke University Medical Center, Durham, North Carolina, U.S.A.*

## INTRODUCTION

Currently, over 140,000 weight-loss or "bariatric" surgical procedures are performed each year in the United States (1). Surgery is considered by the National Institutes of Health (NIH) to be the weight-loss treatment of choice for appropriately selected individuals who are severely obese (2). Surgical treatment of obesity is routinely associated with loss of greater than 100 lb. Hence, it is not surprising that patients who undergo such operations can have substantial amelioration of comorbid conditions because such improvements can be seen with losing as little as 15 to 20 lb.

This chapter will review the indications for bariatric surgery and the evaluation of obese patients who are considering surgical intervention. The types of bariatric procedures commonly performed will be described. Finally, the long-term effects of bariatric surgery, with an emphasis on cardiovascular risk, will be discussed. It will be noted that those who undergo bariatric surgery have not only a dramatic reduction in weight but also a dramatic improvement in cardiovascular risk factors including diabetes, hypertension, and hyperlipidemia.

## INDICATIONS FOR BARIATRIC SURGERY

The indications for surgical treatment of severe obesity are based on the recommendations of the NIH Consensus Development Conference on Gastrointestinal Surgery for Severe Obesity (3). The first criterion that must be met before considering a patient for bariatric surgery is weight. Patients must have class II or class III obesity to be considered for such surgery (2,3). Patients with a body mass index (BMI) of 35 to 39.9 kg/m$^2$ (i.e., class II obesity) must also have severe weight-related conditions such as diabetes or sleep apnea. A list of comorbid conditions, which would allow those with class II obesity to potentially qualify for surgery, is outlined in Table 1. Those with a BMI of 40 kg/m$^2$ or greater (i.e., class III obesity) may be appropriate for bariatric surgery even if they have not developed any comorbid conditions, assuming there are no contraindications to surgery as described below. The NIH consensus panel developed these weight criteria based on evidence that such patients are in the "extremely high risk" category for morbidity and mortality, and therefore aggressive, invasive treatment may be warranted (3).

Once patients satisfy the BMI criteria for bariatric surgery, they can be more fully evaluated to determine if nonsurgical treatment options have been attempted and exhausted and if they have an acceptable surgical risk. Hence, a patient should have an extensive history of previous weight-loss attempts through nonsurgical means over a minimum of five years before considering bariatric surgery. There should be no psychological or behavioral conditions that are untreated or uncontrolled, including substance abuse. Patients are routinely screened for such issues before proceeding with surgery.

Patients should not have severe organ dysfunction, which would make perioperative morbidity and mortality risk unacceptably high. For example, those patients with unstable angina, end-stage pulmonary disease, or cirrhosis may have relative or absolute contraindications to bariatric surgery. Patients should receive the appropriate screening evaluation of organ

**Table 1**  Comorbid Conditions That May Qualify Patients with Class II Obesity for Bariatric Surgery

| |
|---|
| Hypertension |
| Hyperlipidemia |
| Cardiovascular disease |
| Obesity-related cardiomyopathy |
| Severe sleep apnea |
| Pickwickian syndrome |
| Poorly controlled type 2 diabetes |
| Degenerative joint disease |

function prior to proceeding with surgery. Of note, particular attention should be paid to evaluating the cardiovascular system because patients with class II and III obesity are at obvious risk for having dysfunction of this system, which may be "silent." The cardiac workup and management of patients undergoing bariatric surgery is described in more detail in Chapter 15.

One ongoing controversy in the field of bariatric surgery is the appropriate age limits for patients considering such surgery. Adults in the 21- to 55-year age range are generally deemed appropriate candidates for surgery assuming they have no other contraindication to surgery. However, it has been felt that patients older than 55 may have a prohibitively high operative risk and that the "risk/benefit" ratio in "older" individuals does not favor advising surgical intervention. At the other end of the spectrum, several have argued that adolescents and very young adults may not have the maturity to make such a life-altering decision; that once they are more mature, nonsurgical weight-loss treatments may be more effective; and finally that the long-term effects of weight-loss surgery in those who have an additional 55 to 60 years of life expectancy are unknown, and therefore such a "radical" approach to weight loss is too risky.

Several articles have explored operative risk in individuals older than 55 who undergo bariatric surgery (4–9). Although it is generally accepted that older individuals do have a higher operative risk compared to younger individuals, it does not seem prohibitive. Some have argued that operating on severely obese patients up to age 70 to induce weight loss may be appropriate (9,10). One can conclude several things based on review of the various articles on this topic. First, there probably should not be a firm age cutoff in terms of offering bariatric surgery. Older individuals can be operated on safely with good outcomes as a group if individuals in this age category are selected carefully. Secondly, older patients require a more careful and potentially more extensive workup looking for silent organ disease (e.g., echocardiograms and cardiac stress tests) than might otherwise be recommended. Although such workup may not prevent individuals from sustaining primary complications nor identify individuals who may sustain primary complications [e.g., anastomotic leak, intra-abdominal abscess, and pulmonary embolism (PE)], it may aid in identifying those with the necessary physiologic reserve to tolerate and survive such complications if one or more complications were to occur. Finally, the ultimate decision to proceed in older patients should be based on one's assessment of the specific individual's risks relative to the potential benefits, and not just age alone.

Adolescent bariatric surgery is less well studied than bariatric surgery in older individuals. However, recent articles suggest that it may be appropriate in this age population as well (11–14). As with operating in individuals at the other end of the age spectrum, there are special considerations. It is recommended that surgery be reserved for only those adolescents with class III obesity, who have weight-related comorbidities and have failed six months of organized weight-loss attempts. Surgery should not be considered in adolescents until the epiphyseal plates are closed and mature bone length has been achieved because rapid weight loss may adversely affect bone growth due to restricted caloric intake during this critical time of development. This is generally an age greater than 13 in girls and 15 in boys (11). In addition, the family support system takes on an especially important role when operating on younger individuals. It is the extremely rare individual who at so young an age does not absolutely require the full support of the family. Thus, patient evaluation in the very young essentially mandates extensive evaluation of the patient's family and support network as well.

One final consideration of bariatric surgery in adolescents is which should be the "procedure of choice" for such individuals. The relative roles of gastric bypass (GBP) versus adjustable gastric banding (see description of these procedures below) need to be evaluated. The GBP is "more permanent" in that it requires cutting and rerouting of the intestines, permanently altering the patient's anatomy with unknown long-term effects in adolescents. The laparoscopic adjustable band does not permanently alter patient anatomy and can be removed, thereby returning the anatomy to normal if necessary. Thus, this may be more appropriate for the very young, but this has yet to be critically studied (12,14,15). Although there is a great deal to learn about adolescent bariatric surgery, some form of such surgery is likely to take on an important role, given the rapid rise in obesity in this age group and with the emergence of cardiovascular risk factors such as type 2 diabetes.

In general, the decision to proceed with bariatric surgery requires careful evaluation of the patient and analysis of both physical and psychosocial issues. This usually requires a multidisciplinary team with a comprehensive program to support patients preoperatively, during hospitalization, and for a lifetime postoperatively (2,3). Once a patient has gone through a thorough evaluation, bariatric surgery can be done with relatively low morbidity and mortality compared to obese patients who do not undergo such surgery (16). Several procedures are available for the treatment of obesity and are described below.

## BARIATRIC SURGICAL PROCEDURES

Surgical intervention in the treatment of obesity of morbid obesity began in the early 1950s when several different groups (17) proposed shortening the intestinal tract via "bypass" procedures to produce substantial decreases in absorptive area. Surgeons based this proposal on observations made in patients who had massive small bowel resections for other pathological conditions and in whom there was significant weight loss followed by weight stabilization (18). Although bypassing a large segment of bowel is effective in causing weight loss, the side effects associated with such procedures were often debilitating and at times life threatening. Since then, approximately 30 different surgical techniques have been described for treating obesity, and much advancement has been made. The goal has been to limit debilitating symptoms such as diarrhea and malnutrition while causing substantial and durable weight loss. The surgical attack on obesity has been directed toward creating a negative energy balance by (i) reducing caloric absorption by way of a small bowel bypass, (ii) reducing caloric consumption by limiting gastric capacity through banding and stapling techniques, or (iii) producing weight loss through a procedure that combines both malabsorption and restriction of caloric intake. The description of every type of bariatric procedure is beyond the scope of this chapter. However, the three major categories of these operations are described using a few prototype operations for illustration.

## Malabsorptive Procedures

The *jejunoileal bypass* is one of the earlier bariatric surgical procedures, which was described by Payne et al. (Fig. 1A) (19). It is a classic malabsorptive

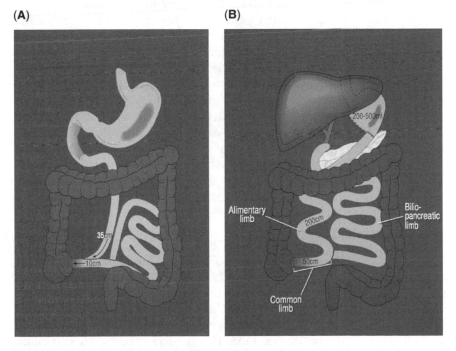

**(A)**      **(B)**

**Figure 1** (**A**) Jejunoileal bypass; (**B**) biliopancreatic diversion.

procedure in that the mechanism of weight loss depends totally on malabsorption of consumed food and not restriction of food intake. In this procedure, the proximal jejunum is divided 35 cm distal to the ligament of Treitz. The proximal segment is then anastomosed to the distal ileum, 10 cm proximal to the ileocecal valve. The long bypassed or excluded segment of the small intestine is vented to the colon or small intestine to prevent obstruction. Of note, no food or biliopancreatic secretions pass through the bypassed segment. Although quite effective in inducing weight loss, the jejunoileal bypass is associated with massive diarrhea, electrolyte imbalances, vitamin and mineral deficiencies, and life-threatening liver dysfunction. This procedure has been abandoned because of its high morbidity and mortality risks and essentially is no longer accepted as an appropriate bariatric procedure (20,21).

More recently, another type of malabsorptive procedure was described by Scopinaro of Genoa, Italy (Fig. 1B) (22). Known as the *biliopancreatic diversion* (BPD), the procedure consists of a subtotal gastrectomy leaving a gastric remnant of 200 to 400 mL. The small bowel is divided 250 cm proximal to the ileocecal valve. The distal small bowel limb is then anastomosed to the gastric remnant. The end of the proximal small bowel limb is anastomosed to the side of the distal small bowel limb 50 cm proximal to the ileocecal valve. This construction results in three small bowel limbs: a long biliopancreatic limb through which biliopancreatic secretions travel, a 200 cm alimentary limb through which food travels after passing through the stomach remnant, and a 50 cm common limb where food and biliopancreatic secretions mix and most of the digestion and absorption of consumed food occurs. The relatively large gastric remnant does little to limit food intake, especially for the long term, and the primary mechanism by which this operation produces weight loss is by inducing malabsorption. Although this procedure is popular in certain parts of Europe, there is limited use of this operation in the United States where malabsorption can be overly harsh and lead to debilitating diarrhea as a result of the typical, high-fat American diet. This side effect seems to be less of a problem in Italy, where the typical diet is higher in complex carbohydrates and relatively lower in fat when compared to the typical American eating pattern.

## Restrictive Procedures

Edward Mason, considered by many to be the father of bariatric surgery, described the *vertical banded gastroplasty* (VBG) (Fig. 2A) (23). In this procedure, a vertically oriented 15 to 30 mL gastric pouch is created along the lesser curve of the proximal stomach. The outlet of this pouch, which leads to the remaining stomach, is encircled with a band of Marlex® mesh to prevent dilatation of the outlet over time. This is a purely restrictive procedure in that it limits the amount of food that one can eat at any one sitting to one

**(A)**                  **(B)**

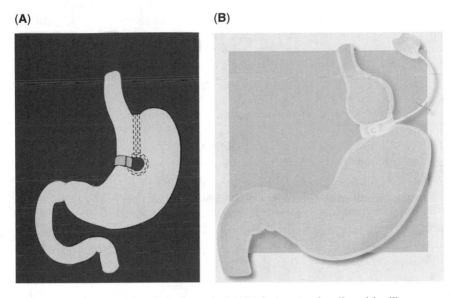

**Figure 2**   (**A**) Vertical banded gastroplasty; (**B**) laparoscopic adjustable silicone gastric banding.

to two ounces of solid food. Any food that is consumed is absorbed in the normal way and to no lesser a degree than that which occurred before surgical intervention. The reduced intake of food, however, results in weight loss. The advantage of this procedure is that it is technically easier and faster to perform than malabsorptive procedures and avoids issues with severe diarrhea, vitamin and mineral deficiencies, and liver dysfunction. However, the long-term weight loss is less effective than pure malabsorptive procedures or procedures that combine malabsorption and restrictive components. Although this operation may be appropriate when a malabsorptive type procedure is contraindicated or not feasible, it is generally agreed that VBG is less effective than other bariatric procedures and therefore infrequently used by bariatric surgeons in the United States (24,25).

    The *laparoscopic adjustable silicone gastric banding* (LASGB), is an emerging restrictive procedure gaining popularity among patients, surgeons, and primary care physicians alike (Fig. 2B). The adjustable silicone band was originally described by Kuzmak et al. (26) and is now almost exclusively placed using laparoscopic surgical techniques (27). The band is a silicone-jacketed, belt-like device that is wrapped around the upper part of the stomach near the angle of His. This results in partitioning of the stomach into a small 30 mL proximal pouch and a larger distal stomach remnant in continuity with the pouch. The inner part of the band has an inflatable fluid-filled sack to which a catheter is attached. The catheter, in turn, is attached to a port, which sits just beneath the skin of the abdominal wall.

The port can be accessed through the skin with a syringe and a needle to either add or remove saline from the sack, thereby tightening or loosening the band, respectively. Thus, the band is "adjustable." Patients have their bands adjusted depending on adequacy of weight loss or symptoms suggesting that it is too tight. The advantage of LASGB is that it is a fast, relatively safe procedure that requires no cutting or stapling of the stomach. The adjustability of the band is also thought to be an advantage, which allows increased durability of weight loss compared to VBG. The downside of LASGB is that weight loss is significantly slower than other bariatric procedures with maximal weight loss taking up to two to three years to be achieved compared to 12 to 18 months with other procedures. In addition, although significant weight loss is achieved with this procedure, the ultimate amount of weight loss may be less than that achieved with GBP (see below) (28,29). This, however, is controversial with some investigators suggesting that although weight loss is slower with LASGB compared to GBP, long-term weight loss is the same (30,31).

### Restrictive–Malabsorptive Procedures

Currently, the gold standard of bariatric procedures in the United States is the *Roux-en-Y* GBP (Fig. 3). In this procedure, a 30 mL pouch is constructed to which a Roux loop of jejunum is anastomosed. This creates a short biliopancreatic limb, an alimentary limb of 100 to 200 cm depending on a patient's weight, and a common limb that consists of the remainder of the small bowel. Thus, the procedure is traditionally said to combine both restrictive and malabsorptive features. However, the importance of malabsorption in contributing to the weight loss produced by GBP has been questioned, as more is understood about how this operation works. It is now thought that the GBP alters the neuro-endocritic environment in a partly understood way, which contributes to weight loss. The procedure can be performed laparoscopically or "open" with equivalent effectiveness (32). This is the operation to which all other bariatric procedures are compared in terms of efficacy, morbidity, and mortality and is the most common bariatric procedure performed in the United States (33).

### POSTOPERATIVE CARE AND COMPLICATIONS

In high-volume centers, hospital stay for bariatric surgery patients varies from one to three days depending on the type of procedure performed. Laparoscopic adjustable silicone gastric band patients are usually discharged within 24 hours of surgery (34). GBP patients who have surgery performed laparoscopically are generally discharged from the hospital in two to three days (34,35). Patients who have an open GBP are generally discharged from the hospital after three days (34).

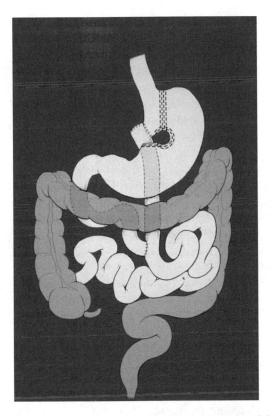

**Figure 3** Gastroplasty with Roux-en-Y gastrojejunostomy.

Routine care focuses on providing adequate pain control and ensuring adequate oral intake. Once achieved, the patient can be safely discharged to home. The diet is advanced through various "stages" over several weeks, and patients receive extensive education about maintaining hydration status and consuming adequate protein. The diet advancement for bariatric patients is detailed in Chapter 11.

The most common "complication" in bariatric surgical patients is nausea and vomiting that may occur in as high as 30% to 40% of patients (36). This can lead to rehospitalization to treat dehydration, despite no identifiable anatomical obstruction of the gastrointestinal tract. Patients usually receive intravenous hydration and are discharged to home in 24 to 48 hours in good condition. Other complications include wound infections, which range from 1% to 2% in patients undergoing laparoscopic procedures to as high as 10% to 15% in those undergoing open procedures (32,35,37–39). Long-term complications include ventral hernia formation, which is more common in the open approach than in the laparoscopic approach. Less common issues include pouch ulcer formation, internal hernia formation, and small bowel obstruction from adhesion formation.

The most common life-threatening complications from bariatric surgery include peritonitis and intra-abdominal abscess associated with an anastomotic leak or iatrogenic, unrecognized perforation of a viscus. Several surgeons (40,41) have noted the paucity of classic signs of peritonitis in the morbidly obese. Instead of abdominal pain and rebound tenderness, patients may complain of back and left shoulder pain and a relatively "benign" abdominal examination until impending death. They may also have tachypnea, tachycardia, and hypoxia without clear etiology. The surgeon should have a low threshold for obtaining radiologic evaluation with water-soluble contrast agents if any of these symptoms should occur without clear explanation. Radiologic studies may be falsely negative given the patient's body habitus and technical difficulties associated with obtaining and interpreting X rays in the morbidly obese. Thus, a patient may require surgical re-exploration even in the face of negative studies if the patient is clinically unstable and without an identifiable source of pathology. The reported incidence of leaks is 1% to 2% and may be higher in those undergoing laparoscopic procedures, especially in the first 100 cases of a surgeon's experience (35,39).

PE, although feared and often discussed, is relatively uncommon in bariatric surgery patients (42). This occurs less than 1% of the time in those who receive appropriate prophylaxis against PE, which is generally "double coverage" (e.g., low-molecular-weight heparin and pneumatic compression boots) (43). PE can be hard to diagnose in the morbidly obese. Persistent tachypnea and hypoxia may be suggestive, but many obese patients have a preoperative history of pulmonary issues with such symptoms, which may lull practitioners into a false sense of security. Hence, there should be a low threshold to work up bariatric patients with ventilation/perfusion scans or spiral chest computed tomography for even subtle changes in pulmonary status.

High-volume centers report a mortality rate of 1 in every 200 to 500 patients for GBP (44). Data from the State of Washington (45) suggest that the rate may be higher, at 1% to 2%, if one collects data from all centers conducting bariatric surgery, which includes those with less experience and higher mortality rates. LASGB has a very low mortality rate of 1 out of 2000 (46).

Overall, several studies now indicate that patients who are severely obese and undergo a bariatric surgical procedure generally have a longer life expectancy, improved comorbid conditions, and decreased medical costs compared to severely obese patients who receive nonsurgical or no treatment for their obesity (16,45,47–49). Hence, although surgery is invasive, the long-term outcome favors performing bariatric surgery in the appropriately selected severely obese individual compared to nonsurgical treatment.

## OUTCOMES AND CARDIOVASCULAR RISK REDUCTION

Several clinicians have noted that there is impressive amelioration of preoperative comorbid conditions in those who undergo bariatric surgical procedures. One of the earlier articles detailing this was that of Pories et al. (50) who noted that GBP surgery "cured" diabetes. This group followed 608 morbidly obese patients for up to 14 years after GBP. Of the 146 patients with type 2 diabetes, who had complete follow-up data available after surgery, 82.9% (121 patients) had normalized blood glucose and glycosylated hemoglobin levels. Patients with impaired glucose intolerance were also monitored; 152 patients had complete postoperative data available for analysis. Of those 152 patients, only two (1.2%) developed type 2 diabetes, and the rest became euglycemic. These results were supported by MacDonald et al. (51), who reported that diabetic patients required significantly less medications (oral hypoglycemic agents or insulin) to treat their diabetes after GBP.

Several articles (52–55) have confirmed that a variety of cardiovascular risk factors are improved in individuals who undergo bariatric surgery. For example, Buchwald et al. (55) recently performed a systematic review and meta-analysis of the English language literature on this area from 1990 to 2003. They identified 136 studies, which included 91 overlapping patient populations for a total of 22,094 patients. They included patients who had a variety of weight-loss operations including GBP, BPD, vertical gastric banding, and gastric banding procedures. Patients lost an average of 40 kg and over 60% of their excess body weights. This weight loss was associated with complete resolution of diabetes in 76.8% of patients and resolved or improved diabetes in 86% of patients. Hyperlipidemia improved in 70% of patients, hypertension was resolved or improved in 78.5% of patients, and obstructive sleep apnea resolved in 85.7% of patients. The authors concluded that effective weight loss in bariatric surgical patients is associated with impressive improvement in several cardiovascular risk factors.

In another clinical study, Lee et al. (56) looked at the effects of weight-loss surgery on the metabolic syndrome. They studied 645 consecutively morbidly obese patients who underwent either laparoscopic GBP or laparoscopic VBG. Over 50% of the patients met the Adult Treatment Panel III definition of metabolic syndrome. (The metabolic syndrome is discussed in detail in Chapter 3.) The patients lost approximately 40 kg one year after surgery, which was associated with marked improvement in all aspects of the metabolic syndrome. They noted that the metabolic syndrome was "cured" in 95.6% of patients within one year of surgery.

The Swedish Obese Subjects Study (57) is probably the best known and largest study looking at cardiovascular risk factors over a 10-year period. In this study, obese subjects who underwent bariatric surgery were contemporaneously matched with "conventionally treated," control obese subjects (i.e., patients who received nonsurgical treatment for obesity).

Ten-year follow-up results have recently been published (16). Weight loss was significantly higher in all patients undergoing surgery compared to that observed in the control patients (Fig. 4). Weight loss was most significant at one year. Weight slowly increased over 10 years, but still was 20% to 30% lower than presurgery, 10 years postoperatively. Weight loss was most significant in GBP patients compared to patients who underwent other surgical procedures and the control group. When the surgical patients were compared to the control patients there was marked, statistically significant improvement in lipid profile, diabetes, hypertension, and hyperuricemia (Fig. 5). The authors concluded that, as compared to conventional, nonsurgical treatment, bariatric surgery results in long-term weight loss, improved lifestyle, and amelioration of a variety of cardiovascular risk factors.

Some may argue that cardiovascular risk factors are just surrogate markers of what is really important—mortality risk. Without clear indication of decreased mortality, surgical intervention may not be justified in the morbidly obese. Mortality data for the Swedish Obese Subjects Study is not currently available. However, other clinical data are emerging, which have examined the effect of obesity surgery on mortality risk. Christou et al. (48) studied 1035 surgical patients who were matched to a control group of 5746 obese patients who did not undergo surgery. As with other studies

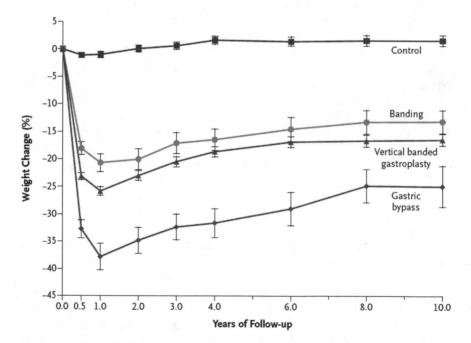

**Figure 4** Weight changes among subjects in the Swedish Obese Subjects Study over a 10-year period. *Source*: From Ref. 16.

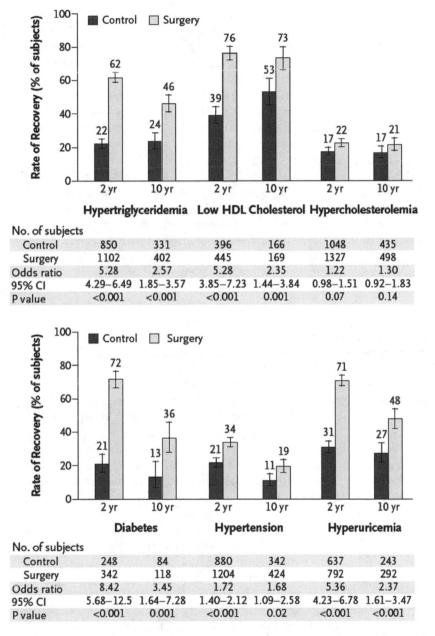

| No. of subjects | | | | | | |
| --- | --- | --- | --- | --- | --- | --- |
| Control | 850 | 331 | 396 | 166 | 1048 | 435 |
| Surgery | 1102 | 402 | 445 | 169 | 1327 | 498 |
| Odds ratio | 5.28 | 2.57 | 5.28 | 2.35 | 1.22 | 1.30 |
| 95% CI | 4.29–6.49 | 1.85–3.57 | 3.85–7.23 | 1.44–3.84 | 0.98–1.51 | 0.92–1.83 |
| P value | <0.001 | <0.001 | <0.001 | 0.001 | 0.07 | 0.14 |

| No. of subjects | | | | | | |
| --- | --- | --- | --- | --- | --- | --- |
| Control | 248 | 84 | 880 | 342 | 637 | 243 |
| Surgery | 342 | 118 | 1204 | 424 | 792 | 292 |
| Odds ratio | 8.42 | 3.45 | 1.72 | 1.68 | 5.36 | 2.37 |
| 95% CI | 5.68–12.5 | 1.64–7.28 | 1.40–2.12 | 1.09–2.58 | 4.23–6.78 | 1.61–3.47 |
| P value | <0.001 | 0.001 | <0.001 | 0.02 | <0.001 | <0.001 |

**Figure 5** Recovery from diabetes, lipid disturbances, hypertension, and hyperuricemia over 2 and 10 years in surgically treated subjects and their obese controls in the Swedish Obese Subjects Study. *Source*: From Ref. 16.

comparing surgery to nonsurgical treatment of obesity, there was markedly greater weight loss in the surgical group. Over a five-year period, mortality was 0.68% in the surgical patients compared to 6.17% in the nonsurgical patients. This meant that risk of mortality was reduced by almost 90% in the surgically treated obese patients.

A final question regarding the use of surgery to treat morbid obesity is concerning the financial costs. Given the high number of patients who potentially qualify for such treatment, the cost of offering it may be prohibitively high for the insurance company industry and the nation as a whole. There could be several very important social implications depending on health care costs. Several studies have begun to examine this question. It is clear that initial health care costs for obese individuals who undergo surgery are higher than that of obese individuals who receive no or nonsurgical treatments. However, it has been demonstrated that approximately three years after surgery, the health care costs of surgical patients is less than that of those who do not undergo obesity surgery. Over a five-year period, number of hospitalizations, total hospital days, number of physician visits, and prescription costs are less in surgically treated obese individuals. This is associated with up to a 25% reduction in health care costs in these individuals compared to obese patients who receive nonsurgical or no treatment for their weight condition (49).

Although it makes intuitive sense that massive weight loss leads to improved health and decreased mortality, the mechanism through which surgery exerts its salubrious affects have yet to be fully identified. One theory is that surgery has a beneficial effect on the inflammatory mediators associated with obesity. Initial work has suggested that inflammatory mediators such as angiotensinogen, transforming growth factor beta, tumor necrosis factor alpha, and interleukin six are all elevated in obesity (58). These mediators may in part lead to the development of several cardiovascular risk factors such as hypertension, diabetes, dyslipidemia, and thrombo-embolic phenomenon. (The association between obesity and inflammatory mediators is discussed in much more detail in Chapter 6.) Weight-loss surgery is associated with reduction of these factors, possibly through reduction of adipocyte mass, and therefore may be the mechanism through which weight-loss surgery so effectively reduces cardiovascular risk and prolongs life (59). Clearly, much more study is needed to examine how weight loss in general, and obesity surgery in specific, improves outcome. However, at present, the evidence is quite strong in favor of surgery for treatment of severely obese individuals compared to prolonged efforts at nonsurgical treatment.

## SUMMARY AND CONCLUSIONS

Weight-loss surgery is the treatment of choice for appropriately selected individuals who have class II obesity with weight-related comorbid conditions and patients with class III obesity with or without comorbid conditions. There have been a variety of surgical procedures designed to treat obese individuals, and current procedures are quite effective in inducing long-term weight loss. However, patients require a careful, comprehensive evaluation before proceeding with such treatment to minimize surgical risks and justify such an invasive treatment. In appropriately selected individuals, there are reduced cardiovascular risks, reduced mortality, and reduced health care costs, making obesity surgery appropriate in this group of individuals until equally or more effective weight-loss treatments are developed.

## REFERENCES

1. Maggard MA, Shugarman LR, Suttorp M, et al. Meta-analysis: surgical treatment of obesity. Ann Intern Med 2005; 142:547–559.
2. Clinical Guidelines on the Identification, Evaluation, and Treatment of Overweight and Obesity in Adults—The Evidence Report. National Institutes of Health. Obes Res 1998; 6(suppl 2):51S–209S.
3. NIH Conference. Gastrointestinal surgery for severe obesity. Consensus Development Panel. Ann Intern Med 1991; 115:956–961.
4. Macgregor AM, Rand CS. Gastric surgery in morbid obesity. Outcome in patients aged 55 and older. Arch Surg 1993; 128:1153–1157.
5. Papasavas PK, Gagne DJ, Kelly J, Caushaj PF. Laparoscopic Roux-en-Y gastric bypass is a safe and effective operation for the treatment of morbid obesity in patients older than 55 years. Obes Surg 2004; 14:1056–1061.
6. Sugerman HJ, DeMaria EJ, Kellum JM, Sugerman EL, Meador JG, Wolfe JG. Effects of bariatric surgery in older patients. Ann Surg 2004; 240:243–247.
7. Gonzalez R, Lin E, Mattar SG, Venkatesh KR, Smith CD. Gastric bypass for morbid obesity in patients 50 years or older: is laparoscopic technique safer? Am Surg 2003; 69:553–574.
8. Cossu ML, Fais E, Meloni GB, et al. Impact of age on long-term complications after biliopancreatic diversion. Obes Surg 2004; 14:1182–1186.
9. Lee H, Stanczyk M, Igwe D, Fobi M. Gastric bypass in patients over 60 years of age. Obes Surg 1999; 9:349.
10. Rossner S. Obesity in the elderly—a future matter of concern? Obes Rev 2001; 2:183–188.
11. Inge TH, Krebs NF, Garcia VF, et al. Bariatric surgery for severely overweight adolescents: concerns and recommendations. Pediatrics 2004; 114:217–223.
12. Horgan S, Holterman MJ, Jacobsen GR, et al. Laparoscopic adjustable gastric banding for the treatment of adolescent morbid obesity in the United States: a safe alternative to gastric bypass. J Pediatr Surg 2005; 40:86–90.
13. Inge TH, Zeller M, Garcia VF, Daniels SR. Surgical approach to adolescent obesity. Adolesc Med Clin 2004; 15:429–453.
14. Widhalm K, Dietrich S, Prager G. Adjustable gastric banding surgery in morbidly obese adolescents: experiences with eight patients. Int J Obes Relat Metab Disord 2004; 28(suppl 3):S42–S45.

15. Dolan K, Creighton L, Hopkins G, Fielding G. Laparoscopic gastric banding in morbidly obese adolescents. Obes Surg 2003; 13:101–104.

16. Sjostrom L, Lindroos AK, Peltonen M, et al. Lifestyle, diabetes, and cardiovascular risk factors 10 years after bariatric surgery. N Engl J Med 2004; 351: 2683–2693.

17. Kim JJ, Tarnoff ME, Shikora SA. Surgical treatment for extreme obesity: evolution of a rapidly growing field. Nutr Clin Pract 2003; 18:109–123.

18. Balsiger BM, Murr M, Poggio JL, Sarr MG. Bariatric surgery: surgery for weight control in patients with morbid obesity. Med Clin North Am 2000; 84:477–489.

19. Payne JH, DeWind LT, Commons RR. Metabolic observations in patients with jejunocolic shunts. Am J Surg 1963; 106:273–289.

20. Livingston EH. Obesity and its surgical management. Am J Surg 2002; 184:103–113.

21. Linner JH. Overview of surgical techniques for the treatment of morbid obesity. Gastrointest Clin North Am 1987; 16:2.

22. Scopinaro N, Gianetta E, Adami GF, et al. Biliopancreatic bypass for obesity: II. Initial experience in man. Br J Surg 1979; 119:261–268.

23. Mason EE. Vertical banded gastroplasty for obesity. Arch Surg 1982; 117: 701–706.

24. Capella JF, Capella RF. The weight reduction operation of choice: vertical banded gastroplasty or gastric bypass? Am J Surg 1996; 171:74–79.

25. Brolin RE, Robertson LB, Kenler HA, et al. Weight loss and dietary intake after vertical banded gastroplasty and Roux-en-Y gastric bypass. Ann Surg 1994; 220:782–790.

26. Kuzmak LI, Yap IS, McGuire L, Dixon JS, Young MP. Surgery for morbid obesity. Using an inflatable gastric band. AORN J 1990; 51:1307–1324 (erratum in AORJ J 1990; 51:1573).

27. Belachew M, Legrand M, Defechereux T, et al. Laparoscopic adjustable silicone gastric banding in the treatment of morbid obesity: a preliminary report. Surg Endosc 1994; 8:1354–1356.

28. Weber M, Muller MK, Bucher T, et al. Laparocsopic gastric bypass is superior to laparoscopic gastric banding for treatment of morbid obesity. Ann Surg 2004; 240:975–982.

29. Mognol P, Chosidow D, Marmuse JP. Laparoscopic gastric bypass versus laparoscopic adjustable banding in the super-obese: a comparative study of 290 patients. Obes Surg 2005; 15:76–81.

30. Jan JC, Hong D, Pereira N, Patterson EJ. Laparoscopic adjustable gastric banding versus laparoscopic gastric bypass for morbid obesity: a single-institution comparison study of early results. J Gastrointest Surg 2005; 9:30–39.

31. Mittermair RP, Weiss H, Nehoda H, Kirchmayr W, Aigner F. Laparoscopic Swedish adjustable gastric banding: 6-year follow-up and comparison to other laparoscopic bariatric procedures. Obes Surg 2003; 13:412–417.

32. See C, Carter PL, Elliott D, et al. An institutional experience with laparoscopic gastric bypass complications seen in the first year compared with open gastric bypass complications during the same period. Am J Surg 2002; 183: 533–538.

33. Buchwald H, Williams SE. Bariatric surgery worldwide 2003. Obes Surg 2004; 14:1157–1164.
34. Fisher BL. Comparison of recovery time after open and laparoscopic gastric bypass and laparoscopic adjustable banding. Obes Surg 2004; 14:67–72.
35. Shikora SA, Kim JJ, Tarnoff ME, Raskin E, Shore R. Laparoscopic Roux-en-Y gastric bypass. Results and learning curve of a high-volume academic program. Arch Surg 2005; 140:362–367.
36. Halverson JD. Metabolic risk of obesity surgery and long-term follow-up. Am J Clin Nutr 1992; 55:602S–605S.
37. Podnos YD, Jimenez JC, Wilson SE, Stevens CM, Nguyen NT. Complications after laparoscopic gastric bypass. A review of 3464 cases. Arch Surg 2003; 138:957–961.
38. Smith SC, Edwards CB, Goodman GN, Halversen C, Simper SC. Open vs. laparoscopic Roux-en-Y gastric bypass: comparison of operative morbidity and mortality. Obes Surg 2004; 14:73–76.
39. DeMaria EJ, Sugerman HJ, Kellum JM, Meador JG, Wolfe LG. Results of 281 consecutive total laparoscopic Roux-en-Y gastric bypasses to treat morbid obesity. Ann Surg 2002; 235:640–645.
40. Alvarez-Cordero R, Aragon-Viruette E. Post-operative complications in a series of gastric bypass patients. Obes Surg 1992; 2:87–89.
41. Mehran A, Liberman M, Rosenthal R, Szomstein S. Ruptured appendicitis after laparoscopic Roux-en-Y gastric bypass: pitfalls in diagnosing a surgical abdomen in the morbidly obese. Obes Surg 2003; 13:938–940.
42. Sapala JA, Wood MH, Schuhknecht MP, Sapala MA. Fatal pulmonary embolism after bariatric operations for morbid obesity: a 24-year retrospective analysis. Obes Surg 2003; 13:819–825.
43. Wu EC, Barba CA. Current practices in the prophylaxis of venous thromboembolism in bariatric surgery. Obes Surg 2000; 10:7–13.
44. Nguyen NT, Paya M, Stevens M, et al. The relationship between hospital volume and outcome in bariatric surgery at academic medical centers. Ann Surg 2004; 240:586–594.
45. Flum DR, Dellinger P. Impact of gastric bypass operation on survival: a population-based analysis. J Am Coll Surg 2004; 199:543–551.
46. Chapman AE, Kiroff G, Game P, et al. Laparoscopic adjustable gastric banding in the treatment of obesity: a systematic literature review. Surgery 2004; 135:326–351.
47. Dixon JB, O'Brien PE. Changes in comorbidities and improvements in quality of life after LAP-BAND placement. Am J Surg 2002; 184:51S–54S.
48. Christou NV, Sampalis JS, Liberman M, et al. Surgery decreases long-term mortality, morbidity, and health care use in morbidly obese patients. Ann Surg 2004; 240:416–424.
49. Sampalis JS, Liberman M, Auger S, Cristou NV. The impact of weight reduction surgery on health-care costs in morbidly obese patients. Obes Surg 2004; 14:939–947.
50. Pories WJ, Swanson MS, MacDonald KG, et al. Who would have thought it? An operation proves to be the most effective therapy for adult-onset diabetes mellitus. Ann Surg 1995; 222:339–352.

51. MacDonald KG, Long SD, Swanson MS, et al. The gastric bypass operation reduces the progression and mortality of non-insulin-dependent diabetes mellitus. J Gastrointest Surg 1997; 1:213–220.
52. Brolin RE, Bradley LJ, Wilson AC, Cody RP. Lipid risk profile and weight stability after gastric restrictive operations for morbid obesity. J Gastrointest Surg 2000; 4:464–469.
53. Carson JL, Ruddy ME, Duff AE, Holmes NJ, Cody RP, Brolin RE. The effect of gastric bypass surgery on hypertension in morbidly obese patients. Arch Intern Med 1994; 154:193–200.
54. Sugerman HJ, Fairman RP, Sood RK, Engle K, Wolfe L, Kellum JM. Long-term effects of gastric surgery for treating respiratory insufficiency of obesity. Am J Clin Nutr 1992; 55:597S–601S.
55. Buchwald H, Avidor Y, Braunwald E, et al. Bariatric surgery. A systematic review and meta-analysis. JAMA 2004; 292:1724–1737.
56. Lee WJ, Huang MT, Wang W, et al. Effects of obesity surgery on the metabolic syndrome. Arch Surg 2004; 139:1088–1092.
57. Sjostrom L, Larsson B, Backman L, et al. Swedish Obese Subjects (SOS): recruitment for an intervention study and a selected description of the obese state. Int J Obes Relat Metab Disord 1992; 16:465–479.
58. Cottam DR, Mattar SG, Barinas-Mitchell E, et al. The chronic inflammatory hypothesis for the morbidity associated with morbid obesity: implications and effects of weight loss. Obes Surg 2004; 14:589–600.
59. Ramos EJB, Xy Y, Romanova I, et al. Is obesity an inflammatory disease? Surgery 2003; 134:329–335.

# 15

# Management of Perioperative Cardiac Risk in the Bariatric Patient

**Zara Cooper, Cesar E. Escareno, and David B. Lautz**
*Department of Surgery, Brigham and Women's Hospital,*
*Harvard Medical School, Boston, Massachusetts, U.S.A.*

## INTRODUCTION

Successful preoperative evaluation requires a careful teamwork and communication between the patient, surgeon, primary care physician, anesthesiologist, and consultants. The initial history forms the most important part of this evaluation and serves as a screen for conditions that can adversely affect outcome. Morbidly obese patients should be assessed for risk of cardiac disease before elective surgery. In the absence of other comorbidities, obesity can cause changes in cardiac structure and function (1). Chronic hypervolemia, elevated cardiac output, and elevations in vascular resistance contribute to left ventricular hypertrophy (LVH), which is a predisposing factor for arrhythmias and ischemia. Although it is well known that morbid obesity increases risk for cardiac disease, there is no data to demonstrate a direct risk for increased perioperative cardiac complications. In a large cohort of obese patients having elective general surgery, obesity alone was not predictive of increased perioperative morbidity, complications, or additional use of medical resources (2). Unfortunately, bariatric patients were excluded from this study and severe obesity was defined as a body mass index greater than 35; so it is unclear if these results could be extrapolated to the bariatric population. There are conflicting studies regarding the effect of obesity on intensive care unit (ICU) mortality.

However, two large studies agree that medical ICU mortality is significantly higher in morbidly obese groups (3,4). Increased perioperative morbidity associated with obesity includes wound infection, pneumonia, pulmonary embolism, and cardiac ischemia and failure.

Anesthetics cause physiologic changes that make cardiac ischemia and arrythmias more likely. Approximately 30% of patients who receive anesthesia for surgery have known coronary artery disease (CAD) or risk factors for coronary disease (5). One million patients will have an adverse cardiac event in the perioperative period. Between one-quarter and one-half of deaths after noncardiac surgery are caused by cardiac complications. High-risk procedures including emergency procedures in the elderly and peripheral vascular procedures may pose a greater than 5% risk of perioperative myocardial infarction (MI). Extensive intra-abdominal procedures with large fluid shifts are also considered high risk. General anesthesia causes decreased systemic vascular resistance, decreased cardiac output, increased myocardial irritability, and decreased contractility, which can provoke decompensation in a previously stable patient. Muscle relaxants, inhalational anesthetics, and commonly used intravenous agents may be arrhythmogenic by sensitizing the myocardium to catecholamines. Endotracheal intubation can cause relative systemic hypertension contributing to significant hemodynamic changes. Spinal and epidural anesthetics block sympathetic outflow, with subsequent vascular dilation and decrease in cardiac output. Patients with cardiac disease are vulnerable in this setting and are at risk for perioperative cardiac morbidity and mortality.

## RISK ASSESSMENT

Perioperative cardiac evaluation is aimed at risk assessment and stratification. A thorough preoperative cardiac evaluation, starting with a complete history and physical examination, is essential in patients with severe obesity, who are at high risk for coronary disease (6). MI, within one month of surgery, and congestive heart failure (CHF) are the most critical perioperative risk factors and are associated with high morbidity. Perioperative reinfarctions occurring one to six months after the initial infarct are associated with almost a 50% mortality rate, making them more deadly than perioperative infarctions in other patients. Morbidity is related to the remaining area at risk of ischemia after the first infarct. Prior revascularization does not increase the risk of perioperative cardiac morbidity. Recent infarct and CHF, along with severe aortic or mitral stenosis, are contraindications to elective noncardiac surgery.

The American College of Cardiology/American Heart Association (ACC/AHA) guidelines serve as a guide for predictors of perioperative cardiac risk in noncardiac surgery (7) (Table 1). The risk of an adverse perioperative cardiac event is related to the amount of underlying heart disease

**Table 1** Clinical Predictors of Increased Risk for Perioperative Cardiac Complications

| Major | Intermediate | Minor |
|---|---|---|
| Recent MI (within 30 days) | Mild angina | Advanced age |
| Unstable or severe angina | Prior MI by history or ECG | Abnormal ECG (LVH, LBBB, and ST-T-wave abnormalities) |
| Decompensated CHF | Compensated or prior CHF | Rhythm other than sinus (e.g., atrial fibrillation) |
| Significant arrhythmias (high-grade AV block, symptomatic ventricular arrhythmias with underlying heart disease, supraventricular arrhythmias with uncontrolled rate) | Diabetes mellitus | Poor functional capacity |
| Severe valvular disease | Renal insufficiency | History of stroke Uncontrolled hypertension (e.g., diastolic blood pressure greater than 110 mmHg) |

*Abbreviations*: MI, myocardial infarction; CHF, congestive heart failure; AV, atrioventricular; ECG, electrocardiography; LVH, left ventricular hypertrophy; LBBB, left bundle branch block.
*Source*: From Ref. 8.

and the type of surgery planned. Cardiac risk factors include a history of CHF, prior MI, diabetes, angina pectoris, heart failure, an age of more than 70 years, or poor functional status (Table 2). Although obesity alone is not a risk factor, the high incidence of risk factors among obese patients makes thorough screening essential. According to the National Hospital Discharge

**Table 2** Factors That Increase Risk of Perioperative Cardiac Complications

| Risk variable | Odds ratio (95% CI) |
|---|---|
| Poor functional status | 1.8 (0.9–3.5) |
| Ischemic heart disease | 2.4 (1.3–4.2) |
| Heart failure | 1.9 (1.1–3.5) |
| Diabetes | 3.0 (1.3–7.1) |
| Renal insufficiency | 3.0 (1.4–6.8) |
| High-risk surgery | 2.8 (1.6–4.9) |

*Abbreviation*: CI, confidence interval.
*Source*: From Ref. 9.

Survey database from 1996 to 2001, hypertension (34%), diabetes (18%), and sleep apnea (22%) were among the most common premorbid conditions among patients having gastric bypass surgery (10). Patients with no risk factors do not require further testing; patients with three or more risk factors or patients with CAD warrant noninvasive testing. Results will dictate the need for preoperative treatment and evaluation should include a cardiologist. Those candidates with one or two risk factors, but no CAD, should receive perioperative beta blockade (11). Perioperative beta blockade has been shown to reduce the incidence of postoperative ischemia and event-free survival for as long as six months after surgery. Beta blockade should be started before surgery and titrated to a resting heart rate between 50 and 60 beats/min.

Intraoperative risk factors include the conditions at the surgical site, unnecessary use of vasopressors, and unintended hypotension. Intra-abdominal pressure exceeding 20 mmHg during laparoscopy can decrease venous return from the lower extremities and thus contribute to decreased cardiac output (9). Trendelenberg positioning leads to exceptional pressure on the diaphragm from abdominal viscera and subsequently reduces vital capacity. Intraoperative hypertension has not been isolated as a risk factor for cardiac morbidity, but it is often associated with wide fluctuations in pressure, and has been more closely associated with cardiac morbidity than intraoperative hypotension.

Preoperative anxiety can contribute to hypertension even in normotensive patients. However, those patients with a history of hypertension, even medically controlled hypertension, are more likely to be hypertensive preoperatively. Those with poorly controlled hypertension are at greater risk of developing intraoperative ischemia, arrhythmias, and blood pressure derangements that may be seen particularly at induction and intubation. Twenty-five percent of patients will exhibit hypertension during laryngoscopy. Patients with chronic hypertension may not necessarily benefit from lower blood pressure during the preoperative period because they may depend on higher pressures for cerebral perfusion. Those receiving antihypertensive medications should continue using them up until the time of surgery. Patients taking beta-blockers are at risk of withdrawal and rebound ischemia. Key findings on physical exam include retinal vascular changes and an s4 gallop consistent with LVH. Chest radiograph may show an enlarged heart, also suggesting LVH.

## PREOPERATIVE TESTING

Extensive preoperative testing may be required to accurately evaluate perioperative risk and should be completed before any elective procedure (Fig. 1). Interviewing practitioners should seek a history of dyspnea on exertion or at rest, chest pain, and syncope, and family history of related disorders. Patients should be asked how long they have had diabetes,

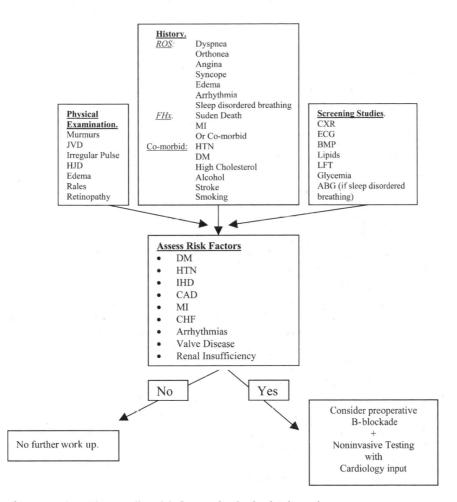

**Figure 1**  Assessing cardiac risk factors in the bariatric patient.

hypertension, and hypercholesterolemia, as well as the number of tobacco pack–years and the extent of alcohol use, if present. Smokers should be counseled to stop before surgery to reduce the risk of cardiopulmonary complications. Laboratory screening is also necessary. One series found that among 300 bariatric patients, 33% of diabetics were undiagnosed and half were untreated. Almost half of the patients with hypertension and just over half of these patients with hyperlipidemia were undiagnosed before their preoperative visit. The cardiac risk is proportional to the amount of time these comorbidites have been present. A focused physical exam should identify signs of cardiac failure, such as elevated jugular venous distention, rales, hepatojuglar reflex, bruits, and murmurs indicative of valvular or wall abnormalities. Obesity may obscure physical findings and further study is often necessary to rule out abnormalities.

Overall functional ability is the best measure of cardiac health. Patients who can exercise without limitations can generally tolerate the stress of major surgery (12). Limited exercise capacity may indicate poor cardiopulmonary reserve and the inability to withstand the stress of surgery.

Noninvasive cardiac testing is used to define risk in patients known to be high or intermediate risk, and with CHF or dyspnea. It is most useful in intermediate-risk patients. 12-Lead electrocardiography (ECG) should be obtained in patients with chest pain, diabetes, prior revascularization, and prior hospitalization for cardiac causes, and for all men aged 45 or above and all women aged 55, with two or more risk factors. High- or intermediate-risk patients should also have screening ECG. A less than normal ejection fraction demonstrated on echocardiography is associated with greatest perioperative cardiac risk, and should be obtained in all patients with symptoms suggesting heart failure or valvular disease. Tricuspid regurgitation indicates pulmonary hypertension and is often associated with sleep apnea.

Exercise testing remains the mainstay of noninvasive cardiac evaluation, and demonstrates a propensity for ischemia and arrhythmias under conditions that increase myocardial oxygen consumption. Numerous studies have shown that performance during exercise testing is predictive of perioperative mortality in noncardiac surgery. ST wave segment ECG changes during exercise, including horizontal depression greater than 2 mm, changes with low workload, and persistent changes after five minutes of exercise are seen in severe multivessel disease. Other findings include dysrhythmias at a low heart rate, inability to raise heart rate to 70% of the predicted value, and sustained decrease in systolic pressure during exercise.

Unfortunately, many morbidly obese patients are unable to achieve adequate workload in standard exercise testing because of related osteoarthritis, low-back pain, and pulmonary disease. In this case, pharmacologic testing is indicated with a Dobutamine echocardiogram. Dobutamine is a beta agonist, which increases myocardial oxygen demand and reveals impaired oxygen delivery in those with coronary disease. Echocardiography concurrently visualizes wall motion abnormalities from ischemia. Transesophageal echocardiography may be preferable to transthoracic echo in obese patients because of their body habitus, and has been shown to have high negative predictive value in this group (13). Transesophageal Dobutamine stress echocardiography has demonstrated value in predicting perioperative and postoperative cardiac risk in a small series of bariatric patients (14).

Nuclear perfusion with vasodilators such as adenosine or dipyridamole can identify CAD and demand ischemia. Heterogeneous perfusion after vasodilator administration demonstrates an inadequate response to stress. Wall motion abnormalities indicate ischemia, and an ejection fraction lower than 50% increases the risk of perioperative mortality. Although studies dedicated to the bariatric population have not been performed, dipyramidole thallium scintigraphy has been shown to have a uniformly predictive value greater than 95% in preoperative testing.

Positron emission tomography (PET) scanning is an alternative to noninvasive nuclear perfusion testing in obese patients. Transthoracic echocardiograms and nuclear perfusion studies may be difficult to interpret in obese patients due to their body habitus. Obesity has been associated with an increased risk of attenuation artifacts, which can decrease the accuracy of nuclear perfusion studies. Even in the general population, single photon emission computed tomography (SPECT) has been shown to have more attenuation artifacts compared to PET, and was shown to have specificity of 64% compared to 84% for PET (15). Furthermore, [82]Rb PET imaging has been shown to have an equivalent prognositic value to SPECT. In 153 patients studied, there was a 94% event-free survival in patients with negative PET studies during three-year follow-up (16). Patients with mild, moderate, and severe defects had 62%, 58%, and 45% event-free survivals, respectively, during the same time period. Despite its efficacy, the use of PET has been hindered by limited availability and limited reimbursement. However, at present most large centers have PET scanning capability and Medicaid reimburses for myocardial PET scanning, making the test more readily available than in the past.

Angiography should only be performed if the patient may be a candidate for revascularization. Generally, fixed occlusions greater than 70% are significant. However, 50% occlusions can cause hemodynamic compromise in the left main artery supplying the left ventricle, and warrant revascularization. Clinical guidelines suggest that coronary revascularization is associated with improved perioperative and long-term (17) outcomes in patients with unstable coronary disease and who would otherwise benefit from coronary artery bypass grafting (18,19). A recent large randomized trial in vascular surgical patients in Veteran's Administration Hospitals did not support prophylactic preoperative revascularization in the presence of stable CAD (20). Weight was not a clinical variable examined in this study, and the majority of subjects were male. Similar studies are needed in other patient groups. The ACC/AHA guidelines recommend that surgeons wait two to four weeks before noncardiac surgery after a patient has received a coronary stent, which allows time for complete endothelialization and a complete course of antiplatelet therapy. Patients who do not receive four weeks of antiplatelet therapy are at risk of stent thrombosis (21).

## PATIENTS WITH PRE-EXISTING CONDITIONS

CHF is associated with coronary disease, valvular disease, ventricular dysfunction, and all types of cardiomyopathy. These are all independent risk factors that should be identified prior to surgery. Even in compensated heart failure, failure may be aggravated by fluid shifts associated with anesthesia and abdominal surgery and deserves serious consideration. Perioperative mortality increases with higher New York Heart Association class and pre-operative pulmonary congestion. CHF should be treated to lower filling pressures and improve cardiac output before elective surgery. Beta-blockers, angiotensin-converting enzyme inhibitors, and diuretics can be employed to this end. The patient should be stable for one week before surgery (22).

Obesity increases the amount of soft tissue in the oropharynx, which can cause upper airway obstruction during sleep. Fifty-five percent of morbidly obese patients may have sleep-related breathing disorders such as obstructive sleep apnea and obesity hypoventilation syndrome (OHS) (23). Symptoms include snoring and daytime sleepiness, and formal sleep studies are employed for definitive diagnosis. Sleep-disordered breathing is associated with hypoxia, hypercapnea, changes in blood pressure, nocturnal angina, and increased cardiac morbidity and mortality including stroke and sudden death (24). Related conditions also include difficult-to-manage hypertension and CHF exacerbations, likely due to increased sympathetic tone caused by hypoxia and sleep deprivation. OHS occurs because the weight of the chest wall impedes excursion during respiration. Symptoms include CHF, shortness of breath, and nocturnal asthma (21). Arterial blood gas with $PaO_2$ less than 55 mm Hg or $PCO_2$ greater than 47 mm Hg confirms the diagnosis. An increased incidence of pulmonary hypertension and right-sided heart failure is seen in patients with OHS, and these patients should have an echocardiogram performed before surgery. In severe cases, intraoperative monitoring with a pulmonary artery catheter may be prudent. Angiographic studies have demonstrated a significant correlation between the severity of sleep apnea and hypopnea, and the degree of CAD. In one series, obstructive sleep apnea (OSA) was a more statistically significant determinant of coronary disease than other risk factors such as hypertension, diabetes, and hyperlipidemia (25). Snoring six to seven nights per week carries an age-adjusted risk of 1.9 to 2.35 for ischemic heart disease, and a relative risk of 4.1 for cardiac-related early morning death (26,27). Studies suggest that oxidative stress in these patients may activate endothelial cells to express adhesion molecules and reactive oxygen species, which may incite coronary atherogenesis (25). Pulmonary management of these patients will be discussed elsewhere in this text.

Patients with valvular disease should receive preoperative antibiotics prior to gastrointestinal surgery to prevent endocarditis. The AHA guidelines stratify patient risk based on clinical condition and history. Prophylaxis includes antibiotics before and after each procedure (Table 3).

Valve disease is particularly important in the bariatric population because of prior exposure to appetite suppressants dexfenfluramine–phentermine and fenfluramine–phenteramine before the Food and Drug Administration withdrew these drugs from the market in 1997. Both were

**Table 3** American Heart Association Prophylactic Regimens for Genitourinary/ Gastrointestinal Procedures to Prevent Bacterial Endocarditis

| | Standard regimen | Allergy to ampicillin/ amoxicillin |
|---|---|---|
| *High risk* | | |
| Prosthetic cardiac valves, including bioprosthetic and homograft valves | Ampicillin plus gentamicin: ampicillin (adults, 2.0 g; children 50 mg/kg) plus gentamicin 1.5 mg/kg (for both adults and children, not to exceed 120 mg) i.m. or i.v. within 30 min before starting procedure. Six hours later, ampicillin (adults, 1.0 g; children, 25 mg/kg) i.m. or i.v., or amoxicillin (adults, 1.0 g; children, 25 mg/ kg) orally | Vancomycin plus gentamicin: vancomycin (adults, 1.0 g; children, 20 mg/ kg) i.v. over one to two hours plus gentamicin 1.5 mg/kg (for both adults and children, not to exceed 120 mg) i.m. or i.v. Complete injection/infusion within 30 min before starting procedure |
| Previous bacterial endocarditis | | |
| Complex cyanotic congenital heart disease (e.g., single ventricle states, transposition of the great arteries, and tetralogy of Fallot) | | |
| Surgically constructed systemic pulmonary shunts or conduits | | |
| *Moderate risk* | | |
| Most other congenital cardiac malformations (other than the above-mentioned) | Amoxicillin: adults, 2.0 g (children 50 mg/ kg) orally one hour before procedure, or Ampicillin: adults, 2.0 g (children 50 mg/kg) i.m. or i.v. within 30 min before starting procedure | Vancomycin: adults, 1.0 g (children 20 mg/ kg) i.v. over one to two hours. Complete infusion within 30 min of starting the procedure |
| Acquired valvular dysfunction (e.g., rheumatic heart disease) | | |
| Hypertrophic cardiomyopathy | | |
| Mitral valve prolapse with valvular regurgitation and/or thickened leaflets | | |

*Abbreviations*: i.m., intramuscular; i.v., intravenous.
*Source*: From Ref. 28.

associated with cardiac valvular abnormalities and pulmonary hypertension. Prevalence of incompetent aortic and mitral valves was approximately 30% in patients taking the drugs, compared to less than 2.1% in controls (29). Higher dose and longer duration of therapy was associated with risk of valve disease. Multiple studies have shown that progression is unlikely within a year after valve abnormality is identified on echocardiogram, and the degree of regurgitation may decrease progressively within two years after discontinuation of the drug (30–32).

Evaluation of patients with a history of anorexigen use does not necessarily require echocardiography. AHA/ACC guidelines do not recommend routine echocardiography for asymptomatic patients who have used anorexigens (33). One series of 189 subjects and 223 controls showed that murmurs detected in prior dexfenfluramine users were predictive of mild or abnormal mitral regurgitation (MR) (34). Overall prevalence of heart murmurs was 14% in dexfenfluramine users and 11% in controls. Furthermore, patients without murmurs had normal valves or only mild regurgitation on echo. Overall, the absence of heart murmur on physical exam predicted clinically important valvular regurgitation in more than 93% of prior dexfenfluramine users. The cardiac auscultation was performed by noncardiologists who were unaware of the echo results.

Aortic stenosis (AS) is a fixed obstruction to the left ventricular (LV) outflow tract, limiting cardiac reserve and an appropriate response to stress. History should elicit symptoms of dyspnea, angina, and syncope; examination may reveal a soft S2, a late peaking murmur, or a right-sided crescendo–decrescendo murmur radiating to the carotids. AS is usually caused by progressive calcification or congenital bicuspid valve. Critical stenosis exists when the valve area is less than $0.7 \, cm^2$ or transvalvular gradients greater than 50 mm Hg, and is associated with the inability to increase cardiac output with demand. Mild to moderate symptoms may present when the valve area in less than $0.9 \, cm^2$. AS is associated with a 13% risk of perioperative death. Valve replacement is indicated prior to elective surgery in patients with symptomatic stenosis (17). Myocardial ischemia may occur in the absence of significant coronary artery occlusion in the presence of aortic valve disease. Perioperative management should include optimizing the heart rate to between 60 and 90 and avoiding atrial fibrillation if possible. Because of the outflow obstruction, stroke volume may be fixed and bradycardia will lower cardiac output. Similarly, hypotension is also poorly tolerated.

Aortic regurgitation (AR) is associated with backward flow into the left ventricle during diastole and reduced forward stroke volume. Bradycardia facilitates regurgitation by increased diastolic time. Chronic AR causes massive LV dilatation (Cor Bovinum) and hypertrophy, which is associated with decreased LV function at later stages. AR is most often caused by rheumatic disease or congenital bicuspid valve. Medical treatment includes rate control and afterload reduction. Without valve replacement, survival is approximately five years, once patients become symptomatic. This is an obvious consideration when planning any other surgical procedures.

Tricuspid regurgitation is usually caused by pulmonary hypertension, secondary to severe left-sided failure. Other causes include endocarditis, carcinoid, and primary pulmonary hypertension. Hypovolemia, hypoxia, and acidosis can increase right ventricular afterload and should be avoided in the perioperative period.

Mitral stenosis is an inflow obstruction, which prevents adequate left ventricular filling. The transvalvular pressure gradient depends on atrial kick, heart rate, and diastolic filling time. Tachycardia decreases filling time and contributes to pulmonary congestion. MR is also associated with pulmonary hypertension with congestion because the pathologic valve prevents forward flow, left atrial dilatation, and subsequent atrial arrhythmias. Atrial fibrillation is associated with emboli. History and physical examination should focus on signs of CHF, such as orthopnea, pedal edema, dyspnea, reduced exercise tolerance, and auscultory findings such as murmurs and an S3 gallop. Neurologic deficits may signify embolic sequelae of valve disease. Perioperative rate control is essential for maintaining adequate cardiac output. ECG findings will reflect related arrhythmias and medications, but will not be specific for valve disease. Laboratory studies should identify secondary hepatic dysfunction or pulmonary compromise. LVH is an adaptive response, which may cause subsequent pulmonary hypertension and diastolic dysfunction.

Patients with atrial fibrillation and prosthetic valves will be on anticoagulation therapy preoperatively, which will need close monitoring in the perioperative period. Anticoagulation therapy should be discontinued for a number of days preoperatively until their coagulation profile is suitable for surgery, and then resumed once safe from a haemostatic standpoint. Heparin can be used as a bridge prior to surgery, and may require preoperative admission. Aggressive management is imperative because thromboembolic risk increases with the amount of time that the patient's anticoagulation is subtherapeutic. Once the use of coumadin is resumed, patients are actually in a prothrombotic state until therapeutic levels are reached; so patients at risk for emboli or deep vein thrombosis should receive anticoagulation therapy until that time. Prosthetics in the mitral position pose the greatest risk for thromboembolism, and the risk is increased with valve area and low flow. Mechanical valves pose a higher risk than tissue valves in patients with a history of valve replacement. Diuretics and afterload- reducing agents will enhance forward flow and minimize cardiopulmonary congestion. Patients with mitral valve prolapse (MVP) should receive antibiotics.

MR may also impair LV function and lead to pulmonary hypertension. Stroke volume is reduced by backward flow into the atrium during systole. The left ventricle compensates by dilating to increase end-systolic volume, eventually causing concentric hypertrophy and decreased contractility. The end result may be decreased ejection fraction and CHF. A decrease in systemic vascular resistance and increase in atrial contribution to the ejection fraction can both improve forward flow and reduce the amount of regurgitation. Echocardiography can clarify the degree of valvular impairment. Medical treatment centers on afterload reduction with vasodilators and diuretics. MVP may be present in up to 15% of women, and is usually associated with a midsystolic click and late-systolic murmur on physical exam. Murmur is indicative of prolapse. Although MVP is associated with connective tissue disorders, it usually occurs in otherwise healthy, asymptomatic patients. Echocardiography is used to confirm the diagnosis and evaluate the degree of prolapse. Chronically, MVP may be associated with MR, emboli, and increased risk of endocarditis. Prolapse may be aggravated by decreased preload, which should be minimized in the perioperative period. These patients are at risk of ventricular arrhythmias with sympathetic stimulation and endocarditis, which can be addressed with pain control and antibiotic prophylaxis, respectively.

Arrhythmias and conduction abnormalities elicited in the history, on examination, or on ECG should prompt investigation into other cardiac disease, metabolic pathology, or drug toxicities. In the presence of symptoms or hemodynamic changes, the underlying cause should be reversed and then medication should be given to treat the arrhythmia. Indications for antiarrhythmic medication and cardiac pacemakers mirror those in the nonoperative setting. Nonsustained ventricular tachycardia and premature ventricular beats have not been associated with increased perioperative risk and do not require further intervention (35,36).

Perioperatively, patients can continue their routine medications except insulin, oral hypoglycemics, aspirin, nonsteroidal anti-inflammatories, and anticoagulants as discussed above. When indicated, beta blockade should be started or continued, to minimize cardiac morbidity and mortality. Intravenous medications can be a bridge to oral beta blockade before patients begin to tolerate oral diet, and are useful in preventing beta-blocker withdrawal.

## ANESTHETIC CONSIDERATIONS

Anesthesia can be complex in these patients because of their formidable body habitus. Special consideration should be given to the airway, which may be obscured by a short, thickened neck, and sites for intravenous access and invasive monitoring. Invasive monitoring can be especially helpful if an appropriately sized blood pressure cuff is unavailable. Falsely elevated pressures can be obtained if the blood pressure cuff is too small. Central venous access is essential when patients are too obese for reliable peripheral access to be obtained. Routine laboratory studies should include chemistries and a baseline arterial blood gas to identify any existing acid–base abnormalities or carbon dioxide retention. In patients with pulmonary hypertension, pulmonary artery catheterization is indicated during surgery, and inhalational agents, which prevent hypoxemia, are recommended. Of course, weight-based dosing of drugs is particularly important in this population, and the anesthesiologist must keep in mind that the volume of distribution of lipophilic compounds is increased relative to normal-weight individuals.

## POSTOPERATIVE CARE

Postoperative management may include heart rate control, judicious fluid management, and aggressive control of pain and anxiety. The use of beta-blockers and alpha-2 agonists and suppression of postoperative pain can reduce myocardial ischemia in the postoperative period. Postoperative epidural anesthetic has been shown to decrease ventricular stroke work and oxygen consumption in the general postoperative population (37). The peak incidence of postoperative MI is 48 hours after surgery and most ischemia during this period is silent. Physicians should obtain cardiac enzymes and ECGs immediately after surgery and on the first two postoperative days in patients with known or suspected coronary disease (38).

Preoperative cardiac evaluation is an opportunity for identification and improvement of short- and long-term cardiac risk. Appropriate intervention can significantly improve surgical outcome and mortality. In bariatric patients, who are often young and healthy appearing, the prevalence of cardiac risk factors requires the surgeon to perform a complete evaluation for such risk factors. This should include a thorough history, including review of symptoms and family history, and focused physical exam looking for signs of cardiac disease. Physicians should be keenly aware of the prevalence of metabolic disorders in morbidly obese patients, including high cholesterol, insulin resistance, and diabetes. Surgeons should be prepared to screen for such disorders because they may have been previously undiagnosed, and refer patients for care as appropriate. A low threshold should exist to pursue noninvasive or invasive testing in those patients suspected of having any risk factors for perioperative cardiac disease, and for involving specialists to help manage patient care. The elective nature of bariatric surgery affords patients time to minimize their cardiac risk factors prior to surgery, and it is remiss to neglect this opportunity.

## REFERENCES

1. Alpert MA, Hashimi MW. Obesity and the heart. Am J Med Sci 1993; 306: 117–123.
2. Dindo D, Muller MK, Weber M, et al. Obesity in general elective surgery. Lancet 2003; 361:2032–2035.
3. Goulenok C, Monchi M, Chiche J, et al. Influence of overweight on ICU Mortality, a prospective study. Chest 2004; 125:1441–1445.
4. El-Solh A, Sikka P, Bozkanat E, et al. Morbid obesity in the medical ICU. Chest 2001; 120:1989–1997.
5. Mangano DT, Golman L. Preoperative assessment of patients with known or suspected coronary disease. N Engl J Med 1995; 333:1750–1756.

6. Shenkamn Z, Shir Y, Brodsky JB. Perioperative management of the obese patients. Anaesthesia 1993; 70:349.
7. Eagle KA, Berger PB, Calkins H, et al. ACC/AHA guideline update for perioperative cardiac evaluation for noncardiac surgery: executive summary: a report of the American College of Cardiology/American Heart Association Task Force on Practice Guidelines (Committee to update the 1996 guidelines on perioperative cardiac evaluation for noncardiac surgery). J Am Coll Cardiol 2002; 39:542–553.
8. Eagle KA, Brundage BH, Chaitman BR, et al. Guidelines for perioperative cardiovascular evaluation for noncardiac surgery. Report of the American College of Cardiology/American Heart Association Task Force on Practice Guidelines (Committee on Perioperative Cardiovascular Evaluation for Noncardiac Surgery). J Am Coll Cardiol 1996; 27:918.
9. Chui PT, Gin T, Oh TE. Anesthesia for laparoscopic surgery. Anaesth Intensive Care 1993; 21:163–171.
10. Livingston EH. Procedure incidence and in-hospital complication rates of bariatric surgery in the United States. Am J Surg 2004; 188:105–110.
11. Fleisher LA, Eagle KA. Lowering cardiac risk in noncardiac surgery. N Engl J Med 2001; 345:1677–1682.
12. Mukherjee D, Eagle KA. Perioperative cardiac assessment for non cardiac surgery, eight steps to the best possible outcome. Circulation 2003; 107:2771–2774.
13. Madu EC. Transesophageal dobutamine stress echocardiography in the evaluation of myocardial ischemia in morbidly obese subjects. Chest 2000; 117: 657–661.
14. Bhat G, Daley K, Dugan M, et al. Preoperative evaluation for bariatric surgery using transesophageal dobutamine stress echocardiography. Obes Surg 2004; 14:948–951.
15. Freedman N, Schecter D, Klein M, et al. SPECT attenuation artifacts in normal and overweight persons: insights from a retrospective comparison of Rb-82 positron emission tomography and TI-201 SPECT myocardial perfusion imaging. Clin Nucl Med 2000; 25:1019–1023.
16. Yoshinaga K, Chow B, De Kemp Robert, et al. Prognostic value of rubidium-82 perfusion positron emisson tomography. Preliminary results from the consecutive 153 patients. J Am Cardiol 2004; 43:338A.
17. Hertzer NR, Young JR, Bevern EG, et al. Late results of coronary bypass in patients with peripheral vascular disease. II. Five-year survival according to sex, hypertension, and diabetes. Cleve Clin J Med 1987; 54:15–23.
18. American College of Physicians. Guidelines for assessing and managing the preoperative risk from coronary artery disease associated with major noncardiac surgery. Ann Intern Med 1997; 127:309–312.
19. Eagle KA, Berger PB, Calkins H, et al. ACC/AHA guideline update for perioperative cardiac evaluation for noncardiac surgery: executive summary: a report of the American College of Cardiology/American Heart Association Task Force on Practice guidelines (Committee to update the 1996 guidelines on perioperative cardiac evaluation for noncardiac surgery). J Am Coll Cardiol 2002; 39:542–553.

20. McFalls EO, Ward HB, Moritz TE, et al. Coronary-artery revascularization before major vascular surgery. N Engl J Med 2004; 351:2795–2804.
21. Kaluza GL, Joseph J, Lee JR, et al. Catastrophic outcomes of noncardiac surgery soon after coronary stenting. J Am Coll Cardiol 2000; 35:1288–1294.
22. Detsky AS, Abrams HB, McLaughlin JR, et al. Predicting cardiac complications in patients undergoing non-cardiac surgery. J Gen Intern Med 1986; 1: 211–219.
23. Flancbaum L, Choban PS. Surgical implications of obesity. Annu Rev Med 1998; 49:215–234.
24. Shepherd JW. Hypertension, cardiac arrhythmias, myocardial infarction and stroke in relation to obstructive sleep apnea. Clin Chest Med 1992; 13:459–479.
25. Hayashi M, Fujimoto K, Urushibata K, et al. Nocturnal oxygen desaturation correlates with the severity of coronary atherosclerosis in coronary artery disease. Chest 2003; 124:936–941.
26. D'Alessandro R, Magelli C, Gambernini G, et al. Snoring every night as a risk factor for myocardial infarction: a case control study. BMJ 1990; 300:1557–1558.
27. Seppala T, Partinen M, Penttila A, et al. Sudden death and sleeping history among Finnish men. J Intern Med 1991; 229:23–28.
28. Committee on Rheumatic Fever, Endocarditis, and Kawasaki Disease. Prevention of bacterial endocarditis: recommendations by the American Heart Association. JAMA 1997; 277:1794–1801; Circulation 1997; 96:358–366; JADA 1997; 128:1142–1150.
29. Cardiac valvulopathy associated with exposure to fenfluramine or dexfenfluramine: US Department of Health and Human Services interim public health recommendations. MMR Morb Mortal Wkly Rep 1997; 46:1061–1066.
30. Shively BK, Roldan CA, Gill EA, et al. Prevalence and determinants of valvulopathy in patients treated with dexfenfluramine. Circulation 1999; 100: 2162–2167.
31. Cannistra LB, Cannistra AJ. Regression of multivalvular regurgitation after the cessation of fenfluramine and phentermine treatment [Letter]. N Engl J Med 1998; 339:771.
32. Gardin JM, Weissman NJ, Leung C, et al. Clinical and echocardiographic follow-up of patients previously treated with dexfenfluramine of phentermine/fenfluramine. JAMA 2001; 286:2001–2014.
33. Guidelines for the management of patients with valvular heart disease. A report of the American College of Cardiology/American Heart Association Task force on practice guidelines (Committee on management of patients with valvular heart disease). Circulation 1998; 98:1949–1984.
34. Roldan CA, Gill EA, Shively BK. Prevalence and diagnostic value of precordial murmurs for valvular regurgitation in obese patients treated with dexfenfluramine. Am J Cardiol 2000; 86:535–539.
35. O'Kelly B, Browner WS, Massie B, et al. Ventricular arrhythmias in patients undergoing noncardiac surgery. The study of perioperative ischemia research group. JAMA 1992; 268:217–221.
36. Mahla E, Rotman B, Rehak P, et al. Perioperative ventricular dysrhythmias in patients with structural heart disease undergoing non-cardiac surgery. Anesth Analg 1998; 86:16–21.

37. Gelma S, Laws HL, Potzick J, et al. Thoracic epidural vs. balanced anesthesia in morbid obesity: an intraoperative and postoperative hemodynamic study. Anesth Analg 1980; 59:902–908.
38. Charlson ME, MacKenzie CR, Ales K, et al. Surveillance for postoperative myocardial infarction after noncardiac operations. Surg Gynecol Obstet 1988; 167:407–414.

# 16

# Obesity and Atherosclerotic Vascular Disease

### Tulika Jain

*Department of Internal Medicine and the Donald W. Reynolds Cardiovascular Clinical Research Center, University of Texas Southwestern Medical Center, Dallas, Texas, U.S.A.*

### Jorge Plutzky

*Department of Internal Medicine and the Donald W. Reynolds Cardiovascular Clinical Research Center, Harvard Medical School, Boston, Massachusetts, U.S.A.*

### Darren K. McGuire

*Department of Internal Medicine and the Donald W. Reynolds Cardiovascular Clinical Research Center, University of Texas Southwestern Medical Center, Dallas, Texas, U.S.A.*

## INTRODUCTION

Obesity is associated with an increased risk of atherosclerotic coronary heart disease (CHD). This fact combined with the rapid increase in the prevalence of obesity in the United States population threatens to reverse many of the advances made in reducing CHD morbidity and mortality and drives major problems with morbidity, mortality, and health care costs (1). Uncertainty remains as to whether excess weight is independently associated with CHD, or whether the association between obesity and CHD is mediated through other risk factors linked to obesity such as physical inactivity, hypertension, dyslipidemia, and abnormal glucose metabolism. If obesity causes or accelerates atherogenesis, the responsible mechanisms remain largely unknown. Adiposity and obesity may exacerbate the development, progression, and destabilization of atherosclerotic heart disease via direct adverse effects on fat and glucose metabolism. Beyond the metabolic effects associated with obesity, adiposity may also contribute to CHD via inflammatory mechanisms mediated by adipocytokines, especially those mediators associated with visceral fat accumulation. All of these issues establish the need for a greater understanding of the complex biologic and clinical interplay between excess adiposity and cardiovascular disease (CVD).


## EPIDEMIOLOGY

The premise that obesity is an independent risk factor for CHD is supported by data from several epidemiologic studies. Independent associations of total body weight, especially when analyzed as body mass index (BMI), with coronary atherosclerosis and clinical CHD risk have been demonstrated in autopsy studies, cohort studies, and clinical trials using noninvasive methods to evaluate intermediate biomarkers of atherosclerosis. In addition, the influence of obesity on clinical outcomes has been assessed in some studies. This data is reviewed below.


### Autopsy Studies

In the Pathobiological Determinants of Atherosclerosis in Youth multi-center autopsy study (2), quantitative assessment of atherosclerosis of the aorta and right coronary arteries was made in 1532 young adults aged 15 to 34 who had died of external causes. The investigators also documented measures of obesity including BMI as well as thickness of the panniculus adiposus. Both of these parameters were associated with subclinical atherosclerosis independent of lipoprotein profiles and smoking status. In another postmortem study, the relationship between coronary atherosclerosis and anthropometric indicators of abdominal fatness was examined in 32 previously healthy men (age<40) and 30 previously healthy women (age <50) (3). In men, age-adjusted waist-to-hip ratio (WHR) was significantly correlated with the severity of obstructive coronary disease, with coronary intima-media thickness (IMT), as well as with cardiac hypertrophy (4). In women, coronary IMT varied significantly across tertiles of WHR and was highest when WHR exceeded 0.87 (5). In a separate retrospective chart-review study that included 599 women, this same Finnish group reported significant age-adjusted associations between severity of coronary lesions and both BMI and abdominal subcutaneous fat thickness greater than 35 mm (6). In this study, the most severe coronary disease was noted in those women with BMI between 24.2 and 27.2 (mild to moderate over-weight), with less severe lesions in the groups with both higher and lower BMI. This upside down U-shaped relationship between BMI and coronary disease has also been observed in other studies using both autopsy assessment and angiographic estimates of coronary artery disease (CAD) burden (3,7).

In contrast to these studies, investigators from the International Atherosclerosis Project analyzed data from 23,000 autopsies and found no independent association between measures of body weight, height, or obesity and precursors of aortic or coronary atherosclerosis (fatty streaks, raised lesions, etc.) (8). The reason for this discrepancy is not clear, although it can be noted that there have been significant changes in national BMI trends between the time the International Atherosclerosis Project was performed and the prior studies. In summary, many analyses from autopsy studies suggest an independent association between obesity and atherosclerosis. Because these studies also offered only limited data with regard to traditional CHD risk factors, it remains unclear whether any of the observed associations are truly independent of established risk factors for CHD.

## Obesity and Intermediate Markers of Coronary Atherosclerosis

In addition to autopsy reports, a number of studies have evaluated the association between obesity and atherosclerosis using intermediate markers of vascular disease. The Muscatine Study evaluated whether BMI was independently associated with electron-beam computed tomography–estimated coronary artery calcification, a radiologic marker of coronary atherosclerosis, in 385 men and 472 women aged 29 to 43 years (9). Using sophisticated statistical techniques that included assessment of receiver operating characteristic curves and multivariable logistic regression, this study reported an independent association between BMI and coronary calcium after adjusting for conventional CHD risk factors estimated by the Framingham risk score (10).

In the Atherosclerosis Risk in Communities (ARIC) study, the association between a number of CHD risk markers and ultrasound-determined carotid artery IMT, another indirect marker of atherosclerotic vascular disease, was assessed in 13,282 men and women with baseline examinations at ages 45 to 64 (11). Both BMI and WHR were independently associated with increased IMT in the overall cohort, even after adjustments for conventional risk factors. The association between change in body weight from young adulthood (age 25) to middle age (ages 45–64) and carotid IMT was also evaluated. A 10-kg increase in weight was associated with higher carotid IMT in black and white men and white women, but not in black women. Whether the differential association between weight change and IMT according to race and sex observed in this study is a real finding, or simply represents a lack of statistical power among the subgroup of black women remains unclear.

The Cardiovascular Health Study (CHS) is a population-based, longitudinal study designed to identify factors related to the onset of CHD and stroke in adults aged above 65 years. Using data from that study, a composite index of subclinical CVD was developed. This index included extent of carotid IMT > 80th percentile; ankle-brachial index ≤ 0.9; carotid stenosis ≥ 25%; major ECG (electrocardiographic) abnormalities; echocardiographic abnormalities of left ventricular wall motion or ejection fraction; and positive response to claudication or angina questions on the Rose questionnaire (12). In analyses including 5201 subjects from the original CHS cohort plus another 672 black participants later added to the study, BMI was associated with the composite index of subclinical atherosclerosis in all sex-by-race subgroups in unadjusted analyses, but in multivariable analyses that were adjusted for blood pressure, low-density lipoprotein (LDL) cholesterol, glucose, smoking, and white blood count, an independent association between BMI and CVD was only seen in white men (13).

Taking all this data together, strong evidence exists for an association between measures of obesity and intermediate markers of atherosclerosis, but these associations are inconsistent between studies, especially with regard to race and sex subgroups. This suggests a complex interplay between obesity and other cardiac risk measures that may vary between sexes and races. For further insight into this relationship, one can also look to cardiovascular outcome studies.

## Obesity and Cardiovascular Outcomes

While the relationship between obesity and CHD clinical outcomes remains controversial despite extensive investigation, several prospective, long-term studies demonstrate an independent association between measures of obesity and CHD death or all-cause mortality.

In the Framingham Heart Study involving data collected from 5209 participants followed over a 26-year period, obesity was an independent risk factor for incident cardiovascular events. Using Metropolitan Relative Weight (MRW) criteria (percentage of desirable weight that is correlated with BMI) as an estimate of obesity (14), an independent association between obesity and incident congestive heart failure and coronary death was observed, independent of age, cholesterol, systolic blood pressure, cigarette use, left ventricular hypertrophy, and glucose intolerance. The association of weight on risk of sudden death was most pronounced (Fig. 1) (15). A subsequent study using data from the same cohort demonstrated an independent association between the MRW (MRW of 110% = ~BMI of 25) and 30-year all-cause mortality for men in the Framingham Study (16). Using MRW measured at baseline, the lowest mortality was seen in the group of men with "normal" weight (100% to 109%). In multivariable analyses, a strong positive relationship was seen between baseline weight and all-cause mortality occurring at any interval. The 30-year mortality rate for nonsmoking, "overweight" (≥110%) men was up to 3.9 times higher than men of "normal" weight. In aggregate, these data from the Framingham Study strongly support an independent association between obesity and cardiovascular clinical outcomes.

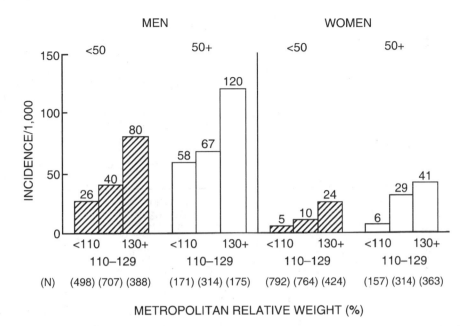

**Figure 1** Twenty-six year incidence of sudden death according to Metropolitan Relative Weight index among those in the Framingham study by sex and age. *Abbreviations*: *N*, number at risk for an event; numbers above the bars, actual incidence rates per 1000. *Source*: From Ref. 15 with permission.

The association between BMI and both total and cause-specific mortality was also investigated in the prospective Nurses' Health Study, a cohort of 115,195 U.S. women enrolled at age 30 to 50 (17). After 16 years of follow-up, multivariable analyses of female nonsmokers revealed a significant linear trend for increasing risk of death with increasing BMI. Compared with the referent group of women with a BMI <19 kg/m², the relative risk of cardiovascular death was: 1.0 for a BMI of 19.0 to 21.9 kg/m²; 1.4 for a BMI of 22.0 to 24.9 kg/m²; 1.7 for a BMI of 25.0 to 26.9 kg/m²; 3.1 for a BMI of 27.0 to 28.9; 4.6 for a BMI of 29.0 to 31.9; and 5.8 for a BMI ≥ 32 (Fig. 2). In this same study, weight gain greater than 10 kg after the age of 18 correlated with increased mortality in middle adulthood. When examining the association between BMI and cardiovascular-specific mortality among nonsmoking women with a BMI ≥ 32 kg/m², the relative risk of death was 4.1 compared with the reference group of women with a BMI < 19 kg/m² (17).

Another prospective study of over one million adults in the United States (457,785 men and 588,369 women) with 201,622 deaths during a 14-year follow-up period found that obesity was strongly and independently associated with an increased risk of cardiovascular death and all-cause

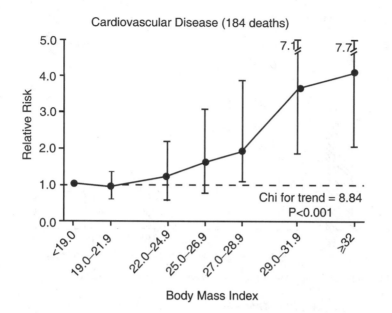

**Figure 2**  Relative risk of death from cardiovascular disease according to body mass index among women who never smoked from the Nurses' Health Study. *Source*: From Ref. 17.

mortality among nonsmokers and those without a history of CHD. The lowest levels of all-cause mortality were seen in men with a BMI between 23.5 and 24.9 kg/m$^2$ and women with a BMI between 22 and 23.4 kg/m$^2$. There was a progressive increase in mortality as BMI increased, and the heaviest men and women (BMI $\geq 40$ kg/m$^2$) had the highest adjusted relative risk of death (2.7 and 1.9, respectively). Increased risk of cardiovascular death was seen among men with BMI $> 25.5$ kg/m$^2$ and women with BMI $> 25$ kg/m$^2$. In multivariable analyses that were adjusted for conventional risk factors of cardiovascular disease, a high BMI was most predictive of cardiovascular death in men (relative risk 2.9) (18). Similarly, among 300,000 patients in the American Cancer Society Prevention Study, high excess body weight was associated with all-cause and cardiovascular mortality but the increment in cardiovascular risk associated with greater BMI declined with age (19).

There are also studies that report an independent relationship between obesity and nonfatal cardiovascular events. Among 504 patients who underwent angiography for stable angina ($n = 226$) or acute coronary syndrome (ACS)($n = 156$) and had evidence of at least 10% coronary artery stenosis, an independent association between BMI and ACS was seen after adjusting for age, sex, blood pressure, lipid levels, insulin resistance, leptin, fibrinogen,

C-reactive protein (CRP), CAD severity on angiography, smoking status, and history of myocardial infarction (MI) (20).

Data also exists in the form of meta-analyses of smaller studies. For example, in one such study of 19 prospective studies including a total of approximately 600,000 white men and women followed for over 15 years, the relationship between BMI and all-cause mortality was examined. In 50-year-old nonsmoking men without evidence of CVD who were followed for 30 years, a U-shaped relationship between BMI and mortality was seen, with the lowest and highest weight subgroups having higher observed risk compared with a group at intermediate weight. All-cause mortality was lowest in the group with a BMI of $24 \, kg/m^2$ and highest in the group with a $BMI \geq 32 \, kg/m^2$ (odds ratio $= 3.49$) (21).

Not all studies have found an association between obesity and CVD morbidity and mortality. The Munster Heart Study (Prospective Cardiovascular Münster) followed 16,288 men and 7325 women for seven years and noted an increase in CHD death associated with BMI, but this association was no longer statistically significant after accounting for major risk factors of age, total cholesterol, LDL, and blood pressure (22). Similarly, in the CHS study discussed previously, there were 646 deaths (11%) during a five-year follow-up period. Although BMI was a significant predictor of sub-clinical disease in unadjusted analyses, none of the measures of obesity (total body weight, BMI, or waist circumference) were significant predictors of total or CHD mortality after accounting for other known predictors of cardiovascular risk (23).

In summary, the association between obesity and cardiovascular clinical outcomes is inconsistent. Possible explanations for the discrepant findings include differences in health status of individuals, varying duration of follow-up among the studies, genetic and cultural differences depending on the location of the study, and inadequate sample sizes to adequately assess the independent associations. While the observed association between obesity and cardiovascular outcomes may be variable, the preponderance of the data from the large, prospective, long-term studies support an independent association between obesity and increased risk for adverse cardiovascular clinical outcomes.

## OBESITY, CVD RISK FACTORS, AND
## THE METABOLIC SYNDROME

The underlying mechanisms through which obesity, particularly abdominal obesity, may induce excessive CHD morbidity and mortality remain largely uncertain although insight has been gained into possible contributors. People who are obese typically manifest associated adverse cardiovascular risk features such as hypertension, diabetes, and dyslipidemia, as well as decreased levels of physical activity. The interactions between obesity and underlying cardiac risk factors are certainly complex, confounding analyses of association and challenging efforts at determining mechanistic links with CVD. In both the ARIC and CHS studies discussed previously, the association between measures of obesity and CVD was attenuated after adjusting for markers of cardiovascular risk and prevalent subclinical CVD; however, hypertension and diabetes were important determinants of CVD, and both risk factors are strongly associated with weight gain and obesity. The overlapping and interconnected nature of these risk factors suggests the notion of a central underlying mechanism that may be at work. The relationship between these risk factors and obesity is thus worthy of closer consideration.

## Hypertension

Weight gain and measures of obesity are important determinants of blood pressure (24–28). Data from several population studies suggest that up to 75% of hypertension may be attributed to obesity (29,30). The Nurses' Health Study, the Swedish Obesity study, and data from the National Health and Nutrition Examination Survey II and III all demonstrated that blood pressure is increased in obese subjects (29). For example, the Nurses' Health Study involving 80,000 women showed that a 5-kg weight gain after age 18 is associated with higher risk for developing hypertension compared with women who gained 2 kg or less. Those women who gained 10 kg or more increased their risk of hypertension by 2.2-fold (28). Thus, obesity is associated with hypertension, which further contributes to cardiovascular morbidity.

## Insulin Resistance, Hyperinsulinemia, and Diabetes

There is a strong link between obesity, insulin resistance, and CVD. Data from population studies suggest that obesity accounts for 50% or more of the variance in insulin sensitivity (30). In a prospective epidemiologic study of 970 men with no history of CHD followed for 22 years, hyperinsulinemia was associated with an increased risk of death or nonfatal MI (31). Central–visceral adiposity, particularly fat in the omental and paraintestinal regions, seems to be the source for a group of cardiovascular risk factors associated with insulin resistance and hyperinsulinemia including dyslipidemia, cardiovascular oxidative stress, coagulation abnormalities, increased markers of inflammation, and premature CAD (32,33). This complex relationship is discussed further in the section on body fat distribution and the biology of obesity and atherosclerosis.

CHD is more common in patients with diabetes, and 80% of patients with type 2 diabetes are obese, which may account to some degree for the increased mortality associated with diabetes. However, among patients with diabetes, the association between BMI and increased mortality is not consistent. This is likely due to a clustering of risk factors associated with the diabetic state that include physical inactivity, dyslipidemia, hypertension, and family history of both diabetes and CHD. Therefore, among diabetic subjects, obesity may simply represent the presence of this atherogenic predisposition, supported by the observation that in analyses that adjust for these covariates, BMI often fails to maintain an independent association (34).

## Dyslipidemia

Obesity is associated with alterations in lipoprotein metabolism including elevations in serum concentrations of total cholesterol, LDL cholesterol, very low density lipoprotein (VLDL) cholesterol, and triglycerides, and a reduction in serum high-density lipoprotein (HDL) cholesterol. Central adiposity and high waist circumferences in particular account for much of the variance in elevated triglycerides and low HDL cholesterol (35). Weight loss is associated with a more favorable lipoprotein profile (36,37).

## Metabolic Syndrome

As discussed above, obesity is associated with many different metabolic perturbations, some of which may be responsible for the observed relationship between obesity and CHD (38). The clustering of metabolic risk factors in obese individuals has been referred to as the metabolic syndrome (and alternatively as Syndrome X) (39,40), and is characterized by five major components (41): Increased waist circumference, elevated triglycerides, low HDL cholesterol, elevated blood pressure ($\geq$130/85 mmHg), and insulin resistance ($\pm$impaired fasting glucose). In addition, a proinflammatory state and prothrombotic state commonly exist in association with this cluster of abnormalities. It remains unclear what mechanisms lie at the core of the metabolic syndrome, although some studies suggest it is the central obesity that plays the most critical role in driving the clustering of metabolic syndrome components, making further discussion of the relationship between metabolic syndrome and CHD relevant here.

　　Several studies have demonstrated associations between metabolic syndrome and CVD as well as all-cause mortality. The Kuopio Ischaemic Heart Disease Risk Factor Study is a population-based, prospective cohort study of 1209 Finnish men aged 42 to 60 years who were initially without CVD, cancer, or diabetes. There were 109 deaths during the 11.4-year follow-up period. Among this cohort of middle-aged men, those who met the criteria for metabolic syndrome had an increased cardiovascular and overall all-cause mortality even in the absence of baseline CVD and diabetes (42). Similarly, in a retrospective analysis of 6447 men with hypercholesterolemia and no history of MI from the West of Scotland Coronary Prevention Study, the presence of the metabolic syndrome predicted CHD events including nonfatal MI or CHD death even after adjusting for conventional risk factors (43). In addition, the predictive power of metabolic syndrome for CVD was further increased among the group of subjects who also had an elevated CRP.

Given evidence supporting the association between the metabolic syndrome and cardiovascular events, the next question is whether obesity contributes to cardiovascular risk independent of the presence of metabolic syndrome. In the Women's Ischemia Syndrome Evaluation Study, a cohort of 780 women referred for coronary angiography to evaluate suspected myocardial ischemia were examined for the influence of obesity on CAD, as well as the incidence cardiac events independent of metabolic syndrome (44). The presence of metabolic syndrome was associated with CAD, but BMI was not an independent predictor of CAD. Further, increases in BMI were not associated with three-year risk of death or with major adverse cardiovascular events, while metabolic status (groups progressing from normal to metabolic syndrome to treated diabetes) conferred an approximately twofold higher adjusted risk of death and major adverse cardiovascular events.

## BODY FAT DISTRIBUTION

Obesity per se is not sufficient to elicit the full-blown metabolic syndrome. Between 75% and 80% of the U.S. population are classified as overweight or obese, yet only 20% to 40% of the population has the metabolic syndrome (45). Thus, some overweight/obese individuals are susceptible to developing the metabolic syndrome, whereas others are not.

One factor that appears to influence this susceptibility is the regional distribution of fat in the body. The distribution of fat among different adipose tissue compartments can be categorized in numerous ways. First, it can be broken down into upper body fat (abdominal obesity) and lower body fat (gluteofemoral obesity) (46). Men tend to accumulate excess fat in the upper body, and women in the lower body. Although persons with upper body obesity typically have excess fat over the whole trunk (47), abdominal obesity is the commonly accepted term to describe this disorder (48). Abdominal fat is further compartmentalized into three regions— subcutaneous, intraperitoneal (visceral), and retroperitoneal. The latter two compartments can be identified and separated by magnetic resonance imaging (MRI), but not by computed tomography (CT) (47,49).

Individuals with abdominal obesity appear to be predisposed to the metabolic syndrome (50–53). It is still not clear if abdominal subcutaneous fat or visceral fat is more highly correlated with metabolic risk factors. Several studies suggest that visceral fat is more "metabolically active" than subcutaneous fat (54–56), and according to some investigators, this metabolic activity of visceral fat accounts for its pathologic role in the development of the metabolic syndrome and atherosclerotic vascular disease

(52,57–59). Other studies however report that subcutaneous fat, particularly abdominal subcutaneous fat, may be the major contributor to cardiovascular risk (47,60–63). On the one hand, although visceral fat is associated with lower adipocyte mass, it may be more metabolically active, releasing mediators directly into the portal circulation and hence the liver. On the other hand, although subcutaneous fat releases its products into the systemic circulation, its larger mass may make it more important systemically in the contribution to atherosclerotic risk.

## Body Fat Distribution and CHD

Studies of body fat distribution and atherosclerosis have generally relied on crude clinical end points and not on direct, quantitative measures of body fat or atherosclerosis. In the past, as seen in earlier cited studies, measurements of skin folds and WHRs or more recently just waist measurements were shown to be strong predictors of cardiovascular risk factors. A waist measurement of greater than 102 cm for men and greater than 88 cm for women defines very high risk. These waist measurements are considered indirect estimates of the amount of intra-abdominal or visceral fat.

Data from several studies have demonstrated that body fat distribution correlates with CHD, and specifically that individuals with abdominal obesity are more susceptible to CHD than are those with lower body obesity (64,65). In a prospective study in men and women from Sweden, the WHR was found to be a predictor of MI and angina (66,67). In studies of men in Hawaii and Paris, subscapular skinfold measurements were used to predict CHD (68). Improved methods of measuring body fatness, body fat distribution, and atherosclerosis will provide better information.

## BIOLOGY OF OBESITY, BODY FAT DISTRIBUTION, AND ATHEROSCLEROTIC DISEASE

It is now well established that adipose tissue, rather than being simply a storage place for fat, is a biologically active, dynamic endocrine organ with ready access to the circulatory system. Moreover, not all adipose tissue compartments are metabolically identical. Different adipose tissue depots vary in many aspects including rates of release of nonesterified fatty acids into the circulation (54), which may have important pathophysiological significance to coronary disease. Indeed, elevated free fatty acids are a characteristic hallmark of type 2 diabetes and often decrease as insulin sensitivity improves. Adipose tissues also release a host of other key mediators implicated in atherosclerosis, such as inflammatory cytokines [interleukin (IL) -6, IL-1, interferon-IIγ] and tumor necrosis factor–IIα. Fat tissue is also thought to contribute to the prothrombotic nature of insulin resistance and diabetes through secretion of plasminogen activator inhibitor-1.

Adipose tissue is also a source of hormones. This has been a recent area of advancement with the identfication of leptin and resistin, two hormones thought to affect energy balance and fat storage (69,70). Although it is tempting to see all these adipocytokines as being pathogenic, this is an overly simplistic view, as clearly established by the fact that individuals as well as mice that lack fat (lipodystrophy) also have diabetes. One fat-derived mediator that may actually protect against atherosclerosis is adiponectin, which appears to have anti-inflammatory effects and may directly influence the arterial wall.

The increased understanding of the basic science of adipocyte biology has not only provided insight into the pathogenesis of problems such as atherosclerosis, it has also offered new therapeutic targets for weight loss, improved diabetic control, and/or decreased inflammation and atherosclerosis.

Peroxisome proliferator–activated receptor (PPAR) -gamma was first identified in the pursuit of adipocyte-specific transcription factors. Serendipitous drug screening led to the identification of thiazolidinediones (TZDs, pioglitazone/Actos, and rosiglitazone/Avandia) as a class of drugs that could increase insulin sensitivity and lower glucose levels. Subsequent studies connected these observations through the recognition of TZDs as molecules exerting their effects by binding to and activating PPAR-$\gamma$, allowing them to carry out their function as ligand-activated transcription factors. More recent studies have implicated PPARs in general (PPAR-$\alpha$, activated by fibrates, and PPAR-$\delta$, for which drugs continue to be developed) as limiting inflammation and atherosclerosis in vitro, in animal models and human surrogate studies. The first of several PPAR-$\gamma$ cardiovascular clinical trials, PROactive, that has now been released continues to suggest that PPAR-$\gamma$ agonists, in this case pioglitazone, may limit cardiovascular events in patients with later stage CVD, although the various metabolic benefits (lower hemoglobin A1C, triglycerides, and blood pressure) leave a direct or indirect vascular effect unresolved. TZDs typically increase weight through a combination of fluid retention but also increased fat. The fact that TZDs increase fat but lower CRP and blood pressure while raising HDL illustrates some of the points made earlier regarding differences in fat depots and adipocyte effects. TZDs may shift fat from visceral to subcutaneous stores. One mechanism that may contribute to TZD effects is their potent induction of adiponectin, a well-established PPAR-$\gamma$ target gene.

## Physical Fitness

The effects of cardiorespiratory fitness and BMI on all-cause and cardiovascular mortality has been evaluated in multiple studies. In 2506 women and 2860 men from the Lipid Research Clinic cohort who were followed for 26 years (71), both fitness and measures of obesity were independently associated with all-cause mortality. Compared with fit/lean women,

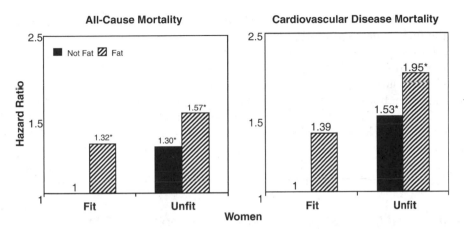

**Figure 3** Relative hazard in women by fitness level and BMI by quintiles. *Abbreviation*: BMI, body mass index. *Source*: From Ref. 71.

adjusted Cox proportional hazard ratios for all-cause mortality were higher for fit/obese women (1.32), unfit/lean women (1.30), and unfit/obese women (1.57). Compared with fit/lean men, the adjusted Cox proportional hazard ratios for all-cause mortality were higher for fit/obese men (1.25) and unfit/lean men (1.44), and unfit/obese men (1.49) (Figs. 3 and 4). Fitness attenuated but did not eliminate the excess mortality associated with obesity. Contrary to these results, in an observational cohort study of 21,925 men aged 30 to 83 participating in the Aerobics Center Longitudinal Study

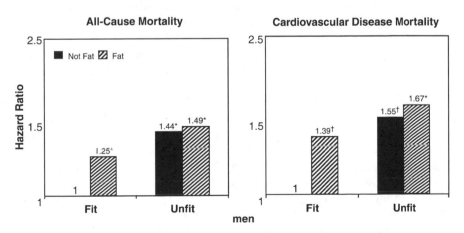

**Figure 4** Relative hazard in men by fitness level and BMI by quintiles. *Abbreviation*: BMI, body mass index. *Source*: From Ref. 71.

(ACLS), with 428 deaths registered during a mean follow-up of eight years, the independent association between obesity and mortality was eliminated after adjusting for various levels of fitness (72). Obese subjects with a high level of fitness at baseline assessments, determined by exercise treadmill testing, had mortality risks that were not statistically different from fit subjects of normal body weight. In a separate analysis of data from 9925 women participating in the same ACLS cohort study with a mean age of 43 at study entry, a low level of cardiorespiratory fitness was a more robust predictor of all-cause mortality in women than was baseline BMI (73). Therefore, at least some if not all of the mortality risk associated with obesity may be accounted for by differences in cardiovascular fitness.

## INFLUENCE OF OBESITY ON PROGNOSIS AMONG PATIENTS WITH CHD

Few studies have evaluated the association between obesity and prognosis once CAD has become clinically manifest. Three studies have reported lower short-term morbidity and mortality associated with greater BMI among patients undergoing percutaneous coronary intervention, the so-called "obesity paradox" (74–76). For example, in the Bypass Angioplasty Revascularization Investigation (BARI) trial, every one-unit increase in BMI was associated with a 5.5% lower adjusted risk for major in-hospital events (75). Data regarding the influence of obesity on prognosis after cardiac surgery are less consistent. In one cohort study of 4372 patient undergoing coronary artery bypass graft (CABG) surgery, underweight patients had a higher risk of death or complications compared with normal-weight patients (77). Data from the BARI trial also demonstrated that in-hospital complications were not adversely affected by obesity in CABG patients; however, higher BMI was associated with a fivefold higher five-year mortality following CABG surgery (75). All of these cohort studies are confounded by the selection bias that occurs in determining which patients will undergo revascularization procedures, with obese patients less likely treated with such therapies, and no study has systematically addressed this question in a prospective fashion.

Previous studies of the association of BMI with clinical outcomes following acute coronary ischemic events have failed to consistently demonstrate an independent linear association between overweight/obesity and cardiovascular clinical outcomes (78–80). In a cohort study of 2541 patients following a first MI, an independent association between increasing BMI and the risk of recurrent coronary events was observed (78). For subjects with BMI of 30 to $34.9 \, kg/m^2$ and those with BMI $\geq 35 \, kg/m^2$, the adjusted relative risk of recurrent coronary events was 1.49 and 1.80, respectively. Other studies, however, have reported a U-shaped relationship between BMI and outcomes similar to that observed in the revascularization studies discussed above, with the lowest adjusted risk observed in the overweight groups (e.g., BMI 25–29.9 kg/m$^2$) compared with low- and normal-weight or with obese subgroups. For example, Hoit et al. reported such a relationship between BMI and one-year survival following MI, with the lowest risk observed in the subgroup with intermediate BMI (BMI = 25–30 kg/m$^2$) (79). A similar U-shaped association between BMI and risk for subsequent major adverse cardiovascular events was observed in the "Sibrafiban Versus Aspirin to Yield Maximum Protection from Ischemic Heart Events Post-acute Coronary Syndromes" (SYMPHONY) and second SYMPHONY trials that included over 16,000 patients with ACSs (80). The most favorable outcomes were observed among overweight and obese individuals after multivariable adjustment for predictors of clinical outcome (including baseline characteristics, clinical parameters, region of enrollment, concomitant medical therapy, and procedures) with the very obese and the normal weight having the highest risk-adjusted mortality at 30 days, 90 days, and one year after ACSs. The explanation for this U-shaped relationship remains unclear, but the consistency of the observation among different populations suggests some validity to the findings.

## EFFECTS OF WEIGHT LOSS

There are no randomized controlled trials that demonstrate that voluntary weight loss has an effect upon long-term outcomes such as cardiovascular or all-cause mortality; however, even modest amounts of weight loss mitigates some cardiovascular risk factors (81). These effects could predict decrease CVD risk in the long run. A study from the Center for Disease Control and Prevention analyzed prospective, self-reported data from 6391 overweight and obese persons aged more than 35. They found that attempted weight loss independent of weight change was associated with lower all-cause mortality (82). Among overweight women aged 40 to 64 without preexisting illness ($n = 28,388$) from the prospective Iowa Women's Health study, intentional weight loss of 20 pounds or more was associated with a 25% decreased risk for cardiovascular, cancer, and all-cause mortality (83). Despite the paucity of data from randomized trials to support long-term cardiovascular benefits of weight loss, given the well-documented comorbidities associated with excess body weight and the favorable effects of weight control on myriad intermediate markers of cardiovascular health, physician prescription for weight control should remain a cornerstone of preventive health care.

### Strategies for Weight Loss as a Goal for CVD Risk Reduction

Successful weight management through comprehensive therapeutic lifestyle approaches including dietary discretion, increased physical activity, and even pharmacologic and surgical therapies may bring with them a decrease in CVD risk. Many strategies of diet modification for the prevention of CVD are being investigated including increasing monounsaturated fatty acids to replace saturated fatty acids, water intake, and the role of meal replacements, diet supplements, vitamins, minerals, and macronutrients. Adding dietary intervention to a more global approach of therapeutic lifestyle modification that includes nutrition education, modification of lifestyle habits, stress management, and relapse-prevention training will need to be investigated.

There are several pharmacologic approaches to weight loss, but the effect of many of these drugs on cardiovascular morbidity and mortality is unknown. Through the inhibition of pancreatic lipases, Orlistat prevents the complete hydrolysis of ingested fat into fatty acids and glycerol. This alteration in fat metabolism results in increased fecal fat excretion. Randomized, double-blinded, placebo-controlled trials have shown that weight loss is significantly higher in groups taking orlistat (84,85). Orlistat has also been shown to improve risk factors for CVD, such as lipids and diabetes, but its benefit in decreasing CVD has not been determined (84–87). Sibutramine has been shown to produce weight loss by its affects on serotonin and noradrenergic reuptake in the central nervous system. As a side effect, it can increase blood pressure and heart rate and probably should be avoided in patients with cardiac disease (88,89). Blocking of the cannabinoid receptor leads to a number of effects including decreased appetite and weight loss. Rimonabant is a cannabinoid receptor antagonist and has been reported to promote decreased body weight and waist circumference as well as improvement in cardiovascular risk factors (90). Metformin has been shown to have beneficial effects on obesity and cardiovascular risk factors (91), and it is the only oral hypoglycemic agent that has been shown to decrease cardiovascular risk when used for the treatment of type 2 diabetes (92). Of note, this data was in a relatively small subset of obese patients. In summary, substantial efforts are being made to develop pharmacologic adjuncts for the treatment of obesity, but the cornerstone of therapy remains therapeutic lifestyle modification. Whether or not gastric restriction procedures (gastric banding, vertical-banded gastroplasty, and vertical-ring gastroplasty), gastric bypass, biliopancreatic bypass, vagotomy, jaw wiring, intragastric balloons, liposuction, and plastic surgery carry with them favorable effects on CVD risk remains unknown.

## CONCLUSIONS

Obesity appears to be an independent cardiovascular risk factor, with the effects of obesity on cardiovascular risk confounded by numerous factors including weight gain, hypertension, diabetes, dyslipidemia, physical inactivity, and factors related to inflammation, thrombosis, and fibrinolysis. Despite the ongoing controversies with regard to the independent link between obesity and atherosclerotic risk, the Nutrition Committee of the American Heart Association has determined obesity to be an independent risk factor for CHD (30,93). The 27th Bethesda Conference identified obesity as a category II risk factor and recommended that intervention is likely lower to the incidence of CHD events based on the accumulated evidence (94). As the biologic basis of obesity and the complex interplay between obesity, fat distribution, and associated cardiovascular risk factors is better understood, management strategies can be devised to help prevent cardiovascular complications of obesity.

## REFERENCES

1. Mokdad AH, Marks JS, Stroup DF, Gerberding JL. Actual causes of death in the United States, 2000. JAMA 2004; 291:1238–1245.
2. McGill HC Jr, McMahan CA, Malcom GT, Oalmann MC, Strong JP. Relation of glycohemoglobin and adiposity to atherosclerosis in youth. Pathobiological Determinants of Atherosclerosis in Youth (PDAY) Research Group. Arterioscler Thromb Vasc Biol 1995; 15:431–440.
3. Kortelainen ML, Sarkioja T. Extent and composition of coronary lesions and degree of cardiac hypertrophy in relation to abdominal fatness in men under 40 years of age. Arterioscler Thromb Vasc Biol 1997; 17:574–579.
4. Kortelainen ML. Association between cardiac pathology and fat tissue distribution in an autopsy series of men without premortem evidence of cardiovascular disease. Int J Obes Relat Metab Disord 1996; 20:245–252.
5. Kortelainen ML, Sarkioja T. Extent and composition of coronary lesions in relation to fat distribution in women younger than 50 years of age. Arterioscler Thromb Vasc Biol 1999; 19:695–699.
6. Kortelainen ML, Sarkioja T. Coronary atherosclerosis associated with body structure and obesity in 599 women aged between 15 and 50 years. Int J Obes Relat Metab Disord 1999; 23:838–844.
7. Adams-Campbell LL, Peniston RL, Kim KS, Mensah E. Body mass index and coronary artery disease in African-Americans. Obes Res 1995; 3:215–219.
8. Montenegro MR, Solberg LA. Obesity, body weight, body length, and atherosclerosis. Lab Invest 1968; 18:594–603.
9. Mahoney LT, Burns TL, Stanford W, et al. Usefulness of the Framingham risk score and body mass index to predict early coronary artery calcium in young adults (Muscatine Study). Am J Cardiol 2001; 88:509–515.
10. Anderson KM, Wilson PW, Odell PM, Kannel WB. An updated coronary risk profile. A statement for health professionals. Circulation 1991; 83:356–362.
11. Stevens J, Tyroler HA, Cai J, et al. Body weight change and carotid artery wall thickness. The Atherosclerosis Risk in Communities (ARIC) Study. Am J Epidemiol 1998; 147:563–573.
12. Rose GA, Blackburn H. Cardiovascular Survey Methods. Geneva: World Health Organization, 1968:56.
13. Kuller L, Fisher L, McClelland R, et al. Differences in prevalence of and risk factors for subclinical vascular disease among black and white participants in

the Cardiovascular Health Study. Arterioscler Thromb Vasc Biol 1998; 18: 283–293.

14. Metropolitan Life Insurance Company. New weight standards for men and women. Stat Bull Metrop Insur Co 1959; 40:1.

15. Hubert HB, Feinleib M, McNamara PM, Castelli WP. Obesity as an independent risk factor for cardiovascular disease: a 26-year follow-up of participants in the Framingham Heart Study. Circulation 1983; 67:968–977.

16. Garrison RJ, Castelli WP. Weight and thirty-year mortality of men in the Framingham Study. Ann Intern Med 1985; 103:1006–1009.

17. Manson JE, Willett WC, Stampfer MJ, et al. Body weight and mortality among women. N Engl J Med 1995; 333:677–685.

18. Calle EE, Thun MJ, Petrelli JM, Rodriguez C, Heath CW Jr. Body-mass index and mortality in a prospective cohort of U.S. adults. N Engl J Med 1999; 341:1097–1105.

19. Stevens J, Cai J, Pamuk ER, Williamson DF, Thun MJ, Wood JL. The effect of age on the association between body-mass index and mortality. N Engl J Med 1998; 338:1–7.

20. Wolk R, Berger P, Lennon RJ, Brilakis ES, Somers VK. Body mass index: a risk factor for unstable angina and myocardial infarction in patients with angiographically confirmed coronary artery disease. Circulation 2003; 108:2206–2211.

21. Troiano RP, Frongillo EA Jr, Sobal J, Levitsky DA. The relationship between body weight and mortality: a quantitative analysis of combined information from existing studies. Int J Obes Relat Metab Disord 1996; 20:63–75.

22. Schulte H, Cullen P, Assmann G. Obesity, mortality and cardiovascular disease in the Munster Heart Study (PROCAM). Atherosclerosis 1999; 144:199–209.

23. Diehr P, Bild DE, Harris TB, Duxbury A, Siscovick D, Rossi M. Body mass index and mortality in nonsmoking older adults: the Cardiovascular Health Study. Am J Public Health 1998; 88:623–629.

24. Stamler J. Epidemiologic findings on body mass and blood pressure in adults. Ann Epidemiol 1991; 1:347–362.

25. Landsberg L, Troisi R, Parker D, Young JB, Weiss ST. Obesity, blood pressure, and the sympathetic nervous system. Ann Epidemiol 1991; 1:295–303.

26. Frohlich ED. Obesity and hypertension. Hemodynamic aspects. Ann Epidemiol 1991; 1:287–293.

27. Folsom AR, Burke GL, Byers CL, et al. Implications of obesity for cardiovascular disease in blacks: the CARDIA and ARIC Studies. Am J Clin Nutr 1991; 53:1604S–1611S.

28. Huang Z, Willett WC, Manson JE, et al. Body weight, weight change, and risk for hypertension in women. Ann Intern Med 1998; 128:81–88.

29. Kannel WB, Garrison RJ, Dannenberg AL. Secular blood pressure trends in normotensive persons: the Framingham Study. Am Heart J 1993; 125: 1154–1158.

30. Krauss RM, Winston M, Fletcher BJ, Grundy SM. Obesity: impact on cardiovascular disease. Circulation 1998; 98:1472–1476.

31. Pyorala M, Miettinen H, Laakso M, Pyorala K. Hyperinsulinemia predicts coronary heart disease risk in healthy middle-aged men: the 22-year follow-up results of the Helsinki Policemen Study. Circulation 1998; 98:398–404.

32. Rimm EB, Stampfer MJ, Giovannucci E, et al. Body size and fat distribution as predictors of coronary heart disease among middle-aged and older US men. Am J Epidemiol 1995; 141:1117–1127.
33. Sowers JR. Obesity and cardiovascular disease. Clin Chem 1998; 44:1821–1825.
34. Bray GA. Risks of obesity. Prim Care 2003; 30:281–299, v–vi.
35. Pouliot MC, Despres JP, Lemieux S, et al. Waist circumference and abdominal sagittal diameter: best simple anthropometric indexes of abdominal visceral adipose tissue accumulation and related cardiovascular risk in men and women. Am J Cardiol 1994; 73:460–468.
36. Sharman MJ, Gomez AL, Kraemer WJ, Volek JS. Very low-carbohydrate and low-fat diets affect fasting lipids and postprandial lipemia differently in overweight men. J Nutr 2004; 134:880–885.
37. Volek JS, Sharman MJ, Gomez AL, et al. Comparison of a very low-carbohydrate and low-fat diet on fasting lipids, LDL subclasses, insulin resistance, and postprandial lipemic responses in overweight women. J Am Coll Nutr 2004; 23:177–184.
38. Grundy SM. Metabolic complications of obesity. Endocrine 2000; 13:155–165.
39. Reaven GM. Banting Lecture 1988: role of insulin resistance in human disease. Diabetes 1988; 37:1595–1607.
40. Groop L, Orho-Melander M. The dysmetabolic syndrome. J Intern Med 2001; 250:105–120.
41. National Cholesterol Education Program (NCEP) Expert Panel on Detection E, and Treatment of High Blood Cholesterol in Adults. Third Report of the National Cholesterol Education Program (NCEP) Expert Panel on Detection, Evaluation, and Treatment of High Blood Cholesterol in Adults (Adult Treatment Panel III) final report. Circulation 2002; 106:3143–3421.
42. Lakka HM, Laaksonen DE, Lakka TA, et al. The metabolic syndrome and total and cardiovascular disease mortality in middle-aged men. JAMA 2002; 288:2709–2716.
43. Sattar N, McCarey DW, Capell H, McInnes IB. Explaining how "high-grade" systemic inflammation accelerates vascular risk in rheumatoid arthritis. Circulation 2003; 108:2957–2963.
44. Kip KE, Marroquin OC, Kelley DE, et al. Clinical importance of obesity versus the metabolic syndrome in cardiovascular risk in women: a report from the Women's Ischemia Syndrome Evaluation (WISE) Study. Circulation 2004; 109:706–713.
45. Ford ES, Giles WH, Dietz WH. Prevalence of the metabolic syndrome among US adults: findings from the third National Health and Nutrition Examination Survey. JAMA 2002; 287:356–359.
46. Bjorntorp P. The associations between obesity, adipose tissue distribution and disease. Acta Med Scand Suppl 1988; 723:121–134.
47. Abate N, Garg A, Peshock RM, Stray-Gundersen J, Grundy SM. Relationships of generalized and regional adiposity to insulin sensitivity in men. J Clin Invest 1995; 96:88–98.
48. National Institutes of Health. Clinical guidelines on the identification, evaluation, and treatment of overweight and obesity in adults—the evidence report. National Institutes of Health. Obes Res 1998; 6(suppl 2):51S–209S.

49. Abate N, Burns D, Peshock RM, Garg A, Grundy SM. Estimation of adipose tissue mass by magnetic resonance imaging: validation against dissection in human cadavers. J Lipid Res 1994; 35:1490–1496.

50. Kissebah AH, Vydelingum N, Murray R, et al. Relation of body fat distribution to metabolic complications of obesity. J Clin Endocrinol Metab 1982; 54:254–260.

51. Bjorntorp P. Abdominal obesity and the metabolic syndrome. Ann Med 1992; 24:465–468.

52. Despres JP. Abdominal obesity as important component of insulin-resistance syndrome. Nutrition 1993; 9:452–459.

53. Bjorntorp P. Body fat distribution, insulin resistance, and metabolic diseases. Nutrition 1997; 13:795–803.

54. Funahashi T, Nakamura T, Shimomura I, et al. Role of adipocytokines on the pathogenesis of atherosclerosis in visceral obesity. Intern Med 1999; 38:202–206.

55. Lemieux S. Contribution of visceral obesity to the insulin resistance syndrome. Can J Appl Physiol 2001; 26:273–290.

56. Vidal H. Gene expression in visceral and subcutaneous adipose tissues. Ann Med 2001; 33:547–555.

57. Matsuzawa Y, Shimomura I, Nakamura T, Keno Y, Kotani K, Tokunaga K. Pathophysiology and pathogenesis of visceral fat obesity. Obes Res 1995; 3(suppl 2):187S–194S.

58. Kissebah AH. Intra-abdominal fat: is it a major factor in developing diabetes and coronary artery disease? Diabetes Res Clin Pract 1996; 30(suppl):25–30.

59. Lemieux I, Pascot A, Prud'homme D, et al. Elevated C-reactive protein: another component of the atherothrombotic profile of abdominal obesity. Arterioscler Thromb Vasc Biol 2001; 21:961–967.

60. Abate N, Garg A, Peshock RM, Stray-Gundersen J, Adams-Huet B, Grundy SM. Relationship of generalized and regional adiposity to insulin sensitivity in men with NIDDM. Diabetes 1996; 45:1684–1693.

61. Kelley DE, Thaete FL, Troost F, Huwe T, Goodpaster BH. Subdivisions of subcutaneous abdominal adipose tissue and insulin resistance. Am J Physiol Endocrinol Metab 2000; 278:E941–E948.

62. Gautier JF, Milner MR, Elam E, Chen K, Ravussin E, Pratley RE. Visceral adipose tissue is not increased in Pima Indians compared with equally obese Caucasians and is not related to insulin action or secretion. Diabetologia 1999; 42:28–34.

63. Cnop M, Landchild MJ, Vidal J, et al. The concurrent accumulation of intra-abdominal and subcutaneous fat explains the association between insulin resistance and plasma leptin concentrations: distinct metabolic effects of two fat compartments. Diabetes 2002; 51:1005–1015.

64. Lakka HM, Lakka TA, Tuomilehto J, Salonen JT. Abdominal obesity is associated with increased risk of acute coronary events in men. Eur Heart J 2002; 23:706–713.

65. Rexrode KM, Carey VJ, Hennekens CH, et al. Abdominal adiposity and coronary heart disease in women. JAMA 1998; 280:1843–1848.

66. Larsson B, Svardsudd K, Welin L, Wilhelmsen L, Bjorntorp P, Tibblin G. Abdominal adipose tissue distribution, obesity, and risk of cardiovascular

disease and death: 13 year follow up of participants in the study of men born in 1913. Br Med J (Clin Res Ed) 1984; 288:1401–1404.

67. Lapidus L, Bengtsson C, Larsson B, Pennert K, Rybo E, Sjostrom L. Distribution of adipose tissue and risk of cardiovascular disease and death: a 12 year follow up of participants in the population study of women in Gothenburg, Sweden. Br Med J (Clin Res Ed) 1984; 289.1257–1261.

68. Donahue RP, Abbott RD, Bloom E, Reed DM, Yano K. Central obesity and coronary heart disease in men. Lancet 1987; 1:821–824.

69. Mavri A, Alessi MC, Bastelica D, et al. Subcutaneous abdominal, but not femoral fat expression of plasminogen activator inhibitor-1 (PAI-1) is related to plasma PAI-1 levels and insulin resistance and decreases after weight loss. Diabetologia 2001; 44:2025–2031.

70. Sakkinen PA, Wahl P, Cushman M, Lewis MR, Tracy RP. Clustering of procoagulation, inflammation, and fibrinolysis variables with metabolic factors in insulin resistance syndrome. Am J Epidemiol 2000; 152:897–907.

71. Stevens J, Cai J, Evenson KR, Thomas R. Fitness and fatness as predictors of mortality from all causes and from cardiovascular disease in men and women in the lipid research clinics study. Am J Epidemiol 2002; 156:832–841.

72. Lee CD, Blair SN, Jackson AS. Cardiorespiratory fitness, body composition, and all-cause and cardiovascular disease mortality in men. Am J Clin Nutr 1999; 69:373–380.

73. Farrell SW, Braun L, Barlow CE, Cheng YJ, Blair SN. The relation of body mass index, cardiorespiratory fitness, and all-cause mortality in women. Obes Res 2002; 10:417–423.

74. Gruberg L, Weissman NJ, Waksman R, et al. The impact of obesity on the short-term and long-term outcomes after percutaneous coronary intervention: the obesity paradox? J Am Coll Cardiol 2002; 39:578–584.

75. Gurm HS, Whitlow PL, Kip KE. The impact of body mass index on short- and long-term outcomes inpatients undergoing coronary revascularization. Insights from the bypass angioplasty revascularization investigation (BARI). J Am Coll Cardiol 2002; 39:834–840.

76. Gurm HS, Brennan DM, Booth J, Tcheng JE, Lincoff AM, Topol EJ. Impact of body mass index on outcome after percutaneous coronary intervention (the obesity paradox). Am J Cardiol 2002; 90:42–45.

77. Reeves BC, Ascione R, Chamberlain MH, Angelini GD. Effect of body mass index on early outcomes in patients undergoing coronary artery bypass surgery. J Am Coll Cardiol 2003; 42:668–676.

78. Rea TD, Heckbert SR, Kaplan RC, et al. Body mass index and the risk of recurrent coronary events following acute myocardial infarction. Am J Cardiol 2001; 88:467–472.

79. Hoit BD, Gilpin EA, Maisel AA, Henning H, Carlisle J, Ross J Jr. Influence of obesity on morbidity and mortality after acute myocardial infarction. Am Heart J 1987; 114:1334–1341.

80. Eisenstein EL, McGuire DK, Bhapkar MV, et al. Moderate obesity is associated with better intermediate-term survival in acute coronary syndromes: results from The SYMPHONY and 2nd SYMPHONY Clinical Trials. J Am Coll Cardiol 2003; 41:387A.

81. Yanovski SZ, Bain RP, Williamson DF. Report of a National Institutes of Health—Centers for Disease Control and Prevention workshop on the feasibility of conducting a randomized clinical trial to estimate the long-term health effects of intentional weight loss in obese persons. Am J Clin Nutr 1999; 69:366–372.

82. Gregg EW, Gerzoff RB, Thompson TJ, Williamson DF. Intentional weight loss and death in overweight and obese U.S. adults 35 years of age and older. Ann Intern Med 2003; 138:383–389.

83. Williamson DF, Pamuk E, Thun M, Flanders D, Byers T, Heath C. Prospective study of intentional weight loss and mortality in never-smoking overweight US white women aged 40–64 years. Am J Epidemiol 1995; 141:1128–1141.

84. Davidson MH, Hauptman J, DiGirolamo M, et al. Weight control and risk factor reduction in obese subjects treated for 2 years with orlistat: a randomized controlled trial. JAMA 1999; 281:235–242.

85. Rossner S, Sjostrom L, Noack R, Meinders AE, Noseda G. Weight loss, weight maintenance, and improved cardiovascular risk factors after 2 years treatment with orlistat for obesity. European Orlistat Obesity Study Group. Obes Res 2000; 8:49–61.

86. Tonstad S, Pometta D, Erkelens DW, et al. The effect of the gastrointestinal lipase inhibitor, orlistat, on serum lipids and lipoproteins in patients with primary hyperlipidaemia. Eur J Clin Pharmacol 1994; 46:405–410.

87. Hollander PA, Elbein SC, Hirsch IB, et al. Role of orlistat in the treatment of obese patients with type 2 diabetes. A 1-year randomized double-blind study. Diabetes Care 1998; 21:1288–1294.

88. James WP, Astrup A, Finer N, et al. Effect of sibutramine on weight maintenance after weight loss: a randomised trial. STORM Study Group. Sibutramine Trial of Obesity Reduction and Maintenance. Lancet 2000; 356:2119–2125.

89. Lean ME. Sibutramine—a review of clinical efficacy. Int J Obes Relat Metab Disord 1997; 21(suppl 1):S30–S36; discussion 37–39.

90. Van Gaal LF, Rissanen A, Scheen A, Ziegler O, Rossner S. Effect of rimonabant on weight reduction and cardiovascular risk. Lancet 2005; 366:369–370.

91. Hundal RS, Inzucchi SE. Metformin: new understandings, new uses. Drugs 2003; 63:1879–1894.

92. UK Prospective Diabetes Study (UKPDS) Group. Effect of intensive blood-glucose control with metformin on complications in overweight patients with type 2 diabetes (UKPDS 34). Lancet 1998; 352:854–865.

93. Eckel RH. Obesity and heart disease: a statement for healthcare professionals from the Nutrition Committee, American Heart Association. Circulation 1997; 96:3248–3250.

94. 27th Bethesda Conference Participants. 27th Bethesda Conference. Matching the intensity of risk factor management with the hazard for coronary disease events, September 14–15, 1995. J Am Coll Cardiol 1996; 27:957–1047.

# 17

# Heart Failure and Obesity: The Risk of Development and the Treatment of Heart Failure in Obese Patients

**Aruna D. Pradhan, Michael M. Givertz, and
Kenneth L. Baughman**

*Advanced Heart Disease Section, Cardiovascular Division, Department of Medicine,
Brigham and Women's Hospital, Harvard Medical School,
Boston, Massachusetts, U.S.A.*

## EPIDEMIOLOGY

Recent estimates of obesity prevalence among U.S. adults (1) suggest that currently, one in two individuals residing in the United States is overweight or obese as defined by a body mass index (BMI) $\geq 25$ kg/m$^2$. In addition, obesity incidence continues to rise such that the prevalence of marked obesity (BMI $\geq 40$ kg/m$^2$) has nearly tripled between 1990 and 2000. Parallel trends have been observed among children (2). Data from the National Health and Nutrition Examination Survey comparing two time periods, 1988–1994 and 1999–2000, demonstrate that among both boys and girls aged 12 to 19 years and across each of three major ethnic groups (non-Hispanic white, non-Hispanic black, and Mexican-American), the prevalence of overweight as defined by a level above the 95th percentile of sex-specific BMI for age has climbed, increasing overall from 10.5% to 15.5%. These data also reveal a disproportionate increase among non-Hispanic black and Mexican–American adolescents for whom the occurrence of overweight has increased by over 10%.

As these alarming trends in pediatric and adult obesity continue, cardiovascular specialists will undoubtedly encounter a rising rate of obesity-related cardiovascular disorders including hypertension, left ventricular hypertrophy (LVH), and heart failure (3). The Bogalusa Heart Study (4) prospectively evaluated 160 children aged 9 to 22 years, to assess factors predicting change in left ventricular mass (LVM). The strongest correlate of increased cardiac growth was linear growth (height); however, excess weight was a significant determinant of LVM after accounting for change in linear growth. This study is in keeping with other cross-sectional analyses showing that measures of body size and adiposity are independently associated with LVM (5–8). Importantly, an increase in LVM in youth may indicate greater likelihood of subsequent cardiovascular diseases (9).

Despite these observations, whether obesity is an independent risk factor for heart failure among the majority of adult patients who may have other comorbidities associated with left ventricular (LV) dysfunction remains uncertain. The well-characterized Framingham Heart Study cohort provides the strongest support for an independent contribution of obesity to the development of heart failure (Fig. 1). Approximately 6000 patients were followed for the incidence of clinically diagnosed heart failure over a mean period of 14 years (10). As expected, the baseline prevalence of diabetes and hypertension was associated with baseline indices of obesity and subsequent heart failure. However, multivariate analyses demonstrated an overall twofold increase in first heart failure episodes among participants with a BMI $\geq$ 30 kg/m$^2$ as compared to individuals with a normal BMI (18.5–24.9 kg/m$^2$), independent of other cardiovascular risk factors. The estimated risk increase associated with a 1 kg/m$^2$ increment in BMI was 7% and 5% in women and men, respectively.

## MECHANISMS OF DISEASE DEVELOPMENT

The pathophysiology of heart failure in obesity is complex and involves several hemodynamic, neurohormonal, and clinicopathologic features (Fig. 2). Hemodynamic studies of extremely obese patients demonstrate a general state of volume expansion with increased total circulating blood volume, stroke volume, and cardiac output, but typically normal cardiac index after accounting for body surface area (11,12). Systemic vascular resistance in these otherwise healthy subjects is low in the absence of overt heart failure. de Divitiis et al. (11) performed right and left heart catheterizations in 10 obese volunteers who did not have any signs or symptoms of heart failure or any confounding risk factors such as diabetes or hypertension. In these asymptomatic individuals, cardiac output, stroke volume, end-diastolic pressures, and atrial pressures were high, and correlated with the degree of obesity. Pulmonary artery pressures were also elevated and significantly associated with weight, although pulmonary vascular resistance and mean aortic

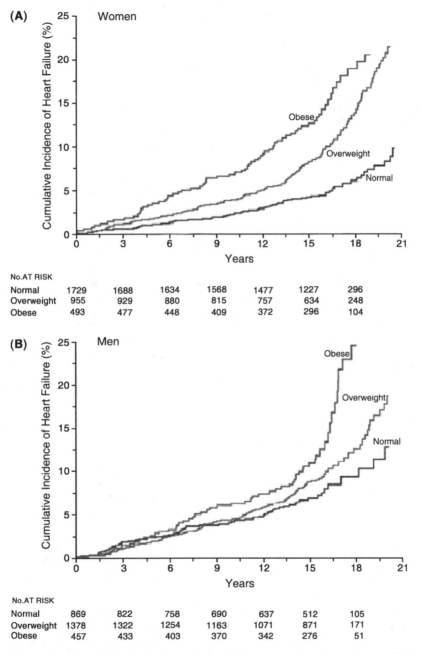

No.AT RISK

| | | | | | | | |
|---|---|---|---|---|---|---|---|
| Normal | 1729 | 1688 | 1634 | 1568 | 1477 | 1227 | 296 |
| Overweight | 955 | 929 | 880 | 815 | 757 | 634 | 248 |
| Obese | 493 | 477 | 448 | 409 | 372 | 296 | 104 |

No.AT RISK

| | | | | | | | |
|---|---|---|---|---|---|---|---|
| Normal | 869 | 822 | 758 | 690 | 637 | 512 | 105 |
| Overweight | 1378 | 1322 | 1254 | 1163 | 1071 | 871 | 171 |
| Obese | 457 | 433 | 403 | 370 | 342 | 276 | 51 |

**Figure 1** Cumulative incidence of heart failure according to category of BMI at baseline examination in the Framingham Heart Study. The BMI was 18.5 to 24.0 in normal subjects, 25.0 to 29.9 in overweight subjects, and 30.0 or more in obese subjects. *Abbreviation*: BMI, body mass index. *Source*: From Ref. 10.

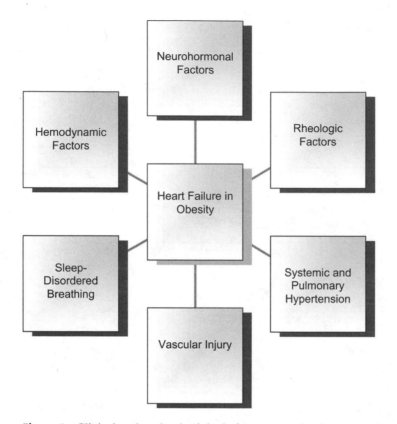

**Figure 2**  Clinical and pathophysiologic factors contributing to the development of heart failure in obesity.

pressure were normal. Measures of LV function such as $V_{max}$ and the ratio of stroke work index to LV end-diastolic pressure were reduced. Thus, even in the absence of symptoms, filling pressures may be elevated and ventricular performance depressed in obese individuals. A report using radionuclide angiocardiography showed similar results; compared with lean subjects, overweight and moderately obese but otherwise healthy individuals had increased cardiac output, stroke volume, end-systolic volume, total blood volume, and total plasma volume with relatively lower ejection fraction (13).

The relationship between obesity, LVH, and noninvasive hemo-dynamics has also been studied. In the Hypertension Genetic Epidemiology Network Study, 1672 participants underwent echocardiography and were evaluated for the presence of LVH (14). Doppler-defined stroke volume was measured, and cardiac output and total peripheral resistance were calculated. Free fat mass, as estimated by bioimpedance, was observed to increase with overweight, and was positively correlated with stroke volume and cardiac output, and inversely related to total peripheral resistance. In addition, increasing free fatty mass was strongly associated with greater LVM.

Pathologic studies have also demonstrated an adverse effect of obesity on ventricular size and coronary artery disease. In a postmortem study of 12 patients weighing more than 300 pounds (mean age 37 years; range 25–59 years), the heart weight and right ventricular size were increased in all subjects, and the left ventricle was enlarged in 11 of 12 (15). Although only two patients had one or more coronary arteries narrowed by greater than 75%, when the arteries were examined in 5 mm segments, virtually all patients had some degree of early atherosclerosis.

Neurohormonal factors may also play an important role linking obesity to heart failure. Insulin resistance and accompanying hyperinsulinemia may aggravate sodium and fluid retention, or directly promote myocardial hypertrophy through activation of insulin-like growth factor-1 receptors in ventricular myocardium (16). In addition, increased sympathetic outflow and inappropriate activation of the renin–angiotensin–aldosterone system are characteristic of obese hypertensive patients (17). Changes in blood rheology including increased blood viscosity, hematocrit, and fibrinogen have been postulated to exert additional stress on the myocardium (18,19). Vascular injury potentiated by an atherogenic lipid profile, coronary microangiopathy, and endothelial dysfunction may also contribute to LV dysfunction (20). Finally, the frequent coexistence of systemic hypertension and obesity is an important modulating factor in adaptive changes in LV geometry (see Chapter 2).

In the United States, the most common etiology of dilated cardiomyopathy is ischemic heart disease, and obesity is a well-recognized risk factor for coronary atherosclerosis. In the Nurses Health Study (21), the relative risk for nonfatal and fatal myocardial infarction adjusted for age and smoking increased progressively from a BMI of $< 21$ to $\geq 29\,\mathrm{kg/m^2}$ (relative risk for extreme categories: 3.3, p-trend $< 0.001$). As described in the previous chapters, obesity is also associated with well-recognized risk factors for ischemic heart disease including hypertension, dyslipidemia, and diabetes. In addition, hypertension and diabetes are independent risk factors for the development of dilated cardiomyopathy. Elevated glucose levels may cause accumulation of advanced glycosylation end products, low-density lipoprotein (LDL) oxidation, endothelial dysfunction, increased thrombogenicity, and altered lipids, which may contribute to atherosclerosis as well as diabetic cardiomyopathy.

A meta-analysis of 61 prospective studies demonstrated that blood pressure is directly related to cardiovascular mortality in a linear fashion, without evidence of a threshold effect to values as low as 115/75 mmHg (22). A number of treatment trials have demonstrated decreased cardiovascular events with treatment of hypertension. In one such trial of subjects who were 60 years of age or older with systolic blood pressure above 160 mmHg, and utilizing a stepped-care treatment of hypertension with a diuretic and beta-blocker, the relative risk of developing fatal or nonfatal heart failure in 4.5 years of follow-up was 0.51 (95% CI, 0.37–0.71; $p < 0.001$) (23). The deleterious effects of high blood pressure are presumed to be magnified in the obese hypertensive population.

Obese patients with glucose intolerance are also at greater risk of developing heart failure. In a cohort of nearly 50,000 men and women, 19 years of age or older, with predominantly type 2 diabetes, each 1% increase in hemoglobin A1C was associated with an 8% increased risk of heart failure, regardless of blood pressure or treatment with beta-blockers or angiotensin-converting enzyme (ACE) inhibitors (24). The Framingham investigators demonstrated that LVM increased progressively with worsening glucose intolerance, with greater effects in women possibly due to obesity (25). In the Strong Heart Study, Devereux et al. (26) found that non-insulin-dependent diabetics had increased LVM and wall thickness with reduced systolic function compared to controls. Therefore, the obesity-associated risk factors of hypertension and diabetes contribute significantly to the development of cardiac dysfunction in this population.

Dietary salt intake may also influence the development of heart failure in overweight and obese patients. In one study, even after adjustment for recognized heart failure risk factors, the risk for heart failure in overweight subjects increased 26% per each 100 mmol rise in daily sodium intake, compared to those with an intake below 50.2 mmol/day (27). In addition, epidemiologic investigations have suggested that there is a significant and independent relationship between dietary sodium intake and LVH. A recent study demonstrated that obese individuals have low circulating natriuretic peptide levels, which may contribute to their susceptibility to sodium and fluid retention and the subsequent development of hypertensive LVH and heart failure (28).

Finally, obesity is associated with obstructive sleep apnea (OSA) and hypoventilation, which may contribute to the development of heart failure and pulmonary hypertension (see Section "Treatment of Comorbidities").

## BASIC MECHANISMS LINKING OBESITY AND HEART FAILURE

Obesity is associated with increased plasma levels of leptin, a 16-kDa peptide produced by adipose tissue. Leptin levels are also elevated in patients with heart failure and correlate with total body fat and insulin resistance (29). There are several lines of experimental evidence that provide a pathophysiologic link between hyperleptinemia and the development or progression of heart failure. In cultures of myocytes obtained from neonatal rat hearts, 24 hours of exposure to leptin increases cell area and markedly increases protein expression. In this model, myocyte hypertrophy is preceded by rapid activation of mitogen-activated protein kinases (30). In isolated perfused rat hearts, leptin increases oxygen consumption and decreases cardiac energy efficiency without a change in glucose oxidation rates. This mechanoenergetic uncoupling is primarily due to activation of cardiac fatty acid oxidation with decreased cardiac triacylglycerol storage (31). Chronic exposure of rat cardiac myocytes to leptin is associated with reduced basal and catecholamine-stimulated adenylate cyclase activity (32). In addition, leptin elicits a dose-dependent inhibition of peak shortening and intracellular calcium exchange. While the mechanisms underlying the myocardial depressant effects of leptin remain unclear, studies have shown that leptin stimulates myocyte nitric oxide synthase (NOS) activity, and that leptin-induced negative inotropic effect can be attenuated by pretreatment with a NOS inhibitor (33,34). There is experimental (35) and clinical data (36) demonstrating that, in human myocardial failure, increased myocardial nitric oxide contributes to impaired contractile function at rest and in response to beta-adrenergic stimulation.

Intact animal studies also suggest a link between hyperleptinemia and heart failure. In adult rats, intravenous leptin infusion increases sympathetic nervous system activity to adipose tissue, skeletal muscle, kidneys, and adrenal glands (37). In conscious rabbits, intracerebral injection of leptin causes a dose-dependent increase in mean arterial pressure and renal sympathetic nerve activity (38). The critical role played by the sympathetic nervous system in the progression of heart failure is well established and serves as the rationale for the use of beta-blocker therapy (39).

Experimental models of hypertension and diabetes also provide evidence linking obesity and heart failure. Isolated ventricular myocytes from obese, spontaneously hypertensive heart failure (SHHF) rats demonstrate attenuated cyclic adenosine monophosphate production and sarcoplasmic reticulum calcium uptake in response to isoprenaline (40). In addition, obese SHHF rats are resistant to the blood pressure–lowering effects of angiotensin receptor blockers (ARBs) (41). Isolated myocytes from prediabetic rats with obesity and hyperleptinemia demonstrate impaired contractile function and prolonged relaxation (42). Finck et al. (43) characterized mice with cardiac overexpression of peroxisome proliferator–activated receptor-α. In this mouse model of diabetic cardiomyopathy, myocardial fatty acid oxidation rates are increased and glucose uptake and oxidation decreased. Furthermore, genetic markers of hypertrophic growth and systolic dysfunction are activated. Transgenic mice with cardiac-specific overexpression of lipoprotein lipase develop dilated cardiomyopathy with increased myocardial fatty acid oxidation, increased expression of heart failure genes, activation of apoptotic markers such as caspase-3, and intramyocyte lipid accumulation. This phenotype can be reversed by targeted overexpression of apolipoprotein B, which causes lipid resecretion from the heart (44).

Finally, there are clinical clues providing pathophysiologic and genetic links between obesity and cardiomyopathy. Alstrom syndrome, a rare autosomal recessive disorder, is characterized by childhood obesity, hyperinsulinemia with chronic hyperglycemia, and dilated cardiomyopathy. The mutant gene (ALMS1) has been identified, but its function remains unknown (45). Heart rate variability studies in nonobese subjects demonstrate that increased plasma leptin levels are associated with a shift of the sympathovagal balance toward a progressive increase in sympathetic activation and an increased response to orthostatic stimulus (46). Obese men with OSA have increased leptin levels compared to obese controls (47), and leptin levels decrease with treatment of OSA with continuous positive airway pressure (CPAP) (48). In hypertensive men, elevated plasma leptin levels are associated with increases in systolic blood pressure (49), BMI, and myocardial wall thickness (50) and impaired LV relaxation (51). In addition, heart rate is faster in hypertensive patients with higher plasma leptin levels, and this relationship is independent of age, BMI, and insulin levels (52). In heart transplant patients with cardiac denervation, plasma leptin levels are independently and positively associated with heart rate (53). Therefore, leptin may increase heart rate by a direct effect on the sinus node, or indirectly via activation of the sympathetic nervous system.

The stimuli for increased leptin production in obesity remain incompletely defined. A recent study found that endothelin-1 induces the expression and stimulates the secretion of leptin by adipose tissue (54). Endothelin is a potent vasoconstrictor peptide with positive inotropic and mitogenic properties. Plasma endothelin levels are elevated in patients with chronic heart failure in association with disease severity, and contribute to disease progression.

With regard to the existence of a distinct dilated cardiomyopathy of obesity, perhaps the most convincing clinical evidence derives from a clinicopathological study of obese patients with heart failure (55). In this large, cross-sectional analysis, 452 consecutive patients presenting for evaluation of heart failure underwent right heart catheterization and endomyocardial biopsy. Hemodynamic variables and clinical diagnoses were compared between 43 markedly obese patients with a $BMI \geq 35 \, kg/m^2$ and 409 nonobese patients ($BMI < 30 \, kg/m^2$), also undergoing cardiac evaluation. Obese patients had significantly higher filling pressures (mean pulmonary capillary wedge pressure 20.8 vs. 15.6 mmHg; $p < 0.001$), suggesting a state of relative hypervolemia. Cardiac output was also increased with no significant difference in cardiac index (2.3 vs. 2.4 liters/min/m$^2$; $p = NS$). Importantly, a final diagnosis of idiopathic dilated cardiomyopathy was more common in obese patients (77% prevalence) than in nonobese individuals (36% prevalence). Mild myocyte hypertrophy was the most common finding on endomyocardial biopsy specimens.

## Ventricular Remodeling and Obesity-Related Heart Failure

Cardiac adaptation to obesity is a heterogeneous process in which two distinct patterns of LV remodeling may occur. Because obesity and hypertension commonly coexist, these morphologic changes are based upon the influence of

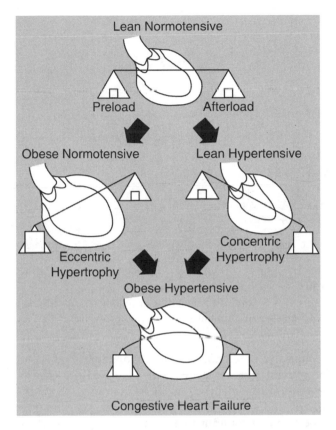

**Figure 3** Adaptation of the heart to obesity and hypertension. *Source*: From Ref. 56.

preload (volume expansion) and afterload (systemic hypertension) on LV geometry. These patterns of hypertrophy have been designated eccentric and concentric hypertrophy, respectively (Fig. 3). Eccentric hypertrophy in more contemporary nomenclature is referred to as a dilated cardiomyopathy. Both are characterized by an increase in LVM.

While not uniformly reported during echocardiographic evaluation, assessment of LV mass may be important in obese patients. A validated method of measuring LV mass utilizes the formula of Devereux and Reichek (57), where end-diastolic measurements of the LV internal diameter (LVID), interventricular septal thickness (IVST) and posterior wall thickness (PWT) are obtained using standard echocardiographic techniques, and LV mass = $1.04[(\text{LVID} + \text{PWT} + \text{IVST})^3 - (\text{LVID})^3] - 13.6$. Using this methodology, the Framingham investigators demonstrated an additive effect of obesity and hypertension on LV remodeling (Fig. 4), each having significant independent associations with LV mass and wall thickness (58). Obesity was also significantly associated with LV chamber dilation in both men and women.

Lean Normotensive
LVM/HT  96:71 g/m
TWT  18:16 mm
LVID  50:45 mm

Obese Normotensive                      Lean Hypertensive
LVM/HT  120:91 g/m                       LVM/HT  102:79 g/m
TWT  20:18 mm                            TWT  19:18 mm
LVID  52:47 mm                           LVID  50:45 mm

Obese Hypertensive
LVM/HT  127:102 g/m
TWT  21:19 mm
LVID  52:47 mm

**Figure 4**  Adaptation of the heart to obesity and hypertension. Age-adjusted least-squares mean values of echocardiographic parameters among subjects followed in the Framingham Heart Study (624 men, 1209 women). Values in black are for men. Values in grey are for women. *Abbreviations*: LVM, left ventricular mass in grams; HT, height in meters; TWT, total wall thickness in millimeters; LVID, left ventricular internal diastolic dimension in millimeters. *Source*: From Ref. 58.

Another study in this cohort evaluated normotensive individuals and found similar results (59). Overweight was associated with increased presence of LVH, particularly in patients with a $BMI \geq 30$ kg/m$^2$, among whom the prevalence adjusted for age and systolic blood pressure was 32% and 30% in women and men, respectively. After adjusting for age and blood pressure, BMI remained a strong independent predictor of LVM, wall thickness, and internal dimension.

## HEART FAILURE IN OBESITY: A DIFFICULT DIAGNOSIS

The signs and symptoms of heart failure are often masked, or at least difficult to appreciate in the overweight patient. Symptoms of heart failure rely on evidence of reduced cardiac output or elevated filling pressures. Symptoms of low cardiac output such as exertional fatigue and weakness are often present in the obese patient due to the increased metabolic work of excess weight. Left-sided congestive symptoms such as shortness of breath, orthopnea, and paroxysmal nocturnal dyspnea are also difficult to decipher in the obese patient. Exertional dyspnea is universal in this group. Symptoms of true orthopnea as well as paroxysms of nocturnal dyspnea are relatively specific for heart failure, but must be distinguished from gastroesophageal reflux, aspiration, and sleep apnea. Signs and symptoms of right-sided congestion include neck fullness, right upper quadrant discomfort, and lower extremity edema. All of these findings may be present in the obese patient.

Elevated jugular venous pressure is often difficult to visualize in patients with obese necks. Additionally, the examiner may not elevate the head of the bed high enough to appreciate the meniscus from an elevated jugular venous pressure. The examiner must look carefully for venous pulsations in the neck, particularly those that are laterally placed and "wiggle" the earlobe, suggestive of a high venous pressure. Hepatic engorgement may be appreciated by tenderness in the right upper quadrant, which should not be present from obesity alone. Lower extremity edema usually indicates total body salt and water excess. However, venous stasis, prior episodes of thrombophlebitis, or the effects of trauma may complicate examination of the legs.

The point of maximal impulse of the left ventricle may be difficult to determine in the supine position, depending on the amount of body weight and pectoral mass present. Moving the patient into the left lateral decubitus position may enhance the ability to feel the point of maximal impulse and determine whether the heart is enlarged and gallop rhythms are present. Murmurs may be similarly difficult to auscultate, and there is increased reliance on noninvasive testing to determine heart size and function in this population. Pulmonary auscultation is relatively insensitive because breath sounds may be diminished due to hypoventilation or the presence of excess soft tissue. Hypoventilation may also lead to atelectasis and/or wheezing.

The chest x-ray is of increased importance for the diagnosis of heart failure in the obese patient. An upright chest x-ray provides an accurate estimate of the size of the heart and suggests specific chamber enlargement including the right ventricle. The chest x-ray may also support the diagnosis of heart failure when there is evidence of pulmonary edema or, more commonly, enlarged pulmonary arteries, vascular redistribution, and peribronchial cuffing. Unilateral or bilateral pleural effusions may be differentiated from atelectasis or elevated diaphragms, while noncardiac causes of shortness of breath such as hiatal hernia, chronic obstructive pulmonary disease, or masses may be ruled out by chest radiography. Pulmonary arterial hypertension, due primarily to obesity-hypoventilation syndrome and/or secondary to chronic LV failure, may be suggested by enlargement of the main pulmonary artery and right ventricle with concomitant tapering of peripheral pulmonary vascular markings (60).

The electrocardiogram may be of some assistance in evaluating patients with obesity and heart disease. Patients with obesity are not protected from supraventricular arrhythmias and may develop atrial fibrillation, atrial flutter, and other supraventricular tachycardias that may exacerbate LV dysfunction. Patients with heart failure and cardiomyopathy are more prone to ventricular arrhythmias and may suffer sudden cardiac death. Ventricular voltage may be increased because of the additional LVM associated with weight gain or may be decreased because of the difficulties of electrical transmission through adipose tissue. In overweight and obese patients, the electrocardiogram remains a gold standard for ischemic findings, particularly Q-wave infarctions or ST-segment depression or elevation during ischemia or injury, respectively.

The echocardiogram is the most sensitive and specific study to evaluate cardiac structure and function in obese subjects. Ideally, transthoracic echocardiography with two-dimensional and Doppler techniques can define chamber size and left and right ventricular systolic function, identify abnormal valvular structure or function, and estimate filling pressures (particularly, pulmonary artery systolic pressure). Newer techniques using pulmonary venous inflow and tissue Doppler imaging can identify abnormal diastolic function, and have been used to estimate LV filling pressure (61). However, as with other noninvasive studies, the echocardiogram is technically more difficult in the obese patient and occasionally cannot be performed due to an inadequate "window" to observe the heart. If necessary, transesophageal echocardiography can be performed to define more clearly cardiac structure and function, although caution must be taken to avoid causing aspiration and/or the need for emergent intubation. When echocardiography is unable to provide adequate information regarding the etiology or severity of heart failure, cardiac magnetic resonance imaging (MRI) should be considered.

## Treatment of Obesity in the Heart Failure Patient

There are several areas in which the clinical management of obese patients with heart failure differs from the standard approach in nonobese subjects. In particular, several studies suggest that weight loss may be an important therapeutic intervention for LVH regression and the prevention of heart failure. Case reports with weight loss induced by biliopancreatic diversion have demonstrated near normalization of cardiac structure and function with losses of between 50 and 146 kg (62,63). Alpert et al. (64) evaluated obese patients before and after substantial weight loss following bariatric surgery. In those both with and without prior heart failure, weight loss resulted in reductions in LV internal diastolic dimensions, end-systolic wall stress and mass, left atrial dimension, and diastolic filling time. In a multivariable analysis these investigators also demonstrated that the duration of morbid obesity was the strongest predictor of heart failure. If the duration of morbid obesity increased by one year, the prevalence odds of heart failure increased by 1.5. For individuals with morbid obesity of 20-year duration, the probability of heart failure was 66%, and 93% for those subjects who were morbidly obese for more than 25 years.

In an observational study of 40 patients undergoing gastroplasty compared with 30 controls treated with dietary strategies alone, weight loss after bariatric surgery correlated with LVH regression, independent of reduction in blood pressure over a one-year follow-up period (65). Average weight loss in the surgically treated group was 33 kg (baseline $117 \pm 15$ kg vs. follow-up $84 \pm 14$ kg), with average decreases in LV mass of 27 g and wall thickness of

2.1 mm. Conventional weight reduction through intensive diet and exercise has also been demonstrated to favorably impact LV mass. In a small clinical trial involving a total of 41 young, overweight, hypertensive patients, LV mass decreased by 20% among subjects conforming to the diet and exercise prescription, who showed an average weight loss of 8.3 kg over a 21-week period (66).

While LVH has been associated with increased cardiovascular event rates (67), no clinical outcomes data are available regarding event reduction with sustained weight loss among obese patients with established LVH. This may be due to the difficulty of maintaining weight loss in these patients and/ or the paucity of long-term outcomes data among patients undergoing bariatric surgery. Furthermore, there are serious risks associated with bariatric surgery, including pulmonary embolism (PE) and respiratory failure, which may be increased in patients with LV dysfunction and/or heart failure (68).

## Treatment of Heart Failure in the Obese Patient

Patients with obesity and heart failure should be treated aggressively with pharmacologic therapy, as recommended by American Heart Association/ American College of Cardiology guidelines (69). Standard treatment includes diuretics, ACE inhibitors or ARBs, and beta-blockers. Spironolactone may be considered for patients with advanced heart failure or LV dysfunction following myocardial infarction. Digoxin and nitrates may be used as an adjuvant therapy to treat symptoms of advanced heart failure. The combination of hydralazine and isosorbide dinatrate has recently been shown to reduce morbidity and mortality in African-Americans with heart failure, and may be considered as an adjuvant therapy in patients who remain symptomatic despite standard therapy (70).

Diuretics are utilized for virtually all patients with evidence of sodium and fluid retention (71). As noted above, assessment of the degree of volume overload is often challenging in this patient population because of difficulties in determining jugular venous pressure, the etiology of pulmonary rales and the cause of lower extremity edema. While B-type natriuretic peptide levels have been proposed as a surrogate marker for volume status in heart failure (72), they are lower in obese patients (Fig. 5) (28,73) and may be falsely normal in severely obese patients with marked congestion. If clinical evaluation suggests fluid retention, patients should be treated with standard loop diuretics to decrease intra- and extravascular volume. The clearest endpoint for therapy is the development of prerenal azotemia or other evidence of excess diuresis, including postural hypotension. Once this level of "dehydration" has been achieved, diuretics can be decreased until these symptoms or signs resolve. Spironolactone or eplerenone can be added to loop diuretics, as both agents have been demonstrated to improve the prognosis of patients with heart failure (74,75). Additionally these potassium-sparing diuretics may lessen the need for potassium

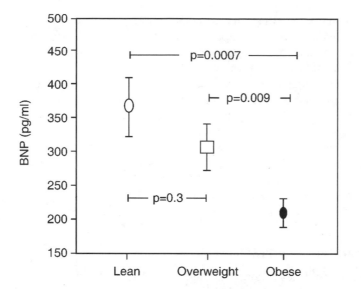

**Figure 5** BNP levels in 318 patients with heart failure were significantly lower in obese patients (BMI $\geq$ 30 kg/m$^2$) compared to overweight (BMI $\geq$ 25–29 kg/m$^2$) or lean (BMI < 25 kg/m$^2$) patients. *Abbreviations*: BNP, B-type natriuretic peptide; BMI, body mass index. *Source*: From Ref. 73.

replacement and save magnesium, therefore diminishing the risk for arrhythmic events.

Both ACE inhibitors and ARBs have been demonstrated to improve the prognosis of patients with heart failure and reduced ejection fraction (76,77). ACE inhibitors should be used preferentially, unless the patient is intolerant due to cough or angioedema. Patients should be diuresed maximally before titrating the dose to target levels, as defined by randomized controlled trials. The maximally tolerated dose of ACE inhibitor or ARB is determined by patient tolerance, particularly the development of hypotension, worsening renal function, and/or hyperkalemia (78).

Beta-blockers improve ventricular performance, decrease the risk of sudden death, and prolong survival in heart failure. Carvedilol or metoprolol CR/XL are currently approved for the treatment of heart failure and have similar beneficial effects on outcomes (39). Because these agents also decrease blood pressure, they must be titrated carefully with other medical therapy, particularly diuretics and vasodilators. The dose should be increased to the maximal tolerated or until the achievement of maximal suggested doses by weight.

Treatment with beta-blockers has long been known to have adverse effects on insulin sensitivity and lipid metabolism, while alpha-1 blockade may improve glycemic control (79). It has therefore been suggested that treatment with carvedilol, a nonselective beta-blocker with alpha-blocking properties and favorable effects on plasma lipids, may be preferred among insulin resistant patients with dyslipidemia or the metabolic syndrome. Two small randomized clinical trials in patients without heart failure have evaluated this hypothesis (79,80). Both studies demonstrated improved glycemic control and favorable changes in lipids among patients treated with carvedilol versus those treated with a selective beta-blocker, metoprolol or atenolol, over a 12 to 24-week period. In a large study of patients with type 2 diabetes and hypertension, treatment with carvedilol for five months was associated with stable hemoglobin A1C, improved insulin sensitivity, and decreased progression to microalbuminuria, compared to those treated with metoprolol (81). Whether these positive short-term effects on metabolic parameters can be sustained long term and are associated with reduced cardiovascular morbidity and mortality remains to be determined.

Digitalis is an agent with a relatively narrow therapeutic window. In 6800 patients with mild–moderate heart failure, the Digitalis Investigation Group trial demonstrated no improvement in survival with digoxin and a potential adverse effect of increased drug levels (82). While digoxin is usually administered with consideration of weight, in view of the relatively limited benefit (decreased hospitalizations for heart failure), most clinicians use no more than 0.25 mg/day, even in the most obese patients. A level should be acquired on at least one occasion after one to two weeks of oral treatment or rechecked in the setting of worsening renal function, to ensure that it is less than 1.0 ng/mL.

## Treatment of Comorbidities

### Diabetes

There are several concerns with regard to pharmacological treatment of diabetes in obese heart failure patients. The thiazolidinedione (TZD) class of oral hypoglycemic agents have gained widespread popularity for the treatment of insulin resistance, because of several advantageous ancillary effects on lipid metabolism, vascular endothelial function, and inflammatory cytokines (83). However, these agents may increase fluid retention and exacerbate heart failure symptoms. In general, TZDs produce a 6% to 7% increase in circulating intravascular volume. In a study of diabetic patients with chronic heart failure, initiation of TZDs was associated with fluid retention in 17% of patients as defined by a 10-pound involuntary weight gain (84). Peripheral, rather than central, edema predominates and usually resolves upon drug withdrawal. Despite this, the U.S. Food and Drug Administration (FDA) has issued a warning that these agents not be used in patients with New York Heart Association functional class III or IV heart failure.

Metformin is another popular oral insulin sensitizer. According to prescribing information provided by the FDA and the package insert, metformin is contraindicated in patients with "heart failure requiring pharmacologic therapy" due to the risk of lactic acidosis (85). While the overall incidence of life-threatening lactic acidosis is low, the FDA assigned a black-box warning in response to postmarketing reports of increased risk among patients with chronic hypoperfusion and hypoxia. Despite cautionary alerts, a review of prescribing patterns among Medicare beneficiaries hospitalized with a primary diagnosis of heart failure in 2000 and 2001 reported that nearly one-fourth of patients were discharged on either a TZD or metformin (85). Given the increased awareness of the beneficial cardiovascular effects of these agents when used in the general population, further data are needed to examine their risk–benefit ratio in patients with heart failure.

### Sleep Apnea

It has been estimated that at least 50% of patients with heart failure have sleep apnea (86). Therefore, screening for this disorder is an important part of cardiovascular care for heart failure patients, in general, and for those with concomitant obesity, in particular. Sleep apnea may be classified into two major forms: obstructive (OSA) and central (CSA). Obesity is the main risk factor for OSA where pharyngeal obstruction occurs in the setting of adjacent fat accumulation and luminal narrowing, with resultant hypoventilation due to complete or partial pharyngeal collapse (86). In isolated obesity, the prevalence of OSA approaches 50% (87). Among heart failure patients, this estimate varies between 11% and 37% (88,89), with the additional burden of obesity linked to a sixfold increase in risk at least among men. Central sleep apnea, unlike OSA, likely develops as a consequence of heart failure. Pulmonary congestion and superimposed periodic arousals stimulate hyperventilation and hypocapnia, triggering a central apnea (90). Central apneas are sustained by recurrent arousals resulting from apnea-induced hypoxia and the increased work of breathing during the ventilatory phase because of interstitial edema and reduced lung compliance. Sleep apnea may also contribute to heart failure progression. Underlying mechanisms include apnea-induced hypoxia and hypercapnea, periodic surges in sympathetic outflow, daytime hypertension, and loss of vagal tone. These adrenergic and hemodynamic loads contribute directly to myocardial ischemia, arrhythmias, adverse ventricular remodeling, and disease progression. Until recently, there was limited data demonstrating the efficacy of sleep apnea therapy in patients with heart failure. In a small randomized clinical trial of patients with mild–moderate heart failure and OSA, Kaneko et al. (91) demonstrated that treatment with nocturnal CPAP for one month is associated with significant reductions in daytime systolic blood pressure (by 10 mm Hg) and LV end-diastolic dimension (by 3 mm), while significantly increasing LV ejection fraction. It remains to be determined whether these beneficial effects of CPAP on cardiovascular function are sustainable and translate into improved clinical outcomes.

### Venous Thromboembolism

Obesity and heart failure are significant risk factors for deep venous thrombosis (DVT) and PE (92). As with heart failure itself, determining the presence of venous thromboembolic disease in the obese patient is more difficult than in nonobese subjects. Obese heart failure patients should be screened for the presence of DVT/PE when they present with unilateral or asymmetric bilateral lower extremity edema, pleuritic chest pain, increased shortness of breath, and/or presyncope. Appropriate diagnostic studies include plasma D-dimer levels, venous ultrasonagraphy of the lower extremities, and high-resolution computerized tomography of the chest (93). Transthoracic echocardiography may show new or worsening right ventricular function and evidence of pulmonary hypertension. Recent studies suggest that measurement of B-type natriuretic peptide levels may also help to risk stratify patients with acute PE (94). Hospitalized patients should be treated with low-molecular weight heparin to prophylax against thromboembolic complications, and consideration should be given to chronic anticoagulation in the obese heart failure population. Obese patients with dyspnea on exertion, out of proportion to their findings of heart failure, should be evaluated for chronic recurrent PE.

### Pulmonary Hypertension

Pulmonary vascular resistance is frequently elevated in patients with chronic LV failure as a result of dysregulation of vascular smooth muscle tone and structural remodeling (95). These abnormalities are due, in part, to pulmonary vascular endothelial dysfunction that results in impaired nitric oxide availability and increased endothelin production. In patients with heart failure, the resulting pulmonary hypertension directly affects right ventricular function and may affect exercise capacity (96), morbidity, and mortality (97). Obesity may contribute to the development of pulmonary hypertension in heart failure by several mechanisms including obesity-hypoventilation syndrome, OSA, and chronic venous thromboembolism. In addition, pharmacologic agents used to treat obesity have been associated with the development of pulmonary hypertension (98) and regurgitant valvular lesions (99).

### Dyslipidemia

Dyslipidemia is common in patients with obesity and cardiovascular disease (see Chapter 4). All patients with heart failure and obesity should have a fasting lipid panel checked at the time of initial evaluation. For patients with ischemic heart disease or significant cardiovascular risk factors, LDL levels should be reduced according to the National Cholesterol Education Program Adult Treatment Panel III guidelines (100). If drug treatment is required to achieve these goals, statins represent first-line therapy (101). Retrospective data suggests that statins improve survival in patients with ischemic and nonischemic heart failure, regardless of the presence of obesity (102). Recent studies with rimonabant, a cannabinoid receptor antagonist, demonstrate improvement in lipid parameters and reversal of the metabolic syndrome with sustained weight loss, and suggest a novel treatment for obese patients with heart failure (103).

## TRANSPLANT CONSIDERATIONS

Consideration of cardiac transplantation is problematic in the obese patient with advanced heart failure. Obese patients have symptoms not dissimilar to heart failure, making it difficult to determine whether heart failure treatment has been effective. In general, obese patients with chronic symptoms of heart failure are often followed up for longer periods of time before serious consideration is given to cardiac transplantation. Cardiopulmonary exercise testing and right heart catheterization provide the most objective assessments of peak functional capacity and hemodynamics, respectively, and can be used to risk stratify potential transplant candidates. Once they have been listed for transplant, these patients may face difficulties in matching with an appropriate donor. The donor pool is relatively small and fixed in the United States, and donors are matched with recipients based on blood type and body weight. The donor pool of an adequate weight to sustain the obese recipient is small. Additionally, large donors who may themselves be obese often have depressed ventricular function, making them suboptimal candidates for organ donation.

Additionally, retrospective and prospective studies demonstrate that transplant recipients who are obese experience decreased quality of life and survival after heart transplantation (104,105). The most definitive study, analyzed over 4500 patients from the Cardiac Transplant Research Database (105). In this analysis, patients greater than 140% of ideal body weight before heart transplant displayed increased postoperative mortality. The authors also evaluated BMI or percent ideal body weight as a better measure of future morbidity and mortality after heart transplantation, and demonstrated that percent ideal body weight appeared to be preferable. Unfortunately, because of the need for corticosteroids as part of routine post-transplant immunosuppression, most patients gain additional weight following transplantation. This added obesity has adverse effects on morbidity and mortality, not dissimilar from the risks of obesity before transplantation.

## Prognosis of Obese Patients with Heart Failure

Although obesity is a risk factor for the development of heart failure and influences its treatment, obese patients appear to have a better prognosis than their lean counterparts if they develop symptomatic LV dysfunction. Davos et al. (106) evaluated 589 heart failure patients to assess the influence of body weight on survival. Cachectic patients were excluded from analysis, and non-cachectic patients were divided into quintiles of BMI. There was no difference in age, exercise capacity, or ejection fraction in the five groups. Survival was greatest in the fourth quintile, with a relative risk of death of 0.91. Comparatively, quintiles 1, 2, and 3 had relative risks of 2.3, 1.7, and 1.8, respectively. In a multivariate analysis, exercise capacity, ejection fraction, and BMI were independent predictors of survival over one year. Horwich et al. (107) also evaluated obesity and mortality in patients with advanced heart failure, by analyzing outcomes in over 1200 patients divided into quartiles by weight. While the obese and overweight groups had higher rates of hypertension, diabetes, and dyslipidemia, there was no difference in survival rates for the four BMI groups. A higher BMI was associated with a trend toward improved survival. Lavie et al. (108) evaluated patients who were less symptomatic (New York Heart Association functional class I–III), and also assessed body composition parameters including lean body weight and percent body fat. Patients with subsequent events had significantly lower body weight and total body fat, compared with event-free survivors.

The mechanisms by which obesity is protective are unclear. It has been proposed that lower body weight may represent a relative catabolic state with an increase in proinflammatory cytokines such as tumor necrosis factor-α causing myocardial depression and ventricular remodeling (109). Additionally, obese patients may have lesser degrees of neurohormonal activation and increased nutritional or metabolic reserves.

## SUMMARY

The increasing prevalence of obesity has important implications for cardiovascular health, in general, and for patients with heart failure, in particular. Given the significant morbidity and mortality associated with heart failure, greater recognition of obesity as a risk factor for the development of LV dysfunction is critical to the formulation of strategies for prevention, diagnosis, and treatment of heart failure in this growing patient population. In addition, clinicians must give special consideration to the treatment of obesity in this high-risk patient population. Novel targets of therapy include metabolic abnormalities associated with obesity and heart failure and other comorbid conditions including sleep apnea and pulmonary hypertension. In addition, research efforts to understand the mechanisms underlying obesity-related heart failure as well as the potential paradoxical benefits of obesity in established heart failure are a major priority in the coming years.

## REFERENCES

1. Freedman DS, Khan LK, Serdula MK, et al. Trends and correlates of class 3 obesity in the United States from 1990 through 2000. JAMA 2002; 288: 1758–1761.
2. Ogden CL, Flegal KM, Carroll MD, et al. Prevalence and trends in overweight among US children and adolescents, 1999–2000. JAMA 2002; 288:1728–1732.
3. Olshansky SJ, Passaro DJ, Hershow RC, et al. A potential decline in life expectancy in the United States in the 21st century. N Engl J Med 2005; 352:1138–1145.
4. Urbina EM, Gidding SS, Bao W, et al. Effect of body size, ponderosity, and blood pressure on left ventricular growth in children and young adults in the Bogalusa Heart Study. Circulation 1995; 91:2400–2406.
5. Verhaaren HA, Schieken RM, Mosteller M, et al. Bivariate genetic analysis of left ventricular mass and weight in pubertal twins (the Medical College of Virginia twin study). Am J Cardiol 1991; 68:661–668.
6. Goble MM, Mosteller M, Moskowitz WB, et al. Sex differences in the determinants of left ventricular mass in childhood. The Medical College of Virginia Twin Study. Circulation 1992; 85:1661–1665.
7. Malcolm DD, Burns TL, Mahoney LT, et al. Factors affecting left ventricular mass in childhood: the Muscatine Study. Pediatrics 1993; 92:703–709.
8. Daniels SR, Meyer RA, Liang YC, et al. Echocardiographically determined left ventricular mass index in normal children, adolescents and young adults. J Am Coll Cardiol 1988; 12:703–708.
9. Mahoney LT, Schieken RM, Clarke WR, et al. Left ventricular mass and exercise responses predict future blood pressure. The Muscatine Study. Hypertension 1988; 12:206–213.
10. Kenchaiah S, Evans JC, Levy D, et al. Obesity and the risk of heart failure. N Engl J Med 2002; 347:305–313.
11. de Divitiis O, Fazio S, Petitto M, et al. Obesity and cardiac function. Circulation 1981; 64:477–82.
12. Kaltman AJ, Goldring RM. Role of circulatory congestion in the cardio-respiratory failure of obesity. Am J Med 1976; 60:645–653.
13. Licata G, Scaglione R, Barbagallo M, et al. Effect of obesity on left ventricular function studied by radionuclide angiocardiography. Int J Obes 1991; 15: 295–302.
14. Palmieri V, de Simone G, Arnett DK, et al. Relation of various degrees of body mass index in patients with systemic hypertension to left ventricular mass, cardiac output, and peripheral resistance (The Hypertension Genetic Epidemiology Network Study). Am J Cardiol 2001; 88:1163–1168.
15. Warnes CA, Roberts WC. The heart in massive (more than 300 pounds or 136 kilograms) obesity: analysis of 12 patients studied at necropsy. Am J Cardiol 1984; 54:1087–1091.
16. Ito H, Hiroe M, Hirata Y, et al. Insulin-like growth factor-I induces hypertrophy with enhanced expression of muscle specific genes in cultured rat cardiomyocytes. Circulation 1993; 87:1715–1721.

17. Ward KD, Sparrow D, Landsberg L, et al. Influence of insulin, sympathetic nervous system activity, and obesity on blood pressure: the Normative Aging Study. J Hypertens 1996; 14:301–308.
18. Carroll S, Cooke CB, Butterly RJ. Plasma viscosity, fibrinogen and the metabolic syndrome: effect of obesity and cardiorespiratory fitness. Blood Coagul Fibrinolysis 2000; 11:71–78
19. Solerte SB, Fioravanti M, Pezza N, et al. Hyperviscosity and microproteinuria in central obesity: relevance to cardiovascular risk. Int J Obes Relat Metab Disord 1997; 21:417–423.
20. Ziccardi P, Nappo F, Giugliano G, et al. Reduction of inflammatory cytokine concentrations and improvement of endothelial functions in obese women after weight loss over one year. Circulation 2002; 105:804–809.
21. Manson JE, Colditz GA, Stampfer MJ, et al. A prospective study of obesity and risk of coronary heart disease in women. N Engl J Med 1990; 322: 882–889.
22. Lewington S, Clarke R, Qizilbash N, et al. Age-specific relevance of usual blood pressure to vascular mortality: a meta-analysis of individual data for one million adults in 61 prospective studies. Lancet 2002; 360:1903–1913.
23. Kostis JB, Davis BR, Cutler J, et al. Prevention of heart failure by antihypertensive drug treatment in older persons with isolated systolic hypertension. SHEP Cooperative Research Group. JAMA 1997; 278:212–216.
24. Iribarren C, Karter AJ, Go AS, et al. Glycemic control and heart failure among adult patients with diabetes. Circulation 2001; 103:2668–2673.
25. Rutter MK, Parise H, Benjamin EJ, et al. Impact of glucose intolerance and insulin resistance on cardiac structure and function: sex-related differences in the Framingham Heart Study. Circulation 2003; 107:448–454.
26. Devereux RB, Roman MJ, Paranicas M, et al. Impact of diabetes on cardiac structure and function: the strong heart study. Circulation 2000; 101:2271–2276.
27. He J, Ogden LG, Bazzano LA, et al. Dietary sodium intake and incidence of congestive heart failure in overweight US men and women: first National Health and Nutrition Examination Survey Epidemiologic Follow-up Study. Arch Intern Med 2002; 162:1619–1624.
28. Wang TJ, Larson MG, Levy D, et al. Impact of obesity on plasma natriuretic peptide levels. Circulation 2004; 109:594–600.
29. Leyva F, Anker SD, Egerer K, et al. Hyperleptinaemia in chronic heart failure. Relationships with insulin. Eur Heart J 1998; 19:1547–1551.
30. Rajapurohitam V, Gan XT, Kirshenbaum LA, et al. The obesity-associated peptide leptin induces hypertrophy in neonatal rat ventricular myocytes. Circ Res 2003; 93:277–279.
31. Atkinson LL, Fischer MA, Lopaschuk GD. Leptin activates cardiac fatty acid oxidation independent of changes in the AMP-activated protein kinase-acetyl-CoA carboxylase-malonyl-CoA axis. J Biol Chem 2002; 277:29424–29430.
32. Illiano G, Naviglio S, Pagano M et al. Leptin affects adenylate cyclase activity in H9c2 cardiac cell line: effects of short- and long-term exposure. Am J Hypertens 2002; 15:638–643.

33. Wold LE, Relling DP, Duan J, et al. Abrogated leptin-induced cardiac contractile response in ventricular myocytes under spontaneous hypertension: role of Jak/STAT pathway. Hypertension 2002; 39:69–74.
34. Nickola MW, Wold LE, Colligan PB, et al. Leptin attenuates cardiac contraction in rat ventricular myocytes. Role of NO. Hypertension 2000; 36:501–505.
35. Kelly RA, Balligand J-L, Smith TW. Nitric oxide and cardiac function. Circ Res 1996; 79:363–380.
36. Hare JM, Givertz MM, Creager MA, et al. Increased sensitivity to nitric oxide synthase inhibition in patients with heart failure: potentiation of beta-adrenergic inotropic responsiveness. Circulation 1998; 97:161–166.
37. Haynes WG, Morgan DA, Walsh SA, et al. Receptor-mediated regional sympathetic nerve activation by leptin. J Clin Invest 1997; 100:270–278.
38. Matsumura K, Abe I, Tsuchihashi T, et al. Central effects of leptin on cardiovascular and neurohormonal responses in conscious rabbits. Am J Physiol Regul Integr Comp Physiol 2000; 278:R1314–R1320.
39. Bristow MR. Beta-adrenergic receptor blockade in chronic heart failure. Circulation 2000; 101:558–569.
40. Hohl CM, Hu B, Fertel RH, et al. Effects of obesity and hypertension on ventricular myocytes: comparison of cells from adult SHHF/Mcc-cp and JCR:LA-cp rats. Cardiovasc Res 1993; 27:238–242.
41. Sharkey LC, Holycross BJ, McCune SA, et al. Obese female SHHF/Mcc-fa(cp) rats resist antihypertensive effects of renin-angiotensin system inhibition. Clin Exp Hypertens 2001; 23:227–239.
42. Hintz KK, Aberle NS, Ren J. Insulin resistance induces hyperleptinemia, cardiac contractile dysfunction but not cardiac leptin resistance in ventricular myocytes. Int J Obes Relat Metab Disord 2003; 27:1196–1203.
43. Finck BN, Lehman JJ, Leone TC et al. The cardiac phenotype induced by PPARalpha overexpression mimics that caused by diabetes mellitus. J Clin Invest 2002; 109:121–130.
44. Yokoyama M, Yagyu H, Hu Y, et al. Apolipoprotein B production reduces lipotoxic cardiomyopathy: studies in heart specific lipoprotein lipase transgenic mouse. J Biol Chem 2003.
45. Collin GB, Marshall JD, Ikeda A, et al. Mutations in ALMS1 cause obesity, type 2 diabetes and neurosensory degeneration in Alstrom syndrome. Nat Genet 2002; 31:74–78.
46. Paolisso G, Manzella D, Montano N, et al. Plasma leptin concentrations and cardiac autonomic nervous system in healthy subjects with different body weights. J Clin Endocrinol Metab 2000; 85:1810–1814.
47. Phillips BG, Kato M, Narkiewicz K, et al. Increases in leptin levels, sympathetic drive, and weight gain in obstructive sleep apnea. Am J Physiol Heart Circ Physiol 2000; 279:H234–H237.
48. Harsch IA, Konturek PC, Koebnick C, et al. Leptin and ghrelin levels in patients with obstructive sleep apnoea: effect of CPAP treatment. Eur Respir J 2003; 22:251–257.
49. Kazumi T, Kawaguchi A, Katoh J, et al. Fasting insulin and leptin serum levels are associated with systolic blood pressure independent of percentage body fat and body mass index. J Hypertens 1999; 17:1451–1455.

50. Paolisso G, Tagliamonte MR, Galderisi M, et al. Plasma leptin level is associated with myocardial wall thickness in hypertensive insulin-resistant men. Hypertension 1999; 34:1047–1052.

51. Galderisi M, Tagliamonte MR, D'Errico A, et al. Independent association of plasma leptin levels and left ventricular isovolumic relaxation in uncomplicated hypertension. Am J Hypertens 2001; 14:1019–1024.

52. Narkiewicz K, Somers VK, Mos L, et al. An independent relationship between plasma leptin and heart rate in untreated patients with essential hypertension. J Hypertens 1999; 17:245–249.

53. Winnicki M, Phillips BG, Accurso V, et al. Independent association between plasma leptin levels and heart rate in heart transplant recipients. Circulation 2001; 104:384–386.

54. Xiong Y, Tanaka H, Richardson JA, et al. Endothelin-1 stimulates leptin production in adipocytes. J Biol Chem 2001; 276:28471–28477.

55. Kasper EK, Hruban RH, Baughman KL. Cardiomyopathy of obesity: a clinicopathologic evaluation of 43 obese patients with heart failure. Am J Cardiol 1992; 70:921–924.

56. Williams GH, Lilly LS, Seely EW. The heart in endocrine and nutritional disorders. *In* Braunwald E (ed): Heart Disease: A Textbook of Cardiovascular Medicine, 5th ed. Philadelphia, W.B. Saunders, 1997, pp. 1887–1913.

57. Devereux RB, Reichek N. Echocardiographic determination of left ventricular mass in man. Anatomic validation of the method. Circulation 1977; 55: 613–618.

58. Lauer MS, Anderson KM, Levy D. Separate and joint influences of obesity and mild hypertension on left ventricular mass and geometry: the Framingham Heart Study. J Am Coll Cardiol 1992; 19:130–134.

59. Lauer MS, Anderson KM, Levy D. Influence of contemporary versus 30-year blood pressure levels on left ventricular mass and geometry: the Framingham Heart Study. J Am Coll Cardiol 1991; 18:1287–1294.

60. McGoon M, Gutterman D, Steen V, et al. Screening, early detection, and diagnosis of pulmonary arterial hypertension: ACCP evidence-based clinical practice guidelines. Chest 2004; 126:14S–34S.

61. Sanders GP, Mendes LA, Colucci WS, et al. Noninvasive methods for detecting elevated left-sided cardiac filling pressure. J Card Fail 2000; 6:157–164.

62. Zuber M, Kaeslin T, Studer T, et al. Weight loss of 146 kg with diet and reversal of severe congestive heart failure in a young, morbidly obese patient. Am J Cardiol 1999; 84:955–956.

63. Taylor TV, Bozkurt B, Shayani P, et al. End-stage cardiac failure in a morbidly obese patient treated by biliopancreatic diversion and cardiac transplantation. Obes Surg 2002; 12:416–418.

64. Alpert MA, Terry BE, Mulekar M, et al. Cardiac morphology and left ventricular function in normotensive morbidly obese patients with and without congestive heart failure, and effect of weight loss. Am J Cardiol 1997; 80:736–740.

65. Karason K, Wallentin I, Larsson B, et al. Effects of obesity and weight loss on left ventricular mass and relative wall thickness: survey and intervention study. BMJ 1997; 315:912–916.

426                                                              *Pradhan et al.*

66. MacMahon SW, Wilcken DE, Macdonald GJ. The effect of weight reduction on left ventricular mass. A randomized controlled trial in young, overweight hypertensive patients. N Engl J Med 1986; 314:334–339.
67. Levy D, Garrison RJ, Savage DD, et al. Prognostic implications of echocardiographically determined left ventricular mass in the Framingham Heart Study. N Engl J Med 1990; 322:1561–1566.
68. Steinbrook R. Surgery for severe obesity. N Engl J Med 2004; 350:1075–1079.
69. Hunt SA, Abraham WT, Chin MH, et al. ACC/AHA 2005 guideline update for the diagnosis and management of chronic heart failure in the adult: a report of the American College of Cardiology/American Heart Association Task Force on Practice Guidelines (writing Committee to Update the 2001 Guidelines for the Evaluation and Management of Heart Failure): developed in collaboration with the American College of Chest Physicians and the International Society for Heart and Lung Transplantation: endorsed by the Heart Rhythm Society. Circulation 2005; 112:e154–e235.
70. Taylor AL, Ziesche S, Yancy C, et al. Combination of isosorbide dinitrate and hydralazine in blacks with heart failure. N Engl J Med 2004; 351:2049–2057.
71. Brater DC. Diuretic therapy. N Engl J Med 1998; 339:387–395.
72. Maisel AS, McCord J, Nowak RM, et al. Bedside B-Type natriuretic peptide in the emergency diagnosis of heart failure with reduced or preserved ejection fraction. Results from the Breathing Not Properly Multinational Study. J Am Coll Cardiol 2003; 41:2010–2017.
73. Mehra MR, Uber PA, Park MH, et al. Obesity and suppressed B-type natriuretic peptide levels in heart failure. J Am Coll Cardiol 2004; 43:1590–1595.
74. Pitt B, Zannad F, Remme WJ, et al. The effect of spironolactone on morbidity and mortality in patients with severe heart failure. Randomized Aldactone Evaluation Study Investigators. N Engl J Med 1999; 341:709–717.
75. Pitt B, Remme W, Zannad F, et al. Eplerenone, a selective aldosterone blocker, in patients with left ventricular dysfunction after myocardial infarction. N Engl J Med 2003; 348:1309–1321.
76. Jessup M, Brozena S. Heart failure. N Engl J Med 2003; 348:2007–2018.
77. Pfeffer MA, Swedberg K, Granger CB, et al. Effects of candesartan on mortality and morbidity in patients with chronic heart failure: the CHARM-Overall programme. Lancet 2003; 362:759–766.
78. Kittleson M, Hurwitz S, Shah MR, et al. Development of circulatory-renal limitations to angiotensin-converting enzyme inhibitors identifies patients with severe heart failure and early mortality. J Am Coll Cardiol 2003; 41:2029–2035.
79. Giugliano D, Acampora R, Marfella R, et al. Metabolic and cardiovascular effects of carvedilol and atenolol in non-insulin-dependent diabetes mellitus and hypertension. A randomized, controlled trial. Ann Intern Med 1997; 126:955–959.
80. Jacob S, Rett K, Wicklmayr M, et al. Differential effect of chronic treatment with two beta-blocking agents on insulin sensitivity: the carvedilol-metoprolol study. J Hypertens 1996; 14:489–494.
81. Bakris GL, Fonseca V, Katholi RE, et al. Metabolic effects of carvedilol vs metoprolol in patients with type 2 diabetes mellitus and hypertension: a randomized controlled trial. JAMA 2004; 292:2227–2236.

82. Rathore SS, Curtis JP, Wang Y, et al. Association of serum digoxin concentration and outcomes in patients with heart failure. JAMA 2003; 289:871–878.
83. Inzucchi SE. Oral antihyperglycemic therapy for type 2 diabetes: scientific review. JAMA 2002; 287:360–372.
84. Tang WH, Francis GS, Hoogwerf BJ, et al. Fluid retention after initiation of thiazolidinedione therapy in diabetic patients with established chronic heart failure. J Am Coll Cardiol 2003; 41:1394–1398.
85. Masoudi FA, Wang Y, Inzucchi SE, et al. Metformin and thiazolidinedione use in Medicare patients with heart failure. JAMA 2003; 290:81–85.
86. Bradley TD, Floras JS. Sleep apnea and heart failure: part I: obstructive sleep apnea. Circulation 2003; 107:1671–1678.
87. Resta O, Foschino-Barbaro MP, Legari G, et al. Sleep-related breathing disorders, loud snoring and excessive daytime sleepiness in obese subjects. Int J Obes Relat Metab Disord 2001; 25:669–675.
88. Javaheri S, Parker TJ, Liming JD, et al. Sleep apnea in 81 ambulatory male patients with stable heart failure. Types and their prevalences, consequences, and presentations. Circulation 1998; 97:2154–2159.
89. Sin DD, Fitzgerald F, Parker JD, et al. Risk factors for central and obstructive sleep apnea in 450 men and women with congestive heart failure. Am J Respir Crit Care Med 1999; 160:1101–1106.
90. Bradley TD, Floras JS. Sleep apnea and heart failure: part II: central sleep apnea. Circulation 2003; 107:1822–1826.
91. Kaneko Y, Floras JS, Usui K, et al. Cardiovascular effects of continuous positive airway pressure in patients with heart failure and obstructive sleep apnea. N Engl J Med 2003; 348:1233–1241.
92. Koniaris LS, Goldhaber SZ. Anticoagulation in dilated cardiomyopathy. J Am Coll Cardiol 1998; 31:745–748.
93. Goldhaber SZ, Elliott CG. Acute pulmonary embolism: part I: epidemiology, pathophysiology, and diagnosis. Circulation 2003; 108:2726–2729.
94. Kucher N, Goldhaber SZ. Cardiac biomarkers for risk stratification of patients with acute pulmonary embolism. Circulation 2003; 108:2191–2194.
95. Moraes DL, Colucci WS, Givertz MM. Secondary pulmonary hypertension in chronic heart failure: the role of the endothelium in pathophysiology and management. Circulation 2000; 102:1718–1723.
96. Butler J, Chomsky DB, Wilson JR. Pulmonary hypertension and exercise intolerance in patients with heart failure. J Am Coll Cardiol 1999; 34:1802–1806.
97. Cappola TP, Felker GM, Kao WH, et al. Pulmonary hypertension and risk of death in cardiomyopathy: patients with myocarditis are at higher risk. Circulation 2002; 105:1663–1668.
98. Fishman AP. Aminorex to fen/phen: an epidemic foretold. Circulation 1999; 99:156–161.
99. Teramae CY, Connolly HM, Grogan M, et al. Diet drug-related cardiac valve disease: the Mayo Clinic echocardiographic laboratory experience. Mayo Clin Proc 2000; 75:456–461.
100. Akosah KO, Schaper A, Cogbill C, et al. Preventing myocardial infarction in the young adult in the first place: how do the National Cholesterol Education Panel III guidelines perform? J Am Coll Cardiol 2003; 41:1475–1479.

101.  Wilson PW, Grundy SM. The metabolic syndrome: practical guide to origins and treatment: part I. Circulation 2003; 108:1422–1424.
102.  Horwich TB, MacLellan WR, Fonarow GC. Statin therapy is associated with improved survival in ischemic and non-ischemic heart failure. J Am Coll Cardiol 2004; 43:642–648.
103.  Poirier B, Bidouard JP, Cadrouvele C, et al. The anti-obesity effect of rimonabant is associated with an improved serum lipid profile. Diabetes Obes Metab 2005; 7:65–72.
104.  Butler J, McCoin NS, Feurer ID, et al. Modeling the effects of functional performance and post-transplant comorbidities on health-related quality of life after heart transplantation. J Heart Lung Transplant 2003; 22:1149–1156.
105.  Grady KL, White-Williams C, Naftel D, et al. Are preoperative obesity and cachexia risk factors for post heart transplant morbidity and mortality: a multi-institutional study of preoperative weight-height indices. Cardiac Transplant Research Database (CTRD) Group. J Heart Lung Transplant 1999; 18:750–63.
106.  Davos CH, Doehner W, Rauchhaus M, et al. Body mass and survival in patients with chronic heart failure without cachexia: the importance of obesity. J Card Fail 2003; 9:29–35.
107.  Horwich TB, Fonarow GC, Hamilton MA, et al. The relationship between obesity and mortality in patients with heart failure. J Am Coll Cardiol 2001; 38:789–795.
108.  Lavie CJ, Osman AF, Milani RV, et al. Body composition and prognosis in chronic systolic heart failure: the obesity paradox. Am J Cardiol 2003; 91:891–894.
109.  Feldman AM, Combes A, Wagner D, et al. The role of tumor necrosis factor in the pathophysiology of heart failure. J Am Coll Cardiol 2000; 35:537–544.

# 18

# Acknowledging and Reversing
# the Toxic Environment

**Andrew B. Geier**

*Department of Psychology, University of Pennsylvania, Philadelphia,
Pennsylvania, U.S.A.*

**Kelly D. Brownell**

*Department of Psychology, Yale University, New Haven, Connecticut, U.S.A.*

## ACKNOWLEDGING THE TOXIC ENVIRONMENT

With the prevalence of obesity being at record levels and showing every indication of increasing descriptors such as "epidemic" and "crisis" seem justified (1). To prevent even more unnecessary death, disability, and damage to the nation's collective well being, an honest analysis of cause is necessary; the factors contributing to the causes must be identified and confronted, and bold action must be taken to change the conditions causing the problems.

This chapter takes the position that the environment is causing the obesity epidemic, that the field has not placed biology and environment in the most constructive context, and that specific actions can be taken to change the food and activity environments. We believe these positions offer the greatest hope of affecting prevalence in both the immediate future and the long term.

Obesity has multiple causes, leading to the default explanation that the problem comes about as a result of a complex web of biological, environmental, and psychosocial factors. This is both illuminating and paralyzing at the same time. Simultaneously it paints an accurate picture of the many factors that affect energy balance while inhibiting the field from examining obesity from nonmedical model perspectives and being creative in crafting solutions.

## The Environment and Obesity

The rapid increase in the prevalence of obesity is explained by the environment, straight and simple. Why the environment has taken shape as it has, and the factors shaping it, are not simple at all, but at the macro level, the environment is responsible. It has evolved in such a way as to make the consumption of excess calories, fat, and sugar a high probability event and discourages the population from being physically active.

There are several layers of "proof" regarding an environmental explanation for obesity. The first is that prevalence has been increasing around the globe. The World Health Organization (WHO) activated an alarm after reporting that every country in the world for which reasonable data are available has reported increasing prevalence of obesity (2). The world's gene pool could not have changed so rapidly to explain the increase in obesity. Barring it being some common agent such as an infectious disease that is affecting the entire world, the cause must be the environment.

A second level of evidence comes from studies tracking individuals who migrate from a less to a more obese country (3). For instance, Japanese individuals who move to Hawaii gain weight, which is more pronounced if they move to the mainland United States. A number of studies demonstrate this phenomenon.

A stronger method of examining this issue is to compare individuals who migrate to a new country with their biological relatives who remain in the native country. Bhatnagar et al. (4) studied individuals who migrated to West London from the Punjab area of India. Their body mass index was significantly higher than that of their close biological relatives who remained in India. Although not a perfect control for biology, such observations suggest that weight increases as people enter a more "obesifying" environment.

One of the most pronounced examples of this phenomenon occurs in the United States (5). The Pima Indians living in Arizona came to the United States from Mexico where their relatives are mainly subsistence farmers. The Pimas living in Arizona have the highest rate of diabetes in the world and one of the highest rates of obesity. Pimas living in Mexico have a much different diet, are more physically active, and have normal body weights.

Added to the these first two levels of evidence is an impressive literature on animals, evaluating the impact of access to a "cafeteria" diet consisting of human foods (chocolate bars, cheese curls, salami, cookies, etc.) (6). When presented with a choice, animals reject healthy laboratory food and choose to eat a human diet in large amounts and, as a result, become obese. Work by Tordoff (7) shows a similar impact by demonstrating that when animals are offered large amounts of sugar and fat, they consume much more than necessary to maintain a healthy weight. Conversely, these same animals will pace their eating in a healthy manner when exposed to similar amounts of more healthy foods.

It is important to place biology and environment in context. Animals in the studies mentioned above have a willing biology, but the biology is activated and obesity occurs when environmental conditions change. Clearly an enabling biology must be in place for human obesity to occur. In the absence of a negative environment, however, biology will almost never produce obesity. Countries where food is scarce are proof. In addition, so many people in the population have a permissive biology that defining who is susceptible may not be an enterprise with a worthwhile end. The answer to who is most susceptible may be "almost everyone."

One danger in pursuing biology with such fervor is that with each discovery and the accompanying media attention it generates, there is risk of diverting attention from the environment, overstating the role of biology as a cause, and commencing a search for medical solutions at the expense of public health approaches.

Work on biology is important, because it may produce help for the millions of people who struggle with their weight, and there is the off chance that some compound will be developed that will make humans immune from the weight gain. This latter possibility seems remote, given that both energy consumption and expenditure are involved and that even a compound able to prevent weight would not offset the independent effects of poor diet and inactivity.

## The Toxic Environment

Environmental influences can be classified most broadly as those that affect food intake, energy expenditure, or both. When added together, these influences create a "toxic environment" that makes an epidemic of obesity predictable, even inevitable (8,9).

Beginning with the food environment, a distorted balance sheet exists with economic and other key factors, adding numerous incentives to modern life that promote an unhealthy diet (Fig. 1). Stated simply, foods high in sugar, fat, and calories are available as never before, and are convenient, engineered to taste good, promoted heavily, and are inexpensive. Taking each of these factors individually, many features of the poor eating environment become apparent.

1. *Accessibility.* The number of eating opportunities has increased dramatically in recent years. Fast food restaurants that are open 24 hours, broad placement of vending machines particularly in schools and work sites, and food available in places not imagined 20 years ago (gas stations, drug stores, etc.) just begin to tell the story.

2. *Convenience*. With humans "on the go" and with little time and incentive to prepare meals, foods available quickly and eaten rapidly have become part of the modern food landscape.
3. *Taste*. Humans are attracted to foods that taste good, and what tastes good are sugar and fat. Agriculture subsidies and national nutrition policy have permitted the food industry to add these to common foods at little cost (10,11); hence there is a tragic intersection of human biology with the profit motive.
4. *Promotion*. The resources devoted to promoting unhealthy versus healthy foods are in remarkable imbalance. Examples are given below.
5. *Cost*. Cost is one of the main driving factors behind food choices (taste being another). There is abundant evidence that a healthy diet costs more than an unhealthy one, that food-buying choices for people in poor neighborhoods emphasize poor options, and that federal food programs designed to feed the poor (Women, Infants and Children, Food Stamps, and Head Start) may be contributing to obesity (12–14).

The picture for healthy foods is the opposite of what it should and must be. Fruits, vegetables, and whole grains are less accessible (no drive-in windows, for example), much less convenient (they often take time to purchase and prepare, spoilage is an issue, etc.), do not have the inherent good taste of the alternatives, are promoted very little, and tend to be more expensive than unhealthy options. It cannot be surprising, therefore, that the country suffers from poor diet intake.

Certainly hunger has been a major world problem, even in developed countries, and the agriculture industry has responded with increasing yields and lowering costs. This is a major victory, but an unintended consequence has been the fattening of the population. The production and promotion of

## Food Balance Sheet

| **Unhealthy Foods** | **Healthy Foods** |
|---|---|
| Highly accessible | Less accessible |
| Convenient | Much less convenient |
| Promoted heavily | Promoted very little |
| Good tasting (sugar/fat) | Less tasty |
| Inexpensive | More expensive |

**Figure 1**   Reality of the current food environment.

highly processed, calorie-dense foods is taking place not to feed the poor, but to maximize profits.

There are numerous examples of the overwhelming nature of the poor food environment. Marion Nestle in her book *Food Politics* (15), Greg Critser in his book *Fat Land* (10), Eric Schlosser in the book *Fast Food Nation* (16), and Brownell and Horgen in *Food Fight* (9) have painted dramatic pictures of the food landscape. Examples are as follows:

1. The primary government nutrition education program is the Five-a-Day Program, which encourages people to eat more fruits and vegetables. At its peak, this program was funded with $3 million for promotion (17). The same year, McDonald's spent $500 million for the "We love to see you smile campaign."
2. Nestle (15) estimated that the entire government budget for promoting healthy eating, added across all agencies, was 1/5th the annual advertising budget for Altoids Mints.
3. The average American child sees 10,000 food advertisements per year on television alone (18). A parent eating every meal of the year with their child, and who delivers a persuasive nutrition message at each meal, would have only 1000 exposures, and would not have cartoon characters, sports heroes, and other celebrities working on their side.

At the same time that the food environment has deteriorated, conditions related to physical activity have also done so. Energy-saving devices, physical activity being subtracted from work and school, people remaining inside because of engagement with computers, video games, and television, less leisure time, and parental concerns with safety when children leave the home are some of the factors contributing to declines in physical activity. Many examples document this point.

1. Fewer than 10% of American children walk or bike to school regularly. Thirty years ago the figure was 66% (19).
2. By the time a typical child leaves high school, she or he will have spent more hours watching television than in school (20). There is a strong relationship between television time and both poor diet and obesity (21,22).
3. In a typical gym class in school these days, a child is aerobically active for 3.5 minutes (23).

Deterioration in either diet or physical activity might be partially offset if there were improvements in the other area, but the two are in simultaneous decline. The problem of obesity is so severe, and the momentum carrying the population weight to higher levels so powerful, that it is a foregone conclusion that both diet and activity must be addressed. A focus on one to the exclusion of the other is likely to have limited impact.

## The Importance of Prevention

Treatment of obesity is difficult (24,25). Even the most optimistic among us will be sobered by the struggle we witness in those attempting to reduce and will not take heart from long-term studies tracking people who undergo even the most intensive treatments (with surgery being the exception).

Long ago the field jettisoned the attainment of ideal weight as a goal, with good reason, but now there is a sentiment that even a small weight loss of 5% to 10% is a clinical "victory" (25). True, this leads to some improvement in risk factors, but by any standard, is not a remedy. Treating obesity must be conceptualized as offering help to those affected, but not as a means for reducing prevalence.

Prevention, therefore, must be a public health priority. Sadly, there is relatively little research on preventing obesity, a deficit in knowledge that must be corrected. The absence of research on this can be explained by several factors. First is the bias and stigma attached to obesity (26). Second is that obesity, until recently, has been under the purview of medical rather than public health researchers. This places the focus on treatment rather than prevention, considers the utility of treatment outside the context of cost, and ignores the public health need to reduce the population burden of a disease. Third, it is true of our culture in general that prevention gets far less attention than needed.

Only now is a scientific base being established for the prevention of obesity. It is logical to focus on children, because this is the group in which brand loyalties are established, food habits become ingrained, and there is the greatest possibility of introducing new eating and physical activity patterns that might be integrated into a person's self-definition.

The most important questions facing the obesity field today are whether obesity can be prevented; and if so, how this might be done. The remainder of this chapter is devoted to our suggestions for environmental interventions designed to prevent obesity.

## REVERSING THE TOXIC ENVIRONMENT

### Medical vs. Public Health Models

Using a traditional medical model, one looks for causes and cures at the level of the individual. From this perspective, biology is an important player—in an individual, it enables or even promotes weight gain. A person's genetic makeup is important in this context, because it helps shape a number of metabolic factors affected by many systems of the body. Biology helps explain why some people are overweight and others are not, given the same environment, and of course, the pursuit of biological remedies becomes a priority.

Using a public health perspective, which has only recently been applied to obesity, one looks for population-level causes of the problem and solutions directed at those causes. Treatment and prevention are both possibilities, with the emphasis placed on the approach that delivers the most cost-effective means of reducing the public health impact of the disease.

There is abundant evidence from which to assess the likelihood that current treatments will have a public health impact. Stated simply, most treatments do not work well or are too expensive to be used widely. The only treatments showing efficacy beyond a one-year period, much less effectiveness, are intensive cognitive behavior therapy (which integrates diet and exercise), some medications, and surgery. Each would be impossible to use on a broad scale because of cost. There is no hope presently that this problem can be treated away. For every person who is subtracted from the population of obese individuals with treatment, hundreds or thousands more are entering because of the environment.

The bias toward traditional medical thinking has had a profound impact on the way obesity has been studied, how funding agencies orient their support, and how the nation deals with this issue. Examples are as follows:

1.  Despite knowing for years how difficult it is to treat obesity, vast numbers of treatment studies have been done (many recent studies with drugs are examples), while little research has been done on prevention.
2.  Government funding from agencies such as the National Institutes of Health on genetics, biology, and treatment dwarfs what has been allocated to study prevention.
3.  An immense industry selling diet books, products, programs, and foods is based on the accepted cultural notion that obesity is the fault of the individual and that the individual must take charge (and pay money) to change. Little concern has been raised, until recently about the factors that promote the overconsumption of calories and sedentary lifestyle.

## Policy Recommendations

Powerful environmental forces are causing the obesity epidemic, and current approaches have little hope of affecting its pervasiveness. There is a dire need for bold action; intervening with public policy offers the most immediate and, perhaps, most powerful means for having an impact. The following policy recommendations have been drawn from Brownell and Horgen (9) and are based on a public health model.

### National Oversight of Nutrition and Physical Activity

Under the current national structure, multiple government agencies supervise nutrition and physical activity programs. A result is that there exists no single department, agency, or person overseeing these vital areas. While the Centers for Disease Control and Prevention offer some funding for nutrition research, so does the National Institutes of Health, the U.S. Department of Agriculture (USDA), and even the Department of Defense, just to name a few. Resulting from having no strategic national nutrition plan, which would organize and direct such efforts, is the simultaneous funding of similar studies by different agencies while other important areas of research are sparsely funded.

As an example of this disconnected web of agencies, one of the authors sought to locate a document that would describe the totality of subsidies relevant to food and agriculture. He wished to learn how pork, beef, and poultry farmers/businesses were supported as compared to the assistance given to the fruit and vegetable sectors of the industry.

Following lengthy searches and multiple phone calls to administrators at the USDA and other agencies, several discoveries were made. First, there are numerous categories of subsidies through which the government is involved with agriculture. A few examples are price supports, purchase of a particular season's surpluses, use of commodities in school lunch programs, and a subsidy for irrigated water. Second, no single authority makes such decisions, and hence there is no logic (such as improving the nation's health) one can discern other than legislators seeking to help certain elements of the agriculture industry. Clearly the goal is probusiness and not pronutrition. Lastly, no document or person was located that could present the big picture—something or someone who has a comprehensive understanding of the complete subsidy issue.

Unfortunately, this subsidy story illustrates a general truth. In the absence of a national plan, the United States has multiple agencies and agendas that regularly conflict. For example, efforts to improve academic performance by using healthier foods by the Department of Education may be undermined by USDA's policies that permit, and sometimes promote, unwholesome foods in schools.

Each of the following government agencies concerns themselves with issues of nutrition: the USDA, the Department of Health and Human Services, the Federal Trade Commission, the Food and Drug Administration, the Federal Communications Commission, and the Department of Education. This just begins the list. A similar logistical problem was identified and addressed with the Department of Homeland Security, created to dispel competing goals, and to prevent duplication of effort, lack of cooperation, communication problems, and inefficiency.

In the absence of a broad oversight, there is a lack of decisive action and the opportunity for special interests to prevail over both science and common sense. Allowing soft drinks and snack foods in schools is a classic example. Other examples are the disparity in research funding for obesity treatment versus prevention and the fact that subsidies paid to the agriculture industry become political rather than public health issues. Further, unlike other issues of child welfare, food advertising aimed at children is essentially unregulated.

This idea is not without risk. Centralizing nutrition programs creates an opportunity to exploit the new system for commercial interests if not done properly. Because there would be fewer officials and elected leaders to woo, the industry could narrow its lobbying focus. Although, if a central nutrition oversight were created correctly, with the aim of maximizing positive impact on public health, buffers could be installed between the decision-making process and the food and agriculture industries.

Encourage Practices Known to Affect Obesity

With all that is known about obesity, there is comparatively little agreement on preventative actions. There are, however, several actions around which consensus is building. It may be sensible to address these immediately (27).

1. *Encourage breastfeeding*: Research from around the world has shown lower rates of obesity in breastfed children than in those who are fed on formula (28–30). Different reasons for this outcome have been proposed. One is that the child, rather than the feeder, decides the quantity consumed during breastfeeding. This may permit food intake to be regulated by hunger rather than by external cues such as the size of the bottle. In addition, breastfed children appear more willing to try a greater diversity of foods, conceivably because breast milk varies in taste while formula does not. This may be helpful in establishing early preferences for foods such as vegetables. Lastly, it also appears that women who breastfeed lose the weight gained during pregnancy more readily (31).

2. *Reduce television viewing and other sedentary activities*: Television viewing is associated with higher rates of obesity, lower levels of physical activity, and all-around poorer measures of health. Promoting less time in front of the television has been proposed as one means for addressing the obesity crisis, especially in children (27,32,33). Ridding dining rooms and bedrooms of televisions, not watching television during meals, and reducing time spent playing video games and on the computer could be helpful in this context.

3. *Enhance opportunities for physical activity*: With declining physical activity being a fundamental contributor to increasing rates of obesity, every opportunity to make physical activity more available, attractive, and rewarding should be taken. In concert with the educational, family, and community interventions being tested, public funding to increase physical activity is needed. Building recreation centers and bike paths, and requiring greater physical activity in schools would be logical places to begin. Alliances among scientists, public health advocates, legislators, and grass

roots organizations around issues of common interest could facilitate this movement. "Rails to Trails" is an example of what can be done when such a partnership is formed.

There is general agreement that declining activity is contributing to obesity, and that increasing activity in the population is a vital goal (34,35). There is little opposition to such a goal, so the objective is finding ways to accomplish this aim and to create a funding source to first generate and then sustain these broad changes. There is every indication that increasing activity is one piece of improving the nation's health, so promoting physical activity should commence immediately.

### Regulate Food Advertising Aimed at Children

As stated above, the average child in the United States sees 10,000 food advertisements per year, 95% of which are for fast foods, sugared cereals, soft drinks, candy, etc. (18). The most intrepid parents have difficulty competing. Efforts were made several decades ago by grass roots groups in conjunction with the Federal Trade Commission to curtail the number of food advertisements during cartoon television hours (Saturday morning), but fierce opposition, particularly from the major cereal companies, scuttled this movement. Owing to the power of the opposition, limiting advertising would be a difficult policy to sell even in the midst of today's obesity epidemic.

An alternative may be to mandate equal time for pronutrition messages advocating healthy foods, which are currently all but nonexistent. A precedent exists for smoking. In the 1960s and 1970s some public health advocates lobbied for a ban on all forms of cigarette advertising. Instead, the fairness doctrine was implemented, which mandated equal time for anti-smoking messages to offset the impact of advertisements from the tobacco industry. The antismoking messages had such a profound effect that the tobacco companies found television advertising to be no longer cost effective. Eventually, the tobacco companies agreed voluntarily to end all television advertising.

We support legislation that would mandate equal television time for pronutrition messages and to provide funds to develop effective advertising campaigns. Additional research would be necessary to find which forms of advertising, in addition to television, should be addressed.

### Prohibit Fast Foods and Soft Drinks in Schools

It is alarming (a) how many schools have fast food franchises in school cafeterias (36); (b) how many schools without such franchises are selling much the same food (37); (c) how many school systems enter into contracts with soft drink companies that provide financial incentives for increasing sales (38); and (d) the extent to which commercial television designed specifically for in-school viewing (e.g., Channel One) has such a heavy concentration of advertising for unhealthy food products (39).

Many possibilities exist for ameliorating these pervasive negative influences. One change, now gaining momentum (see below), would be to prohibit soft drinks and fast foods from schools. A powerful rationale is that poor nutrition interferes with learning. Foods low in nutrition and high in fat and sugar supplant foods that might enhance energy, alertness, mental acuity, and other factors necessary for optimum learning and peak performance.

### Restructure School Lunch Programs

Consistent with the previous point, it is important to restructure school lunch programs in a way that increases consumption of healthy foods. The food service in schools, sometimes run internally and other times subcontracted to large companies such as Sodexo Marriott and Aramark, is considered a support service (such as custodial or grounds) rather than being essential to the educational mission of the institution. If the food service were seen as integral to the development of healthy young people, broad changes would then become possible.

Armed with this new mandate, the totality of schools' nutritional education would involve more than menus. It would include education about nutrition by people trained in this area, engaging both students and their parents, and integration of this learning with other aspects of the curriculum (e.g., health education and physical education). For such education to be effective, the foods themselves must be appealing, and there must be measurable criteria for insuring students acquire basic knowledge.

### Subsidize the Sale of Healthy Foods

Currently, it is easier and cheaper to eat poor and mediocre foods than to eat in a healthy fashion. And because many of the foods low in nutrition taste good because of their high fat, sugar, and salt content, major barriers exist to healthy eating. This present state of affairs must be reversed if obesity is to be curtailed.

If healthy foods were reduced substantially in price, say all fruits and vegetables were reduced by 50%, a number of positive changes could occur. People sensitive to price, who had hitherto found the costs of such foods prohibitive, might increase consumption. Food manufacturers could invest the same technological resources that are currently apportioned to unhealthy foods toward the preparing, packaging, and delivery of healthy foods. This may be possible while maintaining a profit margin similar to what exists now for unhealthy foods. The major fast food chains are resourceful, so a lower price for healthy foods might spark them to develop fast and convenient items that, when priced attractively, could generate significant sales.

A further approach to encourage the retailing of healthy foods is to support their promotion. Because the marketing of fast foods, soft drinks, etc.

so overwhelms the promotion of healthy foods (15), imaginative advertising campaigns should be developed and funded to promote the consumption of healthier classes of products, such as fruits and vegetables.

One possible source of funding to accomplish these goals can be found below in the section "Tax Foods of Poor Nutritional Value."

## Tax Foods of Poor Nutritional Value

A less attractive suggestion at first blush, the proposal to tax foods low in nutrient density was considered highly controversial in the past. But this concept is now appearing more and more apparent and practical.

Although taxes can be conceptualized as a means for reducing consumption of unhealthy foods, the price increase necessary to provoke changes might be intolerable to some. But if a tax, for the sake of accumulating revenues, were to be used in the service of a perceived benefit, such as funding nutrition education programs, supporting subsidies of healthy foods, or building exercise facilities, it might be viewed as having virtuous rather than punitive aims.

In a review of taxes imposed on soft drinks and snack foods, Jacobson and Brownell (40) noted that over a dozen states in the United States have such taxes—in all cases the taxes are small ones. These taxes were instituted to raise revenue and not with the idea of changing consumption, and proved to be acceptable to both the consumers and the food industry. Collectively, these small taxes raise approximately $1 billion per year. In none of the cases noted by Jacobson and Brownell (40) are the funds designated for programs related to nutrition or physical activity. Creative earmarking could provide enormous benefit. Taxes used in the service of a good cause can themselves become good causes, and therefore, might be more generally acceptable.

## Curbing Food Commercialism in Public and Community Institutions

In the latest example of commercialism gone wild, a number of cities have agreed to purchase police cars with ads painted on them, perhaps with logos of companies such as McDonald's (41). As children are taught to respect authority, the exposure of these ads, not to mention their credibility, would be considerable. Sports stadiums, football bowl games, and countless other venues and enterprises have commercial sponsors. How often do we hear that some company or product is the "official sponsor of" some event? For example, Burger King sponsored a Backstreet Boys tour, a band especially popular with young children (42). Through experience and research, these sponsors have developed a solid knowledge of what affects consumer behavior.

In August of 2001, the most visited museum in the world, the National Air and Space Museum of the Smithsonian Institution, began a 10-year,

$16 million contract with McDonald's. The museum contracted to feature McDonald's foods in the cafeteria, creating what may prove to be the busiest McDonald's in the United States. Two of the other new restaurants opening in the Smithsonian are Donatos Pizzeria and Boston Market (43), also owned by McDonald's. Subscquent to this potentially lucrative deal, McDonald's made a $5 million gift to the national museum.

In what may be the greatest irony of all, hospitals have become sales agents for fast foods. Of the 16 hospitals listed in *U.S. News and World Report's* "Honor Roll," 38% contained regional or national fast food franchises, four were contracting with two franchises simultaneously, and one had closed a fast food franchise only to open a hospital restaurant with similar foods (44).

One of the busiest McDonald's in Philadelphia is in the Children's Hospital of Philadelphia—the same children's hospital that *U.S. News and World Report* ranked as the best in the country (45). Seen on its window during a visit by one of the authors was a large advertisement for the "New Cheddar Bacon Sausage McMuffin." Between two halves of an English muffin, starting from the bottom, were cheese, sausage, egg, cheese, and bacon. It is hard to imagine a more efficient way to deliver fat and calories. At some point the nation must say enough is enough.

### Expect More of Celebrities

There is a long, star-studded list of athletes, pop idols, and movie icons endorsing food products. There are the obvious ones such as Michael Jordan, Shaquille O'Neal, LeBron James, and Britney Spears, but endorsements of another kind are becoming more and more common. In 2001, for instance, Coca-Cola paid Warner Brothers $150 million for the global marketing rights for the first Harry Potter movie. Appeals to the author of the Harry Potter books (J. K. Rowling) to stop the use of her characters to promote soft drinks to children were unsuccessful.

Why should we not expect more of celebrities? These individuals would probably not endorse cigarette brands, because this could be a public relations disaster, and they might have reservations about promoting products known to cause harm. This is precisely what could happen in the future with endorsements regarding unhealthy foods. Famous people acting as role models, such as LeBron James who signed a $90 million dollar contract with Nike, perhaps through pro bono work, could have a positive impact by helping promote healthy foods and physical activity.

### Mobilize Parents to Demand More for Their Children

Raising children to understand nutrition, eat a healthy diet, and be physically active has become an increasingly difficult undertaking. On this front, families deserve more help from the nation. Parents fighting to protect their children can be an influential, compelling force inspiring both local and national changes. Parents will be heard if they can be organized and mobilized to advocate for their children on such matters.

A beginning may be to show parents the full extent of how the food companies entice children through advertising, product placements on TV and in movies, and celebrity endorsements. Having been alerted to the ties between food companies and their children's daily lives, parents may demand change. Mothers and father should also be made aware of the connections food and soft drink companies have with schools. As one example, Betty Crocker, maker of Triple Chocolate Fudge Chip frosting, is a "proud sponsor of the National Parent Teacher Association (PTA)" (46). The Betty Crocker Web site proclaims the National PTA a "partner" and links to the National PTA web site for "helpful parenting resources." We assume the PTA receives remuneration of some kind to allow its name to be used in this way.

Armed with this information, parents can declare their protest to school officials and school boards, can organize boycotts of companies they feel are exploitative, and can demand further actions that will be in the interests of their children.

## SIGNS OF CHANGING TIMES

Beginning in about 2002, a remarkable transformation arose. A public health approach began to dominate thinking about obesity, followed by rapidly changing attitudes about what must be done. Examples are as follows:

1. Media articles and news shows on obesity, once dominated by a focus on how to lose weight, have largely changed to emphasize environmental causes, increasing prevalence in children, and prevention.
2. Major institutions are taking action. A prime first move was the elimination of soft drinks from schools by the Los Angeles Unified School District, affecting more than 700,000 children.
3. State legislators in Maine, California, New York, and other states have called for dramatic actions to help reverse the growing rates of obesity. Two of these measures include statewide bans on soft drinks and fast food in schools and a requirement for calorie labeling on restaurant menus.
4. In December of 2003, the WHO recommended taxes on foods as a means of combating obesity, an idea met with blistering resistance when first proposed (8).

These are mostly local, grassroots triumphs, and are more telling and impressive, particularly in the United States, than action by the federal government. The massive influence of the food industry is being felt in Washington, but is less likely to sway state and local leaders. One important priority for the field may be to better understand how local victories are made possible, and then help create the conditions where such victories become contagious.

## CONCLUSION

Obesity must become a national priority and, increasingly, must be a global focus. Prevention is most likely if the environmental causes can be identified and corrected. Children may be the group where the first and most remarkable gains will occur. It is logical to start early and with a group that society historically protects from toxic influences. Impressive actions are beginning to occur in legislative and regulatory arenas. The greatest hope for reducing the prevalence of obesity and the resulting human toll may be to push these public health actions in an aggressive, unwavering manner.

## REFERENCES

1. Centers for Disease Control and Prevention. Obesity and overweight: a public health epidemic. CDC website. Available at www.cdc.gov/nccdphp/obesity/epidemic.htm. Accessed Jul. 21, 2002.
2. World Health Organization. Obesity: Preventing and Managing the Global Epidemic. Geneva, Switzerland: World Health Organization, 1998.
3. Popkin BM. An overview on the nutrition transition and its health implications: the Bellagio meeting. Publ Health Nutr 2002; 5(1A):93–103.
4. Bhatnagar D, Anand IS, Durrington PN, et al. Coronary risk factors in people from the Indian Subcontinent living in West London and their siblings in India. Lancet 1995; 345:405–409.
5. Ravussin E, Valencia ME, Esparza J, Bennett PH, Shultz LO. Effects of a traditional lifestyle on obesity in Pima Indians. Diabetes Care 1994; 17: 1067–1074.
6. Sclafani A. Psychobiology of food preferences. Int J Obes Relat Metab Dis 2001; 25:S13 S16.
7. Tordoff MG. Obesity by choice: the powerful influence of nutrient availability on nutrient intake. Am J Physiol: Reg Int Comp Physiol 2001; 282: R1536–R1539.
8. Brownell KD. Get slim with higher taxes (Editorial). New York Times 1994; A29, December.
9. Brownell KD, Horgen KB. Food Fight: The Inside Story of the Food Industry, America's Obesity Crisis, and What We Can Do About It. New York: McGraw-Hill, 2004.
10. Critser G. Fat Land: How Americans Became the Fattest People in the World. New York: Houghton Mifflin Company, 2003.
11. Pollan M. The way we live now: the agri(cultural) contradictions of obesity. New York Times 2003; 41(3), October 12 (section 6).
12. Besharov DJ. We're feeding the poor as if they're starving. Washington Post 2001; B01, December 8.
13. Besharov DJ, Germanis P. Rethinking WIC: An Evaluation of the Women, Infants, and Children Program. Washington, D.C.: American Enterprise Institute, 2001.
14. Wilde PE, McNamara PE, Ranney CK. The effect on dietary quality of participation in the food stamp and WIC programs. Food Assistance and Nutrition

Research Report No. 9, 2000. Available at http://ers.usda.gov/publications/ Fanrr9. Accessed Nov. 28, 2002.

15. Nestle M. Food Politics: How the Food Industry Influences Nutrition and Health. Los Angeles: University of California Press, 2002.

16. Schlosser E. Fast Food Nation: The Dark Side of the All-American Meal. New York: Houghton Mifflin Company, 2001.

17. Nestle M, Jacobson MF. Halting the obesity epidemic: a public health policy approach. Publ Health Rep 2000; 115:12–24.

18. Taras HL, Gage M. Advertised foods on children's television. Arch Pediatr Adol Med 1995; 149:649–652.

19. Centers for Disease Control and Prevention. Nutrition and physical activity. CDC website. Available at www.cdc.gov/nccdphp/dnpa/physicalactivity.htm. Accessed Aug. 31, 2002.

20. Certain LK, Kahn RS. Prevalence, correlates, and trajectory of television viewing among infants and toddlers. Pediatrics 2000; 109:634–642.

21. Borzekowski DL, Robinson TN. The 30-second effect: an experiment revealing the impact of television commercials on food preferences of preschoolers. J Am Dietetic Assoc 2001; 101:42–46.

22. Gortmaker SL, Must A, Sobol AM, Peterson K, Colditz GA, Deitz WH. Television viewing as a cause of increasing obesity among children in the United States, 1986–1990. Arch Pediatr Adol Med 1996; 150:356–362.

23. Simons-Morton BG, Taylor WC, Snider SA, Huang IW. The physical activity of fifth-grade students during physical education classes. Am J Public Health 1993; 83:262–264.

24. Brownell KD, Wadden TA. Etiology and treatment of obesity: understanding a serious, prevalent, and refractory disorder. J Consult Clin Psychol 1992; 60(4): 505–517.

25. Wadden TA, Brownell KD, Foster GD. Obesity: responding to the global epidemic. J Consult Clin Psychol 2002; 70(3):510–525.

26. Puhl RM, Brownell KD. Psychosocial origins of obesity stigma: toward changing a powerful and pervasive bias. Obes Rev 2003; 4(4):213–227.

27. Dietz WH, Gortmaker SL. Preventing obesity in children and adolescents. Ann Rev Public Health 2001; 22:337–353.

28. Dietz WH. Breastfeeding may help prevent childhood overweight. JAMA 2001; 285:2506–2507.

29. Gillman MW, Rifas-Shiman SL, Camargo CA, et al. Risk of overweight among adolescents who were breastfed as infants. JAMA 2001; 285:2461–2467.

30. Hediger ML, Overpeck MD, Kuczmarski RJ, Ruan WJ. Association between infant breastfeeding and overweight in young children. JAMA 2001; 285: 2453–2460.

31. Rooney BL, Schauberger CW. Excess pregnancy weight gain and long-term obesity: one decade later. Obstet Gynecol 2002; 100:245–252.

32. Dietz WH. The obesity epidemic in young children. Reduce television viewing and promote playing. Br Med J 2001; 322:313–314.

33. Robinson TN. Reducing children's television viewing to prevent obesity: a randomized controlled trial. JAMA 1999; 282:1561–1567.

34. Pate RR, Pratt M, Blair SN, et al. Physical activity and public health: a recommendation from the Centers for Disease Control and the American College of Sports Medicine. JAMA 1995; 273:402–407.

35. US Department of Health and Human Services. Physical Activity and Health. Report of the Surgeon General. Atlanta, Georgia: US Department of Health and Human Services, Centers for Disease Control, National Center for Chronic Disease Prevention and Health Promotion, 1996.

36. Levine J. Food industry marketing in elementary schools: implications for school health professionals. J School Health 1999; 69:290–291.

37. U.S. Department of Agriculture. Foods sold in competition with USDA School Meal Programs: a report to congress. Jan. 21, 2002. Available at http://www.fns. usda.gov/cnd/Lunch/CompetitiveFoods/report_congress.htm. Accessed Nov. 22, 2002.

38. French SA, Story M, Fulkerson JA. School food policies and practices: A Statewide Survey of Secondary School Principals. J Am Dietetic Assoc. 2002; 1785–1789.

39. Brand J, Greenberg B. Commercials in the classroom: the impact of channel One advertising. J Advertising Res 1994; 34:18–23.

40. Jacobson MF, Brownell KD. Small taxes on soft drinks and snack foods to promote health. Am J Public Health 2000; 90:854–857.

41. Christian Science Monitor. Car 54, where's your ad? Nov. 6, 2002. Commercial Alert website. Available at www.commerecialalert.org. Accessed Dec. 26, 2002.

42. Allpop.com. Available at http://www.canoe.ca/AllPop-BackstreetBoys/ 000121_burger.html. Accessed on Dec. 16, 2003.

43. Center for Science in the Public Interest. What's at stake: tell the Smithsonian to say no to Mcdonald's junk food. CSPA website. Available at http://action-network.org/campaign/Smithsoniansaynotojunkfood2/explanation. Accessed Aug. 8, 2002.

44. Cram P, Nallamothu BK, Fendrick AM, Saint S. Fast food franchises in hospitals. JAMA 2002; 287:2945–2946.

45. US News and World Report. Available at http://www.usnews.com/usnews/ health/hosptl/rankings/specreppedi.htm. Accessed on Dec. 16, 2003.

46. Betty Crocker web site. Available at http://www.bettycrocker.com/prodand-promo/partners/part.asp. Accessed Aug. 8, 2002.

# Index